CRISIS IN CHILD MENTAL HEALTH

Crisis in Child Mental Health: Challenge for the 1970's

REPORT OF THE JOINT COMMISSION ON
MENTAL HEALTH OF CHILDREN

Foreword by Senator Abraham A. Ribicoff

HARPER & ROW, PUBLISHERS

NEW YORK, EVANSTON, AND LONDON

1817

Official distribution of this book has been made possible through a grant from the Foundation for Child Mental Welfare, Inc.

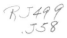
RJ499
.J58

Contents

v

Figures and Tables

PRESIDENT
REGINALD S. LOURIE, M.D.

VICE PRESIDENTS
JULIUS RICHMOND, M.D.
NICHOLAS HOBBS, PH.D.
HARRIET MANDELBAUM

SECRETARY TREASURER
CHARLES SCHLAIFER, ESQ.

ASSISTANT SECRETARY
WALTER E. BARTON, M.D.

EXECUTIVE DIRECTOR
JOSEPH M. BOBBITT, PH.D.

ADMINISTRATIVE OFFICER
D. J. DERISO

Joint Commission
on
Mental Health of Children, Inc.

June 30, 1969

To the Congress of the United States:

This report of the Joint Commission on Mental Health of Children
responds to its mandate to make a report on June 30, 1969, as
stated in Section 231 (d) of the Social Security Amendments of
1965 and 1968 (P.L. 89-97) as amended. The purpose of this report
is to apprise Congress, the Secretary of Health, Education and
Welfare, and the Governors of the several States of the findings
of the Joint Commission on Mental Health of Children and to recommend for their consideration the best obtainable opinions about the
inseparable health and mental health needs of children in this
country.

We are grateful to the Congress, to the National Institute of Mental
Health, the professional and voluntary associations and individuals
who have supported the Commission and its work since its inception.

In addition, we wish to express our appreciation to the Congress
for making possible this timely and much-needed study of one of the
most important problems facing the country, the ability of its
citizens to function as usefully and satisfyingly as possible both
in their personal lives and community functioning. We gratefully
acknowledge the continued support of the work during this study by
the National Institute of Mental Health.

Sincerely yours,

Reginald S. Lourie, M.D.
President and Chairman

Charles Schlaifer, F.A.P.A., Lit.D.(Hon.)
Secretary-Treasurer

NOTE: An earlier version of this report was submitted in June, 1969, to members
of the United States Senate and House of Representatives, to the governors of the
fifty states, the National Institute of Mental Health, the Secretary of Health, Education,
and Welfare, and to participating agencies and members of the Joint Commission on
Mental Health of Children. Those who read the initial draft will find that certain
modifications have been made by the Commission's Board of Directors in the process
of finalizing the report.

See Appendix VII, p. 562, for more details

Foreword

Our children are our future. This report is about them.

It is also about us—their parents.

It asks us how we really feel about our most precious resource. What are we prepared to do to assure that our children grow up strong and healthy, both physically and mentally?

That is the fundamental question the Joint Commission on Mental Health of Children has placed before this nation.

It is a deceptive question.

While most Americans would do "everything" to help their children, the fact is that today millions of children receive little. Some suffer mental and emotional illness. Others live in destructive poverty. Too many are victims of conditions they did not create. Their parents may be doing all they can for their children. But what about the rest of us? What about society at large?

That is the kind of concern the Joint Commission has sought to instill in the American public. The Joint Commission wants us to think not just about sickness and health but about child development and growth, about the environment in which a child lives—his family, his schools, his friends, his community. For this is where the child learns and shapes himself and the world around him.

By offering us this perspective, the Joint Commission on Mental Health of Children has broadened our outlook. For this we are grateful.

When I first introduced legislation in 1965 to establish the Joint Commission, this body was charged with assessing the care this nation provided to emotionally and mentally disturbed children.

This the Commission has done. Its findings are shocking.

During the past forty years, the Commission reports, the situation has not improved. It has become worse.

Only a third of the children who need care receive it. Nearly one million receive no care at all.

The Joint Commission concludes:

"As of today, the treatment of the mentally ill child in America remains uncertain, variable, and inadequate. This is true on all levels, rich and poor, rural and urban. . . . Only a fraction of our young people get the help they need at the time they need it."

Thus, the American public faces a double challenge—the challenge of caring for the child who is already sick and in need of help, and the challenge of preventing sickness by fostering healthy growth.

The Joint Commission has no easy answers for either, because there are none. But it has taken a major first step by forcing us to think in new concepts, to develop new ideas.

I especially commend to the readers of this report the Joint Commission's call that we become advocates—not advocates in behalf of any single program, profession, bureaucracy or theory but advocates in behalf of healthy children and a healthy society.

Societies can be judged on how they care for their children.

The Joint Commission asks us to judge ourselves and to act upon our verdict.

ABRAHAM A. RIBICOFF

Preface

For the last fifty years there has been a growing concern over the number of mentally ill and emotionally disturbed children in the United States and an increasing dissatisfaction with the unavailability of mental health services. When the previous Joint Commission on Mental Illness and Health, for unavoidable reasons, was unable to cover this important area, both professional and concerned citizen groups pressed for a study of the mental health needs of children. The acute necessity for such knowledge was painfully brought into public awareness by President Kennedy's assassin, who had been diagnosed a mentally disturbed child for whom treatment was never obtained. Responsible legislators initiated steps which ended with amendments to the Social Security Act* that made possible the three-year study reported here.

Thirteen national professional associations joined the incorporators of the Joint Commission on Mental Health of Children to form a board of directors. The board, with a grant from the National Institute of Mental Health, developed a fine dedicated staff, headed by Dr. Joseph M. Bobbitt as executive director. More than 500 of the country's leading authorities on early childhood, adolescence, and the young adult were enlisted to work on task forces, on substantive committees, and to collect information in specialized areas. The universal willingness of these persons to contribute their knowledge and energies, and the richness of their contributions, has earned them their country's gratitude.

* See Appendix I.

The background information and the several hundred recommendations made by our colleagues were synthesized by the Commission's staff. Overlap and contradictions were reviewed and ordered with the assistance of board committees. We are grateful to literally hundreds of our colleagues and to our staff, but we have a special debt to Catherine Chilman for her work in preparing the original draft and to Barbara Sowder for preparing the final draft.

The Commission was also greatly assisted by the continually available participation of specialists at every governmental agency level, and particularly by the staff of the National Institute of Mental Health. Many of our affiliate member organizations assisted by providing both funding and professional collaboration. The National Association for Mental Health, for example, held a productive joint conference with the Commission on the needs of mentally ill children in America. A number of national professional associations appointed very useful task forces to review and advise the Commission as it formulated its recommendations. The valuable, often remarkable, reports from which the Commission's recommendations stem will be published in a series of volumes intended for both interested public and professional groups. Many of the findings and recommendations from these various reports have been incorporated into this final document.

In the process of the Commission's study, it quickly became evident that health, mental health, and environmental influences are interwoven and that they are most intricately interrelated in the earliest years of life. Both child development and social action findings and recommendations were integrated because they could not be separated from each other. These recommendations are presented in the opening chapter of this report. The reader who wishes to better understand the rationale for the Commission's proposals may prefer to read the descriptive material in Chapters II through XII before turning to Chapter I.

The struggles in the professions between the clinicians and those concerned with prevention were apparent in the deliberations of the Commission and were not easily resolved. It became obvious, however, that priority could be given neither to curing the sick and relieving pain nor to learning how to achieve the most healthy development for every child. Putting out fires has therefore been given equal weight with fireproofing.

This report is meant to fill the gap between what we know now and the time when new knowledge will make possible greater advances. The future holds promise through such techniques as chromosome manipulation and molecular and biochemical approaches—all of which need to be better defined and controlled if they are to serve the interests of mankind. In the meantime we know enough at least to approach some of the major problems facing our families and our cities. Babies are not born racist, violent, and without respect for law, nor are they born having given up their capacity to learn. All these they acquire. We have learned that we must not miss critical periods of development in the first years of life, that we must provide appropriate experience and corrective help, if we are to deal with the most fundamental aspects of these problems. In our various reports we have attempted to share the latest research information about the developmental needs of children and families so that planning for future human settlements and services will bring about enhanced human functioning and satisfactions and eliminate some of the hazards.

Through its series of reports, the Commission has been provided with up-to-date information on normal and abnormal human development. Scientific knowledge has advanced. We know a great deal about *why* abnormal development occurs, at least enough to allow us to say in these recommendations *what can be done* to prevent or treat much of what goes wrong. We are only on the threshold of learning *how to do it*. We must move in new and innovative directions; however, we must not abandon our current methods for relieving the pain and sickness we see around us.

The interest of many outstanding legislators and governmental officials and agencies and their response to the Commission's findings and recommendations has been especially gratifying. We fervently believe that there should be some continuity in maintaining this high level of involvement in the Commission's work. It has been suggested that national citizens' groups, such as those which worked with the Commission, should function together in a type of consortium to represent a centralized "voice for children." It has also been strongly urged in our studies that a nonprofit, independent strategy and planning group in the child health and mental health field is viable and needed, at both governmental and private agency levels, to think through immediate and longer-range problems. It is hoped that the movement under way to create such a group will allow the rest of the field to keep up with its leading edge.

The problem of estimating costs produced many irreconcilable conflicting opinions from budget authorities and others. It is particularly difficult to project costs in a changing economy, complicated by inflation. Therefore, it was decided to leave this aspect of the Commission's studies to be defined piecemeal as it is seen fit to activate any of its recommendations. It is clear, however, that the child-rearing program of our communities, if properly carried out, will be one of the largest "industries" in the country—one of the largest in manpower utilization and therefore costs.

It is our opinion that this is as it should be. If vast expenditures, both human and monetary, are not made, it will in the long run be more costly in terms of mental illness, human malfunctioning, and therefore underproductivity. In this aspect of our economy we are far behind many countries which give highest priority to the proper shepherding of their most important resource, their children.

This report is therefore dedicated to the children and youth of this country, in the hope that it will create a national awareness of their needs and a prompt call to action.

FACTUM FORTUNA SEQUITUR

CRISIS IN CHILD MENTAL HEALTH

Introduction and Recommendations

We proclaim that we are a nation devoted to its young. We believe that we have made great strides toward recognizing the needs of children and youth. We have enacted child labor laws, established a public education system, created treatment services for our disturbed and handicapped, and devised imaginative programs such as Head Start for our disadvantaged young. Yet, we find ourselves dismayed by the violence, frustration, and discontent among our youth and by the sheer number of emotionally, mentally, physically, and socially handicapped youngsters in our midst. It is shocking to know that thousands of children are still excluded from our schools, that millions in need go untreated, and that many still suffer from hunger and malnutrition. We recognize in these ills some of the sources and symptoms of poverty and racism in which all of us, as a nation, take part. Poverty, in this the richest of world powers, is still our heritage. Racism, in a country dedicated to its people's inalienable rights, speaks as clearly of "man's inhumanity to man" as did slavery.

In spite of our best intentions, our programs are insufficient; they are piecemeal, are fragmented, and do not serve all those in need. Unwittingly, we have failed to commit our vast resources to promote the healthy development of our young. We have yet to devise a strategy which will maximize the development of our human resources. Congress gave national recognition to this need in issuing a mandate to establish the Joint Commission on Mental Health of Children. In fulfillment of its task, the Commission declares:

This nation, the richest of all world powers, has no unified national commitment to its children and youth. The claim that we are a child-centered society, that we look to our young as tomorrow's leaders, is a myth. Our words are made meaningless by our actions—by our lack of national, community, and personal investment in maintaining the healthy development of our young, by the minuscule amount of economic resources spent in developing our young, by our tendency to rely on a proliferation of simple, one-factor, short-term and inexpensive remedies and services. As a tragic consequence, we have in our midst millions of ill-fed, ill-housed, ill-educated, and discontented youngsters and almost 10,000,000 under age twenty-five who are in need of help from mental health workers. Some means must be devised to delegate clear responsibility and authority to ensure the well-being of our young.

This nation, which looks to the family to nurture its young, gives no real help with child-rearing until a child is badly disturbed or disruptive to the community. The discontent, apathy, and violence today are a warning that society has not assumed its responsibility to ensure an environment which will provide optimum care for its children. The family cannot be allowed to withstand alone the enormous pressures of an increasingly technological world. Within the community some mechanism must be created which will assume the responsibility for ensuring the necessary supports for the child and family.

This nation, which prides itself on democratic values and equal opportunity, still imposes on its young the psychological repercussions of poverty and racism. No one is effectively empowered to intercede.

This nation, richly endowed with the knowledge to develop its youthful resources, has yet to fill the gap between knowledge and action. We know, for example, that preventive measures are most essential and effective if taken in the earliest years of life; that during this period there are critical stages of development which, if neglected or mishandled, may result in irreversible damage. Yet, our services are nowhere more deficient than in the area of prenatal and infant care.

This nation, highly sophisticated and knowledgeable about mental health and child development, continues its planning and programming largely around the concept of treating, rather than preventing, mental illness. But no agency has the task and responsibility for assuring that treatment is, in fact, received by those who need it.

This nation, despite its emphasis on treatment, has yet to develop adequate mental health services and facilities for all children and youth, regardless of race and economic circumstances. Many receive no attention. The number of young, particularly adolescents, who are committed to mental institutions continues to rise markedly. Yet, we have not provided the resources and manpower to assist those who are devoted to caring for these children. As a result, any possible benefits of confinement are lost in the tragic waste of the back ward. Even less effort is made to develop coordinated community services so these children can be kept as closely as possible within their normal, routine setting.

The Commission strongly urges better treatment for the mentally ill, the handicapped, the retarded, the delinquent, and the emotionally disturbed. We join forces with those who propose a broader but more meaningful concept of mental health, one which is based on the developmental view with prevention and optimum mental health as the major goal. We contend that the mentally healthy life is one in which self-direction and satisfying interdependent relationships prevail, one in which there is meaning, purpose, and opportunity. We believe that lives which are uprooted, thwarted, and denied the growth of their inherent capacities are mentally unhealthy, as are those determined by rigidity, conformity, deprivation, impulsivity, and hostility. Unfulfilled lives cost us twice—once in the loss of human resources, in the apathetic, unhappy, frustrated, and violent souls in our midst, and again in the loss of productivity to our society, and the economic costs of dependency. We believe that, if we are to optimize the mental health of our young and if we are to develop our human resources, every infant must be granted:

The right to be wanted,
> yet millions of unwanted children continue to be born—often with tragic consequences—largely because their parents have not had access to or knowledge of the benefits of birth control information and devices.

The right to be born healthy,
> yet approximately 1,000,000 children will be born this year to women who get no medical aid during their pregnancy or no adequate obstetrical care for delivery; thus many will be born with brain damage from disorders of pregnancy. For some, protein and vitamin supplements might have prevented such tragedy.

The right to live in a healthy environment,
> yet thousands of children and youth become physically handicapped or acquire chronic damage to their health from preventable accidents and diseases, largely because of impoverished environments. Even greater numbers living in poverty will become psychologically handicapped and damaged, unable to compete in school or on a job or to fulfill their inherent capabilities—they will become dependents of, rather than contributors to, our society.

The right to satisfaction of basic needs,
> yet approximately one-fourth of our children face the probability of malnutrition, inadequate housing, untreated physical and mental dis-

orders, educational handicaps, and indoctrination into a life of marginal work and opportunity.

The right to continuous loving care,

yet millions of our young never acquire the necessary motivation or intellectual and emotional skills required to cope effectively in our society because they do not receive consistent emotionally satisfying care. Society does little to help parents. There are few programs which provide good day care, which aid in developing more adequate child-rearing techniques, or which assist in times of temporary family crisis or where children are neglected or abused.

The right to acquire the intellectual and emotional skills necessary to achieve individual aspirations and to cope effectively in our society,

yet each year almost 1,000,000 of our youth drop out of school and enter the adult world with inadequate skills and with diminished chances of becoming productive citizens; countless others are denied the opportunities to develop to their fullest potential through effective vocational training, meaningful work experiences, or higher education. For all of our children and youth the transition to adulthood is made difficult. We fail to provide avenues for learning adult roles and for acquiring leadership skills or some approved means by which youths' voice can influence a world in which they too must live.

We know that when these rights are granted, development will proceed favorably for most infants. Few children, however, encounter continuously those ideal circumstances that maximize their hereditary potential for health, competence, and humanity. At conception, at birth, and throughout development there are vast variations and inequalities in the life chances of our young. Undoubtedly many will continue to be psychologically damaged. If our more unfortunate are to become functioning and productive citizens, we believe they must be granted:

The right to receive care and treatment through facilities which are appropriate to their needs and which keep them as closely as possible within their normal social setting,

yet several millions of our children and youth—the emotionally disturbed, the mentally ill, the mentally retarded, the handicapped, and the delinquent—are not receiving such care. The reasons are innumerable. Many go untreated because the services are fragmented, or nonexistent, or because they discriminate by cost, class, or color. Other young people are diagnosed and labeled without regard to their level of functioning. They are removed from their homes, schools, and communities and confined to hospital wards with psychotic adults or to depersonalized institutions which deliver little more than custodial care.

As far back as the first White House Conference on Children in 1909, the nation has repeatedly, and with considerable eloquence, announced its intentions to develop a strong, imaginative program to care for emotionally disturbed children. For example, the 1930 White House Conference on Child Health and Protection, composed of several thousand citizens and government officials, proclaimed: "The emotionally disturbed child has a right to grow up in a world which does not set him apart, which looks at him not with scorn or pity or ridicule—but which welcomes him exactly as it welcomes every child, which offers him identical privileges and identical responsibilities."

The 1930 White House Conference estimated that there were, at that time, at least 2,500,000 children with well-marked behavioral difficulties, including the more serious mental and nervous disorders.

In the four decades since the issuance of that report, the care of the emotionally disturbed child in this country has not improved—it has worsened considerably. During the three years of its deliberations and fact-finding efforts, the Commission has gathered together an impressive body of descriptive material on the plight of the emotionally disturbed child in America today.

Using the most conservative estimate from various school surveys, the National Institute of Mental Health estimates that 1,400,000 children under the age of eighteen needed psychiatric care in 1966.

Are they getting this treatment? Surveys of various psychiatric facilities undertaken by the National Institute of Mental Health show that nearly 1,000,000 of those children needing psychiatric care in 1966 did not receive treatment. These estimates indicate that we are providing care to only one-third of our children who are in serious need of attention. An additional 7 to 10 percent or more are estimated, by school surveys, to need some help for emotional problems.

What happens to these emotionally sick children for whom there are no services in the community? Each year, increasing numbers of them are expelled from the community and confined in large state hospitals so understaffed that they have few, if any, professionals trained in child psychiatry and related disciplines. It is not unusual in this year 1969 to tour one of these massive warehouses for the mentally ill and come upon a child, aged nine or ten, confined on a ward with 80 or 90 sick adults. Our present data indicates that slightly more than 27,000 children under eighteen were under care in state and county mental institutions in 1966. On the basis of a trend which has been developing over the past few years, the National Institute of Mental Health estimates that by 1970 the number of children aged ten to fourteen hospitalized in these institutions will have doubled.

The National Institute of Mental Health also reports that thousands upon thousands of elderly patients now confined on the back wards of these state institutions were first admitted as children thirty, forty, and even fifty years ago. A recent report from one state estimates that one in every four children admitted to its mental hospitals "can anticipate being permanently hospitalized for the next 50 years of their lives."

After a two-year study of the situation, the Clinical Committee of our Commission had this to say of the hospitalization of these disturbed children:

> The admission of teen-agers to the state hospitals has risen something like 150% in the last decade. . . . Instead of being helped, the vast majority are the worse for the experience. The usual picture is one of untrained people working with outmoded facilities within the framework of long abandoned theory (where there is any consistent theory), attempting to deal with a wide variety of complex and seriously sick youngsters and producing results that are more easily measured by a recidivism rate that is often 30 to 50%, and occasionally higher.

> What we have, in effect, is a state of quiet emergency, unheralded and unsung, silently building up its rate of failure and disability and seemingly allowed to go its way with an absolute minimum of attention from the public, the legislators, or the clinical professionals. Nor is it difficult to understand why this state of affairs obtains—no one likes a delinquent youth, a bad actor, and when he is sent away the chief wish is just that, that he "go away." Out of sight. Out of mind.

What happens if the disturbed child is fortunate enough to escape the state institution treadmill? There are a few private, residential treatment centers which care for about 8,000 children a year. Since the average cost of such hospitalization ranges from $30 to $50 a day, it is obvious that only those of our citizens who are in the higher income brackets can take advantage of such services. Even among these rarefied income brackets the situation is far from satisfactory; for every child admitted to one of these private facilities, ten or more are turned away because of lack of space. In eight of our states there are no such facilities, either public or private. In many of our states there are no public units to care for children from low- and middle-income groups.

The situation today led the Clinical Committee of the Commission to the following inescapable conclusion:

> As of today, the treatment of the mentally ill child in America is uncertain, variable and inadequate. This is true on all levels, rich and poor, rural and urban. The problems are most widespread among the poor, as are all health problems, but the fact is that only a fraction of our young people get the help they need at the time they need it.

From all of its studies, the Commission concludes that it is an undeniable fact that there is not a single community in this country which provides an acceptable standard of services for its mentally ill children, running a spectrum from early therapeutic intervention to social restoration in the home, in the school, and in the community.

What happens to all our children who receive no help for emotional problems? Here the statistics become much less precise, since a vast majority of these children are literally lost. They are bounced around from training schools to reformatories to jails and whipped through all kinds of understaffed welfare agencies. No one is their keeper. No agency in the community is equipped to evaluate either the correctness of their placement or the outcome of such placement.

If they are sent to a training school, as recent testimony before a Senate committee revealed, they generally receive poorer treatment than caged animals or adult convicts. Appearing in 1969 before a Senate committee, Joseph R. Rowan, an expert on delinquency who is now director of the John Howard Association of Illinois, characterized these institutions for juveniles as "crime hatcheries where children are tutored in crime if they are not assaulted by other inmates or the guards first." Another witness, Arlen Specter, the district attorney of Philadelphia, told the same committee that these so-called correctional institutions for juveniles take a thirteen-year-old and in twelve years turn out "a finely honed weapon against society."

Commenting on the failure of juvenile courts and juvenile correctional facilities to even begin to meet the manifest needs of emotionally disturbed and sociopathic children, Judge David Bazelon, a member of the Commission, noted in a recent talk that although this nation is aware of the problem, it does not support funds to treat and care for these children *because it has really given up on them.*

We must ask ourselves whether we can continue to deny our children their inalienable rights. Can we continue to gamble with our nation's future by allowing children to grow up in environments which we know are psychologically damaging—and compound this by lack of adequate care and treatment?

We have the knowledge and the riches to remedy many of the conditions which affect our young, yet we lack a genuine commitment to do so. We blind ourselves to the fact that we create most of the social problems of our young which we so deplore—infants who fail to thrive, seriously disturbed children in mental institutions, adolescent drug addiction, acts of violence and destruction by youth.

Our lack of commitment is a national tragedy. We know already that it is more fruitful to prevent damage to our young than to attempt to patch and heal the wounds. We know that much of the damage could be avoided in the first three years of life. We know that the basis for mental development and competence is largely established by the age of six. Yet we do not act on this knowledge. Studies indicate that most children, regardless of class or race, whether in the ghetto or in suburbia, do not receive the needed support and assistance from our society. But it is the damaged, the vulnerable, and the poor who are given the least opportunities to overcome early deprivations. They benefit least from our health, welfare, and educational services. Those who are the most helpless are the most neglected.

This Commission proposes a shift in strategy for human development in this nation—one which will deploy our resources in the services of optimizing human development. We emphasize the critical need to concentrate our resources on the new generation and eliminate problems which later exact so high and tragic a price.

In the allocation of these resources, it is the consensus of most of the Commission's task forces and committees that equal priority should be given to the following:

Comprehensive services which will ensure the maintenance of health and mental health of children and youth.

A broad range of remedial mental health services for the seriously disturbed, juvenile delinquents, mentally retarded, and otherwise handicapped children and their families.

The development of an advocacy system at every level of government to ensure the effective implementation of these desired goals.

The services we propose should cover the entire range of childhood, from systematic maternal and infant care to the transition of the adolescent and college-age youth into effective young adulthood.

It should be emphasized that fostering the development of human beings in this country is a means to an end—a means to stem the increasing number of people who have no meaningful role in society. Their services in health, education, welfare, and other human and community services are desperately needed and currently unused.

Commitment, genuine commitment, to our children and youth is, necessarily, the beginning. We must look honestly at the scope of the problem and begin *now* to follow our words by action. We must develop advocacy functions at all levels of government and society, functions which will ensure that the needs of children and their families are being met. This commitment to advocacy means commitment to change. It means that we—as parents, educators, professionals, and legislators—must participate and collaborate in change on national, state, and local levels. We must reorder our priorities so that the developmental needs of children rank first in importance. The commitment requires finding effective ways to link our fiscal resources, services, and manpower so that every infant will be guaranteed the continuous care and the opportunities required for his optimal development. The creation of an advocacy system means that we, at last, will act to ensure the rights of our living and unborn young. For in our children lie our future and our hope for the fulfillment of our national goals. We must not—cannot—afford to do less.

RECOMMENDATIONS OF THE JOINT COMMISSION ON MENTAL HEALTH OF CHILDREN

The Commission's task forces and committees immediately recognized that creative and imaginative changes must be made in our major child-serving institutions if we are to provide adequate services and programs for children and youth. Mere reorganization and enlargement of the existing institutions and agencies will not suffice: new methods, new services, and a new kind of mechanism will be required for this enormous task, as well as the development of new pools of manpower, trained to perform various new roles.

The now poorly coordinated services which are fitted to the needs of professionals must be reworked into a coordinated network of services based on the total needs of the child as he develops from conception to adulthood. The current nonsystem must be made systematic and flexible in ways that will promote and support constructive child development as well as identify, diagnose, correct, remediate, and rehabilitate those youngsters who deviate from normal development.

We believe that the child deserves an advocate to represent him and his needs to the society in which he lives, an advocate who will insist that programs and services based on sound child development knowledge be available to every child as a public utility. Section I proposes the means for promoting national, state, and community responsibility and initiative in developing comprehensive and systematic programs of prevention and treatment, in increasing the accountability of those who minister relevant programs, and in coordinating and organizing resources for supportive, effective, and coordinated programs for our children and youth.

The Commission is indebted to its task forces, committees, and contractors for many of the recommendations presented below. We also wish to extend our gratitude to board members who contributed their energies to this undertaking and to Dr. J. McVie Hunt (1966) for allowing us to liberally use his document as a guideline in our formulation of an advocacy system.

I. A Child Advocacy System

The Commission recommends that Congress provide for the President to appoint at the national level an Advisory Council on Children similar to the Council of Economic Advisors. Advocacy for children and youth would then derive its strength from the highest office in our nation. It would be the primary expression of national commitment to children and youth. The President's Advisory Council on Children would advise the President, the Cabinet, the Congress, and the Bureau of the Budget. It would be charged with the responsibility of studying and gathering information on the problems of children and youth in the United States and with doing long-range planning, policy-making, and programming, both for services and for manpower. This advisory body would be concerned about how well federal agencies concerned with children and youth are working together, competing, or overlapping in providing services. It would advise the President and Congress on the effectiveness of programs, on the state of well-being of children and youth, and would make recommendations for legislative and program changes and on allocation of funds.

The Commission did not make specific recommendations about federal government organization and allocation of program responsibilities. The Commission strongly recommends that the Secretary of Health, Education, and Welfare should have a strong unit, headed by a high official in his office, to give leadership to all programs for children and youth. Included in this function would be policy clearance and development, coordination of efforts, evaluation of results, and recommending allocation of resources to the Secretary. Coordination of federal interprogram relationships to State Comprehensive Plans would rest in this unit.

The Commission recognizes that this basic objective of ensuring delivery of services to children and youth can be achieved and sustained only if the local advocacy function is complemented by strong mechanisms for planning policy development and financing at all levels of government. Therefore, the Commission recommends strong machinery be started at the federal level and that federal funding be provided for the establishment of public advocacy functions at the national, state, and local government levels.

The Commission recommends that the advocacy concept at the state level be carried out by a State Child Development Agency. This agency would be charged with developing a comprehensive state plan for children and youth on an ongoing basis and would be governed by law and regulations not unlike the Federal Comprehensive Health Planning requirements. Its crucial task would be to develop a state plan—in conjunction with broad federal guidelines—and to lay out program goals and operating guides for all the services and programs required to meet the needs of children and youth in the state. It would plan the creation of local authorities and councils and assist them to develop. This agency would have responsibility to review applications from local government Child Development Authorities for the establishment of neighborhood and area Child Development Councils and would periodically evaluate the work of the councils. Local authorities and councils would develop local plans for the state agency. The State Child Development Agency would also have responsibility to advise the governor on all program plans and fund allocations that concern children. The Commission recommends that Congress provide that the State Comprehensive Plan include consideration of all children and youth programs, not solely those that are federally funded. Ideally, as in the case of the Comprehensive Health Planning legislation, there should be one state plan for all federal children and youth funds. Each state should have the prerogative to determine where the State Child Development Agency should be housed. Some states may wish to create an interdepartmental agency; some may place it in the governor's office; some may house it in an ongoing agency. The federal agency would act on the State Comprehensive Plans and, on approval, would fund the state agency and the local authorities and councils. As an incentive for states with comprehensive plans, higher percentages of federal matching could be granted for all federally funded children's programs.

At the local governmental level (city or county, or combination of these), depending on state and local structure, the plan would call for local Child Development Authorities and Child Development Councils. These would be the local guarantors of service for children and their families. The authority would be a government agency. The council would be a neighborhood or area coordinating and advocacy body.

The Commission recommends that federal funding be provided for the establishment of a network of Child Development Councils throughout the nation. These councils would act as the direct advocate for children and youth. They would have the responsibility and prerogative of ensuring that complete diagnostic, treatment, and preventive services are made available to all children and youth in the neighborhoods and areas which they serve under mandates prescribed in the Comprehensive State Plan and state legislation.

At all levels—neighborhood, local, state, and national—participation and representation in the work of the several advocacy bodies would include professionals, laymen, and consumers. The Commission proposes that the state and local bodies be concerned with planning, facilitating, and coordinating services and with ensuring that these services be available to children, youth, and their families. The state agency and the local authority may be housed in any agencies which operate public programs directly. The council would not be responsible for operating services. This would be inconsistent with its advocate role. The Commission hopes that a Child Development Council will be established to serve as advocate for every child and youth in America just as there is a public education responsibility for each child. However, the Commission recognizes that these cannot be funded and established overnight. We recommend, therefore, that the following steps be taken within the next immediate period:

The creation of the President's Advisory Council on Children.

The establishment of a State Child Development Agency in each state to develop the state comprehensive plan for services. Federal funds would be provided to develop the state plan based on federal guidelines.

The establishment of at least one experimental local Child Development Authority in each state.

The establishment of approximately 100 Child Development Councils throughout the nation, with at least one in each state to be funded subject to development of a state comprehensive plan.

The creation, by full federal funding, of approximately ten Evaluation Projects with each being placed in a different type of community. These Evaluation Projects, whether independent of, or related to, the Child Development Councils, would study, test, and evaluate the goals proposed for the councils and would provide data for the establishment of future councils and for improvement of already existing councils.

The establishment of Child Development Councils emerged as the Commission's major recommendation for a number of reasons: foremost, we recognized that our existing services and facilities are not fully meeting the needs of many children, especially the needs of hundreds of thousands of children who already have disabilities which need treatment. In many communities in this country even basic services are nonexistent. Where services do exist, they are frequently poorly staffed, inadequately financed, and unable to prevent or treat disabilities. For any given child, agency activities are poorly coordinated. No agency has the key responsibility for guaranteeing that sick children receive careful evaluation and prescribed care related to the severity of their disturbances. As a result, thousands upon thousands of children are literally lost each year. The same is true for children who are not yet severely ill but who are vulnerable.

Second, the Commission is convinced that one of our major thrusts must be identification of mental and physical disorders in the earliest years of life—ages one through five. We must detect and treat malfunctioning before it freezes into severe disorder. Reaching this objective will require a total commitment, an entirely new set of resources for some and better use of present resources for all. Failure to provide new and reordered resources will most certainly result in another generation of children with large numbers not able to "make it," with increasing numbers destined for juvenile courts, reformatories, jails, welfare institutions, and the back wards of state mental hospitals.

Third, programs and policies in the United States continue to be developed with an orientation toward the individual alone, to the exclusion of familial and social considerations. Many programs designed for children—such as Maternal and Infant Care—have fallen short of their goals because the home and family are not given sufficient attention. Yet our research indicates that—especially in the case of the young child—parents and home remain the most important and potentially effective determinants of psychological development. Where constructive influences in the home are absent, it is usually not because parents are unwilling to provide them. They may be unable to do so for a great variety of reasons such as lack of knowledge, insufficient economic resources, or emotional and physical ill health. Oppressed by poverty and racism, many parents are virtually immobilized by the frustration of their difficult circumstances. Programs which will strengthen the home and the family—in ways culturally and socially acceptable to the family—will do much to enhance the development of the child. Our emphasis on social and cultural congruence takes advantage of the many strengths inherent in our pluralism. The Commission urges that all concerned work vigorously to explode myths about some of our ethnic groups, families, and communities and to explore their strengths. There remain, of course, those parents who neglect and maltreat their children. In such instances, society has the obligation to intervene. Even here remedial work may still be done.

Our efforts in behalf of children have not reflected a sufficient concern for child development. The importance of money, manpower, and remedial and preventive measures cannot be overlooked, and we have not overlooked them in our recommendations. But we emphasize strongly the need to create, encourage, and strengthen types of social institutions which help families and neighborhoods to exercise their untapped and natural power to foster the growth of children into healthy, competent, happy, and responsible members of society.

The need is crucial. Urbanization and industrialization have left the family unit increasingly alienated and isolated, and extended families and close-knit neighborhoods are becoming part of a past heritage. In suburbia, and in the inner city, the mother is often the child's main affective resource, while for many young children, television is the principal contact with the outside world. Preschool social and educational opportunities are limited. The activities of youth are also constricted by the demands of our age-graded and class-structured society. Youth are provided few opportunities to contribute to society, to learn adult roles, or to participate in decisions which affect their own fate. This narrow contact with the adult world and with peoples who differ in social and cultural ways seriously threatens the development of our children and youth. Many parents, too, are alienated. They have little voice in determining policies which affect them and their children, and few outlets for active involvement in their communities.

At every level of society, children, youth, and their parents are in need of additional encouragement, support, and opportunities to become involved in and to contribute to the society in which they live. Society has the obligation to assist families in meeting their emotional, economic, and other needs so they may more effectively support the development of their children. In addition, emphasis must be given to opening opportunities for children and youth to learn the roles necessary to a participatory democracy. Too often citizen roles are denied members of lower socioeconomic groups.

The advocacy system which we propose would stimulate the development of such programs for children and their families. The Child Development Authority and the Child Development Council are designed to ensure needed services and opportunities to children, youth, and their families. The program we recommend is not a cheap one, nor would any program be that is commensurate with the need. But if we choose now not to meet the cost, we shall eventually pay a far higher price, reckoned not only in economic loss but in human misery. We cannot refuse to mount the effort. If we are true to our heritage, we must recognize that we are confronted not merely with the needs of children but with their *inalienable* rights.

In urging action on these recommendations, we are motivated by a concern not only for America's children but for the nation. In the broadest perspective, the major goals of these recommendations are twofold: to ensure proper diagnosis, treatment, and care for mentally ill children and youth who presently receive the lowest priority for service, and, beyond this, to strengthen and improve the quality of all youngsters' lives. Initially, our major efforts should be in behalf of those who are ill and the millions of children whose entire lives are in danger of being dwarfed and scarred by the sequelae of poverty, racism, and indifference.

What we propose is a shift in strategy for human development and human services in this country. We believe it is in the interest of economy to concentrate resources on the new generation and thus eliminate problems that later exact a high price. Even more important, we believe that a rededication of America to the needs of her children and youth and to the realization of their human potential will help not only to increase their competence but also to rekindle that spirit of generosity, of magnanimity, of neighborliness, of gentleness and compassion, and of zest and adventure that are part of the American heritage.

In the description which follows, we will delineate the proposed advocacy at each level of government and program operation. We recognize that a nationwide advocacy system cannot be achieved with one legislative stroke. The ideas need to be made operational, designed, engineered, and tested. Relationships to existing programs, legislation, and governmental and voluntary structure need to be carefully studied and alternatives weighed.

Flexibility and wide experimentation are essential, especially in the neighborhood Child Development Councils. These councils will necessarily differ, according to community needs, resources, and desires. No one design will meet each local need. Our pluralistic society is most successful when different means are available for achieving goals. Testing and evaluation enhance this success so long as the main principles and broad structures are consistent with objectives. In Section II of the recommendations there is a proposal for a fundamental, ongoing examination of all service delivery arrangements.

CHILD DEVELOPMENT COUNCILS

Purpose

Child Development Councils constitute a new kind of institution. They have a four-fold aim. They seek:

to integrate the existing fragmented local services for children and youth and to ensure that each child's needs are met through advocacy and improved interagency arrangements;

to guarantee in every community adequate diagnostic, treatment, care, special education, and social services for children with emotional, mental, behavioral, social, and physical disturbances through leadership in planning new services, reorganizing existing services, and ensuring that children in need receive the necessary care and treatment;

to guarantee every child an adequate education and to develop new and emerging programs for developing competence in children and youth;

to involve parents as citizens in the planning and operating of services on behalf of their children, but not with any neglect of known professional services;

to assist parents, older children, and other members of the neighborhood in realizing their potential for constructive contribution to the lives of children, thereby enriching their own lives as well.

Direct functions of the councils

While models for Child Development Councils may vary to meet local conditions, each council should have the following basic functions:

The council functions as an informational service to guarantee the visibility of every child in need. It will make every effort to become acquainted with all children and families within its service area, to inform them of its roles, and its services and activities, and to urge them to participate. In time, it is hoped that every child in need will be known to the council and that a confidential continuing, longitudinal medical and psychological record can be developed for these children.

We also suggest that a number of councils experiment with developing an adequate information base—data about children which are amassed on an *anonymous* basis—and that we specifically try in several cities to develop a computer base. This would provide needed epidemiological data for purposes of generating appropriate manpower and services.

As an agency concerned with treatment and prevention, the council should be the focal point for continuing interest and concern for all children in its area. As the leadership agency for children in the community, it must gain the confidence of the families and agencies in the area by doing an immediate and effective job of helping them cope with their problems. It must take the *full responsibility* for seeing that each child gets all appropriate helping services—diagnostic, treatment, educational, welfare, and in some cases, full-time residential care. The council must never lose track of any child; it must be the central repository for all information on the progress of the child forwarded from facilities to which he has been sent. It must also accept responsibility for periodic assessment of the value of each individual referral, and it must be equipped and ready to change any referral when it is determined that the child is no longer benefiting from it.

Some councils may be given legal power by state legislatures. Some may give direct service temporarily when it is not otherwise available. While not a basic funding agency, a council should be given funds for experimentation, innovation, and demonstration. Funding and organizational patterns for child and youth programs may vary from state to state, as will state-local division of responsibility. Some states may find ways to fit local authorities and councils into the systems through which child and youth programs are funded, regulated, and operated.

In very simple terms, we see the council as the conscience and action arm of the community with regard to its children. It would devise ways of making services accountable to children and to each other. Where it succeeds, every family in the community will know that this is the one place one can go when a child is in trouble or when advice is needed on some developmental or educational problem. The council would be, with agreement of all concerned, the overall coordinator, planner, evaluator, and guarantor that no child in the community is lost or neglected. The state plan and state law should make this possible.

The council must also be the guarantor of the quality of services for children in the community. It should not undertake to operate services already present—or potentially present—in the area.

Where gaps in services exist, the council can urge the authority to arrange for services at the nearest place where these are available and take steps to see that the service inadequacies of its own community are promptly overcome.

The councils would prepare several periodic reports on the deficiencies in local services. Reports would be presented to consumers and the public, to local service agencies, to the local Child Development Authority, the State Child Development Agency, the Federal Agency, and the President's Advisory Council on Children. These reports would aid in planning at the several governmental levels and help lead to more responsive services.

The spectrum of concerted services to be guaranteed by the Child Development Council covers a wide range of needs—comprehensive physical and mental health care and treatment; day care; welfare services; legal services; a variety of educational opportunities; family consultation services; employment and training services; and recreational activities, including opportunities for children and youth to participate in activities now confined to the adult role. These services are described in some detail in recommendations A through E in Section II.

Organizational structure

The Child Development Councils would be the basic, universal type of neighborhood facility responsive to the needs of each designated individual neighborhood unit. All service agencies would join. Membership would not be mandatory except to the extent that state law and funding made it a requirement. They will perform the coordinating and service functions for children outlined previously. Their particular size and location will be determined by local community planning, and they will be coordinated with the overall state plan to be described below. Their function should be spelled out clearly in state law.

The form which these councils eventually take will vary in such different settings as housing projects in major cities, neighborhoods of individual homes in smaller communities, and rural settings such as Appalachia or Indian reservations. The physical location of these councils will also vary. One neighborhood may choose to locate the council in a factory; another may choose a school or hospital or community mental health center; another may wish to erect a new building. Each council, however, would be responsible for every child in its jurisidiction and would be empowered to obtain and ensure them comprehensive and systematic services.

Governing board

In its organizational structure, each Child Development Council would have a governing board which should include the principals of the neighborhood schools, the neighborhood representatives of government agencies, representatives of the various voluntary agencies for health and welfare operating within the neighborhood, and professional and lay persons interested in and knowledgeable about children. At least 40 percent of the members would be parents and consumers including members of disadvantaged groups.

This governing board would have the responsibility to:

> prepare a constitution and by-laws, consistent with state law;
> establish policy for the operation of the council and also employ the director (with the concurrence of the local authority);
> help enlist the cooperation of parents within the neighborhood in the operation of the council's programs;
> maintain relationships with other organizations and agencies in the community;
> hold elections;
> monitor the work of the council's programs.

Staff

Each council would have a permanent professional staff consisting of the director, appointed by the governing board in consultation with the local authority, and as many professional and subprofessional members as would be required by the program. The council would ensure that all agencies involve, in staff or volunteer roles, nonprofessional people from the neighborhood as well as personnel from interested volunteer and professional agencies. Every effort should be made to tap potential sources of manpower, including parents, elderly citizens, rehabilitated handicapped persons, and youth.

Community participation

The council should see to it that family members are actively engaged in the program of all agencies. There should be maximum decentralization and localization of responsibility for operation of the program at the community and neighborhood level. In the distribution of responsibility, errors should arise mainly from too much rather than too little confidence in the ability of people to manage their affairs wisely, given the resources to do so.

It may be necessary to provide intensive programs in some communities to help people meet this challenge. It is not reasonable to expect those who have long been "second-class" citizens to manage their affairs wisely unless they are given the resources to do so. Although the needs of the more affluent are seldom as great, they, like the poor, are often isolated and alienated. The pattern of alienation is not likely to give way to enthusiastic and active involvement unless the council gives leadership to see that meaningful and interesting opportunities for involvement are provided. Many organizations and efforts already exist. The council will not duplicate or overlap. It should be an instrument that all of the others can use as a base through which to plan for children.

In the initial phases of the council's operation, it may be necessary for permanent staff members to devote much of their time to recruiting citizens into council and agency activities as well as to informing them of the services offered by the council and the agencies. These undertakings should be considered among the most important tasks of the staff, for unless the goal of neighborhood responsibility and participation is achieved, we cannot hope to develop fully our human resources. It is unrealistic to expect all our problems to be solved by a few citizens with specific training and talents. Many of our current problems can never be solved by professionals; the solutions must come from parents and from neighbors and from youngsters themselves.

In the long run the council will need some fiscal and legal basis for assuring its central role.

Training manpower

The crucial problem of manpower and training needs will be discussed in detail in Section IV of the recommendations. The needs and purposes of the agencies served by the council will demand multiple types of training programs, some of which might be provided by the councils in concert with community agencies. It is hoped that the following types will be conducted in most areas:

> training of neighborhood and community leaders;
> training of subprofessionals and volunteers to function in various council programs;
> training of adolescents to work in children's programs and community improvement projects.

Funds should be provided to allow local councils and authorities to employ local educational institutions to develop curricular materials and training programs once the councils and authorities have agreed upon the type of personnel and training required for their needs. In the training function, the programs of the councils and the agencies would provide sources of supervised experience.

CHILD DEVELOPMENT AUTHORITY

Programs to foster child development must deal with children and their parents in neighborhoods. But formal government does not exist at the neighborhood level. The level of activity closest to the people is to be found in counties and cities which contain many neighborhoods. It is at the local political jurisdiction level that programs are ultimately administered and funds expended. Here public personnel are hired to provide the public services required. Purchase of services are arranged by public agencies from voluntary groups, and there is *direct* contact between the consumer and his government—a sharp contrast to the remoteness of both Washington and the State House. At this level of local government, which each state determines is its base of local concern for children, the Commission recommends that the Child Development Authorities be established.

The local Child Development Authority would be a public body. It would serve a number of neighborhood councils. The authority would be composed of: (1) appropriate representation from the schools, police, health and welfare agencies, recreation services, and other officials of both public and voluntary agencies whose activities are directly related to child development; (2) professional persons concerned with children, including representatives from professional organizations; and (3) parents and other citizens including consumers and disadvantaged persons. Representation could be developed through the councils. The authority would be headed by an appropriate high-level official selected by appointment by the board and the appropriate governmental bodies. The authority could be housed in the office of the major local political officer (mayor, county commissioner) or in a local department of government. The method of choosing authority members and the board would be specified in state law following federal guidelines. While the recommendation of the Commission is that federal funding be provided for the planning functions of the authority, some states may decide that the authority should have fiscal, organizational, and program responsibilities in respect to direct program services for children and youth.

Direct functions of the Child Development Authority

The authority would have a director and a permanent professional staff and would:

Serve as a coordinating, planning, and policy-setting body for all human services in its political jurisdiction as assigned by state law within federal guidelines. It would have a major concern with quality of care and treatment, with improving delivery of services, and with the development of local councils.

Develop the local comprehensive plan for submission to the state agency.

Establish a permanent planning section responsible for collecting and integrating information about the community required for effective planning for children and youth. The authority would keep informed about federal, state, local, and public and private programs for children and youth, as well as manpower needs and projects at all levels. The authority would establish geographical boundaries for the Child Development Councils and general but flexible policies for the operation of the councils, in keeping with broad federal guidelines and state law. The authorities, however, would not work directly with children and youth. The goal would be to keep administrative overhead to a minimum and give maximum operating authority and responsibility to the neighborhood councils.

Initiate and organize the Child Development Councils in the neighborhoods and receive requests for local financial support of such councils from agencies which can muster the necessary cooperation to provide comprehensive and continuing services. These would be included in the authority's comprehensive plan sent to the state.

Be responsible for the management, planning, and coordination of all councils under its auspices.

Direct programs and expend funds as mandated by state law.

Funding

Funds will come mainly from federal and state sources. Local funds would be supplied according to state decision. In general, federal grants would be provided in accordance with a state plan developed under the auspices of the State Child Development Agency described later. These funds could be allotted to the appropriate governmental body and allocated according to policies set by the state agency.

States which do not develop comprehensive plans and hence do not develop state authorities would not receive federal planning funds. Federal law should provide that direct local grants for local planning could be made in such instances.

STATE CHILD DEVELOPMENT AGENCY

In planning and developing services for children, local Child Development Authorities cannot operate in a vacuum. In order to avoid unnecessary and costly duplication of services, they must operate within a defined geographical framework. Therefore, planning and policy-making at the state level of government can be an effective mechanism for the overall promotion of child development. It is at this level that a comprehensive plan can be devised to meet those needs which are unique to a particular state. This geographical design would not permit the exclusion of any part of a state's population. The successful establishment of a network of community mental health centers was preceded by two years of careful state planning, authorized and funded by Congress. The planning effort, described by many professional leaders as the most comprehensive and successful in the history of public health in this country, involved 30,000 citizens who actively participated in drawing up local plans for community mental health centers which meshed into a statewide pattern of services for the mentally ill.

We recommend that federal grants be provided to the states for the purpose of developing a Comprehensive State Plan for Children. The size of the federal grant should be related to the number of children within a state, with no state receiving less than $50,000 for this planning effort. To carry out the study, a State Child Development Agency would have to be created. This could be a separate agency, an interdepartmental agency, or an agency housed in an ongoing agency.

In carrying out this study, each state governor would initially appoint an advisory and planning group to advise the new agency, which would include representatives of public and voluntary agencies currently serving children and youth; professional organizations concerned with the health, education, and welfare of children; educational systems; parents and other lay citizens; the parents of mentally ill children, and so on. This advisory group would inventory all existing services for children and youth within the state and would be charged with the responsibility for devising a priority listing of the initial location of local Child Development Authorities and Child Development Councils within a state. Ideally the initial emphasis would be upon the delivery services to poor and minority groups; however, this immediate action would be integrated into the long-range goal of services to all children and youth. Services to the poor and minority groups must reflect the severity and our lack of clear knowledge of their specific and urgent problems. This emphasis need not detract from the long-range goal of service to all children and youth. Action toward the goal will obtain from immersion in the special problems of the oppressed.

Functions of the State Child Development Agency

The planning responsibility for services for children and youth is but the beginning of the involvement and responsibility of a State Child Development Agency. This agency would be a continuing body with a professional staff to update the state's plan, forward it to the federal government, evaluate the councils and authorities, alter state plans as future needs develop, stimulate the development of needed services, coordinate the badly splintered services for children and youth, and advise the governor on allocation of federal and state funds. This agency would assist with local planning, consult with state public and voluntary agencies, and act to improve their working relationships.

The major functions of this continuing agency should be:

To develop a comprehensive state plan which will provide for all children; coordinate, in the most efficient manner, all the services and programs required to meet the needs of the children and youth in the state; and build in protections against inequities for any part of the state's population.

To provide a single place at a high level of authority in the state which will have responsibility for understanding and meeting the needs of children and their families. The agency would make recommendations to the governor and state legislature on allocation of funds and needs for children's programs. It would also advise local bodies.

To plan jointly with the state's agencies for health, education, and welfare, as well as with other agencies concerned with children's needs, to maximize the benefit of federal funds granted for children and their families. This would require the establishment of strong interagency machinery involving all those agencies which plan, deliver, or fund services to children, youth, and their families.

To plan the organization of comprehensive programs for all areas and to monitor authorities and councils in urban and rural areas.

To set standards for councils and authorities, review their applications and decide on their funding, study and evaluate their programs, encourage experimentation in programs, and receive their plans and consolidate them into the State Comprehensive Plan.

To administer funds for child development planning and other funds the state may direct.

To make reports and recommendations to the governor, state legislature, the President's Advisory Council on Children, and the appropriate federal agency.

To act as advocate at the state level for children and families.

PRESIDENT'S ADVISORY COUNCIL ON CHILDREN
AND FEDERAL CHILDREN'S LEADERSHIP AGENCY

This Commission is not spelling out any fundamental change in the basic nature of the organization of the federal government. Such a decision is a Congressional prerogative. Yet, as our analysis has indicated, the needs of children and youth have such low priority currently as to endanger the future quality of American life. We urge the Congress to examine federal organization and funding and make such rearrangements as are needed to carry out our recommendations.

Relatively few citizens grasp the long-run implications of allowing the needs of children and youth to continue in low priority in competition with the other demands of government. We believe that their needs call for special consideration and increased priority at all levels of government—federal, state, and local. Although we believe that many programs and services for children must be operated at the level of neighborhoods, below the level of organized government, we also believe that only the federal government commands the prestige, the expertise, the influence, and the financial power to effect a general increase in the level of priority given to children's needs. We believe that children and youth need an effective "advocate" at each level of government, especially at the federal level. Children who bear the onerous label of poverty or color need their advocacy made sure and their strength exposed. We further believe that a national commitment to children, youth, and their families should begin at the highest level—in the executive office of the President. For these reasons, we recommend the creation of a President's Advisory Council on Children.

President's Advisory Council members

The President's Advisory Council on Children would be based on the model of the Council of Economic Advisors and would derive its strength from the office of the President. In effect, it would operate through the influence of the Administration and would have the authority and capacity to recommend legislation to the Administration. The council would have a direct link with the Bureau of the Budget. Its goal would be to engineer a new national strategy for a major investment in children and youth. This effort might necessitate limiting for a temporary period increases in some technological programs if the issue becomes a matter of resource allocation.

Membership in the President's Advisory Council would be limited to a maximum of ten persons. The membership would be drawn from both professional and lay groups, including consumers. Members would be chosen on the basis of recognized competence in formulating, planning, assessing, and delivering services for children. Some of these members should be persons who have been involved in developing innovative programs for children. There should be full representation of persons having intimate and technical knowledge of minority groups and poor children.

Direct functions of the President's Advisory Council

The advisory council would meet several times a year and would have a permanent staff which would aid the advisory council in carrying out the following functions and responsibilities:

to study the problems of children and youth in the United States and provide long-range planning, policy-making, and programming, for both services and manpower;

to advise the President as to the allocation of money for children and their families; this would include specific recommendations concerning the budgets of all the agencies which provide services for children, youth, and their families;

to provide information about how agencies are working together, competing, or overlapping in providing services for children and youth;

to assess programs, assess relationships between programs, and assess appropriate budgetary levels for programs with the goal of integrating programs and avoiding fragmentation and unplanned duplications of money and service efforts;

to assess the functioning of federal, state, and local agencies and make recommendations;

to devise ways to challenge professional organizations to better exercise their public trust;

to advise the President and Congress with respect to any needed re-ordering of federal programs and funding in order to ensure the efficient operation of state and local programs; and

to act as the advocate, at the federal level, for children and families.

The President's Advisory Council would have available to it a yearly administrative budget. However, this group would not, itself, distribute money, as this might detract from its long-range planning responsibility and would be inconsistent with federal program organization and allocation of functions.

We believe that the Department of Health, Education, and Welfare should have: (1) the responsibility for translating policies of the President's Council and the Congress into a Comprehensive Federal Plan for Children; (2) responsibility for setting guidelines and regulations for comprehensive state plans; (3) the responsibility for distribution of funds to states to implement state plans through state agencies, local authorities, and Child Development Councils; (4) to consolidate and coordinate federal programs for children in ways that will serve to implement the recommendations of the Joint Commission and the Congressional mandate that we hope will flow from them.

II. Community Services and Programs of a Supportive, Preventive, and Remedial Nature

If we conceive of child development as a continuum stretching from the prenatal period through to the beginnings of work and adult life, we are able to identify critical points and periods of development as well as values governing this development. We are able to identify the groups, persons, and social institutions (mother, family, ethnic group, school, community, and the like) which critically affect the well-being of the child in the normal course of his development. We can also identify the social institutions which are concerned with the crises which arise at various points along the lines of development (such as disease, handicap, mental illness, juvenile delinquency, illegitimacy, and the like). Each of these institutions is connected "vertically" through a hierarchy of public and voluntary agencies. Each is related "horizontally" to other agencies providing services to children and youth.

There are, in addition, the organizations that train manpower for this system; the policy-making and funding agencies associated with government; the public and private organizations which influence policy and legislation; and the consumers of services who represent, more or less effectively, the interest of the users of services.

In Recommendations A and C of this section, the Commission addresses itself more fully to the deficiencies of social institutions and agencies which provide services to children who deviate from normal development (that is, mental health, public and voluntary welfare, correction services, and programs for the physically handicapped). All these services deal with crises in the lives of children but do so only in a poorly coordinated manner. Present services fail to take account of developmental processes, fail to provide continuity of care, and fail to serve all those in need. Further, these crisis-oriented services do not consider the total needs of the child, nor are they adequately linked to "normal-stream" institutions (that is, educational institutions, health-care services, recreational services, and the informal system of peer group, family, neighborhood, work, and the like).

To remedy these institutional gaps, the Commission strongly urges the creation of a network of comprehensive, systematic services, programs, and policies which will provide every American the opportunity to develop to his maximum potential. The line between the preventive and the remedial nature of services would be blurred by designing and coordinating services to meet the developmental needs of the total child. The advocacy system which we proposed provides one means of creating this network of services. Three levels of effort are required:

1. *Basic prevention.* We envision basic prevention in the broadest sense, taking into account services which are not ordinarily seen as relevant to normal development—family income maintenance, assurance of adequate housing, improvement of neighborhood conditions, provision of transportation, etc. We foresee preventive programs concerned with continued education of out-of-wedlock girls and with the nutritional well-being of children, programs which will attempt to influence food pricing or concern themselves with the question of availability of food,

transportation to markets, and so forth. We envisage preventive programs based on early intervention at critical stages when the child is most vulnerable; this implies systematic prenatal care and the creation or enlargement of day-care and preschool programs designed for children before the commencement of formal schooling. Basic prevention requires adequate provisions for health, cognitive development, significant interpersonal relationships, and opportunities for all children and youth to learn roles necessary to participatory democracy. Moreover, it requires recognition of the fact that health, cognition, and interpersonal relationships are highly interrelated.

2. *Secondary prevention.* We envision a service network highly attuned to intervening upon signs of *early* warnings or symptoms. Although remedial in nature, these interventions would be designed to prevent the compounded and complex problems in children which are the targets of most of our present-day remedial services.

3. *Tertiary programs.* We envision remedial programs built more on the model of health than on the model of illness. Future programs would provide a new and broader range of services to the seriously disturbed, juvenile delinquents, mentally retarded, and otherwise handicapped children and their families. Services would be designed on the basis of the child's level of functioning rather than on the current basis of diagnostic and social labels. These changes would be accompanied by an increased development of community-based facilities which would permit children to be kept as closely as possible within their normal, routine setting. For those unable to remain in the normal setting, institutions would be designed to provide highly personalized treatment and habilitation and rehabilitation services.

As indicated previously, the creation of a network of child-centered services cannot rest upon the mere restructuring of existing services and institutions which now serve children and their families. We must develop a broad spectrum of services and vast new pools of manpower, each based upon our best knowledge of child development as it applies to a pluralistic society.

In the recommendations which follow, we have not attempted to outline details of administration and funding but to identify some of the problems and to suggest possible and feasible modes of solution. We believe that the components listed from A to E in this section should be given highest priority in the creation of a service network. We believe that whereas many of the services and programs we discuss do exist, most are incomplete. Others could be created. All should be coordinated and provided to children through development of the advocacy system recommended previously.

A. PHYSICAL AND MENTAL HEALTH SERVICES
(AND SUPPORTIVE SERVICES)

Just as emotional well-being is influenced by physical well-being, so is cognitive development related to the course of physical and emotional maturation in the growing child. Any effective network of child-centered services must provide highly coordinated medical and mental health services and relate these, in turn, to the other child services and normal socializing agencies if we are to meet the developmental needs of all our children.

Preventing disorders must begin before conception with provisions for genetic counseling and family planning services. Prevention must include systematic care during the prenatal period and throughout all the developmental stages after birth. Currently, these services are not adequate. The poor, in particular, do not have wide access to these needed programs and often fail to use those which are available. Public services are often depersonalized. The poor feel stigmatized by professional attitudes which equate public service with charity.

The failure of the poor to use public facilities is compounded by poor education which hinders the identification of symptoms, by rigid clinic hours unfitted to the working poor, and by the poor coordination of the services themselves. In urban areas, one out of every four or five babies is born to a family dependent upon hospital outpatient clinics for its *total* medical care. Data from several large cities indicate that between one-fifth and one-half of the women delivered in municipal hospitals have had no prenatal care, or have received it too late for it to be effective ("A Look at Problems in Prenatal Service Programs," 1966). The majority of these mothers have been from deprived groups. These women often come to childbearing with a history marked by chronic untreated illness and malnutrition. The lack of prenatal care increases the chances that their babies will be born with physical and mental defects. Their children are those most likely to receive little or no care after birth. For example, most of the 600,000 children who attended Project Head Start Developmental Centers in 1965 had never been to a physician or dentist and had not received immunizations. Seventy percent of the sixteen- to twenty-year-old youths who enrolled in the Job Corps programs had never been to a physician, and many came from homes where at least one parent had physical and/or mental handicaps (U.S. House of Representatives, 1965). Such service deficiencies must be corrected if we are to optimize the development of children and youth in this nation.

However, we must face the fact that our best and most enlightened efforts at prevention and the promotion of positive, vigorous health and competence in children will never be completely adequate. Children in seemingly favorable life circumstances may falter in development, for elusive reasons. Other children will be victims of harmful experiences in home and school, in spite of our best efforts to strengthen these normal sources of affection, support, instruction, and discipline needed for healthy development. Emergency measures will be required, including hospitalization or placement in an institution. One can observe only with concern the rising rate of hospitalization of disturbed children. We must provide the seriously disturbed child with the same services as moderately or mildly disturbed children, but with important additions of special programs, for there is no one arrangement or type of solution that is appropriate or effective with all kinds of disturbed children.

In the recommendations which follow we propose a wide range of preventive and remedial physical and mental health services and supportive services. We recommend that these be made available to all children and youth through:

the enactment of a system of national health insurance, national health service, or some other alternative to guarantee equal access to service, and that

the federal govenment expand its efforts to establish the facilities and services required to meet the physical and mental health needs of American children and their families, either independently through use of federal funds or through a system of matching funds with state, county, or private agencies. Matching funds should be allocated only where agencies adhere to standards which specify comprehensive and coordinated services which will ensure continuity of care.

In heavily or moderately populated areas, we suggest that each area be completely served by each service system, and that all services offering the components described below be available for all persons living within each area. For sparsely populated areas where the traditional building complexes are unfeasible, we urge extensive expansion of traveling clinic services. These clinics should be equipped with special radio equipment to handle emergency cases. Rural locales would communicate with the clinic through the most feasible existing agency, which may be the school, the law enforcement agency, etc. In cases in which the clinic cannot immediately handle emergency cases, the communication would be relayed to an adjunct helicopter service which would pick up the patient and deliver him to the nearest service system. The helicopter service would also supply crisis personnel to homes in need; e.g., nurses, homemaker aides, etc.

It would be desirable for the appropriate federal authority to set guidelines for the geographical population to be served by a group of services. We recognize that local organizational problems make this difficult. However, it is ultimately desirable and urgent that common human service areas be designated just as we designate school districts.

Other coordinating and linkage mechanisms are also available, such as:

a 24-hour telephone information and referral system in each neighborhood or community;

the utilization of interagency liaison personnel, visiting nurses, and indigenous neighborhood aides;

the training of medical and supportive service personnel in the early identification of mental and emotional disorders and in the detection of early signs of dysfunction in the family which suggest abuse, neglect, or other possible detriment to the child;

systematic and continuous recording of physical and mental health data, beginning with information relevant to the prenatal period (with provisions to ensure the confidentiality of these records);

some coordination of public agencies.

In addition to the health and mental health services to be enumerated below, a number of supportive services must be provided to achieve maximum use of services. The following supportive services are crucial, particularly if the needs of lower socioeconomic groups are to be met:

extensive outreach efforts to identify those in need;

provisions for transportation to service facilities;

adequate child-care arrangements while parents are seeking or using service;

homemaker and nursing services for crisis situations and follow-up care;

programs of broad-scale public education in the area of health care.

Far greater use of the mass media should be made for such purposes.

These supportive services should be a component of all the services recommended below.

1. Family planning

The Commission recognized that the prevention of disorders in children begins before conception. Genetic counseling is a promising new area for family planning, one which can help prevent the birth of defective children. Family planning information will aid parents to limit their families as they desire and to plan for well-spaced births that will increase the chances for giving birth to healthy infants. Among medically indigent women, figures show that more than 5,000,000 desire family planning assistance but that only about one in ten of these women receive such aid from public or private agencies (U.S. Dept. HEW, 1966a).

The cost-benefit ratio for family planning services is extremely positive. It is estimated that for every $10,000,000 expended, up to at least the level of $90,000,000 per year, family planning services would prevent approximately 49,000 unwanted births, 2,000 infant deaths, and 48 maternal deaths (U.S. Dept. HEW, 1966b). Each birth prevented would cost about $200, less than the cost of prenatal care and delivery for that child. Further, because of the high incidence of various types of morbidity among the medically indigent, birth control services would greatly reduce the incidence of mental retardation, neurological handicaps, learning disability, sensory deficit, and emotional disturbance. The psychological costs of unwanted births are great, both to our victimized young and to those many parents who face excessive strains which unwanted children place upon them because of limited financial or emotional resources.

In relation to family planning, the Commission wishes to endorse the recommendation of the Planned Parenthood–World Population Organization that abortion and sterilization as medical procedures should be removed from the criminal law. The Commission also fully concurs with the resolution of the American Public Health Association's resolution that it is the right of every woman to decide whether or not she will bear a child.

To promote the development of our young, we recommend:

Birth control methods should be universally available for voluntary use by all females of child-bearing age; however, birth control programs must take into account the physical and mental health aspects connected with such programs.

Vigorous methods of education and delivery of family planning services are recommended at the highest priority level. Birth control methods and materials should be furnished without cost to the medically indigent and carried to such groups through accessible clinics.

Genetic examinations, genetic counseling, and early treatment of genetic disorders provide promising means of preventive intervention. It is recommended that screening tools for the detection of carriers of genetic and chromosomal abnormalities be evaluated for possible incorporation in premarital examinations and that screening of newborn infants for remediable genetic abnormalities be expanded as appropriate means for treatment become available. Further, genetic counseling by individuals competent in both genetics and mental health should be available in every community.

Federal family planning should be consolidated and central responsibility with high position and visibility should be created in the Department of Health, Education, and Welfare.

2. Systematic prenatal care

The inadequacies of prenatal and postnatal care are highly correlated with the incidence of infant mortality, prematurity, birth defects, mental retardation, and other disabilities. The total amount of prenatal damage is difficult to determine; however, it is greater than it should be and contributes to many mental health problems and to mental illness in children. Babies continue to be delivered in deplorable conditions, and not all newborns are checked for conditions which could be corrected. Some hospitals do not have emergency equipment and trained personnel to handle infants of abnormally low birth weight. More regional intensive care units, including ambulatory transportation services, are needed to care for these infants. Insofar as the women of this country are not given every service and opportunity to produce normal infants, the mental health of our children is being neglected.

Early and systematic prenatal care for all pregnant women should be made possible through a reorganization of medical functions and wider use of paramedical personnel. The 1965 Amendment to the Social Security Act which requires states to make maternal and child health services available to all by 1975 is a great step forward in this direction. Programs instituted under this act have apparently resulted in a reduction of infant mortality. We strongly urge the expansion of such programs. We further recommend:

The design of effective alternatives to the present impersonal, inconvenient, and marginal-quality clinics for the medically indigent. Outreach efforts must be increased, clinic hours must be regulated to meet the needs of the poor, and supportive services must be provided so that the poor can make use of available services. Training of medical and paramedical personnel must include a behavioral science component, so these personnel can better understand peoples of different social and cultural groups.

To complement medical services, we recommend the following as preventive measures to ensure maternal and child health: reduced working hours, paid maternity leave, homemaking services, nutritional supplements, prepregnancy immunizations, extensive testing and strict control of drugs, and education aimed at teen-agers and young adults to emphasize the importance of good health and suitable timing of pregnancies.

Mental health workers should be utilized for prenatal and postpartum services such as: (1) more adequate mental health consultation to obstetrical workers at all economic levels; (2) psychotherapeutic intervention in cases of postpartum psychosis and those in which emotional conflicts may possibly result in complications of pregnancy and delivery.

3. Comprehensive pediatric and mental health services for children under three

Many children disappear from professional surveillance during the period from birth to entry into school or preschool programs. Many families fail to take advantage of existing services, and consequently many problems of development go unnoticed until the child enters school. It is during the earliest years, however, that development is extremely rapid and malleable. Infants and very young children are especially vulnerable to trauma of all kinds: various infections, some with long-range consequences; accidents, including anoxia and poisoning; preventable contagious diseases; experiences related to personality and learning disorders, and so on. Some metabolic errors, undetected in newborns, are still amenable to treatment during the first few years of life. Corrective measures for children with hearing, motor, speech, and visual handicaps can often prevent interference with learning which leads to retardation in mental development and which may be complicated by emotional problems. Estimates indicate that about 20 to 30 percent of chronic handicapping conditions of childhood and later life could be prevented by comprehensive health care to age five, and approximately 60 percent if health care were extended to age fifteen.

Our mental health services are most deficient for the very young, yet there is general agreement among clinicians that the most important time for both remedial and preventive mental health services is during the mother's pregnancy and the very early years of the child's life. It has been estimated that 35 percent of apparently normal children of self-sustaining families show behavioral difficulties as early as age four. The prevalence of disorders is thought to be even higher among poor children. The present tendency is to identify children in need and refer them for services after they have reached the age of six or more and are found to present problems in school adjustment. This is often too late for effective intervention.

The Commission believes that highest priority should be given to the development of comprehensive mental health, pediatric, and supportive services for children under three, and that a major effort should be made to provide systematic care during the neonatal and postneonatal stage. The services should include the following:

Programs which deal with potentially handicapping conditions, with emphasis upon early identification of emotionally disturbed, retarded, and organically impaired children. Care and treatment should be prompt and continuing.

Improved practices for premature infants, including adequate stimulation of these infants and a model for identifying high-risk cases of adverse maternal reaction to the birth of a premature baby. Where such reactions are noted, mothers should be provided mental health consultation, visiting nurse services, etc.

Programs using a mother-substitute therapy approach (e.g., "foster-grandmother" program) for treatment of infants with failure to thrive.

Educational programs, both in and out of the home, which are designed to improve mothering practices, to provide early appropriate stimulation to increase sensory and motor adaptiveness, to improve language abilities, and to enrich a child's experiences with people, places, and things. These programs, together with health and mental health services, might be housed where feasible, in one unit, for example, in neighborhood comprehensive centers, or parent and child centers.

However, if neighborhood centers, and parent and child centers, are to accomplish the complex, multidisciplinary services we have outlined, they need the help and consultation of a fully qualified team of experts. Additional help in community organization and family life education should be available. Programs will need to be rapidly evaluated and new research findings translated into program activities. Failure to provide quality in the administration of such programs can leave local groups adrift and could rigidify well-meaning but inadequate services.

4. School health and mental health programs

Our various educational systems provide one means of reaching and helping many children in need of physical and mental health services and the wide array of interrelated services which buttress positive mental health. While most school programs have health and child service components, these are usually not well developed or well coordinated with community facilities and services.

The school should not be a mental health treatment or social services agency. However, it should have either on, or available to, its staff, personnel who can assist in making the connections among educators, families, and other service programs so that efforts can be coordinated.

Many schools have specialized personnel (guidance counselors, school psychologists, psychiatrists, nurses, social workers, etc.). Too many do not. Too often the school medical, "social services," and pupil personnel function is limited to traditional specialized roles. Such limitations are self-defeating.

School mental health programs should be a coordinated effort of all personnel concerned with children and youth. A number of functions such as case-finding, diagnosis, consultation, liaison roles with community agencies, contact with families, etc., should be conducted on the basis of competence rather than a particular professional identity.

The Commission urges that physical and mental health and other child services for children beyond the age of three be intricately co-ordinated with educational systems. Therefore, the Commission recommends:

Increased funding under the Titles of the Elementary and Secondary Education Act for comprehensive services in preschool programs. Mental health components should include screening and subsequent diagnostic assessment for the early identification and prevention of physical, emotional, and learning disorders. Mental health consultation should be made available to the staff and parents participating in preschool programs. Access to and collaboration between preschool programs and community resources would enable the development of a workable alliance. These programs could be modified appropriately for the elementary and secondary school levels.

Each school system should have available to it specialized personnel to work with educators and with children and their families. School needs will vary greatly. In some instances, a school may need more guidance counselors; in other cases, social workers may better fit the community needs. Many schools will need teams composed of all these workers. Each school system should devise an overall plan for stimulating coordination and integration between various personnel and their relationship to the school and community.

A mental health program should be an integrated part of educational programs and should include programs aimed at primary prevention. Planned programs with teachers, children, and parents which would deal with such areas as family living, human behavior, developmental characteristics and problems, patterns of learning, individual differences, etc., should be encouraged and studied.

Specific mental health programs should be designed to support the emotional well-being of teachers as well as children. Sufficient attention has not been given to the relationship between the teacher's emotional well-being and that of the individual child and classroom behavior. The physical and emotional health care of teachers should be the concern of school health and mental health personnel. Pupil personnel should provide support and consultation to help the teacher to not only deal with crisis situations but cope with everyday classroom problems so that the teacher may work more effectively with children.

Specialized school personnel should function as liaison between the family and the educators and between the school and the health, mental health, and social service programs to guide children and their families to appropriate services and to conduct program interpretation so that families, educators, and helping agencies can derive maximum benefits.

Specialized school personnel should serve to assist teachers in early recognition and referral of children with problems.

Special education programs must be an integral part of the continuum of services to be provided. The types of programs proposed by the Commission are presented below in Recommendation 7 on remedial mental health services.

5. College mental health services

American colleges have failed to recognize the relationship of the emotional life of the student to his academic progress. Higher education must shift its approach to view the academic life and the emotional life of the college student as interrelated. The following recommendations concern the college population:

All mental health services for college students must be expanded— from those providing specific therapy to a system of advisers and counselors who have daily contact with students and who are sensitive to student responses. Some services need not be maintained on campus but can be provided through linkages with various community facilities. Besides specific psychological counseling and crisis intervention, college mental health services should include drop-in clinics and provide opportunities for preventive counseling, dialogues, and group discussions in a variety of settings.

College mental health services must have a clearly defined relationship to the rest of the school. Administration and faculty must recognize that such services can play a major role in the creation of a college climate which can prevent many serious emotional disturbances. Mental health services and personnel must be integrated into college life at many levels, with the object of aiding the college in developing increased sensitivity to student development and of helping to facilitate such development.

The extent of psychological service available to students must be clearly defined in advance of registration in the college.

All student communications with the mental health service must be guaranteed confidential. Records concerning the mental health behavior of students should be made available only to the student himself or to others with the student's consent. Mental health personnel should never serve in policing or authority positions. When this is impossible to avoid, a clear definition of the relation of counseling and treatment role to the grading and policing role must be made.

It must be recognized that there is an increasing need to work with adolescents and youth with or without parental consent or knowledge.

6. *Mental health services of the clergy*

Clergymen serve many mental health roles. Many people with problems turn to their minister, rabbi, or priest for help. In recent years, many clergymen have acquired a professional understanding of mental health and combined this with their ability to impart ethical and religious values to persons who come to them for counseling. To utilize religious resources as a medium of assistance in the areas of prevention, care, and management, the clergyman requires field and clinical experience also.

To make adequate use of religious resources in child mental health development there must be a positive attitude toward the value of religious resources in child mental health development and a concomitant positive attitude toward the role of the clergyman in using these religious resources in child mental health development.

This demands the development of a professional relationship between the clergyman and the mental health worker if the contribution of the clergyman to child mental health development is to have more than tangential value. A meaningful collaborative relationship needs to have the following characteristics:

the acceptance of the clergyman by the hospital or agency staff as a bona fide resource person;

a willingness on the part of the hospital or agency staff to be of direct assistance to the clergyman by making available the agency facilities for training, as well as for the discharge of this function.

Assistance rendered by the agency staff to the clergy training process ought to include the following:

delineation and selection by the mental health worker of those cases in which the clergyman's resources are of demonstrable value with respect to the management of the problem;

apprising the client and his family unit of:

the availability of the services of the clergyman;

the relevance of the clergyman's services with respect to the management of mental health problems;

the importance of the resources offered through the clergyman with respect to the successful resolution or management of the problem for which the client is seeking agency assistance;

determination of the time when the clergyman's intervention with his special resources would be of maximum value toward the management of the client's problems.

7. Remedial mental health services

The Commission considered in its study nearly one-half of the American population—that is, the approximately 95,000,000 persons under twenty-five years of age. Of this number, it is estimated:

Two percent are severely disturbed and need immediate psychiatric care.

Another 8 to 10 percent are in need of some type of help from mental health workers.

Of the approximately 10,000,000 under twenty-five who need treatment and/or care the Commission estimates:

Eighty percent suffer from emotional disorders due to faulty training, faulty life experiences, and externalized situational conflicts, such as difficulties with school, sex, or siblings, parent-child relations, and social problems. These groups can usually be treated by general practitioners or pediatricians trained in mental health; school counselors; child development specialists; social workers; paraprofessionals who have been sufficiently oriented; and other persons working in settings not primarily established for treatment of mental illness.

Ten percent show deeper conflicts which have become internalized within the self and create emotional conflicts (the so-called neuroses). The services needed by this group range from outpatient services to Re-ED (see Chapter VI, Appendix D, for discussion of Re-ED) and/or residential care; however, all these services need to be interrelated in harmonious working referral and treatment arrangements, so the child can easily move from one to another of these services as each is required for his needs.

Five percent show physical handicaps and require specialized facilities and intensive care. Of the estimated 7,600,000 physically handicapped children who need services, 5,600,000 receive some services. The present services, however, require many improvements. Mental health services and educational services particularly need to be increased and improved.

The remaining 5 percent suffer severe mental disorders (for example, schizophrenia, severe mental retardation, etc.) and require more intensive care and often institutionalization.

According to our best estimates, only about 500,000 children are currently being served by psychiatric facilities (clinics, hospitals, private therapists).

We have a multiplicity of federal, state, and local public and private services which overlap each other; singly and together they fail to meet the need. Federal mental health funds are generally restricted to grants for demonstration experimental programs, although limited funds are available for construction, training, and staffing of facilities. In face of the need there is virtually little federal money provided for treatment. Legislation is needed for:

funding which will provide incentives to states and communities to establish a range of coordinated services providing interrelated, continuous care and treatment for children in need;

funding to construct service facilities and to train the manpower required to serve the total population at risk;

provisions for the training and proper geographic distribution of manpower needed to meet the mental health needs of all children and youth. (Recommendations for such provisions appear in Section IV of this chapter.)

A wide array of interconnected services is required. These services should be based on the following principles:

Services to the child should be dispensed according to the child's level of functioning rather than on the basis of social, legal, and clinical labels. A classification scheme based on function/dysfunction appears in Chapter VI, Appendix A, of this report. Using such a classification scheme means that children with many different diagnostic labels will be treated jointly under the same service program.

Children are best cared for and treated in atmospheres more related to health and normal living than to illness. Every effort should be made to keep the child as closely as possible within his normal setting. This means that we must expand nonhospital treatment arrangements, particularly those that could be operated under the auspices of community-based facilities, such as community mental health centers, educational settings, and social service agencies.

Programs for long-term care of the more severely handicapped must not be allowed to become custodial in function but must provide vigorous treatment, rehabilitation, and reeducation experiences, coupled with liaison and follow-up efforts. Access to the wide range of services proposed below should be continuously available to the children who need long-term care.

The Commission recommends that federal funding be provided to develop and expand a wide range of remedial services. The first nine recommendations below were formulated in a joint conference sponsored by this Commission and the National Association of Mental Health, Inc.

1. *Informational-referral services* easily accessible and equipped to direct families to available services, resources, and facilities.

2. *Comprehensive developmental and psychoeducational assessment* of each child's special treatment and educational needs should be made as early as possible by a team that may include a pediatrician, psychiatrist, social worker, neurologist, psychologist, speech and language pathologist, ophthalmologist, audiologist, educational specialist, and/or any other professional disciplines available and considered essential for the proper placement of the disturbed child. Highest priority should be given the development of services for comprehensive assessment of dysfunction.

The assessment service should assume responsibility for following up recommendations and referrals and for ongoing, periodic reevaluations to make certain that the appropriate and adequate community treatment, training, and educational facilities are made available to meet the recommendations of the assessment service.

3. *Treatment* for the child and his family when indicated. Psychiatric, psychological, social work, and other support services should be available as needed.

4. *Special education programs* must be an integral part of the continuum of services to be provided.

a. *Preschool home training programs* for the special training and education of disturbed children and for the guidance and counseling of their parents. Early identification and intervention can reduce and sometimes eliminate the severity of a child's mental and emotional disorders.

b. *Regular nursery schools* can help children who show inadequacies of cognitive and coping skills. For children who are too disturbed or disruptive to be contained in a regular nursery school, special nursery schools offering a variety of techniques and approaches to correct or reduce maladaptive behavior should be available.

c. *Regular public school classes* can provide the best setting for the education of a certain number of mentally ill children so long as there are available individuation of instruction, flexibility of programming, and the acceptance and understanding of the child's educational and behavioral problems and needs.

d. *Special classes* within regular schools offer advantages for those children who need a somewhat more intensive program. Those classes are usually close to the child's home and can be partially integrated with regular classes.

e. *Special schools* should be established under public school auspices or by voluntary agencies with governmental and public support for children who, because of the severity of their disturbances, cannot be accommodated in special classes within a regular school.

5. *Rehabilitation* is needed to provide a planned and purposeful process of restoration, remediation, and psychosocial adjustment. De-

pending on the "trainability" or "educability" potential of the individual, the goals of rehabilitation may involve anything from improvement in self-care or socializing skills to preparation for vocational and professional careers. The programs in such rehabilitational facilities should include special education, individual and group guidance, organized recreational and socializing experiences, sheltered workshops, and prevocational and vocational training for productive work experiences and skills.

6. *Residential care,* which may be provided by foster homes, group residences, residential treatment centers, sheltered villages, or hospital settings. It is essential that these facilities offer milieu treatment and have adequate resources for medical care, psychological and psychiatric consultation, special education, and other support services.

7. *Transitional services* must provide the resources to meet the inability of the family to provide support for adaptive functioning of the child; the inability of the school to provide adjusted educational services; the infrequent availability in the community of intensive outpatient treatment or other services for the child and his family, or some combination of these. Transitional services may include partial hospital care—as in day or night hospitals; halfway houses and hostels; and social habilitation programs.

In offering transitional services to children and adolescents, it is necessary to recognize that hospitalization is usually deemed necessary when the child's maladaptive behavior is acute and overtaxes the supports offered either in the home or in the community, especially the school. The child's inability to assume independence of functioning is often the chief obstacle to early release from hospital care to outpatient status. This highlights the need generally for more adequate community-based services, and most particularly the need for transitional services.

8. *Relief services for the families* of children severely disturbed and mentally ill should be provided. In any plan to provide partial hospitalization and transition services, the goal should be to utilize supportive services to keep the family intact. Examples of the above supportive services are OEO programs, foster grandparents, baby-sitting, homemaker services, public health nursing, and homebound services.

9. Within the system of services there should be *periodic* assessment, evaluation, and follow-up to ascertain that the child is maximizing benefits from the system (National Association for Mental Health, 1968).

10. *Intensive-care units* in pediatric departments of general hospitals to provide diagnostic studies and medical and nursing care for children suffering from physical illnesses accompanied by emotional disturbance. These units would be transitional in nature. The child would be referred to the proper service once the illness had been treated.

11. *Acute and intensive diagnostic and treatment services on an in-*

patient basis, as provided by the psychiatric service of a hospital or a comprehensive community mental health center. These should be short-term residential programs (a matter of days and weeks, not of months) because of their great expense and the great need for such resources. The units should provide a first-quality educational program and liaison service.

12. *Special therapeutic recreational or work programs*, including summer and weekend camping, utilizing the resources and personnel of agencies such as the YMCA and the YWCA, the Boy Scouts, and park departments or creating special programs of recreation or work for mental health purposes.

13. *Special foster homes and small group living arrangements* (hostels) for disturbed children and youth with severely disorganized homes or no homes at all, that will make it possible for them to be involved in therapeutic and reeducational efforts listed here.

14. *Re-ED-type schools* or reeducation centers on both a day attendance and a residential basis, to provide intensive short-term (approximately six to eight months) assistance to moderately and severely disturbed children.

The services listed above should be available to all children. The poor should not have to choose between either treatment or preventive mental health and other essentials of life. Mental health workers should be willing to go into the homes of the poor, when necessary. Procedures such as scheduling of appointments, intake, and the like should be tailored to fit the life style of minority groups and disadvantaged communities. (Further recommendations on clinical services to minority groups and the poor are found in Chapter V in this report.)

Residential care: The Commission holds that the present institutional arrangements for residential care of disturbed children are inadequate in many ways, requiring a critical appraisal of both assumptions and procedures, and the invention of a number of new forms for caring for children when normal arrangements fail.

We assume that disturbed children will require an array of mental health services—special programs in regular schools, mental health consultation to teachers and parents, mental health clinics as well as residential care—but we focus here on the last of these. In 1966 an estimated 35,800 children under eighteen were in mental hospitals. Many of these institutions fall far short of meeting the needs of children and youth. There are a few superb institutions in the country, many that are marginal; however, most are disgraceful and intolerable. And their quality is not related simply to costs or to the level of training of staff. Some costly institutions with highly trained staffs are inadequate; some not too expensive arrangements with unconventional staffing patterns are doing a good job. The more conspicuous inadequacies of residential institutions are discussed in Chapter VI of this report.

The Commission makes the following recommendations concerning residential programs:

Residential treatment programs for disturbed children should be designed with the needs of children and their families the foremost consideration. In addition to space for therapy programs there should be facilities for a first-rate school and a rich evening activity program, and there should be ample space for play, both indoors and out. Facilities should be small, seldom exceeding 60 in capacity with 100 a maximum limit, and should make provision for children to live in small groups. The centers should be located near the families they serve and be readily accessible by public transportation. They should be located for ready access to special medical and educational services and to various community resources, including consultants. They should be open institutions wherever possible; locked buildings, wards, or rooms should only rarely be required. In designing residential programs, the guiding principle should be this: children should be removed the least possible distance— in space, in time, and in the psychological texture of the experience— from their normal life setting.

Disturbed children should be confined on wards in large medical complexes for only short periods required for diagnostic studies or for longer periods for medical and nursing care required by such conditions as colitis, acute epilepsy, or other physical illnesses accompanying the emotional disturbance. Intensive-care units in the pediatrics division of general hospitals should be provided for these purposes. The convenience of the staff or trainees is not sufficient reason to place children in confinement not conducive to normal development.

The practice of placing children and adolescents on wards with mentally ill adults should be stopped.

Psychotherapy should be provided children and adolescents in residential programs whenever feasible and appropriate. Training programs should be expanded to increase the supply of psychotherapists. However, two points need to be made to avoid frequently observed restraints on good programming for disturbed children in residential settings: (1) psychotherapy cannot bear the full burden but must be one part of a total program of rehabilitation and reeducation, and (2) the unavailability of qualified psychotherapists should not be allowed to stand in the way of imaginative—and therapeutic—programming for children.

Institutions for mentally retarded and delinquent chi.dren and youth should be periodically screened to identify children who are emotionally disturbed, for whom other arrangements are more functional.

For children who are placed in an institution for more than 60 days, there should be required a periodic report to a proper authority on what the institution is doing for the child. Such reports should be a requirement for retention of a child under court order. This might be a function of the Child Development Councils.

The Commission, recognizing that a critical criterion for health is the ability of the child to function effectively in home, school, and community, recommends that treatment programs for disturbed children be designed to sustain and enhance the competence of the child in these relationships through (1) the identification of specific sources of discord between the child and his immediate environment; (2) therapy, training, and education to increase the ability of the child to meet specified and appropriate environmental demands; (3) family therapy, consultation, and direct intervention in home, school, and community to assist each to be more responsive to the child; and (4) continuing involvement of the child in home, school, and community to the extent that the contact provides instructive and productive interaction between the child and the normal agents of human development.

Because of its proven effectiveness, in terms of both cost per child served and success in restoring the child to home, school, and community, the Commission recommends that the Re-ED model be adopted and extended as one of many needed kinds of services for emotionally disturbed children. Specifically, the Commission recommends that funds be made available to any state, community agency, or nonprofit corporation for the construction and operation of residential schools for emotionally disturbed children, patterned after the Re-ED plan. Funds should be sufficient to establish at least 100 schools with at least one school in each state to serve as models for other programs. (Recommendations relating to research and to training personnel for the Re-ED type programs are found in Sections III and IV respectively.)

B. ASSISTANCE, EMPLOYMENT, AND ENVIRONMENTAL PROGRAMS

The alleviation of poverty

Although we own almost 50 percent of the world's wealth, about one-fourth of our nation's children are living in poverty or near-poverty. The Commission believes strongly that poverty, like racism, is one cause of major mental health problems. Both racism and inadequate family income compound the difficulties which appear to create the need for mental health and social services. Indeed, the Commission is convinced that the eradication of poverty and the conditions which cause it are essential primary prevention measures. Many mental health and social problems would disappear if poverty and racism were eradicated.

Contrary to much public opinion, poor children are not usually the victims of lazy, shiftless parents. They are the victims of our society's failure to ensure full employment and a guaranteed minimum income—a statement borne out by the following facts:

- Despite continuing economic growth and declining national unemployment rates, unemployment continues to be characteristic of large proportions of our disadvantaged populations.
- In 1966, more than 40 percent of impoverished children were living in homes where the family head held a job all year.
- Less than one percent of the more than 7,000,000 Americans receiving public assistance payments could be self-reliant if employment were available. Over half the recipients are dependent children. Nationwide, payments under programs to aid dependent children average only about $40 a month for each recipient—a sum far below the poverty line. Contrary to general opinion, many thousands of people come on public assistance because they lose employment or are underemployed. Many thousands leave the rolls yearly to become wage earners.

A major consequence of poverty is that large numbers of our young, like their parents, are at high risk to be chronically ill, socially incompetent, and mentally disordered. Malnutrition takes its toll by retarding physical growth, by increasing vulnerability to disease, by lessening the capacity to learn, by stunting emotional growth and—if recent studies are confirmed—by producing permanent and irreversible brain damage in some infants. Crowded, unsafe environments create additional adjustment and learning problems and increase the risk of disease and accident. An incomplete medical assistance program, high costs, and chaotic service delivery systems prohibit many poor families from obtaining the social, health, and mental health services which their children need. Grossly inadequate schools and other public services are usually the lot of the poor—despite the fact that the poor pay 18 percent of the total tax dollar.

Too often, the child of poverty becomes the "functional illiterate" in our impoverished classrooms. By the time of his adolescence, school and home lose their influence; idleness and unemployment become a way of life. With so few opportunities open to these youths, it is not surprising that youth unemployment is correlated with high rates of delinquency and antisocial activities. Arrest records almost assure continuing unemployment.

Unemployment is a serious handicap for all the poor. Idleness and rejection hamper development by lowering self-esteem and a belief in the future. The disadvantaged youth may well become the impoverished parent. The cycle of poverty remains unbroken.

By permitting poverty and racism to continue, we do violence to our young. The costs to society are great—both in the tragic waste of unfulfilled lives and in the economic burdens of dependency. Clearly, we can only benefit by increasing our efforts to eliminate poverty and to provide for the needs of our disadvantaged young. Violence, in all its innumerable forms, can only breed more violence.

1. Employment and training

Although the Commission strongly endorses the concept of a guaranteed minimum income, we believe this should be accompanied by a national commitment to a system which provides guaranteed employment for all who can work and desire to work. However, consistent with the principles of positive mental health, any system designed to maximize employment must also provide the incentive of work satisfaction at wages which are at least congruent with the standard of living provided by a guaranteed income system. Indeed, the work system must constantly challenge the individual and provide him with opportunities to advance himself, as in the "career-ladder" program.

Because the welfare of our young is so dependent upon family income and because the American value of self-sufficiency has so many implications for positive mental health, the Commission recommends:

A greater effort should be made to achieve full employment, through job training and opportunities for all persons who can be absorbed into the labor force, including those with physical, mental, and social handicaps.

We urge that special attention be given to creating training and employment opportunities for disadvantaged youth groups. (We realize that this is a highly complex problem which calls for changes in vocational and academic curriculum; suggested changes for primary, secondary, and junior college levels are recommended elsewhere in this report.)

Legislation should be enacted which will provide all employed persons a minimum wage level and humane working conditions. Wage levels should be congruent with at least guaranteed minimum income levels and with federally determined cost of living standards adjusted for regional differences. (A minimum wage rate for adolescents and youth is proposed below in Recommendation E in this section.)

The various fragmented and uncoordinated manpower and training programs should be redesigned to create more viable arrangements. We urge an expansion of such programs in the human service field, and especially in those which deal with mental health.

Enforcement powers should be exercised to eliminate discriminatory practices wherever they exist, and all federal grants-in-aid funds should be withheld from activities which discriminate on the grounds of color, religion, sex, and age.

Location of business and industry in the slums, Indian reservations, and other economically depressed areas should be encouraged by the federal government through financial incentives, guaranteeing insurances, obtaining support from banks and foundations, and establishment of government offices. In order to qualify for this aid, a business or industry must substantiate that its operation will be consistent with the economic and social needs of the community and that employment practices will favor the advancement of personnel from that community.

Migration to urban areas should be countered by providing opportunities in rural areas, through the fostering of industrial development, setting up marketing cooperatives, the providing of loans for developing truck farms, etc.

2. Income maintenance

The Commission recommends revision of all present income maintenance programs to ensure a *guaranteed minimum income* for all Americans. The Commission did not assume the competence to make specific recommendations on the differential values of various new income maintenance proposals, except for children's allowances. We support the guaranteed minimum income principle because its mental health implications are clear. Poor people need resources; they need to be treated as dignified and worthwhile citizens. Our recommendations are designed primarily to improve existing programs. Short of creating one guaranteed income mechanism, we conclude that the movement toward a guaranteed minimum income must proceed by maximizing the potentials of all present programs.

a. Public assistance

The Commission applauds recent federal guidelines and mandates separating the provision of public assistance grants from the giving of services and replacement of undignified investigations with a self-declaration system. However, we find that the entire public assistance program is administered inequitably from state to state: it does not reach all who should benefit; it tends to keep people in poverty and dependent because it provides neither adequate income nor sufficient opportunities and incentives to motivate people to move out of the system.

With elimination of all eligibility conditions except need, and with constantly adjusted cost of living standards, public assistance, so long as it exists as a system, would then, in effect, provide a guaranteed minimum income.

It appears that the public assistance program, presently and apparently for some time to come, will be the major income bulwark for the very poor. Therefore, we strongly recommend that the following steps be taken to improve the public assistance system:

Establishment, in federal law, of a *national minimum* for public assistance grants, based solely on need, below which no state may fall. Federal law should simultaneously establish cost of living standards which should be adjusted for differences in family size and for regional variations in living costs. States should be required to provide the mandated grants and to adjust benefits periodically using federally designated methods to determine the minimum living standards for health and decency in the area where the recipient lives.

Greatly increased federal financial participation in a uniform, simple plan for federal-state sharing in costs of all public assistance grants, including general assistance. The plan should provide for equitable and reasonable fiscal efforts among states and recognize the relative fiscal capacity of the federal and state governments.

Provisions to assure that all public assistance grant programs receiving federal funds are administered consistent with the principle of *public assistance as a right*. This would include: (1) entitlement to all benefits using a declaration system to ensure prompt, objective, and impartial determination of eligibility. Present case-by-case investigations should be replaced by sampling techniques; (2) prompt fair hearings by an impartial appeals agent, with legal representation provided the consumer and with court review; (3) the obligation of state and local agencies to publicize the conditions of entitlement.

Separation of the machinery for determining financial eligibility from the provision of social services.

Elimination of all categories, consistent with the single criterion of need.

Establishment in law of policies and programs which provide work incentives and guaranteed employment for those able and willing to work. However, mothers of young children should not be required to seek employment.

Reformulation of the goals and policies for the treatment of earnings, contributions from relatives, or other income, in terms of their impact on clients' lives. The desired policy goals would be:

Provision of work incentives by federal subsidy of exemption of a portion of earned income, allowing a net income which does not exceed a realistic "standard of need." As income is increased, one exemption would be decreased until the person is self-sufficient. In effect, public assistance would subsidize the full-time working poor. Present federal regulations forbid federal matching of full-time wage earners.

Exemption of owned homes. Some states now place liens on owned homes. This discourages eligible home owners from claiming public assistance. It also discourages public assistance recipients from becoming home owners. As a consequence, millions of public dollars are used for rental of substandard dwellings. These dollars should be used for construction of new dwelling units.

The fact that present welfare policies and practices are often dehumanizing and tend to discourage self-sufficiency is contrary to principles which foster good mental health. Adults caught in this system develop feelings of hopelessness, despair, and dependency which they pass on to their children. Until the poverty child sees that either he or his parents have some power over their own fate, he will continue to succumb to apathy and defeatism.

For these reasons, we endorse the following propositions formulated by the American Public Welfare Association as means to increase the effectiveness of public welfare as a positive and acceptable force in the lives of the poor:

> Expansion and improvement of various means of communication, mutual understanding, and involvement of recipients and other poor people. This would include employment and training of recipients or members of poorer neighborhoods in various types of jobs (e.g., case aides, members of service units, community aides); encouragement of client participation, organization and representation in matters relating to welfare; and the development of methods of dialogue between administrative heads of departments and organizations of the poor for response to questions, complaints, and interpretation of needs.

> Provisions which recognize the rights of recipient citizens to privacy and control over their personal affairs and provide positive protections for the exercise of those rights.

> Elimination of the infringements and limitations on personal privacy, choice, and achievement which are inherent in the prevalent system of applying for financial aid with attendant investigation procedures.

b. Unemployment compensation

Unemployment compensation is an inadequate insurance-type program. It is supported primarily by federally mandated state taxes on employers with federal funds for administration and is governed by limited federal standards. The program covers only about four-fifths of all wage and salaried workers and provides funds to make up for only part of the wage loss for workers covered during periods of unemployment. Provisions are not uniform. States provide different amounts of benefits. Each sets its own benefit period; each state has its own qualification provisions. Only eleven states provide differential benefits for dependents. As a result of fairly low benefits, limited benefit periods, and no provision for dependents, many persons who receive unemployment compensation also apply for and receive public assistance concurrent with unemployment compensation or after they pass the limit of the benefit period.

This is a burden on both systems, a hardship on the consumers, and an inefficient means of providing sufficient income.

The Commission claims no major competence in this or any other public social insurance field. We are assuming continuance of the system, and our recommendations are consistent with the public assistance ones. Since low incomes are conducive to poor mental health in any program, we merely suggest what appear to be reasonable improvements. Therefore, the Commission recommends:

> that the length of unemployment compensation coverage time be made uniform among the states by federal law;
> that federal law be amended to require that states must include provisions for dependents;
> that benefits be made more realistic in terms of the worker's earnings;
> that exclusions and disqualifications be uniform among the states.

c. Social Security

Our largest social insurance program for children, the national old age, survivors, and disability system known as Social Security, is a matter of concern to the Commission because its benefits do not provide a reasonable minimum standard of living.

Social Security is the basic program for ensuring income to the worker and his family when he retires, becomes disabled, or dies. Nearly 100,-000,000 people pay into this system; more than 20,000,000 receive benefits. The program is financed by employer-employee contributions and benefits which are based generally on formulas which take amount of earnings and length of employment into account. However, the poor pay more in proportion to their income than the more affluent.

Benefits are paid as a statutory right, without regard to need or to how much property or income the individual may have.

The Commission recognizes that this program has been constantly improved. It did not study in any depth the details of what additional improvements are needed. However, it did ascertain that in no instance were the benefits high enough to provide poor consumers with incomes which might be classified as a guaranteed minimum income or ones which met the requirements of a minimum standard of health and decency. Since both the affluent and the poor ultimately receive the same benefits from this program, the inequities are obvious.

The Commission noted that an increasing number of Social Security beneficiaries also receive public assistance in order to meet minimum income needs. Therefore, the Commission recommends:

> Social Security benefits should be increased to make them consistent with current costs and standards of living and with built-in periodic adjustments. This would eliminate the necessity for many people to receive

public assistance and Social Security concurrently. It is important to note that many families with children in which there is no breadwinner receive Social Security payments which carry no stigma, yet many needy children whose families do not qualify for Social Security are excluded from the Aid to Families of Dependent Children Program (AFDC), to which a great deal of stigma is attached. This contradiction is representative of the dilemmas and inconsistencies in our income maintenance programs.

Congress should give serious study to the circumstances which find thousands of aged, disabled, and blind persons concurrently receiving public assistance and Social Security payments or who receive only public assistance payments. While we recognize the actuarial nature of the Social Security program, we suggest that it would be more administratively efficient and less wearing on the mental health of the individual if he did not have to cope with two programs. In addition, moving the aged, disabled, and blind from the public assistance to the Social Security rolls would reduce the size and the cost of public assistance programs considerably, increase its ability to function efficiently, and reduce some of the stigma now attached to it. Public assistance would then be primarily for parents and children, and we would be in a better climate to improve conditions for a primarily child- and family-oriented program.

Consideration might also be given to ultimately administering the Aid to Families with Dependent Children program (public assistance) together with the OASDI (Social Security). Through common administration of both these massive programs for children, the stigma attached to AFDC might be lessened or eliminated. From the mental health standpoint, this type of arrangement would diminish feelings of dependency among poor families and children who need and receive cash assistance.

d. The children's allowance

Because children are our most precious resource and because parents and home remain the most important and potentially effective determinants of a child's development, we recommend that a new federal income maintenance program be established in law to provide an adequate universal system of child allowances.

We believe this program, now used in many other nations, to be an effective way of demonstrating a clear national commitment to our young. Both the poor and the nonpoor would receive these allowances. The more affluent would, of course, return some of these in taxes. The allowances would not solve all of the economic problems of the poor. Many would require additional assistance from existing programs.

The Commission is not opposed to other guaranteed income proposals, such as the negative income tax, which are under study by the President's Commission on Income Maintenance. In fact, we suggest that each proposed scheme be studied and tried on an experimental basis in different areas of the nation and that the effectiveness of each program be determined by systematic feedback and evaluation. Such experimentation should determine which of the programs is the most effective and efficient.

However, we are convinced that the children's allowance, while it would not eliminate poverty, could be a major mental health aid for all American children. Each child and each parent would know and feel intimately that the nation is investing in its children.

3. Food programs

. . . We saw children who don't get to drink milk, don't get to eat fruit, green vegetables, or meat. They live on starches—grits, bread, Kool Aid. Their parents may be declared ineligible for commodities, they have literally nothing. We saw children fed communally, that is, by neighbors who give scraps of food to children whose own parents have nothing to give them.

. . . We do not want to quibble over words, but "malnutrition" is not quite what we found; the boys and girls we saw were hungry—weak, in pain, sick, their lives being shortened; they are, in fact, visibly and predictably losing their health, their energy, and their spirits. They are suffering from hunger and disease and directly or indirectly they are dying from them—which is exactly what "starvation" means. (U.S. Senate, 1967.)

These shocking conditions which a team of doctors found in Mississippi in 1967 have since been observed among millions of children in every part of our nation. Hunger and malnutrition take their toll in the form of organic brain damage, retarded growth and learning rates, apathy, alienation, frustration, and violence; they contribute to high rates of premature birth and low birth weight, and consequently, to high infant mortality rates. In financial expenditures we spend far more to remove food from the market, to limit food production, to retire land from production, and to guarantee and sustain profits for producers than we spend to ensure our children an adequate diet.

The Commission highly commends the federal government's recent efforts to study the problem of hunger and malnutrition in this country and the attempts to upgrade federal food programs. While we believe this problem would best be met by guaranteeing an adequate income to all American families so that people would have sufficient funds to purchase food, we recognize the present need to rely on federal food programs. In considering recommendations to improve these federal programs, we have borrowed heavily, though not entirely, from a report made by the Citizens' Board of Inquiry into Hunger and Malnutrition in the United States

(*Hunger, U.S.A.*, 1968). We have addressed ourselves to improvements in federal food and medical programs and related consumer education services.

a. *Federal food programs*

We recommend that federal expenditures for food programs be increased, so that food is universally available on the basis of need and not dependent on local or state option. However, the federal government should encourage more effective and comprehensive state and local administration of food programs by providing greater financial inducement conditioned on state and local plans that meet both federal criteria and the approval of probable beneficiaries of the program. No plan should be certified unless provisions are made for ensuring provisions of federal food benefits for all areas of severest privation within the state and for expeditious procedure for appeals by an individual from a state or local action to a designated federal authority. Present provisions which exclude some of the poor, make access to the programs difficult, or make eligibility procedures undignified should be eliminated.

A free food stamp program should be the basic federal food plan. The commodity distribution program should function merely as a surplus distribution program. Eligibility for the food stamps should be based on a sole criterion: need. This would mean that persons without sufficient income or available cash would receive free food stamps. Requirements for basic eligibility should be based on income, number of dependents, and medical expenses. Additional revisions in the present program should include:

> Food stamp allotments should be high enough to allow each individual to secure a diet meeting the current standards of the recommended daily allowance. The monetary value of food stamps should be increased to meet the special needs of pregnant women, infants, and the sick; and
>
> food stamp prices, for those with sufficient income to purchase them, should be priced within the means of the individual recipient. These should be provided on a "pay as you go" system with provisions which allow for purchasing less than the maximum amount.

The delivery system should ensure that food stamps—based on adequate levels set by law—are available to all eligible without investigation. The system should be simple and devoid of stigma and excessive bureaucratic red tape. One such system has been suggested by the Citizens' Board of Inquiry (*Hunger, U.S.A.*, p. 86); that is, the use of a simplified federal income tax return to which a perforated voucher could be attached. Eligible individuals could simply present the endorsed voucher to the designated food stamp official in order to receive his stamps. Enforcement of truth-telling would rest—as with the income tax—with the Internal Revenue Service, using sample checks. If the public assistance delivery system is connected, it could serve the same purpose.

The Commission recommends that the food and nutrition programs enacted to improve the health status of all children in preschools, schools, day-care centers, settlement houses, and recreational activities should be universally available and not dependent on adoption by school and other officials. All meals should conform to federal nutritional standards. In addition, these programs should serve as a vehicle for the use of fortified foods.

The universal administration of programs provided for under the National School Lunch Act of 1946 and the 1962 amendment to this Act, the 1966 Child Nutrition Act, and the 1968 special food service program will, no doubt, call for greater financial expenditures by the federal government. However, we believe the benefits outweigh the costs since these programs offer the advantage of using an already existing institution as a delivery system for providing poor children well-balanced, highly nutritious meals. Additionally, the programs are a vehicle for nutrition education.

We also recommend that some feasible partnership among federal, state, and local authorities be devised so that the breakfast and lunch programs can be provided to needy children on a nonstigmatizing basis. This might be accomplished through the use of nontransferable stamps which can be purchased by parents at the issuing office or distributed to food stamp recipients along with their food stamps. The issuing office might well be located in the Child Development Councils recommended by the Commission.

b. *Administration of nutritional supplements by federally supported medical programs*

We urge that the federal government increase financial expenditures for the early identification and correction of health problems related to nutritional deficiencies, both in federally supported medical programs and through subsidies to the private health sector. These programs should focus on:

intensive efforts to identify nutritional deficiencies in pregnant women, infants, and young children and the correction of such deficiencies, either through direct administration of the required nutritional supplements (as provided for under the Maternal and Infant Care projects) or through referral to a federally subsidized agency which would be authorized to provide the needed supplements. This could also be accomplished by utilizing the Child Development Councils recommended by the Commission.

We also recommend:

> that the federal government, either directly or through subsidies, package fortified formulas for infants which can be safely stored for long periods, and that several months' supply of this formula be made available to the poor through both the public and the private medical sector or upon direct application by a needy applicant to any appropriate agency. In making this recommendation, we call attention to the fact that the present federally distributed surplus milk products cannot meet this need because they are deficient in the nutrients required for optimal infant growth.

c. *Consumer education*

Federal efforts to teach the poor how to make optimal use of foods are deficient in many respects. No doubt the effectiveness of these programs will continue to be undermined by the mere realities of poverty. It is unrealistic to assume that poor families can follow the low-cost and economy food plans proposed by the U.S. Department of Agriculture until they are guaranteed the purchasing power to buy in quantity and shop for bargains, both of which are indispensable to the USDA plans. However, because nutritional education services sometimes increase the sophistication of the poor we recommend:

> expansion of nutritional services which provide counseling to families on food preparation, budgeting, and management of therapeutic diets (such as those programs offered by the USDA and the Children's Bureau, Social and Rehabilitation Service);
> involvement of indigenous personnel in planning nutrition education programs and in reaching low-income groups. Indigenous workers can be particularly useful in helping nutritionists deal with the problem of differing cultural food patterns.

However, there is a need for more effective techniques of teaching nutrition education in schools. Because of their training, some nutritionists emphasize types of nutrients rather than types of food—a technique of questionable effectiveness among the poor. To increase the effectiveness of educational efforts, we recommend that the federal government:

> increase expenditures for research designed to carry out experimental nutrition education and counseling programs and to determine the effectiveness of these efforts, such as the evaluative study being conducted at Children's Hospital Foundation in Columbus, Ohio, and funded by the Children's Bureau;
> subsidize curriculum development and training based on the findings of a relevant body of knowledge.

In addition to the above, we urge:

that commodity food packages be stamped with recipes and with directions for use;

that a greater emphasis be placed on nutritional education in schools.

4. Housing

Because the physical and mental health of millions of our children are threatened by poor and/or segregated neighborhoods and housing and by the attitudes and policies which have created and perpetuated these conditions, the Commission urges:

that open housing laws be universally enacted and enforced;

that we commit a portion of our resources to the elimination of the ghetto and to the principle of creating communities—through sound housing and urban and community development—which do not segregate by class, by income, or by other nonrelevant criteria;

that a massive construction and repair program be undertaken to ensure adequate housing to all poor families;

that attention be given to converting the approximately $1,100,000 of public monies spent yearly for housing by welfare recipients—much of which goes into slum dwellings—into a positive program of home ownership and rehabilitation of dwellings;

that the design of urban renewal and similar programs give highest priority to the human needs involved and that every effort be made to minimize the risks of disrupting the family and social constellation of community members by providing for community participation on every level of program development;

that a small percentage of all federal monies allocated for construction and renewal be earmarked for beautification of the inner city, rural depressed areas, reservations, etc;

that greater federal expenditures be granted to communities for self-help and community development programs, including cooperative housing.

C. SOCIAL SERVICES

The Commission concludes from present data that services for children and youth are grossly inadequate, antiquated, and poorly coordinated. For children in need, there is a dramatic mismatch between the character of the services and the needs and rights of children. This mismatch is reflected in the mental health, social welfare, and corrections services and in programs for the physically handicapped. Programs designed to strengthen family life and foster the normal development and mental health of our children are nonexistent in many communities. Our investigations reveal shortages of funds, facilities, and manpower in all services designed for children in need; however, we cannot make a reasonable quantitative analysis of the deficiencies in services because present data are incomplete.

It is the sober conclusion of this Commission that even if our financial investments in the present systems were multiplied several times over, inefficiency and suffering would continue on a massive scale. The system is in need of drastic restructuring. There is a need to redesign the technologies for providing services and the organizational methods of delivery. There is a need for a more humane approach. Our services need to enlist consumers and parents as planners and co-workers in children's services.

In analyzing the service systems—including the psychiatric services noted in Recommendation A—we found pervasive, inherent inadequacies in many aspects of the service systems. Among the more critical of these are the following:

1. Systems tend to be oriented to keeping the professions constant and stable rather than to meeting the needs of the children being served.

2. The systems are oriented toward remedial crises services rather than preventive programs designed to alleviate the causes preceding and underlying crises. Different agencies tend to respond separately to a series of discrete crises which arise in the life of the child. There is often no communication between the different agencies which handle the same child.

3. The systems are ill-coordinated and serve only a small fraction of the population in need and at risk. Poor coordination occurs within and between agencies—between those that give similar service and those which should not compete with each other. Such poor organization prevents the service agencies from providing either comprehensive or continuous care. For example, different agencies, or separate departments within a single agency, may conduct their own diagnoses. Such practices expose the child and his family to multiple visits and tests and often result in different diagnoses of the same child. Also, with few exceptions, the agencies find it difficult or impossible either to step outside of their own specialties or to team up with other agencies so as to respond to the whole child as his needs change developmentally.

4. The systems tend to serve those clients most likely to achieve success on the agency's terms rather than those most in need. Agencies select as points of entry into the lives of children those situations which are easiest of access rather than those in which the child presents the greatest vulnerability or opportunity for change. There is a tendency for

agencies to ignore or repress the informal service systems which do respond to large numbers of those in need. For example, many agencies discourage the efforts of nonprofessionals and parents. Few attempts are made to help them become more effective.

5. Overlap is noted in the systems. For example, both psychiatric and nonmedical social agencies see troubled children and families. While the line between mental health treatment of a disorder and a social adjustment case service is often hard to discern, there is little use of systematic procedures and criteria at the case level. Such procedures could provide operational bases for determining the allocation of responsibility and cooperative service by psychiatrically controlled and nonmedical services; they could assure that an appropriate flow of cases and exchange of significant information occurs between the two systems.

6. The system tends to be highly traditional and conservative, even in the programs it labels as innovative.

In addition to the above deficiencies, we found a series of "second-order" problems relating to management and policy-making at agency, neighborhood, city, state, and national levels. These problems are:

1. Unsystematic methods of data collection which result in an oversupply of fragmentary, confused data and an almost total absence of usable operating and management data directed toward problem solution.

2. Pressing problems in the systems which are defined differently at every level; rarely are these differences examined so that meaningful priorities can be established.

3. No agency takes responsibility for a central overview of services affecting the well-being of children at any level. Even at the national level, little attention is given to policy questions of long-term importance.

4. Research tends to be disconnected from operating practice.

We believe that the various advocacy bodies recommended by this Commission can serve as agents to sort out functions and to eliminate the present confusion, fragmentation, and overlap between and among agencies and systems of services. If we do not sort out and allocate functions in service of the child we may find the problems increasing, and systematic, comprehensive services to children may become impossible to achieve.

We further believe that Congress, or the President's Advisory Council on Children which we proposed, should establish a body which would undertake, directly or indirectly, the following activities:

Ascertain the full range of public and voluntary service agencies and programs which operate in or out of legal or licensing sanctions. Sampling or census techniques should be used to map what these agencies and programs do, where they operate, their legal base, how they are funded, and the range of overlap in their operations.

Identify the actual and presumed goals toward which agencies, programs, or groupings of these operate.

Assess such key problems as manpower, its allocation and training, and the interaction among and between agencies, programs, or groupings of these.

Explore the experience gained in successful arrangements in the United States and those in other countries which represent approaches to total service systems for children.

Explore alternative strategies for attaining service goals, with particular attention to those not restricted by the boundaries of traditional practices and programs; e.g., payments to mothers for raising children as an alternative to public assistance.

Formulate and lay the groundwork for experiments in delivering high-quality child-centered services, based on our best current knowledge. Preferably, these projects would involve community-based service systems. These experiments will tend to threaten established boundaries and vested professional interests; they will need continuing outside overview and support. The range of experiments should be broad, testing out approaches to: useful management of a range of services, clear diagnostic bases for continuity of services, easy access to services, matching of services to population clusters of varying kinds, and means of keeping significant control over services in the hands of users. The experimenters should develop strategies for initiating community-based experiments and then help them to connect and to learn from one another and provide them an overview of their conduct.

Formulate systems of data-gathering and identify analogies with successful service systems which will lead to formulation of models of management information systems which can be implemented, in prototype fashion, at city and state levels.

To perform these analytic, data-gathering, and experimental functions, this body must have:

sufficient resources for analysis, data-gathering program understanding, execution and evaluation of experiments, synthesis of results, generation of model programs, and the like;

access to many different constituencies;

ways of handling resistance to change and methods of ensuring that the changes sought are constructive in nature.

We are not proposing that these functions be combined in one centrally organized institution. The resulting bureaucratization and rigidity would render such an institution incapable of the flexible, action-oriented program needed. We propose, therefore, the formation of a permanent study-action group, relatively small but with substantial funding, and a series of temporary programs which the group brings into being to focus on particular problems at particular times, and then dissolves as those problems are met. Although the boundaries of these temporary programs should remain fluid, they should cover these four areas:

1. Program understanding—collection and analysis of basic information on current happenings in agencies and programs on the local, state, and national levels.

2. Data analysis and program generation—examination of alternative objectives and strategies, utilization of funding, manpower and facilities, analogies with other systems. Systematic research should be encouraged and the results analyzed.

3. Experiment and innovation—testing of new programs in specific communities which would include studies of selected, small samples to determine how programs affect people.

4. Strategies for implementation—placing of issues on the national political agenda and the mustering of support behind broad new programs at the national level. Attempts would be made to gather support from business, government administrators, professional groups, political parties, legislators, and the mass media.

The establishment of such a body as that proposed above would aid in the long-range planning of more effective services for children and youth.

Turning to more immediate solutions, we believe that attempts should be made now to achieve coordination between the various social service agencies. There are presently too many separate public and voluntary social service programs. We do not suggest merging them all, but we do suggest that just as the mental health centers were created with the backing of a clear public responsibility, we should seek one public social service agency to assume responsibility for services to all children and youth in each jurisdiction.

We stress, in particular, the need for coordination of social welfare services and policies (including the assistance programs in Recommendation B) at levels of government and the need for coordination between public programs and voluntary agencies in order to prevent duplication and poor coordination of services and to ensure the availability of programs and services. We also emphasize the need to integrate welfare and other components of the comprehensive services, programs, and policies recommended by the Commission, and the importance of a collaborative alliance among the public and voluntary service systems and the Child Development Councils and Child Development Authority proposed previously.

While fundamental rearrangement of federal and local programs and money arrangements should await results of the study body proposed above, we believe that some reordering could be made on the basis of present information. For instance, the overlapping responsibilities of programs funded and promoted by the social services and child welfare provision of Title IV of the Social Security Act and those provided by Vocational Rehabilitation could reasonably be combined. The several day-care programs now funded by the Department of Health, Education, and Welfare and the Office of Economic Opportunity could be also combined. Programs for children with "categorical" vulnerabilities are often created separately and could easily be incorporated into one local social services system.

The Commission deliberately avoided in-depth analyses of federal and local programs and laws designed for children because the task requires more attention than we could give to it; further, we believe such an analysis should not be attempted without the full participation of the agencies and the Congress. We are firmly convinced that the federal, state, and local laws pertaining to children and youth have developed haphazardly, and they need major revisions if they are to meet the objectives set forth by the Commission.

We believe that the social services listed below—all of which are provided now to some extent in federal, state, and local law and programs—should be available to all American children and families as a *social utility* through service systems which are coordinated. Some should be made available to all children and families as tax-supported services like the public school programs. Others should be provided to the poor without cost; those more affluent should pay for services according to their ability. The available services should include the following:

Day care and other group activities
Specialized services for children with particular psychological handicaps
   (see also Recommendation A above)
Foster care and adoption services
Protective services
Vocational and educational counseling
Probation services
Legal services
School social services
Family, marital, and premarital counseling and education
Homemaker service
Consumer education

We believe that consumer participation in the planning, policy-making, and operating of services is essential if these services are to achieve their desired goals. In administering these services, we urge that agencies be encouraged to make maximum use of volunteer manpower, especially of youths who wish to participate in such programs. We also urge that expenditures be increased for the training of both professionals and non-professionals.

1. Programs for the preschool child

A number of psychological studies indicate that people need periods of relief from situations which require heavy emotional and physical investment, and that periodic relief allows them to function more competently. It is hard to imagine any role which requires a heavier emotional and physical investment than that of child-rearing. Because our nation has consistently refused to take this matter seriously, untrained and over-burdened parents, their children, and the total nation suffer. More than 4,000,000 preschoolers have mothers who work, and it has been estimated that 38,000 children under the age of six are left without any care while their mothers work and twice as many are looked after by a brother or sister only slightly their senior. American women remain almost totally deprived of satisfactory child-care arrangements during their working hours or, for that matter, during times of temporary family crisis.

For these reasons, we recommend that high priority be given to:

the establishment of day-care and preschool programs. These programs should be available as a *public utility* to all children on the following basis: half-day or less, full-day arrangements for the working mother, and round-the-clock short-term or long-term care during periods of family crisis or emergencies.

We are opposed to any mandate which requires mothers of young children to enroll in job training or go to work. We believe these mothers should have free choice as to whether they should work. We believe there is a great danger that forcing poor mothers to work could lead to inexpensive and damaging custodial arrangements, since the primary goal would not be to provide developmental and educational services for children, but to cut welfare costs. Presently, 1,500,000 children under six need day care. We contend that it is imperative that day-care and preschool programs be expertly staffed and programmed—both as parent and as child education centers. This argues against rushing into a nationwide compulsory program which could not be adequately staffed. Therefore, we recommend that:

the establishment of preschool programs be based on a *widespread* distribution of well-planned "startup demonstrations" with plans for expanding the program by helping groups in communities to mobilize their efforts in this direction. Professionals should be assigned to recruit, train, and supervise paraprofessionals and volunteers in every community. The recruitment and training should include mothers and fathers as well as older youth who desire this type of service opportunity for their own growth into career and/or parenthood roles. (The educational components for preschool programs are related in Recommendation D in this section.)

2. Adoption and foster care (including institutional care)

Some parents are unable, unwilling, or unfit to care for their children, on either a temporary or a permanent basis. Sometimes this situation is the result of death or illness of the parent or parents; in other cases, psychological disorders of parents lead to child abuse and neglect. Many children in need of placement services are unplanned and unwanted; the scope of this problem in the future would be greatly reduced by the vigorous extension of birth control methods, including an extensive outreach program to ensure that low-income women receive birth control information and services.

Many children are in need of temporary care because of some temporary family crisis. However, a sizable proportion of children who leave their parental residence for substitute care cannot return to their families. Child welfare services, such as adoption and foster care, are presently unable to provide adequate permanent or temporary care for all children who are in need. Too often, children are shunted from one foster home, or one institution, to another. Their psychological growth is endangered because they lack a continuous, stable relationship with parent figures and—as is too often the case—because they are placed with inadequate caretakers or foster parents. Placement of minority-group children has been particularily difficult.

Within the present nonsystem, children often land in foster care without adequate evaluation of their needs. The present reliance on social, legal, and clinical labels for placement is inadequate. We believe that the Child Development Council can play a major role in ensuring the development of diagnostic classification and evaluation techniques which measure children on the basis of their functioning and dysfunctioning so that placement decisions can be based on the child's treatment needs.

The following recommendations regarding adoption and foster care (including institutional care) are framed primarily to improve existing services, to spread the risks and burdens of child-rearing by offering more alternatives to help families keep children in their homes, and to strengthen the tendency for greater reliance on group programs. Recommendations related to research and manpower in these areas are presented below in Sections III and IV respectively.

a. *Strengthening existing service agencies*

Economic and administrative steps should be taken to improve the partnership between public and voluntary agencies in adoption and foster care. Agencies should be encouraged to extend the range of services available in each community and to plan new approaches in their relationship to families. Purchase of service agreements between public and voluntary agencies should be formulated to encourage experimentation and require adequate evaluation.

Financial and other assistance should be given to the underdeveloped parts of the child welfare system. Specifically, assistance is needed for: (a) expansion of adoptive services; (b) homemaker, day-care, and extended day and baby-sitter programs; (c) full-range foster-care programs; (d) group-care programs (both daytime and full 24 hours) for socialization rather than treatment purposes; (e) community-based institutional care. All of these programs should be available equally to normal children and those with physical and mental disabilities without regard to economic status.

b. *Foster care and adoption programs and services*

The following services and arrangements should be implemented or expanded:

The Child Development Council recommended by the Commission should provide leadership in the development of more effective, formal working arrangements among all agencies, including schools, courts, mental health centers, child welfare agencies, etc. These arrangements should be well publicized. Consumers and parents should be given a voice in policy determination. The family must be protected against the twin evils currently evident in some cases, namely: (1) being forced to care for a child even though the effort to meet the child's needs is beyond familial capability and (2) punitive removal of the child from a nonconformist family in instances in which the child's needs are being met. The Child Development Council should work in tandem with health and welfare planning bodies to see that these requirements are met.

Since a sizable proportion of children receiving substitute care cannot return to their families, professionals involved must identify these children at the earliest posible moment and be prepared to provide long-term familial or peer-group substitution. Continuous assessment of the child and family is always necessary. We believe the Child Development Council can play a major role in protecting children in this context.

Total displacement of the natural family is a drastic and painful procedure to be followed only when it is clearly in the best interest of the child. The appointment of a legal guardian in such cases is advisable when the natural parents are incapable of assuming this responsibility. The court has a major role in many cases and should be involved in program planning and execution.

Extension of substitute family programs to take kinship and friendship patterns into account formally when it is necessary to place children. Maximum use of such patterns should be made; this would be enhanced by removing some of the economic and other burdens of placement from the relatives and friends involved. Payments should be made to relatives as they are made to foster parents; however, payments in both instances should be increased.

Public and certain publicly supported housing developments (e.g., cooperative or condominium housing) might be used for the creation of an integrated supportive-substitutive child-care program. A large housing development should include specifically designated space for a day-care program, for foster children in short-term placements with a designated proportion of the resident families, and for a small residential group program.

c. *Illegitimate children*

Programs and services for children born out of wedlock should include the following:

Services should be extended to a larger proportion of unmarried mothers, with less selectivity based on those intertwined factors of class, color, and income. Services must include social supports to encourage natural mothers to care adequately for their children if they so desire; therefore, services should cover not only the period of pregnancy and child birth but also, where necessary, provision to protect and promote the mental health of the child for several years after birth.

Services should include early identification of children to be placed and assistance to mothers in using placement services.

Coordinated community services, including health, education, counseling, vocational assistance, etc., should be offered in such a way as to minimize the disruption in the life of the unwed mother, so that this additional burden does not make more difficult her adjustment. Comprehensive services are most important for the young, unmarried mother whose schooling needs to be continued, whose identification with a stable social group needs to be strengthened, and who most needs the support of familiar figures if she is to retain her potential to become a successful wife and mother.

Services to unwed mothers from whom children are to be removed should be prompt so as to expedite the early placement of children in permanent arrangements, provided this plan is approved by the mother.

Present services to unmarried mothers, like most other services, are unduly fragmented. The Child Development Council should play a major role in arranging for the continuum of care and services that is needed by the unwed mother and her child.

d. *Mental health services*
For all populations served by Child Welfare Agencies, we recommend:

More mental health services should be provided for unwed mothers, for parents who are neglecting or abusing their children, and for foster and adoptive parents. For some, contact needs to be direct; for others, this need can be provided by supervisory and consultative services to health and welfare agencies and to the courts. There is also a great need for children's mental health services and for individual clinicians to devote time to the large number of children who are served by child welfare agencies.

e. *Institutional care*
The institutional care of children and youth often comes under social agency auspices. Recommendations with regard to institutional treatment are found in Recommendation A in this section.

Social agencies should provide a range of institutional services for children who may not need "treatment." The characteristics of such institutions are not unlike those of the treatment institutions. The same components are necessary in both. The main difference usually lies in the intensity of clinical attention given to children and youth. There is a major need for small-group residences for adolescents for whom foster care is not useful and for some physically handicapped and mentally retarded children and youth who need supervision, and a need for halfway houses for youngsters returning from treatment institutions.

While group care of infants and the use of group care for normal young children has not been considered a desirable choice in most instances, the lack of foster homes has increased the use of such facilities. We need more experimentation in this field to determine whether group living should or should not be used as a primary method of choice for rearing some children.

3. *Protective services*

Protective services represent assertive reaching out to a family in which neglect or abuse of children is alleged. Originally carried out through semi-legal Societies for the Protection of Children, they are now looked upon as a necessary service in public agencies providing child welfare services. We recommend that:

protective services be made available as a public service in every locality through the public service agency, using professional and nonprofessional workers who are especially trained to help families understand the problems which cause the complaint, to increase the parents' ability to understand their children and themselves, and to strengthen family life. Such an agency should work closely with the Child Development Council so that coordinated health, day-care, economic, educational, homemaker, consultant, and counseling services can be made available to these children and their families. Such a range of services is crucially needed to provide intensive treatment to the many multiproblem, hardcore families served by protective agencies. Only after all attempts are made to keep the family together would the agency make a formal recommendation to the court for the removal of the child.

4. *Vocational rehabilitation*

Vocational rehabilitation, while traditionally looked upon as a program for rehabilitation of persons with physical handicaps, has done a great deal to rehabilitate persons with mental handicaps.

Administered in the Social and Rehabilitation Service of the Department of Health, Education, and Welfare, this program shares with the other programs, under provisions of the Social Security Act, the resources to make available complete rehabilitation services to all persons with physical, mental, and social disabilities. Each state is now authorized by the federal government to provide separately for both public vocational rehabilitation and social services. Each can deal with the same families, although Vocational Rehabilitation does not have authority to assist young children. Each uses somewhat similar personnel and techniques and shares common objectives. While the Commission recognizes the fact that many socially and mentally disadvantaged persons are not capable of being rehabilitated to the point of readiness for the work force, it believes that combining these programs would provide the mental health treatment system a partnership with a comprehensive public social services agency. The mentally disabled would then have available to them one comprehensive program which would include family counseling, child welfare services, vocational rehabilitation, etc., in each community. Therefore, the Commission recommends:

that the Congress and the Department of Health, Education, and Welfare consider combining the HEW-SRS programs of Vocational Rehabilitation and Social Services into one local public delivery system of rehabilitative services for persons of all ages;

that the above suggested combined system continue present arrangements which provide for direct public service and for purchase of services and that the present differentials in federal matching be made consistent for both programs;

that Congress and the Department of Health, Education, and Welfare study the present program of the Vocational Rehabilitation and the Medical Assistance Program (Title XIX, Social Security Act) in the field of providing health services to determine whether it is feasible to combine the resources of both programs in the purchase of medical care and treatment.

5. *Probation services*

In three recent U.S. Supreme Court decisions on juvenile court procedures, constitutional rights of children and parents who came before the juvenile court were clarified. These were the only juvenile court cases to reach the Supreme Court since juvenile courts were established in 1899.

These landmark cases clearly established that the juvenile court is primarily a court of law rather than a social instrument or agency. Juvenile courts were instructed that in all cases brought before them, children and families must be informed of their rights to counsel, must be provided with counsel if they cannot afford it, must be given timely and specific notice, must have the right of cross examination and of appeal, and that judgments must be decided on the basis of evidence provided in court.

These decisions have great significance for the role of the juvenile probation officer. It is clear that the court needs probation officers for the purpose of assisting it in carrying out all of its judicial functions. In effect the probation officer, who until now operated to inform the court about the child prior to the hearing, no longer can do so without risking defense allegations of prejudgment.

The probation officer can still act as a social service worker in a presentence investigation or in seeing to it that an order of the court is carried out. The three decisions, however, all emphasize that the court is primarily a judicial agency, and that the concept of *parens patriae* which made most juvenile courts social agencies, no longer applies. All states which have revised or rewritten their juvenile courts acts or youth codes since the Supreme Court decisions have limited the scope of the court's administrative and social functions and increased the procedural, legal safeguards.

The recent report of the President's Commission on Law Enforcement and Administration of Justice, in dealing with this matter, said: "Juvenile courts should make the fullest feasible use of preliminary conferences to dispose of cases short of adjudication. . . . The consent decree . . . would prescribe a treatment plan. The movement for narrowing the juvenile court's jurisdiction should be continued."

In a report on delinquency and youth crime, the President's Commission on Law Enforcement and Administration of Justice (1967) recognized that the court needs professionally trained personnel to make key decisions at intake and predisposition studies to assist in making treatment plans and in ensuring that treatment plans are carried out. It did not call for the court to be a social or treatment agency.

This background leads the Commission to conclude that the juvenile court should be strengthened as a legal and judical instrument and as a protector of children and families. It should not be further developed as a social services or treatment agency, and its range of intervention should be limited. When a child is determined by a court procedure to be delinquent and is found to be dependent, neglected, mentally ill, or mentally retarded, the court should seek care and treatment services but should not necessarily offer them directly.

On the basis of the above, the Commission recommends:

Probation personnel in the juvenile court should be professionally trained. The field of social work has developed specialized training for probation officers at the master's level. Some undergraduate colleges also have special curricula for probation officers. Recently enacted provisions for federal grants to states for probation should require state standards for probation.

The court should not delegate functions of probation officers which are clearly related to the legal process of the court.

Where a court does not have personnel skilled in making social studies required for predisposition purposes, it should delegate the function to a competent social agency.

For children who continue under court jurisdiction, care or treatment should be provided by a competent social service or mental health agency which has adequate resources. In such cases the professional probation officer employed by the court should ensure for the court that the treatment or care is being carried out appropriately in the best interest of the child.

The probation officer should use the Child Development Council to assist in diagnosis, evaluation, and determination of appropriate care and treatment resources and to guarantee that the child receives adequate service.

6. *Legal services*

Our complex society, which is based in law, has been particularly deficient in making legal services available to persons with low incomes.

Legal services are expensive and have been generally accessible to the more affluent, who purchase them in the open market from attorneys. In criminal and juvenile cases the Supreme Court has ruled that there must be public provision of legal counsel. Theoretically all poor persons have legal protection now to represent them in criminal or juvenile proceedings.

In civil matters, legal aid services are not widely available. The Office of Economic Opportunity funded legal services in many communities. While they could not fund services in all communities because of dollar limitations, the program of neighborhood legal services has been extraordinarily effective. Recently the Department of Health, Education, and Welfare, through regulations under appropriate service provisions of the Social Security Act, made legal services for civil matters for the poor possible with considerable federal matching funds. States can now provide legal services to those receiving public assistance, those formerly receiving public assistance and those likely to receive public assistance with federal matching funds.

Since access to legal advice and counsel is of such vital importance to persons who cannot afford to purchase services of attorneys, the Commission recommends:

> that every state be urged to take advantage of the opportunity to develop a legal service program for the poor as part of its public social services program;
>
> that legal services be established in all areas where persons of low economic means reside and that they be operated as a purchase program using existing legal services agencies and creating new ones in cooperation with bar associations and other appropriate groups.

7. School social services

The use of school social workers as members of a coordinated pupil personnel service appears in this section under Recommendation A above. As we noted, community needs and available resources vary greatly; however, as general guidelines we recommend:

> One well-trained social worker, backed up by attendance personnel, aides, and other pupil personnel, should be available for every 1,000 to 1,500 school students.

8. Family, marital, and premarital counseling

Family, marital, and premarital counseling is now provided through a variety of public welfare social services agencies including child welfare and voluntary sectarian and nonsectarian agencies. Such services are not widespread enough to provide the coverage needed. Many communities are without them. Often difficult to distinguish from mental health treatment services, family and marital counseling is considered to be vital in achieving and maintaining sound mental health goals.

The Commission recommends:

There should be provision in each community for high-quality family and marital counseling.

Services should be available to high school and college students as well as to all families using resources of public and voluntary agencies. In high schools and colleges, services could be provided by personnel attached to the school system.

Provision should be made for public funding, including purchase of service for those who cannot afford to pay for services.

Mental health treatment services should have this type of social service easily available, and the Child Development Council recommended by the Commission should ensure the availability of these services through its planning and recommending activities.

These services should be closely coordinated with all services for families and children and should be geographically located for easy access.

9. *Homemaker services*

Homemaker services represent an important instrument for keeping families together in times of stress and for assisting professional personnel in family life education. At the present time, homemaker services can be and are provided through a variety of federal grants and matching programs and are carried out by public and voluntary agencies. We recommend:

that the federal authorities redesign their funding arrangements, so that each locality will have one public homemaker service which can provide services directly or through purchase from voluntary agencies;

that homemaker services be available as a social utility to all social and economic groups, with payment for service being dependent upon the income and free to those in low-income groups;

that efforts be made to coordinate homemaker services and home health care services in those communities where these services could be delivered by a single agency.

10. *Consumer education*

People with low incomes undergo considerable stress as they try to stretch limited resources in the marketplace. Studies show that poor people are under great disadvantage in the field of consumer economics. They need considerable help and education to help them in understanding the constantly changing and complex nature of the world of consumer goods and services. Federal programs of financial assistance make it possible for states to develop consumer education as a public social service. Therefore, the Commission recommends:

that each state be urged to take advantage of federal financial opportunities and develop a consumer education program for all persons of low income. Experimental approaches are needed, with systematic evaluation of program outcomes.

The foregoing list of social services is not exhaustive. We sought merely to emphasize some of the major social service elements that ought to be present in a comprehensive system. Those outlined above appear to be of vital, massive importance as major preventive underpinnings of a mental health treatment system. Each service provides its unique support to the child and his family. However, a total social services system should have many other components which the Commission did not study in detail. These include aggressive case findings and group services of the settlement house type which provide not only recreation but community organization and civil education services. The group services should be designed somewhat like the Community Action Programs in order to maximize participation of citizens in improving their communities.

D. EDUCATION

Our nation has delegated to its schools and colleges a major responsibility in preparing its young people to participate in society. Educators are expected to transmit the knowledge and skills necessary both to individual success and to the successful functioning of our society. In many ways, our schools and colleges have served our society well. They have, in part, made possible the advance from a frontier and rural society to a complex, technological, and largely urban society. They helped to shape the many individuals who experienced success in this transitional phase of American society.

We have many reasons to point with pride to our educational system. Yet, few would deny that there are glaring deficiencies. There are old goals which have yet to be realized. There is the unfulfilled dream of an equal education for all—one fitted to the unique nature, needs, and aspirations of each child, one which develops the competence and skill necessary for an individual sense of mastery and accomplishment. For many children, we have made little or no advance toward these goals. For example:

- Only 13 percent of the 800,000 emotionally disturbed children identified as needing special education currently receive such assistance.
- Of the estimated 5,500,000 handicapped children who need special education because of their disabilities, only one-third receive any educational assistance.

- An estimated 50,000 migrant children must travel each year when they should be in school; many of these children are excluded from attending local schools on the basis of their transient status.
- Millions of poor children and those from oppressed ethnic minorities are still herded into old, inferior, and segregated schools where they lag further behind their more affluent counterparts as they advance into higher grades.

At a time when education is becoming ever more essential, when failure in school may mean failure in society, we need to reaffirm our belief that education is the inalienable right of every child. More than ever before in our history, young people need an education which will prepare them for future roles. Rapid technological advances have made many skills obsolete. Simultaneously, there is a growing demand for people who can cope with complex machines, perform diverse tasks, and utilize professional skills that are far from routine. Opportunities abound for those who can compute, who can use language with skill, who can solve problems, and who are motivated to bear responsibility. The opportunities exceed in number the people who are prepared to fill them.

The innovation and novelty which mark our age promise to be commonplace in the world of tomorrow. The ability to learn and to change with new ideas and innovations will be even more important in the future. In this context, the young face new difficulties. It is no longer enough to teach them a few key skills and a set of static traditions and values. Adaptation in our culture will call for a level of competence never before demanded in the history of the world. Our schools must impart not only the capacity for learning but also a love of learning and the motivation for continual life-long learning. Education, more than ever before, will need to concern itself with human development. It will need to become a primary force in shaping the whole person, his emotional as well as his intellectual development, his power to create as well as to adjust, his inner equilibrium as well as his effectiveness in dealing with the outer world.

Never before have educators been faced with such a complex set of problems, tasks, and responsibilities. There are no simple solutions, as will be pointed out in Chapter IX. Some problems—overcrowded classrooms, teacher shortages, exclusion of the handicapped and disturbed, slum schools, and the like—could be greatly remedied by greater financial investments in education. Other problems—the heritage of racism, the irrelevancy of curriculum, the challenges of the future—cannot be solved solely by building new schools and training more teachers. They will require bold and creative planning and action.

In view of the many critical issues and problems confronting our educational system, the Commission proposes a number of strategies, programs, and services which it believes could lead to constructive changes.

1. *Preschool education programs*

In the preceding discussion of social services, the Commission recommended that preschool programs, as well as day care, be universally available as a public utility. We consider this to be one of our *major* recommendations.

The Commission is not suggesting a mere increase in traditional nursery schools and kindergartens—although these may be adequate for many children who come from homes which provide highly enriched and stimulating experiences. We are asking for services which will help parents enhance, during infancy and early childhood, the development of intelligence, of proficiency in language, of motivation to achieve, and of interest in solving problems.

There is no longer any serious doubt that the environmental circumstances of infancy and early childhood heavily influence the later development of the child. We know that early life experiences are important for later impulse control, for self-concept, and for the development of intellectual competence and motivation to achieve. This calls for a new emphasis on the importance of educational experiences for fostering the total development of children—intellectual, social, physical, and emotional. Educational programs must be provided which impart to the young child the necessary skills and competence.

We know that large numbers of American children experience an infancy and early childhood which deprives them of opportunities to develop social and intellectual competence. Project Head Start was an admirable attempt to improve the school readiness of large numbers of disadvantaged children who were likely to commence formal schooling with cognitive and behavioral deficiencies. The lesson of Head Start itself is that, despite all gains, the efforts were "too little and too late." It is important to recognize, however, that the original objectives of Head Start call initially for changes in the child's environment rather than in the child himself. The Commission endorses this philosophy. Together with provisions to correct hazardous environmental conditions faced by our children, we recommend that high-quality, universally available preschool educational and day-care programs be based on the following objectives:

the creation of continuous, year-round programs based on our best knowledge of child development;

the integration of educational programs with comprehensive health, social, and recreational services;

the establishment of programs for the early identification and prevention of emotional and learning disorders;

provision for the active involvement of parents, including the determination of effective roles and the necessary training for these roles.

We believe these should not only be a part of all preschool programs but that these same objectives should be incorporated into special and supplemental educational programs and resources for all school systems. In particular, such provisions should be made for disadvantaged groups.

Because of the present limitations posed by the lack of availability of trained staff and the paucity of curricula for early intervention, emphasis must initially be placed on research and experimentation with new models of service (see recommendations in Section III, Number 1). The Commission recommends that these initial efforts be directed toward developing programs for disadvantaged and handicapped children, such as the following:

a. Programs for children under three. There are several patterns through which educational programs for children under three can be related to and supplement the efforts of families. These include:

1. *A homebound educational program* which will reach the child in his own habitat. Such programs should include vigorous and systematic efforts to bring the knowledge of the physician, nurse, psychologist, social worker, trained paraprofessional, and early childhood educator into the home. Mothers would be taught the preferred ways of handling infants, providing their nutritional needs, and protecting them from disease and infection, and techniques of teaching and play which have been developed to stimulate intellectual, language, and sensory-motor development.

2. *A comprehensive center,* such as the emerging Parent and Child Centers, which will provide not only a program of basic nutrition and health supervision but also a full program of stimulation, affection, and learning experiences suited to the developmental needs of infants and young children. The centers should be open evenings and weekends so that parents and older children can use them for recreation, continued education, and social interaction. Such programs provide an excellent opportunity for older children and youth to participate in the care, education, and development of younger children.

3. *Day-care centers and nursery schools* can also provide an environment which protects physical health and provides learning experiences appropriate to the child's developmental stage. Modified nursery school education could be used in these facilities for children two and a half and three years old. Programs for infants and toddlers would largely involve experiences with adults through contacts in a variety of activities.

b. Programs for children three to five. Comprehensive program planning for the three- to five-year-old should be similar to and continuous with those devised for younger children. The Commission recommends:

1. *Project Head Start* should be modified and expanded in accordance with its original mandate to provide a more balanced emphasis across the seven objectives set for the program. We recommend the following modifications:

the creation of year-round programs;

the extension downward of the age of entry to at least the age of three, and possibly to age two, with continuous experience in the program until the age of entry into formal schooling;

a greater involvement of males, both professional and nonprofessional, on Head Start staffs;

a far greater utilization of "preadolescent and adolescent models," as urged in the original mandate for the program; this offers a major source of participation by males;

regulation changes which will increase the proportion of children in Head Start programs above the poverty criteria; the advantage of placing lower-class children in groups which include substantial numbers of children from the middle class has been well demonstrated;

the establishment of joint appointments of teachers in Head Start and in primary grades to ease the child's transition from Head Start to kindergarten or first grade;

the provision of mental health consultation, either through staff or through community resources.

2. *Nursery schools and other existing preschool programs* for three- to five-year-olds should be expanded and improved in quality. The following modifications would improve program effectiveness:

provision of mental health consultation and services, including programs of early identification and intervention;

increased individualized instruction in programs;

greater flexibility in age-grouping;

programs based on developmental needs and concepts;

program arrangements fitted to the hours of working mothers;

increased use of paraprofessionals and volunteers.

3. *Preschool classes for the emotionally disturbed* should be available for emergency as well as educational services for handicapped children. Many handicapped children can and should be included in regular preschool classes and programs. Others who are too disturbed, too disruptive, or so severely handicapped that they cannot be kept in regular classes will require *therapeutic nursery schools*. Such children need to be

provided special preschool programs offering a variety of techniques and approaches which may correct or reduce their handicapping conditions. For example, all psychotic preschool children should have a "therapeutic trial" in a therapeutic nursery school, with individual play therapy for the child and therapeutic work with the parents.

The Commission recommends that full funding, as authorized by Congress in the Handicapped Children's Early Education Assistance Act (PL 90-538), be appropriated for preschool programs for the handicapped.

2. Mental health and the school environment

The need for special mental health services and specialized personnel attached to schools has been described in the section on recommendations for school health and mental health programs. It must be recognized, however, that the school has a much greater responsibility for the mental health of children in the middle years of childhood than can be met by special services. To be effective, there must be continuity between the underlying principles of the total educational milieu and the focus of the specialized services. In short, there should be a consistent mental health base for everything a child experiences in his school life. To the extent that this condition can be achieved in the school environments in our nation, it may be possible to foresee less proliferation of specialized services which present, as they do, increasing problems of coordination. We could look forward to more accomplishment, certainly on the preventive level, through the direct functions of the educative process.

For the school to be a mentally healthy environment for growing children there must be a change in the concept of how this institution shall serve society through the children it educates. Its goals must be not only achievement but personality development, not only competence but ego strength, not only intellectual power but self-understanding and feelings of self-worth, not only adaptability but individuality, not only accommodation but initiative. The changes to be enacted involve all aspects of the school milieu—curriculum, teaching methods, teacher-child relations, administrative practices, and architectural design. The Commission endorses the acceptance of the following characteristics and objectives as the basis for applying mental health principles to elementary school education because they represent concrete educational mechanisms and relationships through which the school can serve the goal of contributing simultaneously to intellectual mastery and to personality development.

The Commission recommends:

Federal grants should be made preferentially to programs undertaking responsibility for mental health goals as integral to the educative process, and the selection of a school or a school system, for involvement in grants, or designation as models under the Education Professions Development Act, or in future legislation, should be guided by these criteria and the same criteria should be employed in evaluation projects.

1. The goals for education should be focused on developmental processes in childhood: sensitivity to the world around; cognitive power and intellectual mastery of the symbolic systems; synthesis of cognitive and affective experience; differentiated reaction to people; adaptation to requirements of social situations, self-understanding, and moral judgment. Achievement criteria are partial, inadequate measures of development.

2. Instructional methods and technology should be evaluated before adoption by two criteria: productivity in advancing intellectual power and positive value for associated emotional factors related to personality.

3. Learning activities should be designed for independent pursuit by an actively involved child; should afford varied possibilities to observe, discover, invent, and choose; should avoid complete dependence on verbal-vicarious transmission of information.

4. Learning activities should encompass and integrate thinking and feeling experience; children should have opportunity to express feeling directly in relation to people in school and for indirect re-expression, in symbolic form, through creative activities.

5. The organization of learning tasks should make maximal use of the peer-group process: for evolving codes of social interaction, for working through interpersonal reactions, for experience in being part of a forum for the discussion of ideas.

6. The authority structure should be flexible and rational, not arbitrary, not invested in status and position; it should exclude threat, humiliation, or retaliatory punishment; children should participate in formulating regulations; methods of control should be corrective, relevant, and nonpunitive.

7. Genuine work experiences serving the school and the community should be included as an integral part of the curriculum; the work should be perceived by the children as realistically essential and as a sign of their acceptance into the world of adult concerns. Projects of cross-age teaching are an example of intraschool work activities that have had positive results.

8. The moral climate of the school should be built around attitudes of mutual trust, respect, and "fair play" as the basis for judgment and behavior; children should be exposed to diversity of points of view and helped to build up moral principles for judging and guiding behavior; values openly advocated by school adults must not be violated covertly.

9. Sex education should be included as one aspect of the comprehensive goal to deepen sensitivity to the emotional aspects of human interaction; it should be integrated with moral education as part of the total curriculum, not formalized as an isolated topic; factual information on sex should be integrated with the health education aspects of the curriculum and with consultation with parents.

10. The teacher should hold the pivotal position in the educative process; major responsibilities of the teacher are:

a. to stimulate and guide the acquisition of competence in a variety of skills;

b. to receive the individual child as a person and plan next steps for his learning in terms of his specific strengths and deficits;

c. to support the peer group in becoming an open forum for expression of opinion and for partaking in establishing regulations of school life;

d. to monitor the balances between structured presentation of subject matter and techniques of learning by discovery, between open-ended exploration and disciplined consolidation, between the teacher's position as an advocate in the interest of children and his simultaneous role as a surrogate of adult authority.

To translate these principles into concrete educational programming, it is essential that full attention be given to major contemporary problems that face the schools: (a) the wide diversity of life situations from which children come to school, (b) the rapid production of new instructional techniques which need testing out and evaluation, and (c) the shortage of teaching manpower to carry an expanded role.

The Commission recommends, therefore:

that the U.S. Office of Education establish contracts with diversified school systems in cooperation with university centers to develop pilot programs, specializing in such selected areas as:

1. development of differentiated curricula in the elementary school that are responsive to the particular characteristics and needs of children who have grown up in poverty;

2. development of differentiated curricula oriented toward developmental differences of boys and girls in the middle years of childhood;

3. construction of a plan for continuous evaluation of teaching innovations, including assessment of side effects and their implications for the role of the teacher and teacher-child relationship, such evaluation to be a staff process including teachers, principal, and specialized mental health personnel who are allotted staff time to carry on this work;

4. development of a strategy for recruiting men teachers for the elementary school and developing functions and decision-making roles related to the whole school that will make it attractive for men to build teaching careers in the elementary school;

5. planning administratively for an "open school" design in which housing and grouping of children are flexibly responsive to changed educational goals and in which teachers function in decision-making and as change-making agents;

6. development of patterns of flexible and differentiated use of instructional personnel—for example, coordination of teaching roles to include educational strategist, educational technician, teacher and teacher aide; use of parents and paraprofessionals as special aides and tutors in home and classroom;

7. development of a school as a broad-gauge community center involving parents in formulation of the school's long-range plans, sensitive to salient needs and problems of the community of the school, actively using the experience and talents of parents and community persons for enriching curriculum and strengthening the bonds between the school and the child's world beyond the school;

8. development of in-service training programs for teachers with focus on child development knowledge; utilization of mental health consultation; preparation for understanding and tolerating a wide range of behavior in the classroom (see recommendations, Section IV-E, for fuller statement).

3. Expanding opportunities for higher education

The educational system must prepare all youths more effectively for their occupational and citizenship roles. In order to do this, education must be viewed more as a total interlocking system. A comprehensive program needs to be established throughout the elementary, secondary, and post-secondary levels to provide financial assistance, information and counseling services, remedial programs, and enrichment courses which will more adequately prepare young people for work, informed participation in a democracy, further education and training, and the flexibility to assimilate new ideas and new ways of operating.

Many talented young people are unable to attend institutions of higher education because of limited funds. The ability to attend college or other schools for higher training is highly dependent on the income of the student's family. If our society is to benefit from the talents and resources of all of our young, it must expand opportunities for students to continue their education and training past the high school years. To help meet this need, the Commission recommends:

that free public education be provided at least two years beyond high school;

that higher investments be made in student financial assistance programs such as scholarships, loans, and work-study programs, especially for disadvantaged students and particularly those programs under the Higher Education Act of 1965;

that public-supported junior colleges be expanded to train youth not only in technological occupations but in the various human services fields as well. Particular emphasis should be given to training for service in child mental health programs.

College admission procedures determine not only where one attends college but also whether one goes at all. Many students lack adequate information on which to base their college choice; others are excluded from some schools not because they lack the academic potential but because of current admission policies and procedures. The Commission, therefore, recommends:

that the U.S. Office of Education establish a national clearinghouse of information about American colleges and universities;

that federal support for special assistance programs be expanded to encourage colleges and universities to waive ordinary admission requirements for students with academic potential from deprived backgrounds and substandard secondary schools.

The heterogeneity of today's college students has practical consequences for the role of higher education in student development. Because American college students are extremely diverse in their talents, potential, previous education, interests, and cultural identities, no single plan, curriculum, proposal, or rule is adequate for all students or every student body. Translated into educational policies, this means that student diversity should be matched by equal diversity in curricula, programs, opportunities, and choices. To meet this need, the Commission recommends:

that the Higher Education Act of 1965 be amended to provide funds to assist colleges and universities to develop programs concentrated in the area of student development. Such experimentation should include: new techniques of community organization, instruction, student self-government, and student-faculty-administration relationships; research to determine those learning environments that most effectively foster the integrated development of cognitive and emotional factors; pilot programs to develop varying curricula to enable students to pursue diverse pathways through college which are suitable to their differing educational and developmental needs.

4. Special education

Most states have recognized the right of every child to an education. All too often, however, this right has not been extended to the severely retarded, the seriously disturbed, and the child with severe neurological impairment. Many of these handicapped children are not provided a chance to develop the skills and capacities necessary for a productive and satisfying life.

Too frequently, the education which handicapped children receive is of questionable benefit. Many children identified as disturbed or deviant are excluded from the regular classroom or placed in special classes that are more custodial than educative in nature. Youngsters who are institutionalized may be further impaired by inadequate and irrelevant educational programs, if they receive any education at all. Greater efforts must be made to maintain handicapped children within the regular classroom and to provide an appropriate educational program for those who must be placed in a special setting.

The federal government, by establishing the Bureau of the Handicapped, has expressed its commitment to improve educational opportunities for the handicapped. Although federal legislation has made possible great increases in service, training, and research programs, many handicapped children have not been reached. The major barrier has been the lack of money and manpower.

In view of the need, the Commission endorses the recommendation of the National Advisory Committee on Handicapped Children that Congress should act to reduce the large gap between authorization and program appropriation in programs for the handicapped (U.S. Senate, 1968). Teacher training programs, in particular, need to be expanded to train at least 200,000 more teachers for the handicapped. More than half this number (121,000) are needed to teach emotionally disturbed children.

Planning for educational and rehabilitation services for handicapped children needs to begin at the preschool level and should be continuously provided at all educational levels. (See Part A, pp. 40–41, for special educational programs recommended for the emotionally disturbed.) There is, of course, no prototype or model plan which will solve all or most of the educational needs of handicapped children. Each state and local community must plan a full range of facilities and services for education which will fit the needs of all handicapped children.

In order to facilitate planning and the eventual establishment of a full spectrum of educational programs for children with various handicaps, the Commission recommends that the U.S. Office of Education, Bureau of the Handicapped:

undertake a national survey to assess the quality and outcomes of current programs and determine, from this assessment, what changes are needed and how changes can best be achieved;

establish demonstration districts in both rural and urban areas to develop models or patterns of services most appropriate to the needs of handicapped children living in these areas;

collect and disseminate information related to a broad spectrum of educational programs designed for handicapped children.

5. Crisis conditions

Disruption, disorder, and violence have precipitated crises in schools and colleges across the nation. These events have profound and probably detrimental psychological and emotional effects on students and teachers.

The causes of the present wave of protest and disorder imply a disenchantment and even cynicism on the part of our youth for which the schools may have a partial but not total responsibility. It is clear, however, that students, parents, community members, teachers, and educational administrators are involved in conflict and in a confrontation of power and control. The issues which underlie the struggle between youth and educational personnel call for the development of new and appropriate strategies by the community and school if orderly education is to continue.

In order to help meet these crisis conditions, the Commission recommends:

that the U.S. Office of Education establish three regional resource centers to provide assistance to schools upon request. These crises resource centers would have the responsibility to provide:

trained personnel who would be available for consultation and "on-the-spot" assistance for such crises as school-community conflict, student disruption, and racial disorders;

training for crisis consultants so that assistance can be provided;

institutes, conferences, and training programs for educational administrators in order to develop an understanding of methods which will prevent and manage disruption and disorder and rebuild after such crises have occurred;

the dissemination of instructional materials so that schools and communities may study, initiate, and develop techniques and programs which will deal effectively with the basic issues and dynamics which give rise to disruptive situations.

These centers could also be utilized as a resource for developing programs to help solve other problems, such as drug use.

6. School-community relations

The schools, the community, and the parents need to establish open channels of communication. An elaborate and open communication would facilitate an exchange of ideas which could bring about educational self-renewal at the grass-roots level. The schools have the means to attract a wealth of educational hypotheses from the community; they can become a powerful agent for social reform—a potential that should be recognized by the community.

The Commission recommends that federal funding be provided for model programs to demonstrate the effect of the school's initiation in bringing about closer school-community relations. Programs should aim to:

> involve schools more directly in the concerns of the communities which they serve;
>
> provide or establish channels of communication between parents and community leaders and the school administrators;
>
> utilize community talent resources to enrich the educational experience of children;
>
> utilize the Child Development Councils proposed by this Commission to initiate collaborative efforts between the school and community.

7. Education of minority-group children

Many of the Commission's foregoing recommendations apply to children and youth from oppressed minority groups. However, because the problems of these children and youth are so severe, we wish to add a number of specific proposals taken largely from the report of the Commission's Committee on Children of Minority Groups.

a. Curriculum

The school curricula should be made more relevant to minority-group children through such modifications as the following:

> The school systems of the United States should include in all general education more material about cultural diversity, plurality, and the historical antecedents of *all* groups. Supplementary textual material for specific cultures should be provided.
>
> Culturally specific curriculum materials and school programs to promote healthy psychological development in such areas as family life education and intercultural relationships should be developed. Such programs must reflect the standards of the community and the reality situations faced by the children. The curriculum should include some programs that lead to class discussions of prejudice and the appreciation of difference among cultural and racial groups.

Such subjects as anthropology, social issues, social power systems, public agencies, and current advances in science should be introduced in the elementary school.

Standard English should be taught as a second language in schools attended by large numbers of minority-group children whose basic language differs from standard English.

Technical and vocational education should be tailored to the needs of the community and projected employment opportunities (see also recommendations under E below).

b. *Review and revitalization of schools for minority children*

The physical and psychological setting of the educational institutions attended by minority-group children should be reviewed in detail and revitalized. We recommend:

Experimental approaches to meeting the needs of the minority-group child should include changes in the age of entrance to school, length of the school day and the school year, and the type of school building attended by the minority child.

A variety of approaches to educational integration should be tried on a wide scale, and factors that effect success or failure should be determined.

Study space should be provided for inner-city children in school basements, public buildings, churches, the stores of cooperating merchants, etc. Carrels equipped with automated teaching devices are desirable.

Boarding school placement for American Indian children should be eliminated and quality education in local schools substituted.

To the extent that boarding school placement of Indian students will continue in the immediate future, it is crucial that the importance of competent dormitory aides in the psychological development of the young child be recognized. The number, quality, and training of these parent substitutes need to be increased. The number of students supervised by each aide should be reduced to not more than fifteen.

To the extent that boarding school placement for Indian students is frequently used as a disposition for cases of psychological or behavioral disorders and social or family problems it is crucial that responsibility for providing rehabilitative services be recognized and met, and that the passive custodial role of these institutions be restructured into an active therapeutic one.

In those areas where Indian boarding schools cannot soon be eliminated, because of problems of geography or transportation or because of the need for residential placement for therapeutic considerations, the present large dormitory units should be replaced by smaller cottage-type communities which will offer greater privacy and a healthier setting for individual and group psychological development. Further, there is a clear need for developing active and ongoing communication between the family of the student and the boarding school. This communication should include orientation, regular progress reports, conferences over problems in their early stages, and visits to the school by the parents and to the Indian community by school personnel.

An extensive effort should be made to institute the practice of placing Indian boarding school students in substitute families in the boarding school community. These families, whose close involvement in school activities should be sought, could provide for the student greater opportunity for enhanced development of social techniques, of a sense of personal responsibility, and of familial and cultural identity.

c. *Increasing motivation for achievement*

The motivation for school achievement should be fostered among minority-group children through such means as:

Career-mobiles, travel grants, domestic cultural exchanges, and similar programs should be utilized to alleviate the socially reinforced narrowness of vision by which many majority- and minority-group youngsters limit their personal identities and interpersonal relationships. These means would help narrow the gap of mutual distrust and non-communication which currently contributes to the low aspiration level and sense of alienation in so many adolescents of minority groups.

Experimentation with material rewards for school achievement is recommended. Community groups should be involved in setting up such a system so that personal relationships may develop.

d. *School personnel*

Many factors in the life and school career of minority-group children hinder learning in the school. Therefore, they are less likely to recover from poor teaching. We recommend:

All school policy-makers should deal realistically with the causes of poor morale and the avoidance of inner-city school systems, reservation schools, etc., by many of the best teachers who might otherwise be employed in these schools. The remedies might include greatly increased financial incentives and administrative systems that emphasize flexibility and professionally rewarding interactions.

Civil service and tenure systems of teacher employment should be modified so that meritorious service may be rewarded and maintained.

Training for teachers should include field experience in minority-group communities and continuing supervision by master teachers.

Since the personnel in the Bureau of Indian Affairs and the Public Health Service have such influence on the lives of the Indian people, mandatory continuing education on Indian history, culture, and current and ongoing programs is recommended. Material should be developed by these agencies to be made available to state and local bodies providing education and other services to Indian communities. Such a policy would increase the effectiveness of the professional by enabling him to employ the cultural perspective and value system of the group served in his efforts to enhance the process of identity formation and the development of techniques for problem-solving.

Ways should be found to promote meaningful involvement in policy-making by the Indian communities served by both local and boarding schools.

E. WORK, LEISURE, AND PREPARATION FOR ADULT ROLES

As the self-sufficient family unit of pioneer days disappears, as the small town yields to the megalopolis, and as the time that adolescents and youth remain in school lengthens, unnoticed changes are occurring in the social framework of our society. Children and youth are faced with a great deal of unplanned leisure time. The traditional methods and ways of teaching and learning about adult roles and responsibility have all but vanished. With the growing affluence of our nation, many of our young are provided with comforts and possessions in a quantity and style unknown to many in past generations. Today we pride ourselves that our children are better provided for than we were as children, sometimes forgetting that material possessions cannot guarantee satisfying interpersonal relations and leisure-time activities. We have failed to recognize the disadvantage in "providing for" rather than "working with" our young.

In order to reach maturity and possess the ability to undertake responsibility, each child must work out his own "identity." For children and adolescents, identity formation is an unconscious process, one which is both mental and moral and which cannot be acquired alone. It is acquired in interaction with peers, with those younger, and most importantly, with adults. Identity formation is dependent upon the opportunity to interact and to learn. Play and constructive leisure activities are one essential element in this needed interaction.

With the changing times, we have provided fewer opportunities for children and youth to interact with adults, younger children, and those from differing social and cultural backgrounds. Neighborhoods are both more congested and more isolated; adults and youth move in two separate worlds with little interaction and little real opportunity to learn from each other in mutual ways. Sons are no longer apprenticed to fathers to learn a trade; and, in fact, few children actually see their parents or other adults at work. Children develop a concept of work from television, the movies, or comic books. Increasingly, youth have been removed not only from the world of adult work but from all the worlds of adult concerns. We have thus diminished the opportunity for youth to learn adult roles and to develop their own identity. By excluding youth from adult concerns and the exercise of responsibility, we have removed the traditional training area for adulthood and adult responsibility. Presently, adult roles are becoming more and more complicated, yet we allow less and less opportunity for the young to test themselves and to rehearse what it means to be an adult, before they must assume the roles of wage earner, spouse, parent, and informed citizen.

We need to plan for better leisure activities and for more avenues for youth-adult-community involvement. In specific areas, we need to construct ways by which the young can be more adequately prepared to undertake adult roles. Opportunities for involvement and for constructive leisure activities need not necessarily be separated. Many of the leisure activities and programs suggested below provide ideal environments for children and youth to learn adult roles and participate in meaningful activities. Conversely, we assume that children and youth will find enjoyment in many projects which are more "task" or "goal" oriented. Whatever the basic purpose of these activities, each program should have at least one of the following among its aims:

1. *Citizenship training:* encouraging the young person to understand his society, its problems, how it operates, and how to improve it. Exposure to people of different backgrounds is often the first step—a step that can be taken on the playground as well as in a service project.

2. *Personal development:* learning about oneself and others. Helping a mental patient or participating in team sports, for instance, can stimulate both learning processes.

3. *Vocational readiness and job training:* preparing the young person for the world of work through early observation and participation and through later training for entry into a trade, profession, or paraprofessional role.

4. *Academic improvement:* strengthening the young person's academic skills; for example, through tutoring another person. Often, the whole attitude toward school, authority figures, and the realm of ideas is changed simultaneously.

1. Leisure activities

Play is essential to good mental health. Yet, today, many homes and neighborhoods are so congested or so devoid of play and recreational activities that many children and youth have no playground other than hazardous streets. Young children must either be confined indoors for long periods or be left to roam the streets unsupervised.

Low-income families participate less than other Americans in recreational activities, yet this group generally has more children per family than other Americans. Existing programs and facilities, however, are not provided on a per capita basis. For example, in city after city, ghetto areas have fewer programs and facilities than the city as a whole. Geographic lack of recreational resources together with a lack of transportation to available facilities and a lack of funds necessary to participate in many leisure activities are among the reasons why the poor engage less in recreational endeavors. However, many suburban areas are without ample play space and recreational facilities and programs.

Federal participation in the area of recreation has shown little awareness of comprehensive programming. No single agency or department has provided the needed leadership; planning and training needs have been entirely overlooked; authorized funds are usually the first to succumb to cuts when budgetary demands are greater than available funds. We urge that these deficiencies be corrected. We also urge that federal monies be available to provide incentives and technical assistance to both the public and the private sectors to increase recreational programs and facilities, such as:

There is a need for many more camping programs. These should be available to the disadvantaged as well as the affluent. We recommend that the camping capacity of the country be increased through:

day camps, for which transportation is provided;

summer camps;

camps for year-round use.

New camping facilities are needed. These should be built in areas where present facilities are either inadequate or nonexistent. New facilities should be permanent and for year-round use; they should be small (100 or less) rather than large camps. Quality supervision should be provided. To increase available staff, we recommend:

the establishment of training programs in cooperation with universities and established camping groups. Special efforts should be made to recruit adolescents and youth as potential staff.

There is a need for expansion of teen centers. While such centers should be well supervised, adolescents and youth should be involved in the planning, policy-making, and directing of the activities and programs of the centers.

There is a need for well-supervised, well-equipped playgrounds. Adolescents and youth could be trained for these supervisory roles. We urge that provisions be made for playgrounds in urban and community development programs.

There is a need for community and neighborhood recreational programs which will involve both parents and children, as well as people of different cultural and social backgrounds. We believe the Child Development Councils proposed by this Commission should take initiative in establishing such programs.

The Child Development Councils should also undertake to coordinate the now splintered recreational programs in neighborhoods and communities. The councils should also provide consultation to recreational planners and leaders.

The Commission further recommends that funds be provided for evening, weekend, and summer recreational programs which use available school facilities. Funds would primarily be needed for supervisors, upkeep, etc. Adolescents and youth could be trained for supervisory roles and recruited on both a paid and a voluntary basis.

2. Participatory activities

Many young people are currently involved in helping others, in reaching out into their communities, reforming their schools, and serving in a variety of ways. Space does not permit listing all of the fine programs which involve children and youth in these activities. However, we strongly recommend that such programs be expanded, especially to:

> involve children, from very young ages, in learning about and participating in adult roles, such as decision-making, according to democratic procedures; helping children younger than themselves; taking on roles of leadership, etc.;
>
> involve adolescents and youth in social problems, such as projects to eradicate slums, community development programs, programs for disadvantaged and handicapped youngsters, projects designed to achieve racial harmony, projects for the prevention and cure of drug abuse, or the rehabilitation of addicts, etc.;
>
> involve youth in specific teaching projects, such as teaching English to non-English-speaking children, teaching the emotionally disturbed, tutoring younger children with learning problems, etc.

3. Vocational readiness programs

The Commission strongly believes that ways must be devised to ensure children and youth an adequate knowledge of the work environment. Knowledge of the world of work needs to be personalized through observation and participation in ways that are appropriate to the developmental stage of the child. Among the ways this might be accomplished are the following:

At the elementary school level the child should become familiar with the concept of work and develop rational habits of thought as to his potential future work role. This principle could be incorporated into a number of children's programs. In junior high a greater emphasis could be placed on an economic orientation which would familiarize students with the overall economic and industrial system of goods and services so they can develop an understanding of their own interests in relation to academic or vocational training. High school occupational preparation should be built around realistic, actual, and anticipated opportunities for gainful employment suited to individual needs, interest, and ability. Those outside college preparatory course work should acquire a salable skill while at the same time preparing themselves for the fact that they will need to take post-high school training, and probably eventually retraining in their lifetime.

At all school levels community people with various skills should be brought to the school; conversely, youth should be sent into the community to observe a variety of placement situations. Efforts should be made to bring the school, business community, and public and private agencies together to devise a program of work preparation which is flexible enough to fit the capacities and aspirations of the individual adolescent. The Child Development Council proposed by this Commission should take the initiative in developing vocational readiness programs in neighborhoods and communities.

The scope and variety of combined work-school programs should be increased to allow more youth the opportunity to gain actual work experience while in school. Such an arrangement would allow the tryout period to take place while in school, rather than on the job. Opportunities to earn and learn simultaneously may help some youth to stay in school.

Vocational counseling in both junior high and high school should be increased for all adolescents and youth. Supportive counseling should be available for those in a school work program.

High school graduation should be staggered over the year in order to facilitate the absorption of youth into the labor force.

Publicly supported post-secondary education courses should be available. This would raise the number of free school years from twelve to fourteen and would be particularly relevant to youth interested in vocational education.

Programs which train youth in how to look for a job, how to pass tests for a job, etc., should be expanded.

Data on the supply and demand of various occupations should be amassed on a broader and more accurate basis. A greater knowledge on the range of job-families would permit students, whatever their curriculum, more options in career planning.

4. Vocational education

The Commission supports the 1963 Vocational Education Act which states that admission requirements for vocational education should be based on ability to succeed in a field of work rather than on academic grades or rank in class. In addition, we recommend the following:

The "general" curriculum should be eliminated, and vocational education courses should be integrated with basic skills courses and, where possible, with the academic curriculum courses.

The vocational education curriculum should offer opportunities for students to try out a wide range of vocational-oriented curricula. Emphasis should be on providing a broad background of skills and basic education which will be useful in a range of occupations rather than on training for specific jobs.

Regulations should be revised so that students would not have to choose vocational curriculum in the ninth and tenth grades and then be unable to change to another curriculum.

Federal action should be taken to end the segregation in vocational education facilities, so that minority-group youth will no longer be under-represented.

Ways must be found to raise the prestige of the vocational education curriculum which presently has second-class status and a "dumping-ground" reputation.

Programs should be initiated to involve the work world (businessmen, supervisors, labor officials, professionals, FEES, etc.) through exchange; that is, to bring adult workers to the school and the youth to their places of work. Emphasis should be placed on the need to devise summer work programs for youth.

5. Youth work-training programs

As we shall note in Chapter X, work-training programs such as the MDTA, NYC, etc., have been somewhat successful in training youths who cannot function in the ordinary work situation and who are not eligible for aid under handicapped legislation. Such programs must be expanded. We recommend:

The proposed Child Development Councils should undertake to co-ordinate programs providing semiprotected work situations.

The education component in these programs must be packaged in such a way as to make clear its relevance to the job.

All entry-level jobs must have built-in opportunities for upward advancement.

Such programs should expand on-the-job training and on-the-job training coupled with institutional training.

The federal government should aid communities to develop their own manpower system.

The federal government should provide incentives to industry to establish work-training programs.

The federal government should provide incentives to labor unions to expand apprenticeship programs.

Emphasis should be placed on providing incentives to unions to drop exclusionary policies which bar youth because of educational level, arrest records, and so on.

Pilot programs which give assistance to youth in obtaining bonding should be expanded.

To aid youth in gaining employment, the Commission recommends that police records be based on convictions, not arrests. Further, potential employers should not be allowed to view juvenile arrest records.

6. *Vocational readiness for the handicapped, retarded, delinquent, and severely disturbed*

More programs, research, and evaluation of programs are needed to reasonably determine how handicapped youth can be assisted in entering the job market. The severely disturbed adolescent is in particular need of rehabilitation facilities. The Commission endorses the following recommendation of the Advisory Council on Vocational Education:

We support the concept of residential schools which are authorized by the Vocational Educational Act of 1963 but for which Congress never appropriated funds. We submit that there are those whose home and neighborhood environments make training away from home desirable and which residential schools may serve. This includes a large number of potential students living in isolated areas of limited population. (General Report of the Advisory Council on Vocational Education, 1968, p. 41.)

Training in all institutions for the handicapped, delinquent, retarded, and severely disturbed must be upgraded. Training for outmoded jobs must be abandoned. Administrators of facilities must develop closer relationships with local offices of the State Employment service, local vocation educational facilities, local rehabilitation facilities, and all types of employer groups.

The federal government should provide incentives for developing programs that will involve community employers in all facilities which serve the various types of handicapped youth. Open houses and formation of employers' councils or committees to advise patients about job-finding problems and to involve the community in training and employing the handicapped should be components of such programs.

Professionals treating and caring for children and youth with various kinds of handicaps should become more employment-oriented and include this orientation in their treatment program.

An aftercare service should be available to all children and youth with special problems. These services would include supportive counseling after job placement.

7. *Youth employment*

We have previously noted the relationship between employment and feelings of competence and self-worth and, conversely, the relationship between lack of employment and feelings of rejection, inadequacy, hopelessness, and dependency. Areas of widespread youth unemployment are usually areas of high delinquency rates and poverty. The Commission strongly urges that special attention be given to creating more training and employment opportunities for youth, particularly those in disadvantaged groups. We recommend:

Federal funding should be provided for expanded training and employment opportunities for youth. We particularly urge expansion of training and employment opportunities in the human services field.

The Child Development Councils proposed by this Commission should take the initiative in coordinating and expanding training and employment opportunities for adolescents and youth, particularly in the area of human services.

The Commission also supports the recommendation of the U.S. Chamber of Commerce regarding the establishment of a youth employment-experience minimum wage rate which would help provide young people with opportunities to acquire employment experience, training, and skills in the competitive market. The Fair Labor Standards Act should be amended, setting the minimum wage rate for teen-agers and covered employment at 75 percent of the standard minimum wage for adult workers. A 24-month cumulative total time limit should be placed on the employment of a teen-ager by his employer at the youth employment-experience minimum wage rate. Because employment experiences and training are so important, teen-agers should be eligible for the employment-experience minimum wage rate irrespective of family income (Chamber of Commerce of the U.S., 1966).

III. Research

The mental health field, as we know it, represents a recent scientific endeavor. It has posed questions concerned with the infinite and illusive complexities of man: man in relation to himself; man in interaction with his fellow beings, his culture, and social institutions; and man in relation to a complex natural environment in which he struggles as both the master and the mastered.

The broad scope of our recommendations reflects the complex states of being which we call mental health and mental illness. Although we know a great deal about mental health, emotional disorders, and mental illness, much remains elusive and ill-defined.

In the foregoing pages, we spoke of child development knowledge as a promising basis for the prevention and remediation of mental, emotional, and behavioral disorders. We recommended an advocacy system which will make child development a public utility through effective planning and policy-making at all levels of society and through advocate functions at the neighborhood level which will ensure delivery of services to children, youth, and their families. And we proposed a number of changes in current services, programs, and policies which affect the mental health of our young. We urged that efforts be made to coordinate all the child services into a comprehensive and systematic network. In Section IV we will present recommendations which deal with the crucial problems of manpower and training, as these are related to the various child services. In all these areas, our present state of knowledge makes it possible to define directions in which we should be moving to promote the mental health of our children and youth. Yet, in all these areas upon which we touched, there is a demand for more knowledge, just as there is a demand for more services.

Neither programmatic efforts nor the search for greater knowledge, however, should receive higher priority. Both researchers and practitioners agree that the very best programs and practices are required to alleviate human distress and to enhance human and social potential. On this agreement there can and must be a meeting of hearts and minds, a genuine partnership between activists and researchers who concern themselves with understanding and enhancing human development. We must move ahead with action aimed at prevention and treatment, and we must combine these efforts with related research. There must be a constant interweaving between action and research so that observations and clues from the action field can be referred to research fields for theory building and testing; moreover, basic research must be fed into action programs for hypothesis testing and to authenticate its general applicability.

The Commission strongly believes that the following are among the principles that should guide research programs:

1. Behavioral research is essential to a technological society if we are to narrow the gap between the well-being of the individual and that of the society. Both basic and applied research are necessary. We must increase programs in the research fields related to mental health. To do so, we need epidemiological studies of populations who lack various kinds of services. It is imperative that we know much more about the nature, prevalence, and interaction of problems related to poor physical and mental health, social deviancy, deficiencies in the environment, etc.

2. A high priority must be given to the establishment and preservation of a national research climate which optimizes the productivity and opportunities of individual researchers.

3. Short-range, applied research projects should be planned on the basis of their potential for productivity at a given time in the nation's history.

4. Carefully designed applied research projects need to be increased to evaluate and assess action programs.

5. The role of the universities in carrying out basic research must be preserved. Universities may also wish to contribute to applied and directed research and can do so by using several ways available to assure that these activities will not undermine the independence of research workers.

6. Multidisciplinary collaboration between researchers in both basic and applied fields is urgently needed.

7. There is a drastic need for longitudinal studies of human development that cover the entire life span. We need information on the origins of disorders, their continuity throughout the life span, and the factors that affect these disorders in both positive and negative directions over time. In such studies it is imperative that the following variables be included genetic; constitutional; physical health; life experiences and situations; community characteristics; intellectual development; influences of family, neighborhood, employment, school, occupations, religious affiliation, and other social and economic factors. We need to examine the effects of these variables at different developmental periods and over long time spans; therefore, we need both longitudinal and cross-sectional studies. Cross-cultural studies are also needed in order to distinguish between cultural and genetic determinants of development.

8. Besides studies dealing with a limited number of variables, we need multivariate research which manipulates a number of variables but is capable of examining the effects of each as well as the interaction of all. We must simultaneously study a number of factors in relation to their

interaction, multiple influences, and differential effects on various kinds of individuals and in relation to such components as intellectual, social, physical, and emotional development.

9. We recommend that the NIMH sponsor, in connection with its clearinghouse activities, studies which would develop techniques for evaluating material which should be quickly retrieved and more rapidly disseminated to the relevant professional practitioners.

10. Further efforts are needed to increase the training of research manpower.

11. There is a need for emphasis upon the area of methodology in research on child development and child mental health.

These principles are discussed further in Chapter XI. In the recommendations which follow, the Commission has focused on several areas which are of critical importance in the prevention and remediation of disorders in children and youth. We urge that greater federal expenditures be granted for both basic and applied research in these areas, and for research of both a specific and a multivariate nature.

A. PROGRAM RESEARCH AND EVALUATION

A good deal of time, talent, and other resources is devoted to intervention programs. Many of these are ill-planned, nontheoretically based, and never evaluated. This results not only in a waste of resources but in the continuation of unsuccessful programs. To enhance the potential for successful programs, far more attention and financial support must be given to evaluation of intervention programs.

Some of the issues relating to program research in the clinical field are noted in Recommendation B which follows. We will not reiterate the many intervention programs recommended elsewhere in this report; however, we believe that all the recommended programs should be evaluated as to their success, their effects on the clients, and their efficiency. We wish to call attention here to the need for evaluation of the Child Development Councils which we proposed as our major recommendation.

We recommended that various kinds of models of such councils be tried in different types of communities. One focus of research, then, should be on the relative effectiveness of these models.

The assessment of these councils will be extremely complex. Such assessment should be carried out at predetermined points in time, such as before the council is established and each year thereafter. A number of communities should be studied in a similar fashion, including communities with *no* councils. Assessment should include the following research operations:

1. A careful description of the program components, including the council's location, the nature of its staff, its sources and amount of

financing, the nature of its board, the structure of its facilities, and its program content and goals.

2. A naturalistic history of the founding and operation of the council.

3. The kind of community in which the council is located and the characteristics of the population it is meant to serve.

4. The numbers of people reached and the characteristics of these people in comparison to the characteristics of those who are not reached. Program assessment should not be limited to the overall impact on the total population served by the council. It is also important to look at subgroups in the population.

5. The effectiveness of the services which are given or the services to which the individuals and families are referred in reference to factors in the total population such as: the physical health of children and parents; changes in the rates of psychoses, emotional disorders, learning disorders delinquency, etc.; improvements in employment and income of parents and youth; changes in the community, such as development, coordination and use of services, the nature of community attitudes concerning the councils, etc.

I. MENTAL ILLNESS AND EMOTIONAL DISORDERS

Progress in the treatment, reeducation, and rehabilitation of mentally ill and emotionally disturbed children depends heavily on the acquisition of new knowledge. Well-controlled experimental research is an ideal that can be only approximated in many studies dealing with important clinical problems. One must recognize that ethical considerations that place the patient's needs before the researcher's interest, difficulties in matching cases with diverse characteristics, obstacles to gathering a large number of cases meeting specified criteria, and inevitable differences in the specifics of treatment programs all conspire to make clinical research less rigorous than the scientific ideal would demand. The need for patience, ingenuity, and willingness to define important clinical concepts in objective, measurable terms makes clinical research more difficult and demanding than most laboratory investigations. It is important to guard against facile rationalizations that would make clinical research synonymous with superficial, careless, unsystematic, hence inconclusive studies. We therefore recommend:

that the concept of "appropriate rigor" become the guiding principle of clinical research programs, making it possible to assemble data based on "comparably" diagnosed patients treated in "comparable" ways by "comparable" therapists;

that, as in systems engineering, wherein the abbreviation "R and D" (research and development) describes two-faceted programs, the abbreviation "D and E" be officially promulgated to announce the adoption of the policy that demonstration *and evaluation* are similarly inseparable aspects of projects which seek to test a new clinical stratagem;

that periodic census be taken by investigators trained in assembling clinical data which is comparable in as many significant variables as possible as a way of "measuring" the effectiveness not only of tax-supported programs but also as a way of assessing when and where outmoded techniques might require continuing education, since techniques once taught but presently outmoded have a way of enduring nonetheless.

Recognizing the current limitations on federal funds, but appreciating the urgency of the problem and the economy that knowledge can produce, the Commission recommends that funds be made available through the National Institute of Mental Health, the National Institute of Child Health and Human Development, and the Office of Education for the support of program projects for research on certain crucial problems.

Specifically, *we recommend that ten child mental health special research centers be established* under the auspices of NIMH or NICHD to study issues related to childhood mental health. These research centers should be concerned with both basic research and program projects. The centers should be concerned with such problems as:

1. The development of a more adequate system of classification of emotionally disturbed children that would include, but not necessarily be limited to, an evaluation of assets and deficiencies of the child and of the ecological system of which he is a part. We recommend the support of three to five program projects, with special provision for intercommunication among them.

2. The longitudinal study of the natural history of emotional disturbance in children from the point of earliest identification through the adult years. We recommend the support of two or three program projects at well-established centers for the long period required by the problem.

3. The study of early childhood autism, childhood schizophrenia, and similar severe disturbances from both a biological and a behavioral viewpoint. We recommend the support of ten to twelve program projects. These might well be placed in major medical centers in which the range of resources required is available, and some might be affiliated with mental retardation research centers.

4. The study of the effects of various forms of therapeutic intervention on the course and style of life of the child, including the effects of institutionalization and the prolonged use of tranquilizing drugs. We recommend the support of three to five projects in this problem area.

5. The comparative study of the effectiveness of various kinds of intervention procedures. Ideally, these studies would be multivariate in nature. They would include comparison of children who show comparable levels of functioning at the beginning of treatment and would give appropriate attention to differences in social class, ethnicity, age, and sex. There should be from ten to twelve program projects in this neglected problem area.

6. The development of assessment procedures to facilitate the types of studies noted in 4 and 5 above. These procedures should include: (a) assessment of the special characteristics of individual therapists and patients; and (b) attention should be given to the "rater's" qualifications of competence and independence from treatment outcomes. We recommend the support of three to five projects in these areas.

Other specific suggestions for research on mental illness and emotional disorders are presented in the recommendations which follow.

C. BIOLOGICAL RESEARCH RELATED TO MENTAL HEALTH

The way is open for a new set of advances in the genetics of human behavior and the important interactions between genetic and environmental inputs. But the needed concentration of efforts in this important area of psychological development is lacking. We must increase our efforts to identify the factors that are potentially responsible for damage to the unborn child and follow this by research to develop compensatory mechanisms for any deficiency or disorder. The Commission urges:

> expanded support for research into the identification of both carriers and affected individuals, and for means of treatment. Basic research into the mechanisms of genetic transmission, including polygenic interaction, should be expanded. Research into those modifications of the environment which may be appropriate to the function of the individual child with genetic disorders must be undertaken. The evolvement of compensatory mechanisms for any deficiency or disorder is possible; the outcome of specific genetic disturbances need not be "inevitable."

Priority should be given to genetic and related research on the following questions:

> Is there a genetic component in schizophrenia? If so, how does it interact with various life experiences? What results are obtained when genetic criteria are employed along with the studies of the individual's biochemistry and behavior?
> What is the prevalence of the XYY chromosome aberration? Is it transmitted to offspring? If so, what differences in development can be

observed in babies with XYY constitution beyond the prenatal period? For example: How do they study in school? What is their psychological and neurological profile like? If subjected to some form of therapy, such as child analysis, what are the findings?

Much more research is needed in reference to the functioning and development of the brain, both before and after birth. Studies should focus on both normal and aberrant functions, including the neurochemistry of the brain and the effects of enriched or deprived prenatal and postnatal environments on brain growth.

Further study is required on the interaction of the individual and his environment. We need to know more about the impact of the environment and acquired human behaviors on the individual's physiological functioning, including the functions of the nervous system and the endocrinological functions. More research is needed on the effects of stimulation and sensory deprivation (including maternal deprivation) and the effects of these on development and functioning of the nervous system, including its neurochemical aspects.

Studies on the effects of maternal malnutrition both before conception and during pregnancy need to be combined with careful consideration of possible genetic factors that also may be involved. Multidiscipline field research is also needed to determine the circumstances and manner in which malnutrition influences intellectual and physical development in infants and young children.

Further assessment is needed of the effects of the neuropsychopharmological drugs on the developing nervous system.

In general, it is strongly recommended that biologists, social and behavioral scientists, and clinicians work closely together in these research fields, so that knowledge from the various disciplines can be pooled and tested in laboratory and action settings.

D. BIRTH CONTROL

The Commission recommends that ample support be given to the search for more effective, more acceptable, and easier means of birth control. Research is also needed on attitudes toward birth control. Studies into the relationship between sexual behavior and the maternal role need to clarify an issue that has plagued mankind for centuries.

E. DEVELOPMENT OF INFANTS AND YOUNG CHILDREN

Development during infancy and early childhood is extremely rapid and malleable. There appear to be critical periods in which cognitive, social, physical, and emotional development is most easily enhanced or thwarted.

It seems probable that some forms of pathology established in early life are irreversible. We are in dire need of more studies of the infant and very young child, especially in reference to development between the ages of one to three. Systematic attention should be given to parent-child interaction during these years and to the relationship between this interaction and the development of creativity, interpersonal skills, the ability to learn, etc. Short-term longitudinal studies are badly needed to link the phases of infancy, toddlerhood, early childhood, and school age. In the absence of such studies, we are not in a position to determine the effects of deprivation or enrichment of particular patterns of relationships at particular stages. We are unable to plan the best preventive and remedial programs, yet we know that we could greatly reduce disorders and handicaps among our young if we provided systematic care during the early years of life. An adequate and systematic body of knowledge on infancy and early childhood is urgently needed. Among the areas to be given research priority are:

1. Early detection of disorders

Many disorders in children could be corrected if they were detected early. Further study is needed in a number of areas, including the following:

Research is needed to elucidate the earliest signs of variation from normality (developmental delay; pathological symptoms; high-risk patterns of behavior).

Further investigation is required in reference to the correlations between early variation and subsequent pathology. Studies should include the long-range implications of various indices of difficulty which can be obtained through professional and paraprofessional observation, testing, and parental report.

Evaluative techniques need to be devised to determine the effectiveness and efficiency of personnel other than mental health specialists in screening clinically disturbed children.

Procedures for detection and evaluation of early childhood disorder must be developed if accurate estimates of the magnitude of this mental health problem are to be made.

2. Deprivation

Further study is indicated in several areas. Epidemiological research to document the extent and demographic characteristics of these disorders is necessary for appropriate planning for case-finding, diagnosis, treatment, and rehabilitation. Specific study of each syndrome of deprivation will be required before appropriate diagnostic and preventative measures can be undertaken. These studies should include further investigations of the subtleties of the distortions of the mother-child relationships which result in deprivational syndromes. The relationships of the specific traumas and disruptions of family life to the child's development in different time periods should be investigated. Research is required for the appropriate and most sensible method of diagnostic study of these children and also to evaluate the efficacy of the initial treatment methods. Further study of the outcome needs emphasis if the extent of these disorders is to be recognized.

There is plentiful evidence concerning the general composite picture of the effects of social deprivation on children. Further research should concentrate on particular deficits and motivational patterns, specific parent-child interactions and their consequences, the development and long-term evaluation of programs aimed at prevention and remediation at an early age, and ways of involving parents in parent-education experiences.

3. Psychosis in young children

It is highly desirable that research programs of different orientations currently studying psychotic children be coordinated so as to reduce ambiguities regarding basic definitions of diagnosis, severity, and change.

Regional programs on the model of the Maternal and Infant Health study are necessary. Long-range studies are needed of a large number of children under five representing all (or a known percentage of all) cases in a given region evaluated by the same methods and against the same criteria for psychosis.

Collaboration among studies, including those of deprivation and cerebral dysfunction, should be encouraged. Clarification is needed of the overlap between deprivation and psychosis in the etiological process. It may be that a psychotic state in a child, manifested as withdrawal or as hyperreactivity to stimuli, antedates deprivation and, by stimulating adverse maternal reactions, precipitates a deprivation syndrome such as "failure to thrive." On the other hand, deprivation may be predisposing or precipitating to psychosis. Because of the concomitance of the two, a common or related etiologic factor is likely to be operating.

Children exhibiting psychosis with demonstrable cerebral dysfunction or with mental retardation must be included in the groups needing research attention. Their identifications will enhance the understanding of the roles played in the psychotic picture by the other condition. Such inclusion does not imply the absence of differences; it allows for clarification of what such differences may be.

Many if not all of the attitudes implicit in these recommendations have been embodied in work already begun at different research centers. Research has not, however, been conducted on what appears to be the necessary multicentered collaborative level which could be greatly facilitated by federal support and encouragement.

4. Emotional disturbance

Research is needed to determine the etiology of emotional disturbance. Studies should focus on organic and experiential primary factors and on the role of secondary emotional disturbance resulting from the disability and its effects on the child's self-concept and his interaction with others.

5. Predelinquency studies

Support should be given for developing methods for the very early identification of youngsters who are likely to manifest repetitive delinquency, particularly the maladjusted group. Incorporated into other large-scale longitudinal studies of childhood development and intervention should be measures designed to carefully describe both the child and his family setting, so that antecedent-consequent relationships may be studied in this area. Early childhood longitudinal studies should be continued through the adolescent period so that the emergence of delinquency can be observed; frequently, the child who is legally identified during adolescence as a delinquent has been well known to teachers, school authorities, and even the police during his earlier years.

6. Family support

Because of the paucity of firm knowledge concerning the care of the young child, generous support should be given to a wide variety of studies. Many different models for support of the family in caring for the child of this age should be tried and evaluated. Wherever possible, evaluation of a long-term nature is desirable. Studies should revolve around investigations of the varieties of optimal mother-child relationships and child-rearing practices.

Many mothers are now working. Many more will probably enter the labor force in the future. In addition, there is the necessity for beginning intervention, screening, and family support in the early years.

The increasing need for day-care and preschool programs makes it imperative that research efforts be mounted immediately so that serious mistakes will not be made with infants and children who are extremely vulnerable, so that inadequate facilities will not be allowed to function, and so that ineffective programs will not become permanent arrangements. Perhaps in no other area is there such a pressing need for both basic and applied research, drawing for its direction upon the many disciplines involved in the comprehensive care of infants and children.

7. Learning disorders

Research is needed to develop better techniques for the identification of early signs that the child will be unable to profit in the ordinary way from regular school experiences. Attention must be given to disorders of perception, language, fine and gross motor control, "soft" neurological signs, personality immaturity, and emotional disturbance. Attention should also be given to the possible identification of children differing in etiology or in nature of disability or both.

Research is needed to develop more effective remedial programs for both preschool and school-age children. Model programs of remediation should receive thorough evaluation before they are proliferated; this evaluation will need to be systematic and longitudinal.

8. Language development

Increased funding is needed for research in developmental linguistics to determine more precisely the strategies and tactics that children use in verbal learning and memory. Such knowledge is particularly relevant to educational and remedial programs. The problems which bilingualism poses for minority-group children also need to be studied.

F. EDUCATION

Children and youth spend a great deal of time in an educational setting. Recent increases in college enrollment and in the development of preschool programs indicate that many more children will spend far more time in schools in the future. Thus, the nature of the school experience will be an even greater determinant in the development of cognitive, emotional, and interpersonal skills for many of our children and youth. In Section II-D above and further in Chapter IX, we refer to the problems, the successes, and the failures of current educational practices. Attention is called to the need for greater financial expenditures, for bold and creative thought, planning, and action.

Because the school experience is so crucial to child development, because so few blueprints exist for educational reform, and because great wisdom and much knowledge are needed before we can determine the most promising directions, we need a diverse and large body of research to improve our educational programs. To accomplish this, the Commission recommends:

a. A National Institute for Research in Education

The establishment of a National Institute for Research in Education provides one answer to solving some of the serious problems which educators face today. Such an institute could address itself to the current need for providing alternative reform efforts based on research. This institute should have as one of its principal functions the planning, guidance, and stimulation of demonstration research efforts so that an evaluation of outcomes can lead to the formulation and testing of alternative educational policies. Among the specific areas with which the institute would be concerned are:

1. Basic research in learning within the educational setting.

2. Studies of teacher-pupil relationships which view the classroom as a social unit.

3. Program planning on a long-term basis of research approaches in the educational field, including such areas as:

> student development (e.g., the effects of the school on the psychological development of its students; the routes and pathways currently used by distressed students in seeking help; a frank evaluation of the adequacy of existing facilities that aid distressed students);

> the development of pupil personnel services.

4. The development, assessment, and comparative evaluation of alternative educational strategies, particularly for those children who are high educational and mental health risks. Research efforts might include:

> studies of the roles and functions of new types of paraprofessionals (both adults and adolescents) and new types of professionals (e.g., the *educateur,* child development specialist, etc.);

> assessment of programs which extend educational services beyond the school building into community agencies, for both school-age and post-school-age youth;

> large-scale research and demonstration projects to improve vocational curriculum, vocational guidance services, and related job-training facilities for youth.

b. Educational programs for the preschool child

Before rushing into massive programs of providing services to young children, stress should be laid upon research and training. Slow growth of programs, especially in the beginning, is certainly to be preferred to premature, ill-staffed, and ill-equipped programs which will be likely to be of little advantage to children and may lead inevitably to public reaction against further support for such services.

Particular support should be given to research centers which, in sum, approach the development of comprehensive patterns both from laboratory studies and from applied settings. Existing programs and those being developed in diverse patterns should be carefully and continuously evaluated.

A significant segment of research in this area should be longitudinal in design, continuing to follow during the school years children who have come from different backgrounds, who have experienced various kinds of programs, and who have entered varied public school experiences and programs supplementary to school. Such research is expensive and demands long-term commitments.

Among the research questions to be considered in the development of new educational programs are the following:

The long-range effects of early-childhood learning in a variety of areas; new methods and materials to support such learning; and the effects of early learning on children's motivational patterns and self-concepts.

The assessment of the resources and activities available to children within their homes, and determination of areas which need supplementation in service programs.

Assessment of the ways in which needed experiences can best be provided (in group setting, directly by professionals or paraprofessionals, or indirectly through work with the parents).

Determination of areas in which children need direct instruction and the development of methods of diagnosing assets and deficits. Findings in these areas should lead to appropriate individualizing of instruction.

Determination of differences, if any, in the provisions to be made for boys and girls.

Development of methods of enhancing the children's participation in the world of adults.

Development of methods of providing opportunities for children to incorporate and practice learnings provided in structured situations in which spontaneous play and privacy are balanced with structure and group participation.

Means of providing a suitable balance between direct, immediate experience and vicarious experience through books, television, and mechanical aids.

Delineation of optimal types of locations for educational programs and means of integrating the programs with other services to children.

Development of methods which will provide children a wide range of interpersonal experiences and contacts with individuals of different ages, styles, and backgrounds so that children can learn to identify these people as individuals who care about them, and with whom continuous friendships can be established.

Development of methods of working with parents and other caretakers so that their abilities to provide for the child are both strengthened and supported.

G. ADOLESCENCE AND YOUNG ADULTHOOD

The transition from childhood to adulthood in our society is one of considerable psychological turmoil and upheaval for many adolescents and youth. We lack, as yet, a body of research which will permit a firm understanding of the developmental phases through which adolescents and youth pass. We do not know enough about how these developmental stages vary for males and females or for persons of different social classes and ethnic groups. The role which the family, peer group, school, and other factors play in the formation of identity, ego strength, and personality during these periods is not yet well understood. Nor do we have a clear understanding of the strains imposed by the structure of our modern technological society. Thus, we are in a poor position to assess either the benefits or the adverse psychological effects of youthful rebellion or complacency. Too little is known about the development of psychopathology; thus, the best treatment procedures for adolescents and youth in need remain undetermined. In addition, we have little knowledge about what the adolescent needs relative to the process of becoming a responsible adult. The transition of youth into one or many of a wide range of roles—military, student, worker, spouse, parent—is made more difficult by the lack of adequate preparation to assume these roles.

Many recent events indicate that we must move in new directions. Alienation, apathy, discontent, and unrest are apparent from the junior high to the college level, from the ghetto to suburbia. Further, the number of adolescents admitted to mental hospitals has risen markedly. To meet the many problems faced by our adolescents, youth, and young adults, we need a vast body of research on the many factors which touch on their development, including the following:

Research is needed to determine how the earlier biological maturation of American children affects their emotional maturity and mental health. In particular, means need to be devised to aid adolescents to cope with biological maturity while striving to achieve emotional maturity.

Research is needed to promote a better understanding of early and late adolescence and young adulthood and of sex differences in these various phases of development. Among the important issues to be determined are those relating to the resolution of self-identity and the development of adult roles and identities.

Multidiscipline studies should be undertaken to determine the underlying causes of the sudden upsurge in our society of the incidence of psychoneuroses among females during adolescence.

Systematic research should be undertaken to determine the efficacy of all treatment modalities (psychotherapeutic, somatic, and pharmacological therapies, behavioral therapy, milieu therapy, parental therapy, etc.). Such studies should determine the efficacy of such treatment modalities within psychiatric diagnostic categories, for different types of delinquents, for different types of special populations (e.g., the mentally retarded, physically handicapped), and for the different developmental stages of adolescenthood for the populations noted above.

Biological and behavioral scientists should cooperate in studies related to drug use and drug abuse among adolescents and youth. Further studies are needed on the physical, emotional, and behavioral effects of the various drugs and on more effective ways of treating various adverse reactions to these drugs.

Further examination should be made of the underlying causes of suicide among adolescents and youth. Particular attention should be given to determining the part which student stress plays in the causes of higher suicide rates among college students as compared to peers of their same age in the general population.

A survey of resources, development of resources, and referral and follow-up procedures is needed in relation to such special problems as: school suspensions, social problems, police referrals, family conflicts, abandoned adolescents, and runaways.

Research is needed to determine the factors which differentiate "activist" students, "alienated" youth (e.g., the so-called "hippie" subgroups), and the large majority of adolescents and youth who indicate that they are well satisfied with their homes, schools, and communities. Such multifactorial studies should attempt to determine the impact of each of these adaptations on the development of individuality and personality. Attention should be paid to variances in family characteristics, such as life styles, child-rearing techniques, social attitudes, and parent-child relationships. An underlying question should be the extent to which adolescent rebellion is a function of personal experience as opposed to factors associated with the overall social structure of our society.

Systematic studies should be undertaken to determine the underlying issues leading to student protest and riots in junior highs, high schools, and colleges. Attention should be given to such questions as: How do the issues which give rise to protest activities vary between schools and colleges? Under what conditions do protests occur and escalate, and how are the protests resolved? What are the responses of the schools, the communities, and the mass media?

Extensive experimental programs should be instituted to determine successful ways of including youth in responsible policy-making decisions in schools and colleges.

Research is needed to determine the factors associated with the tendency to marry early. Studies should attempt to determine the factors associated with "successful" and "unsuccessful" early marriages.

H. WORK

Questions related to the development of work orientation, the transition from school to work, and the importance of work to feelings of self-worth and competence have received very little attention from researchers. Future research in this area should focus on such questions as:

How much and what type of educational skill is necessary for a given type of employment?

What kinds of preparation have youth received in relation to the jobs they actually obtain? How is the amount and quality of schooling, kinds of curriculum, and extent of counseling or guidance related to success in initial job entry and later job success? What are some of the linkages between particular kinds of school experience and the first entry into work? What are the linkages between different part-time work experiences and the first entry into full-time employment?

What kinds of testing procedures are the most appropriate for drop-outs and disadvantaged youth in determining success on the job? Which I.Q. and aptitude tests are best suited to this determination?

What type of work program is best suited to a particular type of delinquent exhibiting a particular type of delinquent behavior? The same question should be asked in relation to the handicapped, retarded, and severely disturbed.

What are the various values and expectations of youth entering the labor market and how are these subsequently molded by employment experiences?

I. DISADVANTAGED CHILDREN AND YOUTH

There is ample general information which demonstrates that poverty and discrimination tend to adversely affect the physical, intellectual, emotional, and social development of children and youth. Much more detailed research is needed on the effects of these two variables. Specifically, we need to focus on:

the differential impact of poverty and discrimination on males and females;

the strengths of the disadvantaged as well as their particular problems;

knowledge concerning the life styles and the impact of poverty and racism on various subgroups in the population (Mexican-Americans, Puerto Ricans, Indians, etc.) in both rural and urban settings;

information regarding the impact of poverty and the life styles of various disadvantaged minority groups in such areas as: physical growth and development, language development and learning skills, emotional and social development, achievement and work attitudes, moral development and values, and attitudes toward the disadvantaged individual's own subgroup and the larger society;

adaptation to a bicultural pattern, including the adoption of English as a second language;

factors associated with "upward mobility" of disadvantaged persons and the impact of "upward mobility" on the physical and mental health of those who achieve in spite of the multiple handicaps of their environment;

the extent to which cultural patterns of the various subgroups change, the circumstances under which they change, and the effects of cultural change on mental health and social and family relationships;

delineation of family patterns in both well-organized and disorganized disadvantaged groups, including various patterns of parent-child interaction, and the effects of this interaction upon the child's development;

the impact of other "socializing agents" such as older children and adults in the neighborhood, the school, the church or temple, and youth-serving organizations.

Further recommendations relating to research in the area of racism are presented in the concluding section of Chapter V.

J. FOSTER CARE

There is a dire need for two kinds of information regarding foster care: how much is needed and for what types of children; and determination of the consequences of various foster-care decisions. To meet this need we recommend:

Research based on a national sample census of families should be undertaken in order to arrive at a meaningful estimate of the numbers who need supportive, supplementary, and substitutive services.

Several service and research centers should be established in various regions of the country with the primary objective of innovation and research follow-up; they should determine the consequences of alternative courses of action and serve as demonstration and training centers. Grants should be made specifically to encourage feedback research in foster-care agencies.

K. FAMILY RESEARCH

Throughout this report we stress the importance of the family characteristics and constellation upon the development of the child. We strongly urge that increased funding be made available for research relating to the family. Research efforts should include assessment of the various service programs which we have recommended elsewhere, such as: family planning; family counseling, including personal counseling; premarital and divorce counseling; consumer education; sex education and counseling; and the participation of parents, children, and youth in the Child Development Councils and other programs. Funding should also be available for:

assessing the effect of work training and employment on low-income mothers and their families, especially in terms of one-parent families, different types of family situations, child-care arrangements, and different employment and training settings;

experimentation and research in the area of working with families, including such dimensions as techniques of treatment, ways of working with seriously disoriented families, and the exploration of a number of commonly held assumptions concerning work with the child and family members;

longitudinal studies to establish a baseline for judging deviant processes as they evolve in families;

the development of research and developmental centers which use a multidiscipline team to study the development of children and families.

We further recommend that ways be explored which could lead to a further coordination of federal research activities related to children and families. These are currently being diversely planned and sponsored in a number of federal agencies such as the Office of Education, the Social and Rehabilitation Service (including the Children's Bureau), NIMH, NICHD, the Departments of Labor and Agriculture, and OEO. There is also a need to develop a central information resource about these programs.

L. MANPOWER

Any attempt to formulate mental health goals must give major consideration to the use and training of manpower. No other area is as central to the provision of adequate, high-quality services to our children and youth. Any consideration of the uses of skills must include at least three different aspects of the problem:

1. the community health requirements as defined by the community as well as the professionals;
2. the operations of education and training establishments;
3. the existing service structures that deliver health and related services.

Our recommendations are future-oriented. They demand a reconceptualization of current thinking about manpower recruitment, development, and utilization, not in an ex cathedra manner, but with the aim of developing an informational base which would take into account community attitudes and the three basic requirements as noted above. This calls for an estimation of the state of the national mental health and related professions, as well as the roles of the community, educational resources, and the service structure arrangements. In this exploration the following questions need to be raised: How do people choose their health services and receive them? Which professionals give service? How do these professionals receive their training and how does their knowledge about services affect the recipients of services? The Commission recommends that such queries be the basis of future inquiry into manpower needs and deployment policies. We further recommend:

Investigation of the use of personnel should include an intensive study of present structures (e.g., hospitals, clinics, residential treatment centers, schools, etc.) and of new and emerging structures (e.g., community mental health centers, comprehensive neighborhood health centers, regional medical plans, etc.).

Assessment of the use of manpower should not center merely on the number of available jobs and available people to fill them. We need to know how these are balanced with respect to the functions required to meet community health needs, educational resources, service structures, and the existing manpower, and occupational and professional practices. We strongly urge that studies of traditional and new occupational functions, manpower resources, and their relationships be explored in order to make intelligent decisions on manpower development.

The utilization of both professional and trained paraprofessionals and their relationships to the new service structures should be reconceptualized with an emphasis on the new ways of delivering skills. This means that trials of these new manpower resources would be made in both traditional settings and new community-based service organizations. We recommend that research in these areas guide the development of new careers and new service settings. The Child Development Councils should be intensely involved in such efforts.

People involved with therapy should move to intervene at a broader level of social organization rather than be restricted solely to the individual therapeutic intervention. Large-scale intervention would involve epidemiological, social, and political considerations. In light of this we recommend that NIMH focus its child health activities in the direction of the collecting of literature around the leading edges of treatment and the quick dissemination of this information, so that the most up-to-date information is readily available for the practitioner and the therapist.

If the base in treatment is the social-psycho-therapy of the individual, then we should develop a new set of psychiatric criteria which involves an extension of our traditional taxonomic schemes. The concept of indications and contra-indications should be made the central core of this process, and rethinking should include at the central governmental level a formalization of the interdisciplinary dialogue, which is now in process. This could also include a recommendation that NIMH explore the experimental mental health programs by using both HUD and NIMH resources in devising new teams to develop evaluation methods. Mental health experiments should be tried in experimental communities. One experiment which might be tried in conjunction with the promotion of an interdisciplinary dialogue would be the development of a demonstration using the new health teams. This would be one way to work toward common goals, across administrative lines.

We need to identify those elements of professional curricula which are, in fact, useful and relevant to the professional's work. Most curricula are relics, emerging out of tradition, inter- and intra-departmental power balances, and untested hypotheses. It would be feasible to collect data which will make possible realistic professional training.

We need to do something about the institutionalization of the "Peter Principle" and learn alternatives to our present tendency to reward excellent clinicians by removing them out of clinical work and into administration, where they may no longer be excellent. The role of the hospital administrator is a possibly applicable model.

In Section IV below, we will deal more fully with the need for training paraprofessionals. To maximize the potential value of this source of manpower, there are a number of things we need to know, such as:

If we are to identify useful paraprofessional positions, we need to know, in industrial detail, what concrete activities professionals actually spend their time doing—and how much time they spend at each task. The techniques of time-motion study, for example, could well identify a large number of time-consuming activities which could be assigned to less-trained people, freeing time for the professional to do those things for which his training is essential. Much of the existing experience of Florida's and Illinois' mental health technician programs could be directly useful in such studies.

We need to develop realistic and reliably observable criteria and goals for mental health service if we are to make any sensible evaluation of the effects of either training or service programs. All the health, education, and welfare occupations need to be reanalyzed and separated into component parts in relation to the levels and nature of education and skill required for adequate performance so as to maximize the potential use of volunteers, paraprofessionals, and professionals.

Professionals are acutely aware of what they cannot do. We need to identify what kinds of things many people who are not professionals can effectively do. Sensitivity, empathy, warmth, and respect for others are potent and widely distributed characteristics which can be identified and focused outside the professional curriculum.

Time-motion studies and the use of such new tools as PSYCHE (the Reiss-David Clinic's technique for computer analysis of case history and anecdotal records and psychotherapy notes), transactional studies of patients and helping agencies may suggest whole new progressions or rearrangements of curricula which could make significant increases in the effective use of scarce people with unusual talent. The British model of the doctorate in medical psychology is an example of what may be a far more relevant combination of learning than is provided in our present degree programs. Accompanying such studies must be vigorous incentives to break through the parochialism and territoriality so often present in our separated professional departments and schools. The present federal training grants programs could play a major role in this task, instead of simply continuing to strengthen professional separatism.

We need to develop systems of rewarding people for what they do—in service—as well as for the degrees they earn and the papers they publish. The new paraprofessional will not be likely to function well or for long if the job he enters is a dead end, with no opportunity for growth or for vertical or lateral mobility.

IV. Manpower and Training

The services our children so urgently require cannot possibly be provided within our existing mental health care network. The needs seem certain to increase with time, unless we seriously seek new directions. In medicine (particularly psychiatry), in social work, in clinical psychology, and in all the related subspecialized fields the manpower shortage is acute. The increased demands for services in recent years has not been matched by the increase in manpower. This problem is further compounded by the poor distribution of available personnel. Clinical psychologists, and particularly psychiatrists, have tended to move into urban centers and into private practices where services are limited to a small and usually more affluent segment of the population. Children's services are neglected in favor of services for adults. Meanwhile, public institutions languish for lack of personnel.

In providing services to children and youth, the present mental health care network is largely oriented toward providing diagnosis and treatment for the severely disturbed 2 or 3 percent and crisis care for the less severely disturbed. The present system, however, cannot even meet the needs of these children. Preventive measures receive only scant attention from the overburdened and harried professionals.

Clearly, we must seek new solutions to meet the need for both preventive and therapeutic services. The Commission's proposals for achieving positive mental health for our nation's children and youth depend upon ensuring their inalienable rights. This can be done only if we devise new ways of organizing, delivering, and ensuring comprehensive and systematic services at the local level; merely increasing services is not enough.

Nor can we expect the mental health professionals to assume total responsibility for the mental health of our children and youth. It is apparent that all of us—parents, legislators, teachers, urban planners, professionals, etc.—are ultimately involved in the development of our young. Those who are expert in mental health and related fields must expand their areas of influence. They must reach out to all of us and advise us as to the ways in which each of us may enhance the development and mental health of our children and youth. They must provide mental health training throughout the community so that all those who come into contact with children, or are sought to advise on their behavior, can establish a series of "helping relationships" in which one person can aid others in developing their talents and capabilities. Those in the mental health field must also help in the creation of a societal milieu which fosters healthy child development. Increasing the involvement of mental health personnel in these ways is essential to achieving the ultimate goals of the Child Development Councils proposed by this Commission.

But those in mental health and related professions must do more than advise and train in the community. They must also listen. They must be sensitive to the needs of the time, and they must understand the socioeconomic, cultural, and geographic factors that determine the expectations of various communities and their demands for and acceptance of mental health care for their children. They must define the needs of any population they intend to serve. Only in this way can the proper personnel and services be provided to meet the particular needs of either normal or deviant children. Because of their importance to the well-being of children and youth, those in the mental health professions must look honestly at the shortcomings of their own particular professions. Each profession must devise new ways of evoking in its members a genuine sense of the responsibility which underlies its public trust.

The traditional answer to our manpower problems has been to train more professionals. But the traditional solution, with its inherent limitations, cannot possibly be implemented—for reasons which are discussed more fully in Chapter XI. There is little doubt that we need to expand our training efforts to increase the supply of traditional professionals. But precisely because the traditional answer to our manpower problems has not worked well enough, we must look more systematically and creatively at what we have and what we need. We must create new roles and functions which will make better use of traditional professionals, such as those alluded to above. We must also find new sources of manpower and ways of training this needed manpower, if we are to provide for the mental health needs of our nation. But because we must open ourselves up to new ways of thinking and acting on these problems we may, in the end, provide a better system of mental health care than the patchwork quilt that has been our traditional pattern.

A. FEDERAL PROVISIONS FOR MANPOWER AND TRAINING

The first essential step in the process of manpower planning for mental health is to specify the general goals for which manpower is needed. In addition, subgoals must be identified with sufficient clarity and specificity to permit manpower tasks and requirements to be determined. Present deployment of financial and human resources is largely unplanned. Rational planning for future change is difficult, if not impossible, by our present standards. Typically, conflicts arise between our desires for children and vested interests, between the familiarity of tradition and the need for innovation, between our belief in free enterprise and our recognition that federal funds, and often federal coordination, can spell the difference between good intentions and actual social change.

The Commission recognizes that training manpower for mental health is a problem of such magnitude that it warrants extensive public concern and financial commitment, both federal and local. Federal funding for manpower training in the past has not been adequate to the national need. To confront the more basic issues underlying any manpower planning, the Commission recommends:

An effective manpower policy which will grapple with the priority problems of the various professions should be developed. It is only by such an effort that any ability can be acquired to ensure that one profession or another can be increased in size.

To meet the urgent manpower crisis, we urge that the federal government subsidize the expansion of training facilities and training personnel for both professional and paraprofessional training, so that the intake of students can be greatly increased.

We further recommend that the federal government subsidize students throughout their training. Such subsidies should be adequate to meet the student's life situation so that poverty youths will not be forced to decline or withdraw because of some immediate economic crisis, and so that middle-aged and retired persons can be recruited for training or retraining. Special efforts should be made to recruit persons from lower socioeconomic strata and from ethnic minorities in order to help fill the service gaps among these groups.

The National Institute of Mental Health, and any other federal agency which elects to provide training grants, should institute a requirement that recipients of its training grants serve for an equitable period in a public agency or in a nonprofit agency devoted to service, training, or research in mental health.

A minimum of 50 percent of the training funds of the National Institute of Mental Health should be committed to the education of psychiatrists, psychologists, social workers, psychiatric nurses, teachers, counselors, and other mental health specialists for work with children and youth.

The federal government should undertake to provide tax incentives to mental health professionals to work in areas that are presently receiving few or no services. The federal plan should attempt to ensure proper distribution of mental health personnel, so that adequate services will be provided to children, to the poor, to ethnic minorities, and to persons in all geographic regions.

The federal government should establish some form of National Service which would allow young people of eighteen and older to participate in service programs such as projects in urban ghettos, in the Appalachian region, among migrant workers, or in psychiatric hospitals or welfare agencies. We recommend that a number of National Service pilot programs be established in different regions of the country to determine the amount and type of participation desired by youth and young adults. National Service would not only add to our source of manpower but would serve to develop an effective sense of community as an integral trait of youngsters moving into meaningful adult roles.

In the recommendations which follow, the Commission addresses itself to more specific areas of concern. It is hoped that the federal government will provide both technical assistance and financial support to increase the manpower, and the effectiveness of personnel, in the various professions and paraprofessions which are mentioned below.

B. MEDICAL PERSONNEL FOR SERVICES TO THE
MOTHER AND YOUNG CHILD

The capacity of specialists and paramedical personnel to provide the necessary care to every mother and her child calls for both an increase in and a reorganization of medical manpower. Training support for new professional and paramedical personnel is urgently needed. Further, changes in training and curriculum are required so that all those who deal with the mother and young child will be able to identify high-risk, or potential high-risk, cases. Specifically:

Support is needed for training programs for all personnel involved in rendering obstetrical care. Only about 850 obstetricians are currently being admitted to the board of qualified specialists each year; this number exceeds only slightly the number of obstetricians who retire. In 1966, there were only 415 nurses enrolled as students in graduate programs in maternal and child health (National League for Nursing, 1966) and only 29 graduate programs that prepared nurses in this area or in obstetric or pediatric nursing (National League for Nursing, 1967).

Although there is some controversy surrounding the advisability of heavy reliance on nurse-midwives, it is clear that some such solution will be required in order to provide the necessary services. Since presently only 10 schools offer such training, and fewer than 1,000 trained midwives practice now in the United States (American College of Nurse Midwifery, 1968), research should examine the efficacy of the use of well-trained individuals in various kinds of settings.

In addition to obstetric and pediatric physicians and allied personnel, there is need for specialist neonatologists, practicing in large centers but serving primarily to train other pediatricians and to continually bring to their attention current findings in the field.

All professional personnel who will be involved with young children should receive training in the basic aspects of child development: motor, emotional, social, intellectual, moral, and motivational facets; age-appropriate expectations, both growth and natural "problem behaviors," and cognizance of the needs of children. Such training should enable a large number of persons who have contact with children and families to enhance their sensitivity to possible disordered patterns of development and thus to serve an initial screening function, which would be followed by referral for more specialized evaluation. Their common training should also facilitate communication and cooperation among them.

Insofar as possible, paraprofessional personnel should likewise receive training to permit them also to become sensitive to distortions in development and symptoms of emotional disorder during early childhood, so that children with questionable problems can be more closely observed and appropriate referrals made.

Each facility offering medical surveillance and screening might involve individuals whose primary responsibility is follow-up of referral and treatment prescriptions with families who are likely to need special assistance with carry-through. Competent individuals with only short-term training might be supervised by public health nurses; these individuals might well be selected from social-ethnic groups similar to the target families.

Workers in many disciplines concerned with mental health have insufficient experience with the preschool child, especially during the first three years of life. While there are many nonprofessional people who can participate in programs of early child care, we will need specialized, trained persons at both professional and paraprofessional levels for work with emotionally disturbed young children. At the present time there is an increasing gap between the need in this field and the very small number of trained personnel. In spite of the insufficient attention paid to this age group thus far by such workers, persons with sufficient skill are able to make early diagnosis of such disorders as infantile autism, schizophrenia in childhood, depressive states, psychosomatic conditions, developmental deviations, and the children who belong in the aytpical group. The number of persons with such skills must be greatly increased by training if the extent and severity of emotional disorders during early childhood are to be discovered.

C. MANPOWER FOR SERVICES TO ADOLESCENTS

Like the preschool child, the adolescent is a target population whose clinical and other service needs are especially acute at present. We recommend increased training to prepare professionals and paraprofessionals to deal with adolescents. Manpower specifically trained to deal with adolescents should be available for:

provision of more adequate mental health consultative and other services to courts, detention centers, correctional institutions, etc.;

provision for emergency services to adolescents in clinics and hospitals;

provision of services to adolescents who are not patients—this involves professionals going out of the clinics to the young people.

We further recommend:

Youth should be involved as both volunteers and paid workers in all service programs. For example, healthy well-adjusted adolescents should be involved in clinical services for other adolescents.

Youth should be involved in planning community services and in the evaluation of all projects aimed at serving youth.

Adolescents of the poverty community and those from oppressed minority groups should be involved in mental health programs by playing leadership roles in both planning and operation. Professionals should promote this involvement by functioning as consultants.

D. FAMILY SPECIALISTS

Increasingly, mental health professionals have placed a greater emphasis on treating the child in the family context. We recommend:

that funds be provided for the training of family specialists. The overwhelming number of families to be dealt with makes it obvious that large numbers of professional and paraprofessional personnel will be required for the many programs which will be developed in this area. Individuals who work with families and children under stress generally need training, but short-term training courses for sensitive and warm individuals without specialized backgrounds is often sufficient (see the recommendations on paraprofessionals below).

E. TEACHERS

The public school system is a major community resource which has a responsibility for education of all children wherever they may reside. There is a need for understanding this responsibility in that it necessitates correlated training of educational personnel to work in the public school, preschool, special classes, and institutional centers. Since it is evident that educational aspects are a major condition of treatment for all seriously disturbed children, this represents one of the major areas of manpower shortage. Frequently the current trend of educational personnel stops short of an appreciation of the potentials of the seriously disturbed child. A reexamination of the training programs in this area is in order. Often they are designed for training personnel for children with minor difficulties, and personnel are encouraged to rely exclusively on nondynamic approaches.

1. Training programs

The Commission recommends that the U.S. Office of Education provide high levels of support to teacher training programs which:

include the study of child development to promote an understanding of the drives, conflicts, and capacities characteristic of successive stages of learning;

prepare teachers to deal with a wide range of behavior in children so that more children can be maintained within the regular classroom;

place heavy emphasis on practical experience in all types of communities and provide regular mechanisms for students to engage with faculty in a critique of the student's experience as a novice teacher;

establish built-in guidance and counseling provisions which will help students integrate mastery of skills and knowledge of child development with personal values and with the personal experiences of frustration and problem-solving encountered in the actual teaching role;

provide training which allows appropriately motivated teachers to deal openly with the life stresses which destroy the minority-group child's ability to participate in the calm atmosphere of the classroom;

incorporate the real problems of the school into actual teacher training curriculum. This could be accomplished by establishing portions of "clinical professorship" in which key school personnel and key faculty members have joint appointments in the university and in the school system.

In addition the Commission recommends:

That the U.S. Office of Education establish a Center for Advanced Study in Education for the training of educational statesmen for the public schools and for teacher education. We suggest that the Center provide for 100 Fellows for advanced training in the behavioral sciences, administrative leadership, and the dynamics of change. Each Fellow should be chosen on the basis of potential leadership, from either the public schools or teacher education, and must agree to return to his position following training in the center.

That provisions be made through the Education Professions Development Act (PL-9035) to increase training funds for teacher-counselors, liaison teachers, and administrators for schools modeled after Re-ED; for doctoral-level programs for preparing research and graduate-level training personnel; for the training of consultants from relevant disciplines, and for cadre training for the staff of projected Re-ED schools.

2. School mental health services

The Commission recommends that a Center for Pupil Development Services be established in the U.S. Office of Education. This center would have the responsibility for:

conducting an ongoing assessment of the manpower needs for pupil development services;

coordinating and developing training programs in (a) professional areas inclusive of pupil development services and (b) the use of paraprofessionals, in keeping with knowledge of needs, school staffing patterns, and emerging concepts of new roles and functions.

F. FOSTER CARE

Personnel is a major problem in foster care and in the supportive and supplemental services which may help prevent extended separation of children from their natural parents. The following steps are recommended:

Introduce a new semiprofessional position: the child-rearer for both full-time and part-time work. This position will require courses and experience in child care which can be acquired through on-the-job training at the junior college level. Persons with such training will occupy important positions under professional supervision in foster care, day-care centers, group-care programs, and as mothers' aides in certain supplementary services.

Reexamine the use of professional personnel working on the adoption of infants, the recruitment and selection of foster homes, services to children in and out of foster-family care, and in the review of eligibility for economic assistance. By using higher salary as an incentive, move staff to child and family centers, to supportive day-care programs, to intensive treatment arrangements whether in group care or foster-family care, and to intensive work with families whose children are to return to them.

Under competent supervision, involve foster parents in the formulation of agency policies and the recruitment of new homes. Move older and more experienced foster parents into positions of responsibility for child care in the homes of others by giving them supervisory and advisory functions vis-à-vis new foster families, and possibly by shifting to them the task of screening and approving new applicants. Foster parenting should be considered as a career. Foster parents should be paid more and treated with all usual benefits, including vacation leave, salary raises, etc.

G. CHILD-CARE WORKERS FOR INSTITUTIONALIZED CHILDREN*

A ten-year plan should be conceived and implemented on a nationwide scale to develop and uplift child-care work. This plan, if successful, will provide child-care workers who can realistically occupy the significant position they need to hold in institutions for children and youth. Presently, many institutions can offer little more than custodial care.

In order to increase the effectiveness of child treatment institutions, it is essential to:

* M. F. Mayer and J. M. Goldsmith (1968).

1. Upgrade the present group of child-care workers to make them more effective.

2. Create a new resource of personnel by a systematic professionalization of the child-care work within the next decade.

To accomplish these objectives, we make the following recommendations:

1. Upgrading of present staff

a. Salaries should be commensurate with comparable work in industry and comparable professions (i.e., practical nurse, etc.).

b. Working conditions should include a work week of forty hours to encompass time for training, supervision, recording, and direct practice.

c. Adequate arrangements should be available for fringe benefits such as hospitalization insurance, sick leave, retirement, death benefits, etc., as accorded to the social work and teaching professions.

d. Housing and living quarters should be so arranged so to permit maximum ability to pursue normal life with opportunities for privacy. Wherever possible, arrangements should be made for child-care workers to live off campus and be provided with a salary which makes the arrangement feasible.

e. Working schedules should be established to allow for continuity of free time and not spread over the day, thereby splitting the worker's free time into unusable fragments.

f. Supervision should be provided on a differential basis for each child-care worker. The supervision should be realistically provided in terms of regular allocation of supervisors' and workers' time for that purpose, and in terms of the number of supervisees. We would suggest not more than five child-care workers to one supervisor in order to ensure availability and continuity.

g. In addition to individual supervision, institutions should establish group in-service training sessions to cope with the common practice problems of child-care work.

h. Recognizing differences in ability, child-care workers should be offered maximum opportunity to participate in clinical and administrative conferences.

i. The communication system in the institution should include channels from the child-care worker to the administration.

j. A program of learning outside the agency should be established to teach new concepts of child care to the child-care worker, to enable him to see his work not only from the parochial confines of his agency experience but as a part of a total system of child treatment. Federal financing should be provided on a regional basis throughout the country for university-based institutes and workshops for the child-care workers. These should continue for an academic year with opportunity to earn college credits. Agency budgets should include funds to release staff time for participation in these training programs. Where fiscal resources do not exist, government grants should be made available to encourage these training efforts. These courses should have a systematic long-range objective, including field work in other than the worker's own institution.

k. Tangible encouragement should be given to the development of regional and national associations of child-care workers. These organizations should be initiated mainly through the efforts of the child-care workers themselves with the help of the administrators of the child-care institutions and the local community and welfare councils. Local federal and national federations and foundations should assist in the development of such child-care workers organizations.

2. Professionalizing the child-care worker

a. The primary professional commitment of the child-care worker should be to the field of child care rather than to any particular institution. The recruitment of child-care workers therefore should be directed toward candidates for training in child-care work rather than toward applicants for one institution.

b. A major effort should be developed to attract students attending junior colleges to this field.

c. A specialized recruitment leading to an associate degree in child care should be developed in community colleges and/or the first two years of regular colleges.

d. Recruitment offices should be located in the community college and/or university. Special committees should be established for selection and admission of new recruits. Committees should include representatives of public employment offices, college counseling bureaus, and the representatives of the institutional centers themselves.

e. A campaign of public information should be conducted to provide knowledge about child-care work and opportunities for training and employment.

f. Through government aid, stipends should be provided for the child-care student, including tuition and subsistence. These stipends should be sufficient to allow the student with a family to undergo training without undue economic pressure.

g. Such programs should be developed throughout the country. The courses should include a combination of didactic and practice work. The didactic work should include courses in child development, deviant behavior, understanding of the functions of other disciplines, concepts of group processes, play and recreation techniques with children, and training to express observations and recommendations orally and in writing. At least one half of the training should be field-work practice.

h. All qualified institutions should be committed to provide placement facilities for the field-work practice of the students to make available to the students sufficient time with a qualified supervisor and to permit the student to participate in all other forms of learning available to child-care workers at the institution.

i. Eligible child-care workers employed at the present time and interested in undergoing training leading to the associate degree should be released by their employers for such training.

j. The programs should be organized in such a way that a good number of the didactic courses could be taken as evening and summer courses to hold to a minimum the interruption of the vocational life of the students.

k. For many child-care workers in institutions remote from centers of learning, it might be more practical to develop a system of intensive academic training for a three-month period to be followed by a period of internship under the school's supervision.

l. At the completion of training, the college placement bureau and the professional sections of the state employment offices should assist the graduates in finding positions in residential care.

m. Child-care workers with an associate degree should be encouraged to acquire a bachelor's degree if they are capable and willing to do so.

n. A leave of absence from the institution should be given to such child-care workers for two years if they so desire, with the understanding that they can come back after they have achieved their bachelor's degree.

o. Full or partial stipends should be made available for child-care workers studying toward their bachelor's degree as supplements or substitutions for their loss of income through such studies. To the degree that such stipends are not available within the institutional budget or within special funds, federal and state grants should be given for such purposes.

p. Facilities for graduate training for child-care workers, which is only in its infancy at the present time, should be increased. A combination of adequate training in the field of human relations, child development, psychopathology, group interaction, and group dynamics on one hand with supervised graduate field work on the other hand, should be the basic content of such training. Students with a bachelor's degree and with at least two years of practical experience as child-care workers should be eligible for such training.

q. Graduate training is considered as two-year training with at least two field-work placements, one of which should preferably be in a residential treatment center.

r. The availability of stipends for the students is particularly important since it is assumed that many of the students will be already at a relatively advanced age (from the middle twenties on) and may have family obligations.

s. It is recommended that ultimately many of the supervisors and administrators of child-care institutions should be graduates of such programs.

H. CLINICAL MANPOWER AND TRAINING

The traditional triumvirate of clinical professionals—i.e., psychiatrists, psychologists, and social workers—seems now to be experiencing, in addition to changes within its own ranks, changes in the number and kinds of professionals and paraprofessionals who are joining it in the tasks of treating the nation's children. For this reason (and for others), the trend we observe is that clinical roles are increasingly being redefined, partly reflective of and partly causing a redefinition of the nature of therapy. As new responsibilities emerge, new staff roles are called for, which, in turn, alter the responsibilities clinicians and their newfound partners share. The trend toward the inclusion of social relations in therapy brings with it a set of new tasks, which do not always harmonize with traditional ones. The best strategy is not always increasing specialization, since cooperation, coordination, consultation, and integration are not thereby facilitated. We therefore recommend:

Primary priorities should be allotted *after* a census of mental health needs has been taken, after which allocation of functional responsibilities may be made in proportion to manpower availabilities; remuneration for service should not be given highest priority.

Deficits in manpower discovered in the above procedure should be translated into training mandates, deliberately encouraging enrollment in understaffed professions by offering subsidized educational grants and/or draft deferments, as third-order priorities.

Education and training of paraprofessionals should *not* be undertaken on an ad hoc "crash" basis but, instead, be translated into an appropriate number of paraprofessionals' civil service ranks for which standardized educational procedures ought to be devised (e.g., assistant nurse, assistant doctor, assistant psychologist, assistant teacher, assistant social worker, etc.).

Work study programs for graduate students should be devised, using the NIMH fellowship program as a model for the development of assistant professionals.

New interdisciplinary teams should be assembled and tried out on a demonstration-evaluation project basis.

A design and staffing breakthrough should be deliberately sought to replace as quickly as possible the present asylums called mental hospitals, which should be charged with the responsibility to approximate the therapeutic situations in which therapy is known to work best, i.e., small patient-to-staff ratios.

Deliberate efforts should be made to reconstitute the specialties of community organization workers in social work, and counseling psychologists in psychology, these having apparently suffered a dilution over the years until they reached their present condition.

Conflicts between clinical and civic roles among so-called "indigenous workers" should be mediated by an elected board of clinicians and such workers in equal representation, on the premise that freedom in one role is contagious for the other.

Crisis therapy teams, mobile in nature, should be established under the aegis of the community mental health facilities now in process of construction. Such teams should *not* be seen as merely primary prevention efforts but as legitimate forms of emergency treatment, whose priorities should be calculated accordingly.

Rates should be established and partial subsidies offered to psychotherapists whose fees presently prohibit all but the relatively affluent from availing themselves of this mode of therapy. Specifically, we call for reexamination of the Medicaid policy which permits nonmedical therapists to enjoy the benefits of this program only when specifically supervised by medical personnel. "The poor" should enjoy the right to select the therapist of their choice. We extend the range of this recommendation to include provision for "home visits" by therapists (Gioscia *et al.*, 1968).

Further recommendations in this area have been made by the Commission's Clinical Committee. Included in these are the following:

Specialty training should extend from the nursery school teacher's aide to the child analyst. In particular, training emphasis must be given to the first three years of life, both for those directly concerned (e.g., nurses, obstetricians, pediatricians, etc.) and for those with more general interests (e.g., child psychologists, social workers, child analysts, etc.). The clinician will be crucial in terms of his functions as consultant, educator, resource, and back-up person. However, he too will need additional preparation in work with the first years of life.

Clinical training should include a great deal of specialized preparation to deal with minority groups. Also, more trainees need to be recruited from minority groups. (For further recommendations regarding minority-group personnel, see Chapter V.)

Training at the professional level has been critically influenced by the shift of interest toward community work. Many of the younger people in the field are far better prepared in community organization than they are in clinical skills. We emphasize that basic to all mental health work is a thorough grounding in the dynamics and techniques of individual encounter.

Since the trend in all mental health professions is a return to observing people in their own settings, it is best not to select any one criterion or special domain for one profession—psychiatrist, psychologist, or social worker. The needs are so great that professionals cannot do the job themselves and must work indirectly as consultants. Therefore, we recommend maintenance of an elite group with a rich experiential background—the people needed for supervisors and consultants.

Clinical work can best be learned in clinical settings, whether they are attached to a university or are on their own in the field. Future manpower programs should incorporate the principle of dispersal of training and built-in evaluation programs.

Clinicians should be directly involved in curriculum planning with junior colleges and community colleges—particularly in the core content of what the students learn about behavior.

Federal funding should be available for agencies which want to develop paraprofessionals; this would involve a relationship with junior colleges and community colleges regarding curriculum (official credit given) and personnel placement.

Federal subsidies should be granted for medical students to continue their work in the behavioral clinical fields; some form of encouragement should also be given for persons with a bachelor's degree trained in an assistant capacity to remain in that capacity.

Regarding standards, incentives must be developed to keep top people in supervisory and consultant posts.

The host of paraprofessional roles developing demand constant clinical supervision on many levels. The more untrained the paraprofessional the greater will be the degree of clinical sophistication needed to guide and support him.

The question of too much training vs. too little is a critical one for the paraprofessional. Evaluation programs must constantly look at these issues in order to determine the best path.

Clinicians must be intimately involved in recruitment programs which extend to high school, community college, and undergrad students of every socioeconomic level. Particular attention must be paid to recruitment programs among minority groups.

One of the Commission's major concerns has been the youngster who is so severely disturbed as to require residential care. To salvage a severely sick child who must be sent to a public residential institution, we must reverse our present indefensible order of priorities and place the greatest emphasis on vastly increased funding, so that we can recruit and hold our best-trained mental health manpower. We cannot plan intelligently for the number and kinds of manpower needed until we develop a comprehensive working model of the kinds of settings best suited for the various graduations of childhood mental illness. At the present time, the provisions of trained services seem seldom related to community needs. Frequently the child psychiatrist is located in the affluent part of the big city, and even the child guidance clinic is often located in a chosen community, usually in suburbia, where educational and income levels and psychiatric sophistication tend to be high. Regarding personnel in residential facilities, we recommend:

> Where training is part of the function of a long-term treatment setting, it is desirable to have permanent staff in senior clinical positions rather than to have trainees occupy all the direct roles with the children; thus, if a psychiatric resident is assigned as psychotherapist and ward doctor, there should also be a staff psychiatrist attached to that ward. Every effort needs to be made to limit the turnover of therapists and to maintain the stability of the child's residential experience for as long as necessary. Various methods should be utilized to fit the turnover of trainees into the needs of sick children.
>
> In the residential treatment setting, the ratio of one therapist to ten patients is potential and critical—and should not be exceeded.
>
> The long-range goal of current practice must be to develop a core of child-care staff adequately trained to perform life-space interviews as a therapeutic tool. The therapist has a vital role to play in unit life—he needs to be available as a consultant and instructor for on-the-spot handling of patient crises, so that he can perform life-space interviews while at the same time teach the child-care staff this technique.

I. MANPOWER AND TRAINING FOR REEDUCATION-TYPE SCHOOLS

The Commission has elsewhere recommended the establishment of a large number of day-care and residential centers based on an educational, rather than a strictly psychiatric, model. (See Section II-A, recommendations, pages 40–44.) Although this recommendation does give access to a large manpower pool, there will still be need for training of teacher-counselors and related personnel. To provide personnel for these special schools, to increase our national capacity for training and for research, and to prepare psychiatrists, psychologists, and social workers for their special consultative roles in such programs, the Commission recommends, with respect to training, that a special appropriation be made jointly to the National Institute of Mental Health and the United States Office of Education to make possible long-term grant support for the following purposes:

1. The establishment of reeducation training centers at several universities that have access to Re-ED schools and similar programs. These centers should provide:

a. Special continuing education institutes of approximately two months' duration for the purpose of introducing mental health and special education training program directors and staff (psychiatrists, psychologists, social workers, special educators, and others) to the concept and practices of reeducation with the expectation that these established mental health and education professionals would become qualified to set up or staff training programs for teacher-counselors and other personnel needed for Re-ED-type schools.

b. Cadre training programs of approximately nine months' duration, which will provide a thorough grounding in the principles and practices of reeducation for small preselected groups (four to eight) of center staffs who will return to their home communities to establish reeducation programs and to provide on-the-job training for the remainder of the required staff.

c. Instructional materials and other learning and teaching aids required for reeducation programs.

The Commission recommends further that funds be made available to the several reeducation training centers and to the additional training centers which would be established through the program provided for in paragraph 1a above, for the following purposes:

1. The training at the baccalaureate or junior college level of personnel to work as aides and assistants in reeducation programs.

2. The training at the master's degree level of teacher-counselors, liaison teachers, special educators, physical education and arts and craft specialists, and other personnel to provide core staff for Re-ED-type schools.

3. The training in a two-year post-baccalaureate program of experienced teacher-counselors for supervisory positions in Re-ED-type schools.

4. The training at the doctoral level in psychology, education, and related fields of personnel for instructional positions in universities, for research on the processes and outcomes of reeducation, and for admin-

istrative posts in statewide or other programs involving a number of Re-ED-type schools.

J. PARAPROFESSIONALS

To the historian of the helping professions, our present concern for the utilization of paraprofessionals must seem like a paradoxical full circle, for all the professions concerned with people started *with* concerned people who were *not* professionals. Medicine has only recently become a licensed art requiring special and extensive formal education; social work and nursing both emerged from the volunteer efforts of concerned laywomen. Clinical psychology came from the efforts of a few people seeking to put laboratory measurements to practical use in the alleviation and prevention of personal distress. In many ways the mental health professions are much newer than society's recognition of the need for their service.

From the days of the shaman who kept the secret of the fire stick to modern times, we have seen men seek to retain as exclusive property the power which comes from specialized knowledge. The guilds of the Middle Ages were not very different from their progenies of today, and from all indications their apprenticeships were no less crowded with materials irrelevant to the tasks for which they trained people than are today's professional curricula.

The gradual growth and lengthening of training programs for the helping professions, both for reasons of increased technology and knowledge and for reasons of status and control, have brought us to our present dilemma. We cannot possibly provide the urgently needed services our people require with our present supply of professionals and the present capacities of our professional schools. Nor are we likely to be able to do so in the foreseeable future.

Professionals do not have the option of shrugging their shoulders and saying "too bad." The only real options are whether the professions will take responsibility for developing new sources of help or be supplanted by groups who will.

The options—and feasibility—of developing new helping manpower have been amply demonstrated. Medical men long ago discovered that they could readily "slice off" parts of their work and rapidly teach other people to do these portions. Few patients today expect the physician to give routine injections, to run the X-ray machine, or to perform laboratory tests. These portions of his professional work have been assigned to technicians— paraprofessionals—who work under the physician's supervision. This successful model is applicable to the mental health professions as well as to general medicine. Such recent demonstration projects as the Mental Health Aides Project at Lincoln Hospital in New York and the Family Agent

Program of the Neumeyer Foundation in Los Angeles have shown us that people without specialized formal education, carefully selected for their personality traits, can be rapidly trained to take on effective responsibility in direct service to troubled people. In these projects, ongoing professional supervision and back-up ensured a high level of care, and scarce professional time was significantly amplified. Many of the burgeoning programs for paraprofessionals do not have the safeguards of careful selection and adequate supervision, and much of the potential value for service of the new paraprofessional positions has been lost in the rush to create new employment, with service quality a secondary consideration.* As we point out in Section III, if we are serious about increasing the supply of effective mental health workers, then it becomes clear to the thoughtful person that there are a number of things that we need to know about, some important research that needs to be done.

The Commission urges that particular emphasis be placed on training and employing paraprofessionals and that both training and functions be carefully determined by systematic research (see Section III on manpower research). No doubt a number of new careers will emerge from research efforts. At present we need to concentrate on the seriously limited supply of trained and professional personnel in the existing human services occupations. The severe shortages in the field of health, education, and welfare can be alleviated by increasing the training and career opportunities for such positions as teacher aides, child-care specialists, vocational training aides, home visitors, roles in mental health agencies and associations, liaison workers between services, recreational companions, and so forth. There are large groups of underemployed and unemployed persons in this country who, in all probability, might be employed and trained in significant numbers to perform necessary functions in these occupational fields. Such employment has other possible advantages: (a) neighborhood people are most apt to understand their own neighborhoods and can contribute to the vitality and relevance of a local service agency, and (b) through the employment of parents and young people in public programs there is a greater likelihood that they will acquire important new learning and identification with the goals of these programs. To accomplish these goals, we recommend†:

The development of a hierarchy of new careers and the restructuring of old ones. These careers should range from trainee positions to fully professional ones. The concept of progressive development of the

---

* Dr. Irving Lazar, written communication, May 19, 1968.

† A number of these recommendations have been drawn from a study by the Task Force on Parent Participation of the Department of Health, Education, and Welfare. For further discussion see *Parents as Partners in Department Programs for Children and Youth,* Washington, D.C., Office of the Secretary, Dept. HEW, August, 1968.

individual must be a central component of any such plan. The principle of the career ladder is crucial and calls for a structuring of job levels so that an employee may move both vertically and horizontally within public programs; that is, an employee should be able to move upward to increasingly responsible work levels and increasingly high rates of pay. He should also be able to move from one field of work to another. Wages must be adequate to meet the basic needs of the employee and to conform to the minimum wage laws and the wage scales of the organization. Supplementary assistance should be available when necessary.

Generic education and training in the field of health, education, and welfare ought to provide a base for occupational movement into various sectors of the human service family of occupations. Specific training, related to specific job techniques, can be added in specific occupational settings.

It is essential that specific jobs be planned before employees are recruited and trained.

The employee selection process requires the application of new understandings and methods. Educational requirements for any job should be carefully reexamined and lowered for all jobs for which this is possible. Many of the tests which have been used for occupational placement lack relevance and validity for the selection and placement of disadvantaged people, and there is no evidence that these tests necessarily predict job success in the paraprofessional human service occupations. We recommend such alternatives as oral tests, use of short-term job placement opportunities, rotation through a variety of work experiences so that both employee and supervisor can assess employment potential for various job functions, etc.

Counseling and assessment as to an employee's work potential and occupational opportunities are appropriate after he has been placed in a job. This should be a continuing process as part of a longer counseling program.

Recruitment and employment should be based on the interests of the potential employee and the requirements of the work to be done. It is important that persons seeking such employment have full information about new career possibilities so that they can more nearly match their interests and needs to the job. Some communities have found it useful to establish a central job center so that the employment opportunities of all the human service agencies, both public and private, may be registered in one place. This plan is helpful to the agencies and to persons seeking employment.

Provision for planned, well-supervised in-service training is essential. Group supervision, democratic and informal staff meetings, work opportunities to increase self-esteem through "quick success," and counseling are among the seemingly successful methods for in-service training for disadvantaged people. These principles suggest the need for a director of on-the-job training programs. Experience shows that such a director needs to be a flexible, informal person who is open to experimentation, keenly interested in working with paraprofessionals, and able to withstand pressure and strains.

It is necessary to coordinate the educational and job programs. This involves working closely with schools in the development of curricular materials. It is essential that poor people be paid for the time spent in in-service education as well as for in-service training.

K. FUTURE MANPOWER AND TRAINING NEEDS FOR LOCAL SERVICES AND CHILD DEVELOPMENT COUNCILS

As Child Development Councils move from the initial pilot stage to full-scale operation across the nation, the proposed goals will require an immense increase in manpower. In fact, the manpower problem is so important that it constitutes a major argument for a federal advocate agency which would be given the specific challenge to acquire the people needed for staffing both the councils and the service institutions with which the councils collaborate in ensuring service. Expert sources indicate that several categories of personnel are needed:

People from existing professional groups and especially from the newer technician levels being developed, such as those in pediatrics, psychology, etc. If social service were to be separated from payment of money in welfare programs, a great source of trained personnel would become available for retraining for new programs.

A new professional group trained in child development. These should be trained at a number of levels (BA, MA, PhD, EdD, etc.) for varying degrees and types of responsibility in the services to be obtained by the councils. These professional child workers would include:

administrators of Child Development Councils;

educationally oriented child-care specialists to supervise day-care and preschool facilities in the community;

child-parent counselors to visit homes, to demonstrate new strategies of child care in homes, and to train and supervise paraprofessional workers in home visiting.

A new paraprofessional group of child-care workers, aides, "upbringers," etc., approximately at the level of the high school graduate, who might make a life career of work with children or who might with further education move into the professional roles. A large corps of these workers is needed to serve as caretakers in various institutions and service facilities, to serve as "teacher's aides," and to serve as home visitors.

Adolescents, in large numbers, for both service and training, to work with children in various types of programs and to perform other services for the community.

Volunteers, paid and otherwise, who are employed as full-time or part-time people. These might be drawn from a number of different groups: parents; foster grandparents; college men and women; retired teachers; hobbyists; "indigenous workers"; Junior League; church groups; ex-alcoholics; rehabilitated mental patients, delinquents, and criminals who are purposefully seeking a centering point for their lives.

Contemporary American Society: Its Impact on the Mental Health of Children and Youth

Our nation must make a new and major commitment to its future—to the healthy development of its children and youth. Our greatness rests with our oncoming generations.

A nation can be of no higher quality than its people. We have reason today to be deeply anxious about the quality of our society. On all sides we see signs of breakdown: violence, rioting by the disenchanted and dispossessed, distrust and hatred between groups, voluntary exile on the part of some of our brightest and most principled young people, hunger and despair among the poor. There is a frantic race on the part of most of us, not so much toward a goal but in pursuit of escape—escape from the fear of loneliness, boredom, the physical ugliness and human misery of the blighted areas of our cities and sprawling suburbs, a desperate and dragging sense that we have permanently and irretrievably lost the American dream. We have cherished this fading dream, this noble dedication to the ancient but forever-new belief in the inherent power of each individual to grow, to learn, to create, to love and live in peace with self and fellowman.

Our nation has been founded on this belief. This has been a land dedicated to the ideals of opportunity, freedom, and justice for each child and each adult. Throughout our history, we have clung to a fundamental faith in the magnificent potentialities of all human beings, especially the potentialities of children and youth. It has become fashionable to point out that we, as a nation, have failed over and over again: that our years have been torn by violence, injustice, exploitation, oppression, and discrimination

—that poverty, inhumanity, and human failure are nothing new in our land.

Of course, all this is true; we have failed in countless ways. But we have succeeded in just as many ways. This *has* been a country in which the poor, the persecuted, the dispossessed from many lands have found an opportunity to rebuild a life for themselves and their children. This country has been a living laboratory, offering dramatic proof that there is indeed a magnificent potential for human development *if* the opportunities for this development are provided.

Today, there is a growing disbelief in the inherent goodness and potential of our people and in the society which we have created together. It is said that we have run out of solutions, that we are a sick society with an incurable disease—and the definitions of that disease are many, depending on the age, color, neighborhood, job, and bank account of the diagnostician.

It is the belief of the Joint Commission on Mental Health of Children that we, as a nation, have *not* run out of solutions, that this country does not have an incurable disease. The Commission is convinced that solutions are at hand to resolve or significantly reduce many of this nation's problems—severe though they may be. What is needed is a rededication and recommitment to the power and promise that lie within each human being for healthy growth and development.

This rededication and recommitment requires more than an effort of will and purpose. It demands an investment of knowledge, manpower, and money. It calls for a reassessment of priorities and of national goals. It requires a major investment in our children and youth and the families to which they belong and a greater emphasis on improving the human aspects of the society in which they live.

These are priorities that we as a nation can, and must, assume. We are the richest of all large nations, yet we have fallen shamefully behind most other industrial countries in our programs for children and families. Other nations far less endowed than ours with resources of all kinds have developed comprehensive programs to insure the health and well-being of their people, from birth to old age. These countries recognize and act upon what we, as a nation, have failed to comprehend: that life truly begins at conception, that the developmental potential of the individual's total life is critically and pervasively affected by the care his mother receives before he is born and by the services that are available to him and his family during the first few years of his life and thereafter. Because of the very demanding and complex nature of our society, each individual needs a wide range of services throughout the life cycle—educational, physical and mental health, and social welfare. The provision of these needed services is most crucial at the very beginning of life.

Our society has the capacity to create the most splendid life experience that man has ever known. We have conquered most of the scourges that have hounded mankind in the past—famine, flood, drought, and uncontrollable disease. We have virtually eliminated the blight of ignorance and the necessity for hard physical drudgery. We stand within sight of the summit which has represented man's aspirational dreams over the centuries: the control of nature for the health, well-being, and enlightenment of all people. And yet, within sight of this summit, we are overtaken by many perplexities and hazards. We are in danger of entrapping ourselves in an avalanche of failure.

Building Mental Health

What does all this have to do with the child's mental health? The answer is: everything. A child's mental health is dependent upon the many societies and systems which make up his life. A child's mental health depends on the functioning of his own body, the state of his physical health, the health and well-being of his family, and the kind of home, neighborhood, and community in which he lives. It depends on the medical services he receives, the schools he goes to, the church or temple and other organizations to which he belongs—or doesn't belong. It depends on the food he eats, the air he breathes, the water he drinks, and the loving (or unloving) care that he receives while he is growing up. It depends on his family's income, the kinds of parents, brothers, and sisters he has, and the work they do—or the work they cannot find. It depends on the kind of a society he lives in, on whether that society believes and acts as if children and young people are valuable and important—standing in need of tenderness, guidance, investment, and respect—or whether that society neglects, disvalues, and distrusts its young.

Mental health is not an individual trait haphazardly given to some and not to others. It is not "all in the mind." It is not a contagious disease. Nor is it a condition that parents can bestow upon their children solely through their own efforts of care and good will, or one which can be provided exclusively by treatment from such specialists as pediatricians, psychiatrists, psychologists, and social workers. A child's mental health is formed throughout his development and is influenced and determined by all that goes into his existence. His mind and body are not separate but function together and in interaction with his outer environment. He is a complex system within a series of systems. His nervous, muscular, digestive, and other inner systems interact with one another and with a host of other interrelated dynamic systems—the family, the neighborhood, the school, the religious, the recreational, the economic, the employment, and the political systems. These living, dynamic systems are unlike man-made systems, such as machines, in that they cannot be adjusted by a knowledgeable manipulation of parts, by a "turn of the screw." They cannot always be repaired by finding and treating "the cause of the problem."

A child's mental health has many causes; a child's mental illness or emotional disorder likewise has no single cause. Because the child is a complex, growing, changing system interacting with many other dynamic systems, his mental health can be promoted only by appropriate attention to him, as an individual, and to the systems to which he is related.

If we are to promote the mental health of our children and youth, to prevent mental disabilities, and to treat and care for those who suffer from these disabilities, we need to concern ourselves with all aspects of the child's care and all aspects of the social systems in which he lives.

Definition of Mental Health

Mental health is exceptionally difficult to define, partly because it is a complex state of being. The mentally healthy person is able to see and generally deal with the realities concerning himself and his world; he is able to relate to other people in ways that are satisfying both to him and to them; he is able to accept and control his impulses for sexual and aggressive expression; he is able to learn and to apply what he has learned. He has confidence in his competence. He has acquired a set of values upon which he builds his life; he has a sense of community with others and a sureness of his own identity. The mentally healthy person continues to grow throughout his lifetime, building on earlier foundations of strength and flexibility as he meets new tasks and situations.

A child grows and develops gradually into a mentally healthy adult. During this growth he is affected by what has happened to him in the past, what he is experiencing at the present, and what he hopes or fears for the future. He gradually builds his capacity for seeing and knowing what is real, for relating to other people, for controlling his feelings, for learning, for competence, for knowing and acting upon his own values, for becoming a self-confident and flexible individual. If, from the earliest years, he has been denied the opportunities to participate in decisions which affect his life and environment, he will not be prepared for mentally healthy involvement as an adult. His life will be thwarted by isolation. If he is handicapped by physical, social, educational, or economic adversities, he may become mentally ill or emotionally disturbed.

Prevention and Treatment

Individuals vary in their capacity to weather adversities; however, no child can fulfill his inborn potential unless society provides the wide range of services and opportunities that make this possible. We cannot promote the mental health of our children and youth and prevent mental and emotional disabilities simply by providing more treatment services. Important as these services are for those who are already afflicted, we will constantly fall short of our goals if we only provide treatment for the ill and disturbed.

We must press forward on many fronts. We must provide high-quality care for those with disabilities. We must build upon our knowledge that developmentally critical periods occur during rapid growth and development—especially in infancy, childhood, and adolescence—which, if not taken advantage of, or if adversely affected by physical and psychological trauma, can impede and seriously affect further growth and development throughout life. From this point, we must begin to develop and coordinate preventive services which will maximize the mental health potential of *all* children and youth. We must restructure our society so that it no longer plays such a great part in the causation and perpetration of mental health problems. These goals require a massive investment in services, organization, and coordination of these services, development of mental health and related manpower at many levels of skill, and continuing research—both basic and applied.

At present, our society is falling far short of meeting these important goals. Much has been accomplished by public and private groups, especially in the last half century and particularly in the last decade. However, much more remains to be done. To understand the nature and magnitude of this task, let us take a look at the situation of children and youth in our society today.

THE WORLD IN WHICH OUR CHILDREN AND YOUNG PEOPLE LIVE

A Society of Both Promise and Threat

Today's young people live in a world of splendid potential and of terrifying threat. There are vast opportunities for many of our children and youth, but it is a time of tremendous pressure for all of them. If they are to take advantage of these opportunities and to withstand these pressures, they must have great emotional and physical stamina. We must provide them the strengthening experiences which will enable them to humanely and productively use the abounding technology, rather than misuse it or be overwhelmed by its potentially harmful effects.

This is a time of multiple stimulation, a time when the whole world can virtually enter the living room. The impact is probably greatest on the highly impressionable minds and feelings of children. Although the communication media are potentially enriching, they may mean in effect that many of our children and young people have been everywhere by eye and ear and almost nowhere in the realities of their self-initiated experiences.

This is also the age of prepackaged "magic for the millions." The blessings of push-button ease, however, threaten to undermine the individual's sense of mastery over his environment, partly because so little is required of him in actual skill and participation. Luxuries, once the province of a tiny aristocracy, are available now to one-fourth or more of our citizens. Many of our children and youth have been surfeited with things but starved for significant interpersonal experiences. In this era of materialism, parents respond to social pressures to "buy the best" for their youngsters. They frequently become so preoccupied with earning and buying that they have little time or energy left to be with their children in a person-to-person relationship: to talk with them, listen to them, work and play with them, love and guide them.

Although our standardized mass society offers a high material level of living to about 40 percent of our population, it also threatens the individual's sense of unique significance. Fathers—and frequently mothers—are likely to work in huge organizations where they may be identified mostly by their Social Security numbers; college students are often recognized most readily by their IBM identifications; even young children may be virtually unknown as individuals as they attend huge schools and mass recreation programs.

Our massive, impersonal, complex technological society presents not only psychological but also physical dangers. In many metropolitan areas, youngsters cannot explore or adventure safely on their own. This situation makes it difficult for boys and girls to develop a sense of independence and self-responsibility. It has become so necessary to protect children and young people from dangers that, for many of them, life becomes a packaged tour, seen as through a plastic bag.

The Rush of Social Change

In a relatively few years we have changed from a predominantly rural society to a complex, interdependent urban one in which much of our highly individualistic, do-it-yourself tradition is no longer very appropriate. All of our customs and values are in a state of upheaval associated with the tremendous velocity of technical change. We are hurtling through history, and in the course of this rush, old values are being reexamined and new ones are being sought. This may be particularly upsetting for children and young people who have yet to find the principles upon which they can base their lives.

Separate Worlds

We are rapidly becoming a separatist society. We have lost our former sense of community and the experience of diverse peoples living close to one another and working in the pursuit of common interests and goals. Our people have come to live in many separate worlds—rural versus urban, metropolis versus suburb. A sense of polarization exists between the more affluent and the disadvantaged. Rural unemployment and poverty has driven millions into urban areas, swelling our city slums with poorly educated, unskilled, and semiskilled workers whose urban circumstance is often as critical as was their rural dilemma. The majority are low-income, minority groups who tend to have large families.

The plight of the cities has led to the exodus of upper-income families to the suburbs. Only a sprinkling remain—a few persons of wealth, some single individuals, and families who are middle-aged or older. High land costs and taxes hasten a parallel migration of industry, which reduces the tax bases of the cities. Industrial relocation increases the problem of already inadequate mass transportation for low-income city dwellers. Thus, our urban poor become more and more trapped within the depressed areas of our cities. To a growing extent, the only children living in central cities are the children of poverty and/or discrimination. These children, like those in our rural slums, experience the multiple disadvantages of overcrowding, poor services, deteriorated housing, and encapsulation in a society of frustration and defeat. They and their parents are shut off from the "good life" except through the distorted images wafted to them through the mass media.

The outer reaches of the metropolitan districts sprawl with unplanned suburbs—the separate world of the more privileged, stable working class and middle-class families, the majority of whom are white. The insular and standardized nature of many suburban neighborhoods is well recognized. Suburban children tend to grow up knowing only persons like themselves, unaware of the many social classes and races outside suburbia. The suburbs tend to have a centrifugal effect on families, with fathers being preoccupied with the downtown job and mothers becoming "organization moms" as they are consumed by the complex organizational life of the suburban community. Suburban children and adolescents are apt to be following age-specific mazes of their own through the school, special lessons, and organized activity complexes.

"He Who Has, Gets"

This is a society which rewards the high achiever and the socially adept. These rewards usually go to children and young people who have been fortunate enough to be born into more privileged families and/or communities where life experiences are enriching and services are of high quality. Today's race is to those with quick minds rather than strong backs. Advantages accrue to those who are facile and flexible, to those with strong verbal skills, and to those who are highly trained and adaptable technicians. The ability to adjust readily and smoothly to the group is becoming an increasingly valuable asset as the large organization grows more dominant. All the while, the gulf seems to grow steadily wider between the advantaged who can generally make it and the disadvantaged who frequently cannot. As this gap widens, more and more disadvantaged children simply accept the reality that their chances for "making it" are slim. They see little value in education. Their developing sense of futility is strengthened by schools that seemingly see little value in helping them. Out of this sense of hopelessness and frustration come higher rates of nonlearning and delinquency.

Never before has the individual amounted to both so much and so little. Even though mass destruction is possible, we still hold, albeit feebly and ambivalently, to the ideal of the extreme importance of the individual. If the individual is in some special trouble which is well publicized by the mass media, virtually the whole nation may be stirred to rush to his aid, especially if this help requires little personal sacrifice or direct person-to-person interaction. On the other hand, we have learned to live, with relative calm, in an age in which increasingly powerful weapons can destroy thousands of people, merely by pushing a button.

Problem Versus People

We tend to be a pragmatic people who want to know how much programs cost in dollars and cents. We like to attack one problem at a time, especially if it doesn't cost too much. Whatever it costs, we want to know exactly what measurable benefits we are getting for our money. This pragmatic, problem-specific, measurement approach has played into an emphasis on social programs that are overly specific and tied to particular identifiable human problems. This has brought about a proliferation of separate pieces of legislation and a burgeoning of programs which are becoming more and more chaotic at the community and individual level. The programs are often confusing, disjointed, and short-lived, and many of them fail to meet the needs of those whose problems are most acute. Specific services—both public and private—have proliferated partly because we would like to think that relatively simple, one-factor, short-term, inexpensive remedies will solve human problems. This thinking overlooks the fact that human behavior—including mental health—is a product of the long-term, continuous interaction of a multiplicity of factors within the person, his family, and the community. It also overlooks the fact that healthy human growth and development cannot be promoted unless all of its aspects are recognized and treated simultaneously in a coordinated way throughout the life-span, but particularly in the very early years of life.

Future Trends

The enormous baby boom that took place between 1948 and 1958 has endowed us with a large youth population. Even if the birth rate goes down and these young people have only two children per couple, our population will still reach alarming proportions in the future (Campbell, 1968).

It is probable that our nation will become increasingly urbanized as agriculture becomes more highly mechanized and there are fewer and fewer employment opportunities on the farms. No doubt our society will become even more complex and offer even more choices and temptations than it does at present. It is also likely to become more highly technological. Longer and longer periods of education will be required to prepare for specialized jobs which will be available mostly in large organizational settings. Reeducation and retraining in vocational fields may be necessary a number of times over the life cycle so that people can remain employable.

The families of tomorrow are likely to be smaller. They will probably tend to live in large, multiple dwelling units, partly because of dwindling space for private homes. More and more wives and mothers will go to work. This will bring about an even greater crisis in the need for child-care facilities—services which at present are alarmingly inadequate.

The future promises increasing leisure time for many members of the population; however, those who are in the specialized scientific and professional fields may work harder than they ever have before. There will be an accelerated trend toward a consumer economy and a high demand for personal services.

It is probable that the future will bring with it an increasing lack of differentiation in the sex roles of males and females. New patterns of relationships are already emerging between the sexes, bringing anxiety and confusion to males and females alike. Out of this current upheaval may come greater freedom and honesty in this important area.

There are other, more critical problems which face us all and which are likely to be with us in the next generation. These include the issues of war and peace; of racial conflict and the myriad disadvantages that our society has heaped upon ethnic minority groups; the crisis of our urban centers; and the violence, hostility, and negativism which have swept over our society.

These issues and the total nature of our society require high levels of individual psychological and physical strength. Perhaps more than ever our society demands of the individual a sturdy sense of self-confidence and self-respect, an ability to withstand numerous temptations, steady impulse control, a well-developed intelligence and capacity for continuous learning, and a healthy body free of handicapping conditions. Perhaps it is unrealistic to expect any society to assure all of these attributes to all of its children and young people, but certainly our nation can do a far better job in this respect than it has done in the past or is doing at present.

CHILDREN AND YOUTH: A POSITIVE SOCIAL RESOURCE

A Profile of Our Young Population

One of our country's greatest assets is its very large population of children and youth. Although it has been customary to think of adulthood as beginning at age nineteen, society today often demands long periods of educational and vocational preparation for the full shouldering of adult responsibilities. Moreover, there is an increasing body of evidence that human beings do not actually complete their physical, social, and psychological development toward adult status until they are twenty-four or so. For these reasons, the Commission believes it is important to include young people up to age twenty-five in developing programs of positive mental health for children and youth.

A national program designed to promote positive mental health for all our citizens is most likely to succeed if emphasis is placed on providing coordinated health, education, social, and vocational services (combined with research and training) for our young. Such a program must start prior to an individual's conception and continue through the young person's twenty-fourth year. Of course, this does not mean that services are discontinued after that time. The great majority of today's youth will found families of their own. Their well-being as parents will be critical to the healthy development of *their* children. In fact, about half of today's youth will become parents before they reach age twenty-four, as will be discussed in the next chapter.

Number of Young People by Age Groups

In July, 1967, the U.S. Bureau of the Census reported that there were more than 93,000,000 young people in this country under age twenty-five (more by now, of course). This is well over twice as many young people as we had in 1950. The accompanying chart shows how the youth population was divided by age groups in 1967.

About 85 percent of these young people are white. Children and young people—like the rest of our population—tend to live in urbanized, densely populated areas of the country. At present, well over two-thirds of whites live in areas that are classified as urban. This includes small cities as well as many of the suburban and exurban areas. Most minority groups fit into a similar pattern. More than two-thirds of both blacks and Spanish-speak-

Fig. 1.—Children and Youth in the United States
by Age Groups, 1967

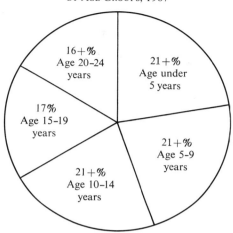

ing Americans live in urban areas. The most urbanized of all ethnic groups are Chinese and Japanese youth, 90 percent of whom were living in cities in 1960. Only one-fourth of American Indians, however, live in urban areas. American Indians, like families of migrant workers, tend to cling to rural areas (U.S. Dept. of Agriculture, 1967).

As shown in the map on page 148, large numbers of young people live in certain far Western states, such as California, and in the highly industrialized sections of the Midwest and Eastern coast. These areas, as well as others shown on the map, are experiencing great increases in the number of persons under twenty-five. In part, these increases are due to the fact that older youth have been migrating to cities in search of greater opportunities at a steadily growing rate. As a result, farms and small villages tend to be disproportionately populated with children, young adolescents, and older people. This trend shows every indication of continuing, unless some means is found to counter the complex of serious problems which beset our rural areas. The mechanization of agriculture and mining and the resulting reduction of employment opportunities, particularly for unskilled or semiskilled labor, offer little hope to the rural youth. The general lack of quality education and health and social services also plays a part in the migration of young people to the cities.

Poverty and Family Income

The paradox of extensive and continuing poverty in a nation as wealthy as the United States has been widely publicized in the past few years. (Details concerning this matter will be discussed in some depth in Chapters IV and V.) Currently about one-fourth, or *19,000,000,* of our children

Fig. 2. — Estimated Population Age 0 to 24 by State in 1965 and Percent Change Since 1950
(Population Shown in Thousands)

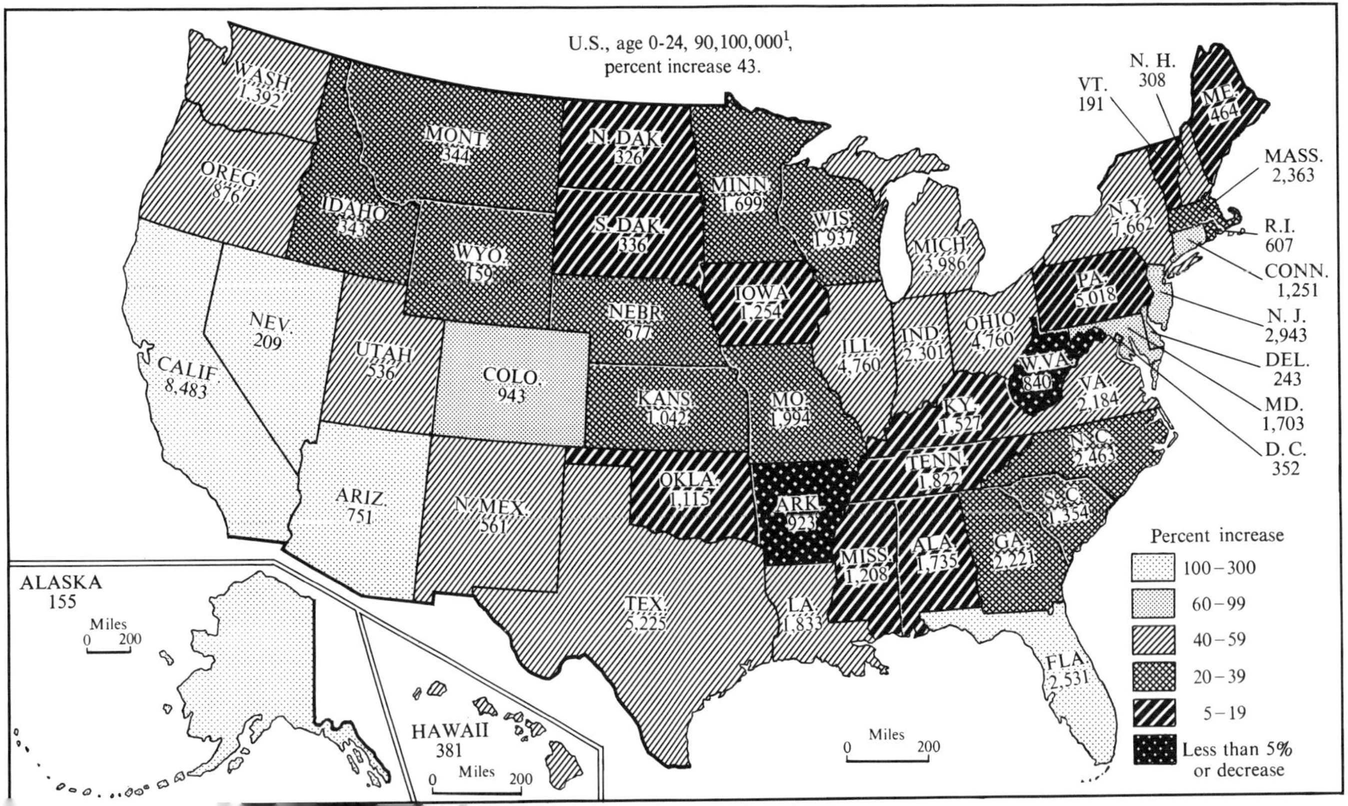

U.S., age 0-24, 90,100,000[1],
percent increase 43.

Percent increase

100–300
60–99
40–59
20–39
5–19
Less than 5%
or decrease

Miles
0   200

MASS. 2,363
R.I. 607
CONN. 1,251
N.J. 2,943
DEL. 243
MD. 1,703
D.C. 352

N. H. 308
VT. 191

N.Y. 4,601
PA. 5,018

OHIO 4,169
IND. 2,301
ILL. 4,106
MICH. 3,598
WIS. 1,637

VA. 2,184
N.C. 2,169
S.C. 1,354
GA. 2,221
FLA. 2,531
TENN. 1,822
ALA. 1,733
MISS. 1,208
KY. 1,357
W.VA.

MINN. 1,699
IOWA 1,255
MO. 1,954
ARK. 975
LA. 1,831

N.DAK. 326
S.DAK. 336
NEBR. 617
KANS. 1,042
OKLA. 1,115
TEX. 5,225

MONT. 342
WYO. 159
COLO. 943
N.MEX. 561
UTAH 536
ARIZ. 751
IDAHO 341

WASH. 1,392
OREG. 876
NEV. 209
CALIF. 8,483

ALASKA 155
Miles 0 200

HAWAII 381
Miles 0 200

under age eighteen are living in or near poverty, as measured by the Social Security Index.

Poverty means that millions of children are at high risk in health and mental health. It means hunger and malnutrition which may cripple intellectual and physical development and undermine a child's belief in his parents and the world in which he lives. It means a crowded, meager home which can offer little to overcome the child's increasingly reduced potentialities. It means life in a neighborhood which probably offers little opportunity for healthy play, privacy, or safety but many opportunities for danger, brutality, and exposure to deviant behavior. It means a stunting of hopes and prospects, a feeling of exclusion and rejection, a sense of rage at injustice, or surrender to defeat. It too often means that the child receives little or no medical and dental services, that he attends schools of inferior quality, that his life prospects are constricted and darkened even before life is barely begun. The wonder is not that so many of the poor continue to have critical mental health and related problems throughout their lives but that they manage to do as well as they do and complain so little, especially when they are continuously exposed to the rich and exotic life patterns that are advertised as being "the American way."

Many Kinds of Young People

There is a tendency to speak of children and/or youth as being a monolithic whole. We speak of "the youth culture," "what youth wants," or "the youth problem." Our children and young people, like their elders, are highly various. They vary in age, race, and the region in which they live. They differ in national background, religion, and the language they speak. Because each person differs from all others in terms of his heredity (except for identical twins) and his life experiences, each child, adolescent, and young person is specifically and uniquely himself. But because he belongs to a social group, he also reflects in his own special way the group to which he belongs. Thus, services and programs, to be truly successful, must be designed with due regard both for group and for individual characteristics.

Our rapidly growing and mobile youth population has strained our established resources: the schools, medical services, housing, transportation, and all the rest. We have tended to emphasize these strains and to casually ignore the potential wealth that young people bring to a society. We tend to fear the rebellious ways of youth, forgetting that these young people have much to offer our society with their idealism, their search for significance and commitment, their energy, and their capacity for change. Even at a very young age, children show great flexibility and a great drive to grow and learn. Both for the sake of our children and youth and for the sake of our society, we need to provide them and their parents a climate in which each individual can grow and in which each can enhance his own life and contribute to the needs of the larger community.

Emotional and Mental Disorders

Research shows that 10 to 12 percent of children and youth have major psychological problems. According to the best available estimates, 2 to 3 percent suffer from mental illness, including psychosis. Another 8 to 10 percent have serious emotional disabilities. Data derived largely from teachers' assessments of maladjustment in elementary school children indicate that about 10 percent are identified by teachers as having behavior problems that are serious enough to require clinical attention. Considerable agreement is noted between teachers' ratings of maladjustment in children and clinicians' and parents' assessments. Only about 4 percent of elementary school children are referred to clinical facilities or would be referred if facilities were available (Glidewell and Swallow, 1968).

As can be seen from the above figures, large numbers of our children are in need of professional attention, yet it is estimated that facilities exist for only about 7 percent of the child and youth population who need them (*Report of Task Force V*, 1968). Moreover, we have a severe shortage of mental health manpower as well as facilities. This situation will become even more critical in the future, with the growth of our child and youth population and the demands and pressures placed on them by society. (See also Chapter VI, "Emotionally Disturbed and Mentally Ill Children and Youth.")

Educational Problems

A larger proportion of young people are graduating from high school than was true in the past. However, as shown in Figure 3 below, about a fourth still fail to graduate. The dropout rates are far higher for poor children and for those who are members of disadvantaged minority groups.

Although national data are not yet available, reports from various localities indicate that perhaps the majority of seriously disadvantaged children fail to learn to read at more than the fourth- or fifth-grade level. The crisis in many of our inner-city schools has been widely publicized. Many of our rural schools are also inadequate. The fact that so many of our children do not attain essential basic and higher-level skills condemns them to a future of total or semi-exclusion from many facets of society: as workers, consumers, citizens, and family members. The causes of these problems are multiple and reflect not only on the schools but on the

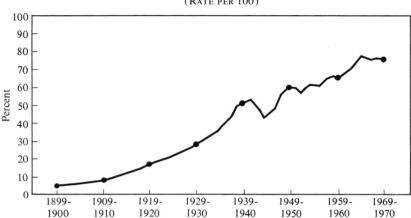

FIG. 3.—PERCENTAGE OF THE POPULATION 17 YEARS OF AGE
GRADUATED FROM HIGH SCHOOL, 1899–1900 TO 1966–67
(RATE PER 100)

crippling conditions that society has imposed upon many of these young-sters from the time of their conception onward.

Delinquency

The officially recorded delinquency and youth crime rates have shown an alarming increase in the past ten years, particularly in our inner-city slums and especially in those which have become racial ghettos. The rise is due, in part, to the increase in the youth population, to better police reporting of crime, and perhaps to the arrest and adjudication procedures of the authorities (see Fig. 4). Whatever the true incidence, delinquency *is* a serious problem—both for the youth involved and for society.

FIG. 4.—POLICE ARRESTS OF JUVENILES,
JUVENILE COURT DELINQUENCY CASES
(EXCLUDING TRAFFIC), AND CHILD POPULATION, 1940–1966

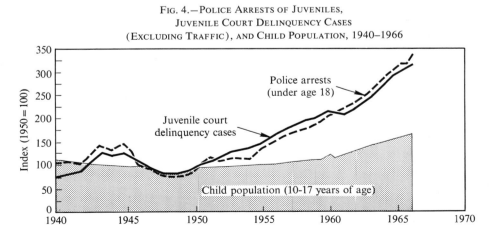

It cannot be said with certainty that juvenile delinquency is always caused by poor mental health; however, many delinquents do suffer from mental and emotional disorders which require treatment. Many who were born and raised in poverty have been denied the opportunity to achieve their full developmental potential or to participate in legitimate activities in our society. Many, if not most, represent the problems of a nation that has become disorganized and lacking in humane concerns. Treatment programs for delinquents are shamefully deficient. The great majority of institutions for delinquents provide few, if any, services that are rehabilitative in nature. These are the young people whom we punish for the deficits of society and the adult world; our failure to help them is revealed by the fact that more than half who are committed to institutions are recommitted in later years (*Report of Task Force VI,* 1968). (See also Chapter VIII, "Adolescents and Youth.")

Medical Care: Failure to Serve a People

Increased facilities and manpower are needed to meet the physical and mental health needs of the American population in general. The need is particularly acute for those in low-income families. There are innumerable examples of the serious lacks in adequate medical care for poor children and youth. For instance, about one-fourth of the babies born each year in the United States are born to women who get little or no medical care during their pregnancy or who receive inadequate obstetrical care at delivery. This lack of medical care is highly related to defects and injuries to the child that occur during pregnancy or at birth. Such damage may seriously affect all aspects of the child's development, including his capacity to learn (*Report of Task Force I,* 1968).

The deficiencies in our medical services also take a toll in infant lives. The perinatal death rates of children born in poverty areas are about 50 percent higher than is the average for the country. Overall, the United States has one of the highest infant death rates of any of the industrialized nations.

Illegitimacy

In 1967 more than 300,000 illegitimate babies were born in the United States. They constituted almost 10 percent of all babies born, one-fourth of those born to girls between the ages of fifteen and nineteen years, and almost one-fifth of those born to young women between the ages of twenty and twenty-four (U.S. Dept. of Health, Education, and Welfare, 1968). There is great concern about the high rates of teen-age illegitimacy. Actually, these rates rose rather markedly between 1948 and 1958, along with the general rise in the birth rate. Since that time they have tended to level off. The present annual rate per the total population of girls between the ages of fifteen and nineteen is between 2 and 3 percent; rates for women over the age of twenty are somewhat higher.

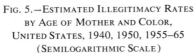

Fig. 5.—Estimated Illegitimacy Rates
by Age of Mother and Color,
United States, 1940, 1950, 1955–65
(Semilogarithmic Scale)

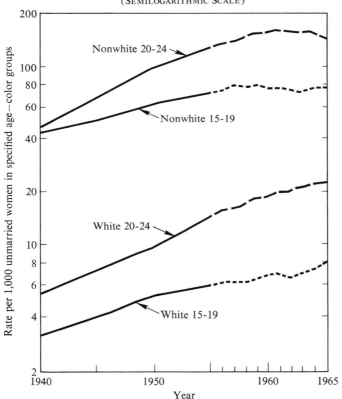

However, illegitimacy is still a serious problem, partly because of the large numbers of girls and babies involved. Although the annual rates of illegitimacy are not markedly high, the ratios of illegitimate to legitimate births is disturbing indeed. For a number of complex reasons, illegitimacy is closely linked to poverty. Moreover, unmarried mothers and babies, especially those who dwell in poverty, are less likely than others to obtain high-quality medical services. It is estimated that perhaps one-fourth of the babies in the poverty enclaves of our central cities are born out of wedlock. Unless we provide coordinated social, medical, educational, and related services to these mothers and their babies, we shall more than perpetuate the poverty and poor health that are so frequently at the root of this problem. Along these lines, there is evidence that the higher rates for non-white illegitimate births are almost entirely the result of poverty rather than race (see Fig. 5).

Premarital pregnancy often leads to an early and forced marriage. Some estimate that nearly half of the marriages in this country occur after the girl is pregnant. Statistics show that early marriages, especially when complicated by early pregnancy, have a much lower rate of success than do later marriages and later births of the first child (Glick, 1964; Freedman and Combs, 1967). One reason for these findings may be that early marriages and early pregnancies occur more frequently at lower socio-economic levels where there are multiple pressures against the success of marriage.

Venereal Disease

Venereal disease rates have risen considerably in the past ten years or so among our youth, particularly among those in low-income groups. The incidence of syphilis in the population rose from .2 cases per 100,000 individuals to 11 between 1956 and 1966. During this same time period, the rates for adolescents rose from 10 to 22, while those for the twenty-to-twenty-four-year-old group climbed from 18 to 47. Rates were *far* higher for gonorrhea, although the overall increase was relatively unchanged for fifteen-to-nineteen-year-olds (415 per 100,000 in 1956; 436 in 1966). A greater increase in incidence of gonorrhea occurred among the twenty-to-twenty-four-year age group (781 in 1956; 994 ten years later) (U.S. Dept. of Health, Education, and Welfare, 1967). Clearly, we must make a greater effort to educate our young people in this important area.

Youth Unemployment

Youth unemployment continues to be a grave problem, especially among our disadvantaged and nonwhite youth. This has serious implications for mental health, as will be noted in Chapter X. Although the situation has improved slightly since 1962, rates continue to be distressingly high (Fig. 6).

Adolescence: A Time of Crisis?

With the onset of adolescence there seems to be a rise in the severity and rate of problems. For instance, available evidence indicates that diagnosed mental illness increases at this time, as does delinquency. This trend is also found for attendance at psychiatric clinics and placement in treatment centers and mental hospitals (*Reports of Task Forces III and V,* 1968).* There are a number of reasons why problems appear to increase during the adolescent period. Among the reasons is the fact that higher standards are held for adolescents than for younger children, and their deviant behavior is regarded as being more serious. Their problems are considered more severe because they are capable of getting into greater difficulty and the consequences of their acts tend to be more serious. Parents tend to become increasingly alarmed about the characteristics of their adolescents as they are forced to recognize more and more that their sons and daughters are not going to "simply outgrow" certain difficulties.

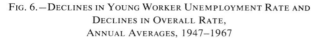

FIG. 6.—DECLINES IN YOUNG WORKER UNEMPLOYMENT RATE AND
DECLINES IN OVERALL RATE,
ANNUAL AVERAGES, 1947–1967

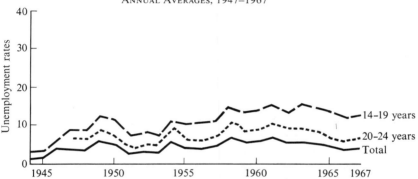

There are differences of opinion among the behavioral and social scientists as to whether deep psychological upheavals are inherent in adolescence. Whether or not these upheavals are manifested seems to depend, at least in part, on the society in which young people live and the prohibitions and expectations of that society. American youngsters, particularly those in urban and suburban areas, seemingly encounter many more pressures as they reach adolescence than do young people in simpler agrarian societies. The task of adolescents in our society includes coping with a growing reality of the modern world and its problems. Our adolescents face increasing achievement pressures for educational accomplishments; the imperatives and difficulties of "getting into college," the shifts in sex behavior and values, and the stresses of the draft. The tragedies and violence that have occurred in this country over the past five or six years certainly must have left a deep impact. Many young people have lost their

* Determination of rates of mental illness and emotional disturbance is a complex topic. See Chapter IV, "Poverty and Mental Health," and Chapter VI, "Emotionally Disturbed and Mentally Ill Children and Youth."

heroes through the assassinations of the Kennedy brothers and Martin Luther King.

Most of our young people are far better educated than their parents' generation. Most are more sophisticated and more urbane than their parents were.They are a different group, with no memories of a Depression but an uneasy feeling that society thinks there are too many of them. We have much to gain from a partnership with youth. Our country needs their re-vitalization and optimistic hopefulness. Young people are able to infuse our society with much-needed qualities of trust rather than distrust, and active hope rather than defensive fear. The problems and promise of our adolescents and youth are discussed further in Chapter VIII.

SUBGROUPS: SPECIAL PROBLEMS AND SPECIAL PRIVILEGES

Up and Down the Socioeconomic Ladder

This is a country of many social classes. However, upward movement from one social and economic level to another is still quite possible, espe-cially if one moves one rung at a time, and particularly if one is white and does not begin at the bottom of the socioeconomic heap.

Broadly speaking, this ladder may be conceptualized as having three upper-class rungs, three rungs in the middle class, and three in the lower class. Class position is generally determined by the father's education and occupation and the family's income.* The attitudes, values, and behavior of children and young people are importantly affected by the socioeconomic level, or social class, to which the parents belong—and to which they and/or their parents aspire. The effect of class membership is related both to the cultural patterns generally held by the various social classes and to the social and economic situations in which they live. Of course wide variations in individual behavior and personality occur *within* social classes because each individual is uniquely himself as well as a member of a certain cultural group.

Upper-class Groups

Relatively little is known of the society in which upper-upper-class youths live. This is a relatively small class, involving only about 2 percent of the population. It tends to be an exclusive and closely guarded private world which gives little encouragement to the would-be scientific investiga-tor. It is a society in which emphasis is placed on inherited money which

* This matter of social class, its determinants, and its characteristics is a specialized, complex subject. A detailed presentation is far beyond the scope of this chapter. For further references see, for example, Cavan, 1964; Hollingshead and Redlich, 1958; Rainwater and Weinstein, 1960; O. Lewis, 1961; Komarovsky, 1964; Sewell and Haller, 1959.

has been in the family for a number of generations, on family name and prestige, on marrying within one's own social class, on education in private schools, and on an acquisition of the "social graces" (Cavan, 1964).

The middle-upper and lower-upper social classes involve about 8 percent of our youth. These classes are somewhat better known to social scientists, although neither group has received very much research attention. Members of these groups (especially the lower upper) may be recent arrivals from the middle class or, in rare instances, the working class. A major passport to this place on the ladder is advanced education beyond college graduation and outstanding achievement in a profession, especially the more prestigeful professions such as medicine or law. Another route to this relatively lofty position is via high-level achievement at major executive levels in industry, business, or finance.

Membership in these upper classes is a goal for many middle-class families who are likely to push both themselves and their children for the achievements and social contacts that may make this possible. Because the growing population and expanding economy of recent years has particularly benefited those near the top of the ladder, further upward movement has become possible for more people. The results of this upward climb have been mixed. Mobility has brought gratifying rewards in financial and status terms; however, it has also created severe strains in the climbers and their families. Some of our most vocal, critical, and rebellious youth come from families of the middle-upper and lower-upper classes. These young people have generally had "all the advantages" of life in the more exclusive suburbs or exurbs—cars of their own, private schools and camps, excellent health care, and plenty of spending money. But many of them feel that their parents are more interested in their own social and occupational lives than in their children. Of course, these comments do not apply to all, or perhaps even most, of the families in the lower-upper and middle-upper classes. On the positive side of this picture, available data suggest that children in these classes tend to achieve exceptionally well in schools, to move into the high-level occupations, to provide community leadership, and to have low rates of family breakdown (as revealed by divorce, separation, and out-of-wedlock birth statistics) (Glick, 1964). Such seemingly positive outcomes are associated, to an unknown extent, with the many social and economic supports and the medical, educational, recreational, and other special services available to these relatively affluent children and youth.

The Great Middle Class

Middle-class families have been studied more intensively than those in the higher social classes, probably because there are greater numbers of them and because they are more readily available for study. However, there is no available research on any social class group which is based on national samples or which pays sufficient attention to regional, ethnic, and religious differences within social class groups. The middle class has long been the dominant group in the United States. Until fairly recently, it was mostly a white Protestant group of Anglo-Saxon origins. Increasingly, primarily through the processes of education, acculturation, changing occupational structures, and a growing economy, the middle class has come to include members of a wide diversity of national, ethnic, and religious groups.

The upper-middle class mainly consists of successful members of the somewhat less prestigeful professions, middle-management personnel, and the like. Most are college graduates or the equivalent and many have postgraduate degrees. A good proportion come from lower-middle-class or middle-middle-class origins, and some have climbed upward from the working class. Advancement has been attained largely through higher education. Perhaps the majority cherish ambitions to move up to the next socioeconomic level.

Those who are in the middle-middle class may also be college graduates and most have at least finished high school. Although somewhat lower in occupational status than the upper-middle class, they have achieved at higher levels than the white-collar clerical workers, salesmen, and the like who generally belong to the lower-middle class.

As noted, most of these various middle-class groups live in suburbs, where both the advantages and the disadvantages of this environment affect them in positive as well as negative ways.

Middle-class parents tend to stress such virtues as educational achievement, impulse control, social adaptability, independence, and a verbal rather than a physical action style. These parents are inclined to be self-conscious about rearing their children well and try to take a rational approach to child-rearing (Cavan, 1964). They read books on the subject, attend classes, and seek the help of counselors. Motherhood often becomes a semiprofession. It is frequently regarded by mothers with considerable anxiety, especially when they find that their emotional needs and those of their children and husbands come into conflict with rational approaches to child-rearing. Compared to working-class and lower-lower-class families, middle-class parents tend to be more democratic in their child-rearing behaviors. They are likely to regard each child as an individual, with his own timetable of development. They generally value close, loving relationships and open communication within the family, even though the demands of the larger society and their own limitations may make such relationships difficult. Parents find this ideal relationship particularly strained by potentially conflicting values, such as those of achievement and social acceptability for themselves and their children.

So-called "middle-class anxiety" has been noted frequently. This anxiety is related most closely to striving for further advancement up the social class ladder and a concomitant fear of moving downward. Parents often set unrealistic achievement goals for themselves and their children. Each mark of economic, educational, and occupational success is likely to be exhibited with pride and each indication of failure to be hidden and worried about. This achievement orientation is thought to lead to particularly high rates of anxious, fearful behavior among those middle-class children who, for one reason or another, cannot come up to parental expectations. On the other hand, there is evidence that stimulus for achievement plus moderate associated anxiety is related to effective learning. Thus, for middle-class children who are able to meet parental goals, moderate pressure from home and school may be helpful.

It may be that middle-class families are affected most by the current upheaval in values. This class has traditionally cherished such traits as individualism, exclusiveness, and conformity, and to a great extent our society has been fashioned by the middle-class value system. In our mass, urban, impersonal, consumer-oriented society, these and some other middle-class values do not appear to be as operationally successful as they were previously. Middle-class parents, as well as their children, are in a state of confusion as to what kind of behavior is acceptable and "moral" in the new world which is erupting about them. This confusion may be one important factor in the apparently increasing rates of delinquency and other kinds of deviant behavior (such as use of alcohol and drugs) among middle-class children and youth.

Of course, middle-class youngsters generally enjoy at least moderate economic security, and most of them live in areas where the educational and health services are fairly adequate. Their predominantly suburban existence, for all of its drawbacks, usually provides them with many enriching developmental experiences. In spite of the various stresses that society and middle-class membership impose upon them, most middle-class children (particularly those of the middle and upper-middle class) would seem to be getting along fairly well. However, there is little doubt that much carefully hidden misery and emotional distress affects large numbers of these families.

Lower-class Subgroups

Lower-class socioeconomic groups have received a great deal of research attention in the past ten years or so, but there is still considerable misinformation and confusion about their cultural patterns and situation. Perhaps the greatest fallacy is to link the various groups together and dub them all "working class" or "blue collar." As a matter of fact, the so-called upper-lower-class group, who are members of the skilled and stable working class, are far more like the middle class in their goals and aspirations than they are like the severely disadvantaged chronically poor who comprise the lower-lower socioeconomic group (Herzog, 1963). Particularly in the past few decades, this skilled group of workers has moved up rapidly in income and job security. Their earnings frequently outstrip those of middle-class white-collar workers. Thus, working-class members have also made the move to the suburbs and the "nicer things of life." Parents in this group are eager for their children to join the "solid middle class." This aspiration leads them to stress conformity, neatness, self-control, respectability, security, deference, and obedience. They tend to be more authoritarian than most middle-class parents and less tolerant of individual differences among their children (Kohn, 1959; Gans, 1962).

Some social scientists see today's relatively prosperous working-class families as being in a particularly complex and perplexing situation. Many have middle-class incomes but have not yet acquired all the cultural patterns of the middle class. This conflicting situation frequently leads to feelings of resentment and envy toward white-collar and professional workers. The stable working class is also particularly antagonistic toward lower socioeconomic groups, partly because they are most apt to feel the pressures from those immediately beneath them and partly because, having managed to rise to a higher place in society themselves, they fail to recognize the lack of opportunities for others to do likewise. Members of this class tend to have little sympathy for the rising aspirations and demands of ethnic minority and poverty group members.

These stable working-class families are also less likely to be equalitarian than those in the middle class in their attitudes toward the sex roles of men and women (Komarovsky, 1964). The sexes tend to live in two separate worlds with relatively few shared interests and little open communication. The concept of companionship in marriage has little meaning. Wives generally see their main function as that of homemaker and mother. If they take jobs outside the home, and many of them do, the motivation is usually economic rather than a means of self-expression. Family breakdown is more likely to occur than in the higher socioeconomic groups but is not nearly so common as it is for semiskilled workers and their families (middle-lower class) or for the lower-lower class of unskilled, chronically poor families (Glick, 1964).

Semiskilled workers are apt to live near the poverty line. They may move in and out of the work force and have relatively little job security. Although less stably organized than the skilled working class, they still have a greater tendency to escape from the attitudes of extreme despair so frequently found among the very poor of the lower-lower class.

Families in Poverty

Families classified as being lower-lower class make up the largest sector of the "poverty population." They tend to adopt life styles which grow out of the poverty situation itself. These life styles are often referred to as "the culture of poverty." However, it is far more appropriate to talk about the cultures of the very poor, because this group represents many ethnic, regional, and national groups and reflects a variety of life styles. It is also more accurate to speak of *sub*cultures, since very poor people— like others—generally aspire to such goals as good jobs, advanced education, a happy marriage, a home of their own, and the material advantages that many of our people enjoy. Because of the poverty situation itself, very poor people are forced to change and adapt these goals to the realities of the deprivation in which they live (Chilman, 1966; Rodman, 1965).

Escape from Poverty and Institutional Change

It is fallacious to assume that all lower-lower-class people can be neatly pegged into the so-called subcultures of poverty. However, the research that is available indicates that the very poor, more than others, tend to hold such attitudes as fatalism, apathy, rigidity, alienation from society, antiscientism, a physical action style, lack of long-range commitment to middle-class goals, and authoritarian attitudes.

These patterns, together with others, tend to lower the capacity of very poor people to escape from poverty (Miller and Reissman, 1961; Chilman, 1966; Pavenstedt, 1965; Minuchin *et al.,* 1967). Moreover, the rejecting attitudes of other social classes toward the poverty group serve to reinforce low-income styles. All of the attitudes and patterns which grow out of poverty tend to interact with the effects of poverty to prevent upward mobility. For instance, very poor people have the highest rates of poor health, educational and vocational failure, delinquency, and mental retardation. However, they also have less access to the services which they in particular so desperately need: mental and physical health services, child care, education, and vocational, legal, and emergency aids. If we are to aid our disadvantaged young, it will not be sufficient, as Miller and Rein (1964) note, simply to provide our *"institutions of failure* with more funds—to continue doing what they have always done in the past. *It is necessary to change social institutions so that they are more effectively responsive to the needs of the poor . . ."* italics in the original).

THE CHALLENGE

This recognition of the failure of our institutions to serve not only the poor but *all* our children and youth led to the Commission's recommendations for an advocacy system and our proposals for the creation of a network of coordinated child-oriented services, and additional facilities and manpower.

We have the riches and technology to accomplish these goals. Our greatest challenge is that of humanizing our technologically advanced society. To this end, we must commit ourselves to an investment in all our young people, their families, and the communities in which they live. We must turn from impersonality to personal concern, from fear to positive action, from distrust to trust, from separatism to cooperation, from dismay to belief in human potential, and from hostility to love and compassion. We must create new values which are closely tied to the emerging knowledge relevant to our postindustrial society, a society that offers so much if we can but commit ourselves to an enlightened investment in the well-being of our children and youth. Their mental health should stand as our highest national priority.

SUMMARY

Our men can walk on the moon. Our children and youth must be able to walk with equal pride in our land. Opportunities to develop all possible human potentials for all children are essential in these times of vast complexities, pressures, and rapid change.

Most definitions of mental health include the following elements: the capacity for control over one's own human impulses coupled with the ability to assess realities with considerable accuracy and to act appropriately on this assessment; the ability to form satisfying human relationships; and the ability to learn and to use what one has learned in useful work and self-renewing play.

These abilities and capacities are largely acquired. Development proceeds throughout life, but its foundations are laid in the child's first few years. Many of our children's lifetime chances for development are seriously undermined in the earliest days and years of life. Many children are deprived of nutrition and physical care as well as uncrowded and sanitary housing, intellectual stimulation, emotional guidance, and opportunities for creative and safe play. There is evidence that damage may be irreversible in some cases. To ensure the development of maximum positive mental health for each child, we must provide a wide range of coordinated services —medical, economic, educational, and social—for each child and his family.

Today's mental health crisis is reflected in delinquency, nonlearning, and mental illness. Our inadequate statistics indicate that 2 to 3 percent of our young population are afflicted with mental illness and another 8 to 10 percent with serious emotional disorders. Unknown numbers of children and youth are falling far short of their developmental potential, and alienation from society is widespread. Mental health services in this country exist for only about 7 percent of the identified population in need.

One-fourth of the nation's children and youth—the very poor—have few, if any, services. Prevention, the key to developing mentally healthy productive members of society through attention to the needs of the very young, is a major concern of this Commission, because it is not yet even in sight. Mental illness, delinquency, and underachievement are problems at all socioeconomic levels. Research indicates that a significant proportion of our young people are adversely affected by stresses associated with today's fast-growing, impersonal, and technological society.

In this, the world's richest large nation, these needs can be met. Many other industrialized nations much less wealthy than ours have moved far ahead of the United States in providing a network of developmental and protective services for their young people. We have fallen seriously behind in failing to provide the coordinated, preventive, public programs in health, education, and welfare found in many other countries.

Our new programs in education, health, manpower training, and employment show promise, but they have been poorly coordinated one with another, meager in kind, and frequently short-lived. Often they have failed to reach those most in need. Too frequently they have been directed to special and separate problems rather than to the whole child and his family.

To promote the mental health of children and youth, we must also promote the overall well-being of their families and that of the communities in which they live. Thus, action for the mental health of children and youth must incorporate many programs which start at national levels and move out to states, communities, and neighborhoods. To be successful, these programs must reach each child and his family and do so in ways that will allow families opportunities to participate in the planning and carrying out of services as involved citizens.

We must have clearly designated advocates for the positive mental health of children and youth at all levels of government. An effective advocate function requires the coordination of existing services and the launching of new ones in both preventive and treatment programs in medical, social, educational, vocational, legal, and community planning fields. Our technological and financial resources now make these goals possible. The basic human resource of our land, our children, must have our highest national priority.

Contemporary American Society: Its Impact on Family Life

THE FAMILY SYSTEM AND MENTAL HEALTH

Any commitment to children is a commitment to the family unit. Most children grow up in the context of the family or in some family life group. Their parents exert a tremendously important influence on their growth and development. The role of the parents and its effects on children, however, is far more complex than has generally been assumed. The family has been looked at by many scientists as a system almost like a reverberating electrical system in which actions and interactions in one part of the circuit affect the total function of the system as well as the individual parts. The nature of this intimate system is also molded by the many conditions which define the family's social and physical environment (*Report of Task Force II*, 1969).

The implications are clear. The child's mental health cannot be considered as separate from that of his parents, nor can the parents' mental state be disassociated from that of the child. Sound mental health programs for children and youth must include services and programs which will strengthen and support the entire family.

These child-centered services and programs must retain a family focus. We must not lose sight of the fact that any service or lack of service which affects one member of the family affects all members—brothers and sisters as well as parents. Services and programs should be planned jointly with parents to the maximum extent possible. Family-focused programs involving the participation of parents should help to reduce the sense of

164

isolation, powerlessness, and separateness which threatens the strength and unity of so many families in today's rapidly changing, impersonal, and splintered society (*Report of Task Force II*, 1969).

There is overwhelming evidence that weak and disorganized families are a threat to the healthy growth and development of children in every way—physically, intellectually, socially, and emotionally. The overall health of the parent also affects and is affected by family disorganization (*Reports of Task Forces I, II, V, VI*). Some observers of the contemporary scene claim that the family is no longer needed, because society has assumed so many of its former obligations. However, the majority of social and behavioral scientists hold that the family is still of central importance and that there are responsibilities which belong primarily to the family, even though it now shares some of its functions with other systems in the society.

It is apparent, however, that families must change many of their attitudes, values, and behaviors and also reshape the ways in which they perform their functions if they are to adapt successfully to the revolutionary changes of today. This demand for change exposes families to a host of stresses and strains. How well families manage to deal with these strains depends on the inner strengths of their members *and* on the capacity of society to make changes which are constructively adapted to the needs of families. The Commission believes that its recommendations for a child advocate system and Child Development Councils provide a much-needed mechanism which can lead to the development of needed services and social changes which will help children and families adapt successfully to today's—and tomorrow's—society.

The Commission's recommendations have grown out of an examination of the multiple factors that affect the mental health of children and parents. In this and following chapters we present an overview of this evidence as it relates to families in general, families in poverty, minority-group families, and families of emotionally disturbed and mentally ill children, respectively. The more detailed presentation in Chapters VII and VIII on the growth and development of children and young people also includes a wealth of material on the numerous functions of parents throughout the child's developing years.

The Importance of Marriage and the Family to Its Members

The family is almost the only small, intensely personal, long-lasting group left in our mass society. As such, it is extremely important to the mental health of all its members. Potentially, the family provides an emotional storm center for parents and children—one which allows each member considerable, but not complete, freedom to express both his positive and his negative feelings. Ideally, the family provides warm, supporting, personal relationships as well as the needed opportunities for interdepend-ence. An affectionate family life can give individual members an immensely important sense of their personal significance and uniqueness.

Although most American families provide both economic support and continuing physical care for their children, their major functions are becoming increasingly those of a psychological nature. Parents, ideally, give the psychological support necessary for their children to develop the social, intellectual, and emotional strengths and skills to cope with the many agencies of the larger community, such as the schools, youth or-ganizations, and the like.

One major function of marriage today also lies in the psychological realm. With the advent of the newer and simpler contraceptives, the acceptance of women in the work force, simplified homemaking and food preparation, and changing values, many men and women need each other in a mar-riage relationship as much for emotional and interpersonal support as for economic, social, and cultural reasons.

Although parents are critically important to their children, especially to their very young, their significance is not so direct, simple, and specific as generally portrayed. For instance, social and behavioral scientists are finding that children, from earliest infancy, exhibit individual, partially inborn characteristics which play an important part in determining the be-havior of their parents. In effect, it would seem that children influence the development of their parents just as parents influence their development (see also Chapter VII).

In brief, a child's development is the product of many factors, both within and outside the family. The manner in which a child interacts with his parents depends both on himself and on the characteristics of his parents and their relationship with each other. Indeed, parents bring their whole life history to parenthood. How the parents themselves were treated as children, the quality of their own parents' marriage, their physical health, their education, and their cultural styles all play a part in parental behavior (Stolz, 1967). Parents, like children, are also affected by the present situation in which they are living and by their view of the future. Mothers and fathers are not static in their growth and development but are affected by their own age and their own stage of personal development.

The "Blame-the-Parents Syndrome"

There is a tendency in our society to hold parents responsible for all aspects of their children's behavior and to show little compassion for parents as fallible human beings. Although we hold fairly permissive atti-tudes toward children and regard youth as still being in need of help, parents are usually seen as being fully developed adults who should be able to direct their lives in well-controlled and rational ways. There is considerable disagreement among the social and behavioral scientists as to whether human beings are able to direct their own behavior on the basis of information and their own self-determined motivation. Space does not permit an exploration of the pros and cons of this issue. It seems clear, however, that social and economic arrangements have a strong effect on the behavior of both children and parents. Although there is still an important—often crucial—capacity for change in adolescence, the capacity for fundamental changes in behavior is laid in early childhood and is significantly limited after the age of twelve or so. We have very little systematic evidence of the extent to which adults can change in later life; however, it seems apparent that desired changes are unlikely unless the adult's life situation is modified favorably and a wide range of services is made available to him. In blaming parents for their own deficiencies and those of their children, we overlook known facts about the family as a total interaction system, as well as our knowledge of the dynamics of human development and the ways in which it is affected by the larger environment. We also ignore emerging evidence concerning the importance of biological factors and the effect of these factors on human behavior (see Chapters VII and VIII).

In summary, the question is not one of blame but one of understanding the many factors which affect the mental health of the total family and all its members. Appropriate and effective planning of programs and services depends on such understanding.

THE DATA PICTURE OF MODERN FAMILIES

National statistics provide one basis for understanding our nation's families. These statistics give a numerical count of certain kinds of trends. Although such data can be useful and illuminating, they offer limited insight regarding the complexity and quality of human behavior. Despite such limitations, however, statistics do provide a panoramic view of our families.

Many Marriages, Fewer Youthful Ones

The United States has one of the highest marriage rates in the world. As of 1967 about 94 percent of the men and women in this country had been married at least once at some point in their lives. Young people, however, are not marrying at quite as young an age as was true in the mid-1950's (U.S. Bureau of the Census, 1968a). In 1967 the median age for marriage for men was 23 and for women 20.6. Although the trend of earlier marriage noted during the 1940's and early 1950's no longer holds, it is still customary to hear about "the increase in teen-age marriages."

However, it *is* true that one-fourth of our young men marry before the age of twenty and one-fourth of our young women before the age of nineteen. There is a slight tendency, however, for this age group to marry at somewhat older ages than was true in 1962. By age twenty-six, almost 70 percent of young men are married. Two-thirds of American females are married by the age of twenty-three. Although the trend toward deferment of marriage until a slightly older age is encouraging, there is still reason to be concerned about the large number of teen-age marriages today. As pointed out in the previous chapter, such youthful marriages have particularly high rates of breakdown.

Family Size

The birth rate has been steadily declining since about 1960. At present it has dropped to a low of 18 per 1,000 population. A major reason for this decline is that a relatively small proportion of the total population is now in the child-bearing ages. In the near future, as our large youth population increases in age, the birth rate may begin to rise again (U.S. Bureau of the Census, 1968c). At present our population is still increasing, largely because the birth rate exceeds the death rate.

Average family size in this country is between two and three children. Studies indicate that this is considered the ideal number of children by the great majority of people in all socioeconomic and ethnic groups (Whelpton, Campbell, and Patterson, 1966). Not all parents are able to achieve their ideal of small family size, however. This is particularly true for low-income people with little education. For example, in 1960, families with an income higher than $7,000 per year had an average of 2.5 children, whereas families with less than $2,000 annual income had an average of 3.7 children. In a similar vein, family size is related to educational status. The largest families are noted for women of no education, who average 4.7 children. In contrast, women who have had more than five years of higher education average only 2.5 children.

These figures clearly show that those parents who can least afford to care for many children tend to have a large number, despite their desires for smaller families. The pressures of raising such large families tend to undermine the physical and mental health of mothers and children alike. These are major reasons for the Commission's recommendations that free, high-quality family planning services should be readily available, along with many other services, to all individuals who need and desire them.

Family Income

Family income in the United States increased, on the average, during 1967. When family income is adjusted for changes in consumer prices, the actual average income has risen about 4 percent in recent years. Table 1 shows income changes for various groups of families.

As can be seen from these figures, the greatest increases in income were made by the proportion of families who earned more than $10,000 a year. Only a slight gain was made among that quarter of the nation's families who earn less than $5,000 annually. The adverse effects of inadequate income on the mental health of families is discussed further in the next two chapters.

Table 1.—CHANGES IN FAMILY INCOME LEVEL, 1966–67

| | PERCENT OF FAMILIES | |
INCOME	1966	1967
Under $3,000	14	12
$3,000–$4,999	14	13
$5,000–$6,999	18	16
$7,000–$9,999	24	24
$10,000–$14,999	21	23
$15,000 and over	9	12

SOURCE: U.S. Bureau of the Census, *Current Population Reports on Consumer Income,* Series P-60, No. 59, "Income in 1967 of Families in the United States," April 18, 1969. Adapted from Table 1, p. 21.

Family Breakdown

Although it is often claimed that the American family is in a state of crisis, as indicated by the very high divorce rates, this is not exactly the case. In both 1960 and 1967, about 3 percent of women and 2 percent of men aged fourteen years and over were classified as divorced. Separation rates were also about 2 percent (U.S. Bureau of the Census, 1968a). However, these figures do not reveal the fact that a large number of couples have been divorced at one time and later remarried; thus many children and youth are living in homes with stepparents. Moreover, there has been a gradual though slight increase in divorce rates since 1958 and a more marked increase in the proportion of divorces involving children. A minor numerical increase in homes broken by separation is also apparent.

In 1967, 13 percent of families with children were one-parent families. Six million children were in fatherless families (U.S. Bureau of the Census, 1968a). Of the nearly 5,000,000 families headed by a woman, almost one-half include one or more children under age eighteen and one-fifth include three or more children. Such families are far more likely than male-headed families to have incomes below the poverty line. Family breakdown is far more prevalent among Negro families than among other families in this country. This is especially true in urban areas and is related to the stresses encountered by low-income rural families as they migrate to cities. Family breakdown is also related to the high rates of poverty for Negroes. It is estimated that about 40 percent of Negro families in urban slums are female-headed families (Herzog and Sudia, 1968; see also Chapter IV).

These figures regarding divorce and separation portray only part of the family breakdown picture in this country. There is no way of knowing, in exact terms, the prevalence of strained, unhappy marriages which are held together for a variety of complex social, economic, and psychological reasons. Various studies have been designed to determine "marital happiness," chiefly by asking couples to rate their own marriages. The data indicate that about one-third of the marriages are rated as being unhappy. Ratings of unhappy marriages are more prevalent among very low-income groups and are most likely to be given by people who grew up in homes where there was conflict between parents and between parents and children.

According to themes of current novels, plays, and movies, marital conflict is rampant in the United States and other industrialized nations. Moreover, mental health professionals report that they are encountering a growing number of families in which the marriage relationship is fraught with complex problems. Neither the viewpoint of writers and dramatists nor the experience of marriage and family counselors is necessarily a true indicator of the exact extent of marital and family problems. Other factors may account for the apparent increase in marital problems, such as a freer and more open cultural climate in which individuals are more ready to reveal their hitherto secret marriage problems. Then, too, these problems may be felt more acutely in a society which has such high aspirations for personal fulfillment and well-being.

Be that as it may, there is ample clinical and research-based evidence to show that the mental health of children and young people is adversely affected by serious conflict between parents. In fact, the effects of marital conflict on children can be more severe than the effects of divorce or separation. Therefore, services designed to promote the well-being of children and youth must include services designed to strengthen the marriage relationship as well as the relationship between parents and children. Where breakup is inevitable, services are also needed to help the parents and children cope with their changed situation.

Family Structure

Because of early marriage, smaller families, and greater life expectancy, the average married couple today can expect to spend more than one-third of their married life without children in the home. In contrast, because of older age at marriage, larger families, and shorter life expectancy, there was no time that the husband and wife of 1890 could expect to have a home together with no children present except perhaps within the first years of marriage. During the 1960's, the average woman married at a little over age twenty and had three children by the time she was twenty-six. Her last child went to school when she was thirty-two and married by the time she was forty-seven.

These figures indicate the marked change that has occurred in the nature of marriage and parenthood responsibilities since the end of the nineteenth century. Husbands and wives now have much more time for a "second honeymoon" after the last child has left home. Since the average woman today lives past the age of seventy, she still has about twenty-five years left in her life when there are relatively few demands upon her as a mother. In fact, it might be said that the average mother today has only part-time employment in the home after she is thirty-two years old and her last child has gone to school. In effect, the average woman spends only about ten years of her life as a full-time mother. In spite of these changes, the majority of girls are brought up today with the expectation that their major life function will be as wives and mothers. Since, in actual fact, there is an increasing tendency for women to enter the labor force, especially between the ages of thirty-five and fifty-five, it appears that a different life preparation is in order for our young people, both males and females. Males need a life preparation which includes the probability that their wives will work outside the home for at least a portion of the marriage years, and females should be prepared for different major role functions at different stages in the family life cycle.

This shift in family structure also brings about different expectations about the functions of marriage. At an earlier time, marriage was seen as being primarily for the protection of the young. Now that one-third of a couple's married life is likely to be childless, the marriage relationship, in and of itself, may be potentially strengthened or weakened when the children are gone, depending on whether the couple have seen themselves as being mainly oriented toward parenthood or whether they have also seen themselves as being committed to their own interpersonal marriage relationship.

Brothers and Sisters: Small Families

The smaller size of families today is probably a positive factor in the development of children. Although research evidence is sketchy, it appears that children in small families at all socioeconomic levels tend to have higher tested intelligence, on the average, and to achieve at higher levels both educationally and occupationally (Clausen, 1966; Duncan and Blau, 1967). Evidence is emerging that families with four or more children are less likely to produce reliant, outgoing youngsters or to be viewed as happy families by the children themselves. These findings are also applicable to all social classes (Moore and Holtzman, 1965; Douvan and Adelson, 1966). Among families of five or more children, parents tend to resort to a higher level of authoritarianism and use of physical punishment. Both methods are thought to be detrimental to a child's mental health (Clausen, 1966). Such evidence further supports other findings which indicate that small families are conducive to family well-being.

Families on the Move

About 20 percent of the people in the United States changed residences in 1967. Nonfarm families were more likely to move than farm families, and nonwhites moved more frequently than whites. The unemployed also tend to move more than the employed because of the need to find work. Mobility is highest when people are very young and are marrying and founding their own families. The great majority of moves by a family are made within the same county. Only about 3 percent involve moves from one state to another. In 1967 the greatest amount of movement between states occurred in the Southern region, but this accounted for only 1.3 percent of the population (U.S. Bureau of the Census, 1968b). After parents are older than thirty-five, most families move very little. These figures lend little support to the common assumption that families are frequently uprooted and moved to totally new areas.

However, it is likely that many young families will move at least every three years or so. Even if this move is within the same county, it may cause a fairly drastic shift in friendships, cultural patterns, schools attended, and the like. There is conflicting research evidence as to whether or not this family mobility has adverse effects on children and parents. Common sense would suggest that whether or not such moves produce strains would depend on many factors, including the nature of the move, the reasons for it, and the kinds of situational shifts that are involved. Common sense, plus the apparent success of the well-known "welcome wagon," also suggests that many families need help in reorientation when they move. Aid is especially needed among disadvantaged families with few resources. Unfortunately those families who are most in need of help and who move the most frequently are least likely to receive services such as those provided by welcome wagons, sympathetic school personnel, active churches, and other community organizations. Outreach workers from Child Development Councils might be extremely useful in helping disadvantaged families who have moved into their neighborhoods. Perhaps the most severely disadvantaged group of "families on the move" are migrant workers who follow the crops. Because they face so many dire difficulties, migrant families need a special set of services and programs to help them solve their employment, housing, health, and educational problems.

Mothers at Work

Over the past twenty-five years or so, there has been an increasing tendency for mothers to work (Women's Bureau, 1967), particularly those aged thirty-five years and older. However, this trend has also increased recently for mothers of young children. Almost 40 percent of all women older than fourteen were in the work force in 1966. A large proportion—more than 75 percent—of divorced and separated mothers are employed; however, many wives who are living with their husbands are also working outside the home. A great percentage of families with annual incomes of $8,000 to about $14,000 owe this fact to the employment of the wife as well as the husband. Women at the lowest income and educational levels are not as likely to be employed, largely because it is so difficult for them to find a job. However, women at slightly higher income and educational levels are particularly apt to be in the labor force, because it is often necessary for them to supplement the family income. In families in which the husband earns more than $10,000 a year, the wife is somewhat less inclined to work, partly because her earnings are not so greatly needed. Nonwhite mothers are far more likely to work than white ones, a fact probably associated with the higher rates of unemployment for Negro men as compared to white men.

The lack of day-care facilities for the children of working mothers is rapidly becoming a problem of crisis proportions. In 1967 there were 4,500,000 children under the age of six in this country who had working mothers (Women's Bureau, 1968). Yet American women remain almost totally deprived of satisfactory child-care arrangements during their working hours. According to Department of Labor figures, only about 2 percent of the children of full-time working mothers were in regular group day-care facilities in 1965. Informal arrangements are made for some of the rest of these children, such as leaving them with other family members or friends, but thousands of children under the age of six are left without any care while their mothers work, and others are looked after by a brother or sister only slightly their senior (*Report of Task Force VI,* 1968). It is estimated that licensed day-care facilities are available for only about 200,000 children. Thus, to an unknown extent, more than 4,000,000 young children are endangered by inadequate and inconsistent care. Their mothers are faced with enormous difficulties when trying to work and also provide for the care of their children.

Maternal Employment: Does It Help or Hurt?

Available research evidence indicates that maternal employment, in and of itself, does not necessarily have an adverse effect on children; in fact, in certain instances, it may be of actual benefit to them (Herzog, 1960; Hoffman, 196_).

There is no evidence that maternal employment impedes the development of children at any stage of their growth *if* an adequate, permanent maternal child-care substitute is available. The evidence further shows that maternal employment may be relatively beneficial to children if the mother prefers to work and is frustrated when she does not. On the other hand, if a mother is forced to work against her wishes this may have an adverse effect on the children.

Studies also indicate that the employment of wives does not adversely affect the marriage if the husband acquiesces to such employment. There are some indications that the daughters of working mothers are more likely to be employed themselves when they become adults.

Automation at Home

In the past quarter-century there has been a major shift from home as a producer unit to home as a consumer unit. A great deal of the drudgery has been taken out of homemaking, thanks to "miracle fabrics," frozen and prepared foods, automatic washing machines, and all the rest. Whether mothers and fathers now have more time and energy available for other occupations is open to question. Many couples seem to have far more elaborate notions of homemaking, as indicated by the recent emphasis on gourmet cookery, extensive home decoration, and so on. Higher standards and expectations seem to have accompanied the mass production of goods. Automation has become an accepted way of life for many families. However, this equipment is very expensive and is probably a factor in making it possible and imperative that mothers go to work. It frees them to do so, but at the same time they need to seek employment so they can pay for it. As homemaking becomes more and more a technical specialty, including the manipulation of machines, fathers have taken on many of the homemaking roles—at least in middle-class families.

The automated household, however, means fewer jobs for children and youth in the home. This is partly because their efforts are not needed and partly because parents are reluctant to allow their children to use expensive and complicated equipment. To an unknown extent, the lack of tasks for children in the home may adversely affect the development of their sense of responsibility, importance, and mastery of skills. The fact that children are not needed for the contribution they can make to family work and income may threaten their sense of being valuable assets to the family. In today's home, children are largely an economic liability. Their chief value to parents is largely psychological and social. Therefore, parents may make larger demands on them for affection, gratitude, and achievement.

Family Islands

Today's family is relatively isolated. Although the average contemporary American family keeps in touch with the older generation and other relatives (Sussman and Burchinal, 1962), this is not the same as having relatives readily available in or near the home to help with day-to-day family needs. One might say that today's family is *semi*nuclear. It does have some contact with the extended family, and it also has many other organizational affiliations. But these relationships do not reduce family isolation significantly because most of them are not oriented toward the family and are usually rather distant and superficial.

Although isolation is common among families living in poverty, as will be noted in the following chapter, it is not limited to the poor. Many new suburban areas have developed without regard to family needs. Many have no sidewalks and no public transportation systems. The car becomes a necessity to reach the school, shopping centers, recreational areas, and medical services. It becomes almost impossible for any member of the family to engage in community life without a car to get him there. There is a great dependency on the superhighways that have been developed to speed commuter traffic. For the suburban family the concrete network of highways has become the primary link to work and other essentials of life. In effect, many suburbanites have become slaves to the freeways and the automobile. These concrete barriers, together with mounting social anonymity, breed a sense of alienation and distance from neighbors and a sense of fear and distrust of the surrounding community. While this situation poses problems of isolation for families, it also provides the advantage of allowing them to enjoy greater freedom of life styles. There are no longer the strict social controls from a tightly knit community, nor are these families limited in space. The new transportation systems make it possible for family members to broaden their horizons, to travel far from their communities in short periods of time. The important task is to learn how to adapt these emerging community systems to the needs of families and for families to develop adaptive behaviors to make use of them.

In the newer style of life the father is likely to commute from suburb to city and to be away from the home for long periods of time. This frequently leaves the mother to carry both male and female roles, and she often becomes a much closer companion to both her sons and her daughters than does the father. But as mothers also go to work, and possibly commute, the children are likely to be seriously deprived of support and supervision, especially in the newer, isolated communities.

Such problems are intensified by the fact that the majority of today's families lack readily available and inexpensive services. As communities have become separatist in terms of social and economic groupings, aids such as homemakers, nurses, baby-sitters, home mechanics, and other assistants to family life have become increasingly distant, geographically, from many of the families who need their services.

Family Fantasies and the Mass Media

The mass media are often criticized for presenting a standardized picture of the "nice, average, middle-class family" and for not taking sufficient cognizance of all the other kinds of families in the United States. But what the mass media tend to present, in actuality, is a fantasied picture of an enchanted family life that does not exist anywhere. Advertisements, in particular, play into the dreamlike yearnings of many of our people. They present a vision of glamour, ease, and romantic magic that bears little resemblance to reality. These messages appeal to the inevitable disenchantment that arises in human beings as they gradually abandon the search for magic that has been with them since early childhood. Much of growing into maturity involves coming to terms with reality and recognizing that magic solutions to life's problems do not exist.

Parents also contribute to the fantasy world that surrounds today's children. They tend to transfer their own dreams to fantasied wishes for their young and to set goals for them to be and do all of the things that they themselves had always wished for but never quite achieved. Yet children must grow up in their own ways and in their own worlds and, like their parents, live through hardships and frustrations as well as successes and delights. Parents cannot weave an enchanted existence for their children any more than they can for themselves. Parental fantasies, added to the messages of the mass media, may reinforce overly simplistic and primitive thinking about what life should be for families and their members.

Television, particularly, has been blamed for undermining family life. It is claimed that family members have forgotten how to speak and relate to one another because so much time is spent silently and passively watching TV. It is also claimed that parents regard television as a handy "baby-sitter" which frees them from taking care of their children. On the other hand, family members in former generations escaped to the radio, movies, books, and the like. It seems that, historically, an outcry is always raised against a new form of mass communication. In actuality, it is almost impossible to assess objectively the impact of television on children and families. Comparable population study samples are not available to determine any possible differential effects on one sample of people who have been exposed to television and a comparable sample who have not been so exposed.

It is probably impossible to know the extent to which the mass media shape the culture and to what extent they simply reflect it. All art forms—drama, art, music, literature—achieve popularity and wide public acceptance because they speak to basic psychological needs of many people: needs for love, sex, personal significance, adventure, and aggression. While art forms may stimulate human responses, it is highly improbable that they *cause* basic drives and interests.

Some forms of the media probably have contributed to a greater popular understanding of family life. A number of widely distributed magazines, books, pamphlets, and newspaper columns have presented a good deal of very sound information on the subject of child development and family life. However, almost none of this material is presented at a simple reading level which is understandable to people of little education. Most of it is filled with assumptions about the middle-class situation and life style. The same criticisms apply to the educational films in the field of child development and family relationships. Almost none of these media speaks to poor people in terms with which they can identify or of goals which they can readily achieve. This is but one among many examples of how disadvantaged people are overlooked in our society and only one illustration of the communications gap between the poor and the nonpoor.

Religion and the Family

Religious organizations frequently play a central and vital role in promoting the mental health of families. Studies show that religious counselors are among the chief professional groups to whom young people and adults bring their personal and family problems. Moreover, most of the religious groups conduct an extremely active program in family life education. There is a growing trend for ministers, priests, and rabbis to take special advanced training in marriage counseling and pastoral psychology. Then, too, a number of religious organizations have taken the lead in recent years in pressing for social reforms in areas that immediately affect the family.

Precrisis and Crisis in Families

The strains, separatism, and isolation of today's society place heavy burdens on parents. All but the very prosperous find that they must solve most complex family problems, whether chronic or acute, almost entirely on their own. Although professional helpers, such as doctors, teachers, and counselors, may be available, they generally provide problem-specific and short-term assistance. Moreover, professionals are usually far removed from the family scene. Other forms of family assistance, such as homemakers and the like, are scarce, expensive, and rarely close at hand, as already noted.

These deficits in supporting services for family life create a host of small and large problems. The accumulation of small problems is often likely to mount over time into an increasingly heavy load of frustration and fatigue.

When minor and major crises are added to this burden, family members may develop severe physical or emotional illnesses that are far more difficult to treat than would have been true if services had been available earlier.

For most families, burdens are probably heaviest early in the marriage and during the middle years of married life when adolescent children undergo growth crises and make financial demands.

Early intervention with young families is greatly needed. It is probably the most promising means of strengthening marriages and promoting the healthy development of children. Early assistance to the family may, in many cases, significantly reduce the potential problems of the later, middle years.

Critical periods, large and small, beset most families at many points in the family life cycle, and for the most part, families usually must meet them alone. There are the common short-term illnesses which are not physically severe but which may leave permanent psychic scars because of the strains they impose. For example, all family members may become ill at the same time and have no one to tend to family needs; or the mother may be hospitalized and have no one to look after the children.

There are the long-term chronic problems that can eat away at the financial, social, and psychological foundations of any family. The problem may be a handicapped child, a chronically ill mother, an alcoholic father, a senile grandmother, or an emotionally disturbed or mentally ill family member.

No study has been made of the extent and kinds of problems that even financially secure and generally well-organized families are likely to experience. Common observation would suggest, however, that at least at some time in the family development cycle, one or more of these severe debilitating problems is likely to occur. In some instances, a problem may represent a precrisis, rather than a crisis, situation, which a strong family is able to handle fairly well (Hill and Rodgers, 1964). In less fortunate families, such crises may lead to generalized family and individual breakdown. The full responsibility need not be placed on the family. More social supports in the form of homemaker service, child-care facilities, the required short-term and long-term treatment resources, special financial aid, and the like can often prevent the personal or family disorganization that can occur even in the strongest families if strains are borne alone for too long.

More attention has been given to providing emergency services to families in crisis, such as at the time of death, attempted suicide, acute illness of a family member, and the like. These services are extremely important, but they are apt to be short-term and problem-specific. Living with a complex and continuing problem over a long time period is often more detrimental to overall good mental health than coping with an immediate, specific crisis. There is an understandable preference on the part of the community and its professionals to provide specific, immediate help in a short-lived, dramatic critical situation. But this selectivity leaves the family with the nondrama of chronic problems which cannot be readily resolved but which certainly can be more readily mitigated than they are in most communities today.

Coordinated Services Needed for Families

As we pointed out in the previous chapter, there are severe deficiencies in our services for children and youth. Many needed services do not exist, and many existing ones are lacking in quality, quantity, and coordination. Obviously this situation strongly affects families as well as children and youth. Beyond this, services tend to be focused on individuals rather than on the family as a unit. Parents are frequently asked to carry out a host of sometimes conflicting operations related to specific requirements for their individual children. Thus family life itself may become further disorganized by the very services that are meant to help; and our good intentions merely amplify the forces already present in society which tend to undermine the unity of the family. Families are generally asked to adjust to the many diverse requirements set up by educational, health, and social service agencies. Little thought and recognition is given as to how these various service systems can adapt to the requirements of the family as a dynamic whole (Vincent, 1967). Neighborhood Child Development Councils recommended by this Commission can play an important part in working with parents to obtain coordinated services for their children, and they can do so in ways that are related to the needs of families as a whole. As parents have more of a voice in the development and procurement of services, they can see to it that these services are more flexibly adapted to their needs and less rigidly fitted to the needs of the systems themselves.

SUMMARY

Stable, well-organized families are of crucial importance to the mental health of children and youth. Ideally, the family provides much-needed warm acceptance and long-lasting personal supports to both parents and children. This is vastly important in an age when the family's major function lies in the emotional and psychological realm. These supports are needed so that family members can cope effectively with the harsh requirements of our technological, complex society.

Family life in this country shows signs of strain. Thirteen percent of our children are being reared in one-parent families. A large number are being reared in families in which stepparents are present, largely because of earlier divorces and remarriages. One-fourth of our young people marry before the age of twenty—a fact that greatly increases the risk of later breakdown.

All our families face the stresses of our modern automated and depersonalized society. One-fourth of all families still live in, or near, poverty, with incomes of less than $5,000 a year. About one-fifth of the nation's families move each year. Mobility is particularly high among very young, nonwhite, and low-income families.

There are few services to aid our highly mobile, isolated, and fragmented families in times of crises.

Matters threaten to become more acute with the "population explosion" that seems sure to occur as our large youth population reaches marriage age. Birth rates, at present, are high for poorly educated, low-income families, despite the fact that such families, like others, aspire to having no more than two or three children. Shifts in family structure and in the functions of mothers, along with high costs of living, are factors which contribute to the increasing number of women who enter the labor force. Although maternal employment apparently does not adversely affect the child's physical and mental health if good substitute care is available, there is presently a severe and critical shortage of high-quality day care available for children of working mothers.

The specialized services that have been developed in many communities are a potential aid to families. However, these services have become so overspecialized, frequently so expensive, so poorly coordinated, and so centered on individuals rather than families that very few parents have the resources that are needed to mobilize these services for the well-being of each family member or for the family as a unit. There are enormous gaps, especially in day care, relevant education, and physical and mental health facilities.

These service gaps must be filled. It is far wiser and more economical to protect and promote the well-being of families in general than to focus only on families in which a member or members have serious emotional problems. Specialized, but splintered, services must be coordinated. The physical, social, and economic structures of communities must be better adapted to the mental health of individuals and families. The planning and administration of these services and programs should be directed toward the strengthening of the family so that it can adapt to today's society and carry out its important functions. Since the family is a dynamic system, interacting with agencies and individuals, programs and services should be family-focused and should include parents as partners in administering and carrying out programs. The child advocate system, the Child Development Authorities, and the local Child Development Councils recommended by the Commission should afford the needed mechanisms for the development and coordination of these needed family-focused programs and services.

Poverty and Mental Health

"Listen, it's hell to be poor"

"It's nothin' less than nothin' that we got. For me it isn't so bad, it's for the kids I can't stand it. When you can't even feed your own family, you know you're really down.

"We get by, by the hardest. It's beans and coal off the railroad track and hoping the luck will change. But it doesn't. I keep asking—where will it all end for the kids? Boys get big, you know, and they get so's they won't take it any longer.

"I don't know, I just don't know. All my life I work and work—take anything that comes my way. But it just doesn't add up. Can't even send them to school—no shoes, no money for books. And you don't go anywhere without you get education.

"I brought you my baby. You can see for yourself she's dead. The relief killed her: no milk, no doctor, us out in the street in the snow. That no-relief killed her—just like it's killing us all—only slower.

"You sit there in your nice office and your good clothes and say you understand. You *can't* understand. You have never lived with rats running over the babies and biting them at night. You have never told your kid he couldn't go to the movies this week or next week or any week because there isn't any money. You never lived on a street where junkies and tramps pestered your kids. You never tried like I've tried to raise your boys decent, and lost—with John sent upstate and Dick gone, God knows where, and Joan fighting with me and her teachers all the time. I say there's no justice to it—no justice at all. What are you going to do to help? There's been enough sitting and talking.

"We want help. We want it now. And we don't want any more studies. Things have got to change. You don't need a study to find out that being poor is no damn good for anybody except maybe the rich.

"I worry and worry about what's going to happen to us. Sometimes I think I'm going crazy with it all. I can't sleep, I can't rest. It's those questions all the time in my head—how can we get out of this trap? People are against us; they want to get rid of poor people like me and the wife and kids."

These words portray more vividly than the figures of poverty the sense of hopelessness, despair, and hostility felt by many of the poor. Yet the figures of poverty have much to reveal. Studies and surveys show that poverty brings with it more family breakdown, more school failure, more illegitimacy, more infant deaths, more sickness and handicaps, more emotional and mental disorders, more crime and delinquency, more rage, more despair, and more mistrust of the larger society which permits these things to happen.

Perhaps many of the poor would say there is little point in telling the story "like it is," in a way that the more powerful and advantaged are used to hearing it, and they have ample reason to doubt whether the nonpoor will listen, no matter how you tell it. Nevertheless, we believe there is merit in relating the facts that "scientifically" tell it "like it is." No society that truly understands the price that must be paid for poverty will allow it to continue.

THE IMPACT OF POVERTY ON MENTAL HEALTH

While there is wide agreement that poverty is one of our major mental health problems, it is hard to prove with facts and figures that poverty is bad for mental health. There are many intricate reasons why this is so. These reasons include the following:

a. Although specialists agree that psychoses and other severe disorders are pathological, there is considerable disagreement about what constitutes poor mental health. This matter becomes especially complicated when the question is raised as to whether poor mental health can be defined in the same way for people who are living in different kinds of environments. Does "good adjustment" call for the same behaviors in an inner-city slum as it does for life in an exclusive suburb?

b. Difficulties in carrying out surveys of large populations in order to reliably find out the true rates of emotional disorders and mental illnesses among children and youth of many social and economic backgrounds.

c. The difficulty of determining whether poverty itself causes emotional and mental disabilities or whether people with these disabilities are more likely to drift into poverty.

d. The middle-class bias of most mental health professionals which leads to differing ways of diagnosing and treating different socioeconomic groups (Hollingshead and Redlich, 1958).

e. The greater reluctance of poor people to seek help from psychiatric facilities (Hollingshead and Redlich, 1958).

These difficulties are complex and important. There *is* a need to refine research and survey techniques so that we can obtain more exact knowledge about the association between poverty and poor mental health. However, while we are awaiting the development of this more precise knowledge, we can use our own powers of observation—eyes that are willing to see, ears that are ready to listen, "hearts" that are ready to become informed.

One has only to visit low-income neighborhoods and their schools and clinics to know that poverty undermines the physical and mental health of its children, young people, and parents. There are the pinched, wary faces of little children; there is the boisterous, defiant behavior of older ones, who hide their inner sense of helplessness and fear with a mask of swaggering bravado. There are the exhausted faces of the mothers and the embittered expressions of the men. There is dirt, noise, and a general atmosphere of despair and disorganization. There is the steady erosion on people and things which comes from the grinding, instinctual struggle for sheer personal survival.

Can one doubt that such conditions are abrasive to mental health? Can one doubt that such an environment adversely affects the child's desire and ability to learn the lessons unrelated to the realities of his life, taught in a school planned and operated without adequate sensitivity to the problems of poverty and its damaged children? Mental health experts and spokesmen for the impoverished agree that such an environment undermines a child's sense of trust, self-confidence, and ability to cope with the larger world. Can one believe that babies born into this handicapped atmosphere have an equal chance with the more privileged to grow and develop toward their maximum capacity to learn, to believe in themselves and others, to put off the possible pleasures of the moment for a distant and tenuous reward?

These are some of the facts for those who would continue to doubt, facts which affect the lives of nearly one-fourth of our nation's children and youth.

1. Although a number of factors other than psychological ones play into the incidence of school failure, early school dropout, unemployment, juvenile delinquency, drug addiction, family breakdown, and illegitimacy, the far higher rates of these problems for poor people indicate,

among other things, the corrosive impact of poverty on the mental health of children and youth in low-income families.

2. Studies suggest a close correlation between premature birth and low socioeconomic status, and between low birth weight and high rates of serious handicaps such as brain damage, mental retardation, blindness, and other disabilities. Data further show that a large proportion of poor mothers, particularly nonwhite mothers, receive no prenatal care and inadequate obstetrical care at delivery.

3. Of the estimated 3 percent of children and youth who are mentally retarded, 75 percent show no obvious brain damage and have few physical handicaps. Typically, these nonorganic cases come from census tracts where the median income is $3,000 per year or less (*PCMR Message*, 1968).

4. Poor and nonwhite children show high rates of physical disabilities —tuberculosis, chronic diseases, blindness, etc. In many instances, institutionalization for these disorders could have been prevented by early diagnosis and treatment.

5. Malnutrition takes its toll by retarding physical growth, increasing vulnerability to disease, lessening the capacity to learn, stunting emotional growth and—if recent studies are confirmed—by producing permanent and irreversible brain damage in many infants.

6. Analysis of Head Start children showed that at least 10 percent of them were judged to be crippled in their emotional development by the age of four years (National Committee Against Mental Illness, Inc., 1966). In some cities, this figure is estimated at 20 to 25 percent.*

7. One study found that 70 percent of several thousand first-graders in a typical Negro district of Chicago were mildly, moderately, or severely maladapted to the psychological requirements of the first grade. Compared to a well-adjusted white group, these Negro youngsters ran a 9-to-1 risk of developing psychiatric symptoms by the end of the school year. In the same district, some 10 percent of the youngsters in the seven-to-seventeen age range come to the attention of the public or court authorities each year because of delinquent behavior (Kellam and Schiff, 1967).

8. The early results of a current study of children in Manhattan between the ages of six and eighteen show that 13 percent of them are judged to be markedly "psychiatrically impaired." Rates are much higher for poor children and for children who are members of oppressed minority groups than for others (Langner *et al.*, 1967).

9. Disadvantaged children, particularly those from minority groups, show high rates of cumulative educational retardation. It is estimated, for example, that 85 percent of the eighth-grade students in Harlem are "functional illiterates." Typically, such youngsters know only dilapidated, understaffed, and ill-equipped schools.

* Personal communication, Dr. Eveoleen Rexford, August 6, 1969.

10. There is a consistent correlation between poverty and the number of school dropouts. Of the million youths who will drop out of school this year, about 65 percent will come from families with incomes of less than $5,000; about 85 percent from families with incomes of less than $7,500. The dropout rates for certain minority groups run as high as 60 to 70 percent.

11. The problems of unemployment are particularly acute for youths between the ages of sixteen and nineteen. For white youths the 1967 unemployment rate was double the overall national average, while for nonwhite youths it was seven times higher.

Data indicate that the very poor from disorganized communities tend to lack the developmental experiences which Erik Erikson proposes are essential to a child's healthy personality development. Such environments seem to produce in children attitudes of mistrust rather than trust, doubt and a sense of powerlessness rather than autonomy, indecisiveness instead of initiative, a sense of failure rather than mastery, isolation instead of intimacy, and despair rather than ego integrity (in Beiser, 1965).

In terms of program planning, it is important to distinguish between the poor who have retained the social and psychological characteristics of well-functioning societies and the poor whose family and group structure has typically been highly unstable and disorganized for generations. Generally, the former have experienced poverty for years or decades rather than for generations. They often understand how to achieve collective action, to utilize indigenous or outside leadership, and they share the principles, values, and attitudes of the larger society. The disorganized poor, on the other hand, are apathetic, lack strong emotional attachments to values of the larger society, and exhibit a great deal of aggression and hostility as well as a sense of powerlessness. Alexander Leighton (1968), whose work with disorganized groups has been extensive, feels that these people may be motivated to respond to programs on the basis of at least two commonly felt needs. One such need is health care; the other is programs that promise help for their children. Research findings indicate that the disorganized poor are in need of both such programs far more than any other group.

THE FACTS OF POVERTY

One-Fourth of Our Children and Youth Impoverished

One-fourth of American children under age eighteen live in poor families. Nonwhite children are almost four times as likely to be disadvantaged as white children. Nearly one-half of the families in this country have incomes which fall short of meeting a basic standard of economic self-sufficiency. *More than* half of our nation's families—and considerably more than half of our children—live on incomes which are too low for a "modest, but comfortable way of life." The majority of families need additional supports to promote the healthy growth and development of their children. Although our nation owns almost 50 percent of the world's wealth (Golenpaul, 1966), we fail to provide half or more of our children and youth with services and environments which are basic to the full development of human potential. The public services which are available are generally neither of equal quality nor conducive to easy access. The programs and services which are needed include: high-quality education, adequate medical care, relevant vocational training, good housing, and wholesome community conditions and recreational facilities. Although we know that the lack of such services and conditions in the early years of life is very apt to impose life-long, frequently irremediable handicaps on our children and youth, we persist in taking small, halfway measures to change this dangerously short-sighted public policy, a policy which is particularly perilous in an age requiring higher and higher levels of personal competence for the security of our people and the survival of our country as a democratic, technologically advanced nation. A more exact look at the nation's family income figures shows that many cannot afford to pay for needed services, even when they are not officially classified as "poor."

There are varying levels of measured poverty and inadequate income in the United States, largely depending on what one defines as poor. These definitions vary, depending on the criteria used to define a minimum standard of living, whether standards for various parts of the country have been adjusted to varying living costs, whether variations in family size are taken into account, and other factors. In general, families today are classified as living in poverty (lacking money for minimum basic needs) if their incomes are less than about $4,000 a year. According to other definitions, a family is considered living in poverty if its income is not sufficient for essential routine medical care and some educational costs, added to money for basic shelter, food, and clothing needs. By these latter criteria, the family "poverty line" may be set at an income of about $8,000 a year (and higher for large families, especially in cities). This figure is certainly below the annual income figure of $9,150 which the U.S. Department of Labor (1968) estimated was required for an urban worker with a wife and two children to maintain a "modest but adequate"* living standard in 1968. One might roughly set guidelines for "family poverty" as shown in Table 2.

Using these guidelines, one can see the distribution of family income in the United States in 1966 in Table 2. As shown, half of the nation's

* $8,000 would be barely enough for a family consisting of a father, mother, and two children living in an urban area. Therefore, the term "adequate" would depend on size of family, where the family lives, and whether the family is nearer the $10,000 income.

families have less than adequate incomes and almost one-fifth might be classified as being seriously or critically poor! Another two-thirds have less than adequate incomes to pay for other than the most basic family needs. This situation points to the need for guaranteed employment and guaranteed minimum income levels.

Table 2.—STATUS OF FAMILIES BY INCOME, 1966

Status	POVERTY GUIDELINES Annual Income	DISTRIBUTION OF FAMILY INCOME IN THE UNITED STATES IN 1966
Critically poor	Less than $2,000	6.4%
Seriously poor	$2,000 to $4,000	12.2%
Marginally poor	$4,000 to $6,000	14.2%
Inadequate income	$6,000 to $8,000	17.1%
Adequate income	$8,000 to $10,000[1]	15.4%
Highly adequate income	$10,000 to $12,000	11.9%
Comfortable income	$12,000 to $15,000	10.6%
Prosperous income	More than $15,000	12.2%

SOURCE: Adapted from Consumer Income, Current Population Reports, Series P-60, No. 55, August 5, 1968.

Nowhere is the economic plight of American families more apparent than among some of our minority groups. Indian families had an average annual income of only $1,500 in 1967 (Association on American Indian Affairs, 1968). More than half of all persons in poverty in New York City in 1964 were Puerto Ricans, although they represented less than 10 percent of the population (Fitzpatrick *et al.*, 1968). Mexican-American families are in similar economic straits. Black children, who make up the largest majority of our disadvantaged young, are very likely to live in families who cannot afford the minimum essentials for their healthy development. For instance, about 75 percent of black families, compared to 47 percent of whites, in 1966 had annual incomes that would be rated as inadequate, that is, less than $8,000 a year. Three times as many blacks (15 percent) as whites had critically low annual incomes (less than $2,000 a year), and more than twice as many (40 percent) had "poverty incomes" of less than $4,000 a year. At the other end of the income scale, only about one-third as many blacks (4 percent) as whites (13 percent) were in the prosperous groups who average more than $15,000 a year income. Overall, about 15 percent of black families might be rated as having comfortable or prosperous family incomes.

Although the average income of black families has grown somewhat in the past twenty years, it has not risen as rapidly as that of white ones (*Report of the National Advisory Commission on Civil Disorders,* 1968). Since low-income black families, like white ones at that income level, tend to be large, one could estimate that the *vast majority* of black children suffer from poverty or near-poverty. Some progress has been made in recent years in opening up better economic opportunities for blacks. But the progress is painfully slow, and the plight of black children and youth is still critical. This plight is reflected in the higher rates of mental and emotional problems found in the Langner and the Kellam and Schiff studies cited earlier in this chapter. Since many of these young people suffer the cumulative health, mental health, and related deficits of many generations of poverty and discrimination, services are necessary for the remediation of these conditions. These disadvantaged children are particularly in need of intensive enriched human service and associated programs. From the mental health viewpoint, it is equally important that full and equal participation in society be provided. All these comments are also applicable to children and youth in Indian, Mexican-American, and Puerto Rican families.

Some gains have been made in reducing family poverty in recent years. Since 1960 the proportion of families below the poverty line has decreased at an average of about one percent each year. However, in 1967, the number of persons living in proverty was still estimated, by government criteria, at about 26,000,000. More than 10,000,000 of these were children under the age of eighteen (U.S. Dept. of Agriculture, 1968). While the poor, like other families, have benefited from the recent rise in family income, they have been touched most by the fact that some of the gains have been offset by rises in prices. It has been the well-to-do families that have benefited most from the expanding economy.

Although urban poverty has received a great deal of attention, rural poverty is both more extensive and more severe. For example, the median income for rural nonfarm families in 1964 was slightly more than 80 percent of the urban average. The median figure for farm families was only about half the urban figure. In mid-1965, one-third of all persons living on farms, and one-fourth of the rest of the rural population, were living within the borders of poverty (U.S. Dept. of Agriculture, 1967).

As shown in Table 3, family income varies in different regions of the country, as does the comparative position of black to white income. It should be noted that these government figures are based on a very conservative estimate of the income level required to be classified as living below the "poverty line."

Figures in this table show that the highest levels of family income are found in the Western region, the lowest in the South. Furthermore, nonwhites in the West and in the North Central states are in a better comparative position to whites, on the average, than in other parts of the country. Both comparatively and absolutely speaking, nonwhites in the South are the poorest group. Negro incomes reflect the nonwhite trend.

Table 3.—MEDIAN FAMILY INCOME IN 1967 AND COMPARISON OF NEGRO AND WHITE
FAMILY INCOME BY REGION

	WHITE	NONWHITE	NEGRO INCOME AS A PERCENT OF WHITE
United States	$8,318	$5,177	59%
North Central	8,414	6,633	78%
West	8,901	7,525	74%
South	7,448	4,020	54%
North	8,746	5,936	66%

SOURCE: Herman P. Miller and Dorothy K. Newman. *Recent Trends in Social and
Economic Conditions of Negroes in the United States.* Current Population Reports,
Series P-23, BLS Report No. 347, July, 1968.

FACTORS ASSOCIATED WITH POVERTY

Eight major factors are strongly associated with poverty: little education,
the poverty environment, chronic unemployment, life styles which are a
product of poverty, low income, poor physical and mental health, large
families, and broken families. These factors interact with one another in
ways that keep poor people entrapped in the intergenerational cycle of
poverty.

Poverty Life Styles

As we have noted, families who live in long-term extreme poverty are
often disorganized and unstable. Although the life styles of such families
may vary among the "subcultures" of poverty, these patterns share the
common feature of being different from the dominant values of our society.
Like all youngsters, children in very low socioeconomic groups are strongly
affected by the social situation in which they live, by the cultural patterns
of the people in their environment, and especially by the life styles of their
families.

The child-rearing and family life patterns of very poor disorganized
families differ not only from those of the more affluent classes but also
from those of the more stable poor. For example, Pavenstedt (1965) found
that very young upper-lower-income children experienced a good deal of
order and stability in their environment. Although their homes were not
intellectually stimulating, later testing in school revealed no great language
or behavior problems. Among very low-income families, however, activities in the home were impulse-determined and consistency was totally
absent. Parents often failed to discriminate between children or failed to
discriminate between the child's role and their own. Communication by
words was almost nonexistent. Behavioral problems among these children

were noted upon their entrance to kindergarten or grammar school. Self-perception was low, and language achievement was seldom attained. They became "immature little drifters" who, without anyone to relate to, failed to learn to communicate effectively and came to grips with only certain circumscribed areas of their existence.

The inconsistency in discipline, the lacks in verbal communication between parents and children, and the real environmental dangers which put pressure upon the young to grow up fast are factors which interfere in various ways with a smooth and relatively progressive development. The discontinuity in development is a striking feature of the disadvantaged child's life. Malone (1966) notes that the pressures put upon these children to grow up fast result in an early independence and premature coping and defensive ability; this does not lead to full independence in later life, and "genuine mastery and flexible adaptability are forfeited." Malone earlier (1963) described many behaviors of children from disorganized slum families which predispose them to later chronic acting out and impulse disorders. Such children exhibited low frustration tolerance, impulsivity, and unreliable controls, dominant motor discharge, marked use of imitation, limited use of fantasy and constructive play, language retardation, and a tendency to concrete thought.

Deutsch (1963) suggests that disadvantaged children are subjected to "stimulus deprivation" in the home and that this accounts, in part, for their later difficulties in school. However, Minuchin *et al.* (1967) note that, in some areas of the environment, sensory stimulation may be more intense for slum children than for the more protected middle-class child. This over-stimulation may lead some children to develop a tendency to block out the environment and withdraw into their own private thought. But certainly the slum child's perception is not faulty when he roams the street—which makes difficult any explanation as to why such children do poorly on tests of figure-ground spatial relations. Lowered performance on many types of tests, however, may be attributable to the child's different development in language, verbal, cognitive, and attentive skills, as well as to deficiencies in our testing methods.

Much more research remains to be done on learning, behavior, and emotional problems among disadvantaged children. However, one thing seems clear. The child-rearing and family life patterns of the unstable poor are not the same as those which have been associated with a child's later success in school achievement, employment, or establishment of a stable family life. Nor are they associated with ratings of being "mentally healthy," especially in the broad sense of the term (Chilman, 1966; Irelan, 1966).

Table 4 shows, in highly summarized form, the child-rearing patterns which are indicated by research to be more closely associated with successful adaptation to various aspects of today's society.

Table 4.—CHILD-REARING AND FAMILY LIFE STYLES MORE PREVALENT AMONG THE
VERY POOR COMPARED WITH PATTERNS ASSOCIATED WITH EFFECTIVE
ADAPTATION TO THE DEMANDS OF TODAY'S SOCIETY[1]

Patterns Reported to Be More Prevalent Among the Very Poor	Patterns Conducive to Adaptation to Today's Society
1. Inconsistent, harsh, physical punishment.	1. Mild, firm, consistent discipline.
2. Fatalistic, personalistic attitudes, magical thinking.	2. Rational, evidence-oriented, objective attitudes.
3. Orientation in the present.	3. Future orientation, goal commitment.
4. Authoritarian, rigid family structure; strict definition of male and female roles.	4. Democratic, equalitarian, flexible family structure.
5. "Keep out of trouble," alienated, distrustful approach to society outside family; constricted experiences.	5. Self-confident, positive, trustful approach to new experiences; wealth of experiences.
6. Limited verbal communication; relative absence of subtlety and abstract concepts; a physical-action style.	6. Extensive verbal communication; values placed on complexity, abstractions.
7. Human behavior seen as unpredictable and judged in terms of its immediate impact.	7. Human behavior seen as having many causes and being developmental in nature.
8. Low self-esteem, little belief in one's own coping capacity; passive attitude.	8. High self-esteem, belief in one's own coping capacity; an active attitude.
9. Distrust of opposite sex, exploitive attitude; ignorance of physiology of reproductive system and of contraceptives.	9. Acceptance of sex, positive sex expression within marriage by both husband and wife valued as part of total marital relationship; understanding of physiology of reproductive system, effective use of contraceptives.
10. Tendency not to differentiate clearly one child from another.	10. Each child seen as a separate individual and valued for his uniqueness.
11. Lack of consistent nurturance with abrupt and early granting of independence.	11. Consistent nurturant support with gradual training for independence.
12. Rates of marital conflict high; high rates of family breakdown.	12. Harmonious marriage; both husband and wife present.
13. Parents have low levels of educational achievement.	13. Parents have achieved educational and occupational success.

[1] This table, because it is so condensed, may be misleading since several topical fields have been merged (i.e., mental health, educational achievement, social acceptability, conscience formation, and family stability). For data differentiating these fields, see Catherine Chilman, *Growing Up Poor*, U.S. Dept. of Health, Education, and Welfare, Washington, D.C.: Government Printing Office, 1966.

There is a great deal of argument today as to whether or not low-income and minority groups should be encouraged to adopt the patterns of the dominant white middle-class culture. It is argued that middle-class life styles are "phony, corrupt, and neurotic." However, these patterns have evolved from the historical conditions in this country and have been associated with successful adaptation to the social and economic demands of our society.

Basically, the question is not whether one set of cultural patterns is "morally" better than another. The question revolves around the pragmatic judgment of which set of values and behaviors are the most conducive to effective coping with contemporary society and its economic and social systems and arrangements. In our society those who have been financially able, and who have lived "the middle-class way," have been far more able to achieve educational and vocational success than those in lower socio-economic groups who have had different cultural styles. Questions can easily be raised about the desirability of such a "success" orientation and the sacrifices that go with it. "Success" does require such sacrifices as commitment to long-term goals; impulse control; competitive striving interlaced with conformity to the group; emphasis on verbalization rather than physical action; deference to time, order, detail, and one's "boss." These requirements affect mental health in the sense that they are restrictive to individual self-expression and freedom. Yet these limitations do seem to be the required price for attaining such commonly stated goals as: "a good education; a steady, well-paying job; a nice home; and a stable family life." Poor people are obviously aware of these requirements, since it has been noted that most persons who escape from poverty tend to identify with middle-class values. These limitations and requirements appear to be necessary for achievement of "success" goals in our relatively open society in which "the good life" depends largely on individual conformity to the demands and framework of our dominant institutions. Individual initiative is still a strong factor within this framework. Inexperience in today's larger society, fantasies born of this inexperience, and the adverse experience of living in the separated world of poverty understandably lead to the belief of many disadvantaged people that economic success depends on sheer magic, that is, "getting the breaks" and "knowing the right man."

However, there is clear evidence (Blau and Duncan, 1967) that acquiring an advanced education is still the major route to occupational success in this country, although this is less true for Negroes and other people in oppressed minority groups than it is for whites. A sizable number of lower-income and "non-middle-class" people still move into relative prosperity via education. Fewer of them manage it than those of higher-class origins because there are still many obstacles. But the way is still open. Although very poor people, like those in the working and middle class, would have a better chance of escaping from poverty if they had the kinds of values and behaviors presented in Table 4, they cannot suddenly adopt these, as by magic. Nor can adherence to these life styles ensure escape. Such escape requires income supports and other services, plus the *opportunity* to acquire a good education, job training, high wages, and all the rest.

The suggestion that individuals should commit themselves to the "middle-class way" is not popular with some social scientists or with many disadvantaged people. For instance, there is ample evidence that individual hard work and devotion to middle-class patterns frequently has not paid off for people who are disadvantaged by long-term poverty and/or discrimination. This is why some poor people have adopted life styles that include elements of alienation, magical thinking, impulsivity, personalism, and all the rest.

Some of the disadvantaged, disillusioned by the total system, have joined in movements which seek to reform and redo the economic and political system. They, like some nonpoor, believe strongly that full economic and social justice are not achievable within our present highly competitive socioeconomic arrangements.

The cynicism of the poor is justified, and indeed some are surprised that the anger and violence of the civil and poor people's rights movements were so long in coming. We also know that simply "changing the system" to provide better education, jobs, and so on will not, automatically and by itself, assure a better education and a better job to any individual. "Success" depends in part on individual effort, which in turn depends on motivation. The child's upbringing and the opportunities provided by society both have an effect on individual motivation. Changes in our society's dominant institutions and changes in individual life styles should come simultaneously, and hopefully in ways that will maximize sound mental health.

In any society, under any political or economic system, individual effort is needed to achieve "success." Poverty, its causes, and its by-products include many mental health hazards, among which is poor motivation. This, in turn, has multiple causes and in itself is a mental health hazard. It is important to recognize that no simple, single-factor solution will make poverty or its problems disappear. Poverty, if thought of only as lack of finances, can be cured easily through the simple expedient of giving poor people money. Some social scientists claim that this is all that is needed. They argue that if poor people have more money they will readily adapt to the majority culture. There is a great deal of cogency to this argument, although there are those who do not highly value adapting to the majority culture. The position is taken here that adequate income for poor people is fundamental to the solution of their other problems. On the other hand, many of the poor people in this country have been badly handicapped by the corrosive effects of poverty and prejudice for many generations. These handicaps are particularly crippling in a modern society that demands so much individual initiative, stability, and flexibility. Therefore, although poverty, in and of itself, can be cured simply by giving people enough money, the problems that have been caused by poverty, and which continue to handicap many of the poor, require a wide range of remedial services. It is likely that services in the health, educational, environmental, and employment areas need to be particularly enriched because poor people and poverty neighborhoods have been without them for so long.

Although cultural patterns are likely to change in response to altered situations, these changes tend to come about slowly. The demands of today's society are so high-powered that rapid, rather than gradual, changes may be necessary. This does *not* mean that middle-class culture patterns should be imposed on the poor. It surely does not mean that the life styles of the poor should be judged as "wrong" or "inferior." It does imply, however, that members of the helping professions and others concerned with eliminating poverty and mitigating its effects need to help the poor to understand the alternatives and to find bridges, should they want them.

This suggests, among other things, a family-centered approach in which one works with parents as well as children. This approach has long been taken by Child Guidance Clinics, child and family welfare agencies, some therapeutic agencies, and some educational institutions. Children and young people need help to withstand the conflict-ridden situations they encounter, situations in which patterns of their parents and those of "the other world" in which the teachers, doctors, and social workers live clash in ways impossible to hide or avoid. It further suggests that members of the helping professions need to be trained to understand the life styles of the poor and those of oppressed minorities. They also need to be trained to work with so-called paraprofessional aides who are members of subcultural groups. The fact that these aides have been observed, in many settings, to improve communication and understanding between the professionals of the middle-class community and the people of the often separate world of poverty is only one of the advantages of employing paraprofessionals, as will be noted in Chapter XII.

We noted in the foregoing section that changes in some life styles associated with poverty might be useful in helping some poor people escape from their situation. It is equally, if not more, important that the "more advantaged" members of our society—the white population, primarily—change their cultural attitudes and their hostility toward the poor. It is essential that racism be eliminated, since racism perpetuates poverty and is, of itself, extremely detrimental to mental health. Equal privileges in, and easy access to, all aspects of American life are basic ingredients in eradicating the discrimination which many believe is our nation's number one mental health problem. Whites will have to change their life styles, as will some middle-class and upper-class nonwhites.

Technique and policy are important elements in solving poverty problems. The poor who need financial help want and deserve aid with dignity. Those who are being trained or who want to be trained for employment should be guaranteed a job. Those who need decent housing should not have to wait for a millennium. The giving of money should be done because people need money, just as services should be provided because they are necessary to the well-being of our citizenry. Financial support, while it may not solve all problems, should not be granted with conditions that force services on people.

Poverty presents us with one basic issue: that of supporting life at a level comfortable to individuals and to the society. The right to life should not be conditioned by moral judgments. Any other approach will not be conducive to bringing about alternative opportunities for the poor so that they may wish to consider changing life styles. In fact, any other approach may simply perpetuate and rigidify those aspects in life styles which make poverty more difficult to eliminate.

Little Education

It is well known that poverty is closely associated with relatively low levels of formal education. Very poor people are likely to have had less than an eighth-grade education. Statistics show that the high school dropout rate increases as parental income decreases and that it is consistently higher where poverty is most concentrated—among urban slum, rural, and non-white populations (U.S. Bureau of the Census, 1966a). Unemployment rates are far higher for people with little education; conversely, the data clearly show that occupational success and high income are directly related to completion of four or more years of higher education (U.S. Bureau of the Census, 1967).

In general, children and young people who come from poverty backgrounds tend to do less well in school and on intelligence tests, as we have noted. Preschool learning conditions leave many poor children unprepared for entrance into kindergarten or elementary school, since the expectations of educators are usually founded upon middle-class norms. Educators, for example, rely heavily on verbal skills, which are not highly valued in disadvantaged homes. Unable to cope with the demands made upon them, many disadvantaged children develop negative feelings toward the school. The fact that schools have not successfully met the challenge of educating such children is indicated by the large numbers of poor children who lag further behind their more affluent counterparts as they advance into higher grades.

The poverty environment, moreover, does little to provide motivation or resources for a child's continuing education. Added to the low-quality schools is the fact that there is little in this environment to encourage the young person to finish high school and go on to college. The poor child sees few people who have completed formal education, and all too often he sees little evidence that such efforts have resulted in high-status, well-paying jobs. His experience more often teaches him that those who "make it big" are engaged in the "rackets" or in some other form of illegal behavior.

Our most recent antipoverty programs have opened the doors to some new approaches. Many of them promise to break the educational barriers, to increase educational exposure and achievement, and to open new career lines, but the efforts are not massive enough.

The poverty environment is generally a constricted one. Commonly, children and youth raised in such a setting have had little experience outside their immediate neighborhoods. Frequently they are hemmed in by lack of money for transportation, fear of the unknown, parental cautions to "keep out of trouble," ignorance of the larger community, distrust of others, lack of appropriate clothing, and inexperience in dealing with complex situations. Thus, low-income children and parents often do not, or cannot, avail themselves of the opportunities for enriched experiences even when they are offered free of charge to the public, as in many of our urban communities. Poor children often show an almost phobic anxiety about venturing out of their own familiar world. Recreational facilities are drastically needed in low-income neighborhoods, as are programs which will provide the disadvantaged with enriching experiences with people and places outside their communities.

Poor Housing and Poor Neighborhoods

Highly defective housing and deteriorating neighborhoods are an added handicap of the poverty environment. Both racial prejudice and low family income keep poor families in slum areas and in dilapidated housing. Much of this housing is substandard, overpriced, and seriously overcrowded. Commercial and residential areas are generally mixed together in poverty neighborhoods so that children are surrounded by every form of commercial enterprise, rather than the green lawns and playgrounds so often featured in schoolbooks and by the mass media. Living in deteriorated housing and slum neighborhoods, being surrounded by drabness and a debilitating climate, adds to the lack of motivation noted in some poor children. A detailed discussion of the many adverse effects which these conditions have on the physical and mental health of children and their parents will be noted in the following chapter.

Federal housing programs have benefited the nonpoor far more than the poor. In thirty-one years, public funds have financed 800,000 units for the poor. In thirty-four years, tax monies have been used in the construction of 10,000,000 units for the middle class and the rich (Harrington,

1968). Most families who have been displaced from condemned or substandard housing move into other substandard dwellings because nothing else is available. Urban renewal programs have generally concentrated on constructing commercial and luxury facilities and have neglected the community and housing needs of the poor. Further, many public housing units consist of high-rise buildings which are not conducive to the development of a community or to parental supervision of young children at play. Policies that set income limits as to which families may live in public housing tend to bring together in one place an overly large number of disadvantaged families. In effect a new slum may be created by such a policy. Developing children are surrounded by other people who are caught in poverty, and they have little opportunity to learn other ways of life. Scattered site housing, a wide range of supporting services, rent subsidies, planned communities, and a mixture of socioeconomic groups in public housing neighborhoods are among the strategies that have been recommended to remedy the situation.

The poverty environment is often one of disorganization and despair. Compared to more advantaged neighborhoods, city sanitation, fire, police, legal, and public transportation services are usually highly inferior. Such communities provide an explosive situation. Available information indicates that impulse to violence is high and hard to control when human beings are brought up in deprivation, experience little humanity at the hands of others, and grow into adults of limited competence who are unable to find work and are forced to live in poverty while the majority of citizens enjoy prosperity (Bronfenbrenner, 1969).

The poverty environment usually represents encapsulated poverty. In urban areas this environment has become particularly explosive in the past twenty years or so, with the rapid in-migration of very poor people from rural areas. The majority find, when they come to the city, that their poverty and unemployment continues. They do not have the skills, information, or cultural patterns to deal with the increased complexities and temptations of urban life. While it is somewhat common to overromanticize the supposedly stable communities from which they came, the problems of many become intensified and certainly more visible when they move into the city.

Broken Families

The shift from a rural to an urban environment plays an important part in the higher rates of family breakdown that are found for poor people, especially for nonwhites. The most important single factor associated with family breakdown is poverty itself. There is clear evidence that illegitimacy (Campbell, 1968), divorce, and separation rates increase as one goes down the socioeconomic scale (Glick, 1964). Other factors strongly associated with family breakdown include: the high unemployment rates of low-income men, the life patterns of the very poor which tend to foster hostility and poor communication between the sexes (Rainwater, 1967; Komarovsky, 1964), large family size, low education, poor health, inadequate housing, and the public assistance policies in many states which have denied AFDC payments to families when the father is present in the home.

There is a large association between being poor and living in a family headed by a woman. For instance, three times as many white families with a female head had incomes below the poverty line in 1964 than was true for white families with a male head. Somewhat the same situation held for black families, with more than twice as many broken families living below the poverty line as for those where the father was present (see Table 5).

Table 5.—INCOME DISTRIBUTION FOR ALL FAMILIES BY SEX AND COLOR OF HEAD, 1964 (PERCENTAGE)

| Total Money Income | WHITE | | NONWHITE | |
	Male-Headed (N=39,200,000)	Female-Headed (N=3,881,000)	Male-Headed (N=3,629,000)	Female-Headed (N=1,126,000)
Less than $3,000	13%	38%	29%	65%
$3,000 to $5,999	25	33	37	27
$6,000 to $9,999	36	20	24	6
$10,000 and more	26	10	10	2

SOURCE: Special tabulation by U.S. Bureau of the Census of data from March, 1965, Current Population Survey for the Social Security Administration (Figures rounded).

It is clear that many poor children grow up in families with no father in the home. A number of researchers and clinicians hold that children inevitably suffer from the fatherless situation per se. However, a careful analysis of available studies fails to reveal that this is always the case.

In a careful review of the related research, Herzog and Sudia (1968) point out many methodological weaknesses in most of the studies on this subject. The majority of studies consider only one aspect of the child's behavior and not the whole complex of family interaction and the life situation. For instance, not enough attention has been paid to the fact that broken homes are highly variable in and of themselves. One should, for example, take into account the social and economic situation of the family; the reasons why the home was broken (such as whether by death, divorce, separation); how the mother has reacted to the situation; and subsequent events in the life of the child and his family.

Moreover, as the authors point out, it does not necessarily mean that boys and girls grow up without a close association with an adult male simply because they do not live in a home where there is an intact marriage. These children may well have helpful close contacts with male relatives, friends in the community, teachers, and the like.

There are indications, furthermore, that children develop better in a home that has been broken by divorce or separation than in one which is torn by marital discord. All in all, it is important that a fresh approach be taken to the subject of broken homes and their impact on children. The female-headed family should not be seen as necessarily a deviant pattern of family life. Since there are a large number of these kinds of families in this country, it would be more helpful to regard them as one type of family organization. For instance, Rainwater (1967) observes that as many as two-thirds of black children in areas of urban poverty probably will not live in families headed by both a mother and a father. It would seem to be important, therefore, to consider what supports and services might be provided for homes in which there is not a male head, rather than to focus on attempts to create and maintain the two-parent family as the only possible pattern for healthy family life.

Large Families

On the average, poor people are far more likely to have large families than persons at high socioeconomic levels. Large family size is particularly associated with low income, little education, low occupational status, and rural residence or origins (Whelpton, Campbell, and Patterson, 1965). Nonwhite families are especially likely to be large ones, and this is most closely related to poverty itself. Nonwhite families at higher educational and income levels are likely to be similar in size to white families of the same socioeconomic status.

A number of studies have shown that low-income families of all ethnic groups aspire to having no more than two or three children. Their aspirations are similar to those of people at higher income levels (Whelpton, Campbell, and Patterson, 1965). Some hold that the outstanding reason for the higher fertility rates of the very poor is that they lack access to family planning facilities (Jaffe and Polgar, 1968). Available evidence shows that when free, readily accessible, well-run family services are established, and the information disseminated, a large proportion of poor people of all races quickly make use of them. There are, of course, some religious objections to man-made contraceptive devices. There is also some opposition among nonwhites to the dissemination of family planning to the poor nonwhite on the theory that proponents seek to reduce the nonwhite population, particularly the blacks.

Some advocates have particularly espoused family planning for the poor. Some stress it for humanitarian reasons because of the close relation between large family size and such adversities as poor maternal and child health, continuing poverty, family breakdown, and less successful development of children. However, economic arguments of a tax-conscious nature are advanced by some people as the chief reason for making family planning services available to the poor. It appears that arguments of the latter sort are lacking in humanitarian consideration for the well-being of disadvantaged people as human beings. It seems unlikely that poor families would want to control the size of their families just to save their more fortunate fellows tax costs associated with aiding people in poverty. A lower birth rate is necessary in this country for people at all socioeconomic levels, not for the poor alone. Studies all over the world show that family planning appeals to parents because it offers an opportunity for them to achieve a better way of life for themselves and their children. Poor people, like others, are chiefly motivated by personal rather than public goals. Studies also show that small family size and effective use of contraceptives is associated with high income, high occupational status, and higher levels of education. Therefore, it appears that people are most likely to adopt contraceptives and use them effectively and continuously if other opportunities for parents and children are simultaneously available. Family planning programs alone are unlikely to solve the problems of poverty, but when they are combined with other services and supports, they offer important assistance to low-income parents whose problems are made more complex and pressing because of uncontrolled family size.

Poor Physical Health

Many aspects of the poverty situation operate together to create higher rates of poor physical health for the poor. Among the outstanding causes for this are: inadequate housing, lack of high-quality and readily available medical and dental services, poor nutrition, insufficient income, and little education. Research also indicates that poor people tend to adopt patterns which, together with these other factors, inhibit their effective use of medical services (Irelan, 1966).

It is well known that poor people are particularly likely not to receive adequate medical or dental care. In general, lacks are apt to be especially acute for rural people and members of such minority groups as Negroes, Indians, and Spanish-Americans. To a large extent, people in poverty are dependent on free services offered through clinics. These clinics are often overcrowded, impersonal, and understaffed. Many offer services only for specific conditions. Some provide services only for mothers and young children who are in generally good health (the maternal and child health programs funded by the Children's Bureau, for instance). Often services are located far from the homes of the poor and do not include provisions for transportation. Particularly in rural areas, medical and dental clinics may be totally unavailable.

Many poor children do not receive any health care at all. For instance, among children whose family income was less than $2,000 in 1963, only 7.5 percent under age seventeen visited a pediatrician, as compared to 33 percent of those in the $10,000 and above income level (U.S. Bureau of Census, 1966b). Black children receive about half as much attention from doctors as white children. Among poor Negroes, only one out of ten children is likely to see a pediatrician as often as once a year (*Health Care and the Negro Population,* 1965).

Most of the 600,000 children between the ages of three and five who attended Head Start programs in 1965 had never been to a physician or dentist and had not received their immunizations (U.S. House of Representatives, 1965).

Many clinics provide help only for the very poor; the near-poor, who cannot afford medical services but who are rejected because they are not in abject poverty, have extremely serious problems in getting medical care. Other problems associated with lack of medical care for the poor are related to their own informational deficits and, in some cases, such attitudes as distrust, alienation, and antiscientism. These attitudes are often reinforced by clinic practices and by the rejecting attitudes of some professionals. The move toward community and neighborhood health centers has not provided any guarantee of service or of effective delivery of services.

A number of advances have been made in providing medical care for the poor, such as the recent Medicaid legislation (Title XIX of the Social Security Act) and the Comprehensive Health Services Planning legislation. However, the implementation of Medicaid legislation has proved to be extremely difficult and expensive. Moreover, a number of states drastically restrict eligibility for these services to those who are in extreme poverty.

Health services for low-income mothers and young children have been available in some localities of this country for more than thirty years under the Maternal and Child Health provisions of the Social Security Act. Such programs have been funded by the Children's Bureau on a grant-in-aid basis upon the application of states. These programs have been limited in that they have not been statewide and they have offered services only to well mothers and their young children. Recent legislation provides that these programs must be statewide by 1975. It also provides for special medical care projects for mothers and infants who are in the so-called high-risk areas of poverty. About 54 of these special projects have been launched, and it appears that they have had an impact in reducing the infant and maternal mortality rates in the areas where they are located. All of the health programs described above have been seriously handicapped by lack of adequate budget appropriations. There is increasing belief that only fundamental shifts in service delivery methods and financing will correct America's health service inequities.

Chronic Unemployment and Underemployment

Chronic unemployment and underemployment of disadvantaged members of society has been a continuing problem even in times of general prosperity. Although many jobs are available, they require far higher levels of education and skill than the long-time poor generally have. This is particularly true for oppressed minority groups. Since this subject will be covered in greater depth in Chapter X, only a few highlights will be given here. Problems of unemployment are particularly critical for youth between the ages of sixteen and nineteen. In 1967 the unemployment rate for blacks in this age group was almost 30 percent compared to 10 percent for whites.

These rates, however, are misleading because they refer only to those persons who are known to be in the labor force and looking for a job. Large numbers of unemployed youth and adults do not actually register the fact that they are searching for employment, mostly because they feel that such registration is useless. The Department of Labor refers to this factor as the subemployment rate and estimates that one out of every three slum residents has a serious employment problem. In 1967 the subemployment rate of disadvantaged males was estimated to be about 34 percent in a sample of cities throughout the country. The combination of a booming economy, federal programs in job training and job placement, and efforts by the private sector has brought a considerable decline in the youth unemployment rate since 1961. However, efforts to cut the unemployment rate have not been on a large-scale basis, nor have they always accomplished their aim. For example, many youths finish training programs only to find they can't get jobs. Discriminatory practices still exist in many employment sectors, such as in the exclusionary policies set by some labor unions. Despite all efforts, the youth unemployment rate is still high, especially for nonwhite youth. As noted in Chapter I, the Commission believes that guaranteed employment is essential to the well-being and mental health of our nation's citizens.

Underemployment of disadvantaged youth and adults is a pervasive, but less obvious, problem. People with little education and few skills are likely to find only seasonal or part-time jobs if they find work at all. Many of these jobs are not covered by minimum wage provisions, and some are not covered by Social Security legislation. Furthermore, too many of these jobs are nonunion and do not provide employees the protection of organized labor. Even if a parent works full time at the minimum wage, he will not be able to move his family out of poverty if he is a city dweller and has two or more children. In order to earn a minimally adequate income, it is estimated that a father must work full time and a mother at least half time if both work at the minimum wage, have several children, and live in a city (Carter, 1968).

On the average, women are paid lower wages than men. This is particularly true for black women. For example, in 1965 black women who worked full time throughout the year earned a median income of about $2,700 compared to $3,700 for white women. Comparable figures for black men were $4,000 and about $6,200 for white men. The situation in terms of annual earnings has improved markedly for all groups since 1939, with the sharpest increase being from that date to 1955. Despite this increase, it is clear that, on the average, women cannot hope to earn enough, even if they work full time, to support a family of two or three children, and it seems certain they would not earn enough to pay for the care of their children while they work. We have already noted that a very large proportion of disadvantaged women with low earning potential have children under the age of six, and that free high-quality child-care facilities, such as day-care centers, are desperately needed.

The employment problems of poor people, especially of the nonwhite poor, have a severe impact on the well-being of children and youth in a wide variety of ways. Not only are they condemned to growing up in poverty or near-poverty and all the disadvantages that this brings, but they are accustomed early in life to frustration and failure. They lack the experience of having parents who cope successfully with the field of work. Even if they do have a father in the home, his employment problems are likely to lead his children, both boys and girls, to the conviction that he is a failure. This may lead them to reject their father as a male model. If his sons do identify with him, they are not apt to develop adequate patterns for coping with education and employment. Nor are they likely to find successfully employed men in their neighborhoods with whom they can identify and after whom they can pattern themselves. Of course the same principle applies to the problems that the mother is likely to have with employment and the impact that this has on both her sons and her daughters, psychologically as well as economically.

Inability to find work has a seriously adverse effect on a young person's overall sense of self-esteem, identity, and personal significance. Furthermore, unemployment is a major factor in the high rates of illegitimacy, desertion, and divorce found among low-income youth. For example, if a young man cannot find a job, both he and his young woman may believe that there is not much point in getting married, even though a baby has been born or is on the way. If they do marry, the strains of unemployment and little or no income are likely to weaken or destroy the marriage.

The unemployment problems of disadvantaged youth play a large part in their high rates of deviant behavior: delinquency and crime, alcoholism, and drug addiction. Unemployment problems of low-income young people interact with the other poverty factors to drastically reduce their opportunity for all aspects of positive development—physical, intellectual, emotional, social, and vocational.

The complex of factors which cause and perpetuate poverty are for the most part beyond the control of the individuals who are poor. In effect, the fault is largely in the system. Chronic and continuing poverty in a society such as ours might be viewed as a kind of fall-out resulting from the rapid pace of technological advances that have been made in our economic system. The majority of people in this society have reaped a host of benefits from this change. It is both unjust and irrational that poor people should not share in these benefits along with the rest of the population, and that the more affluent should hold them responsible for their own plight. This attitude is also irrational because the presence of extensive poverty burdens our entire nation, not just the poor. Guaranteed employment for those who are willing and able to work, and adequate subsistence for those who cannot work, are far more rational policies for our national interest. An all-out "war on poverty" may indeed be initially costly, and it seems inevitable that it would bring about rises in taxes at least for a time. However, tax investments to substantially reduce poverty would prove less costly over a period of time—in both human and economic resources.

Especially since 1962, there have been a number of federally financed programs aimed at reducing and preventing poverty and its problems. At present, a number of other approaches are under discussion. These programs and related issues will not be discussed in detail in this report because they relate to a highly specialized field on which a number of reports and publications are available. However, a few basic principles will be suggested here.

A number of diverse approaches to the solution of poverty and its problems have been tried under both private foundation and federal stimulation and financing in the past eight years or so. Until fairly recently, the major helping principle accompanying the chief public financial assistance program for children and families (AFDC) was that of individual counseling and social services.

This was based on the premise that poor people, as individuals, had personal problems which prevented their adjustment to society. The individual counseling program, however, was not well funded or staffed in most localities. With the development of the Federal Office of Juvenile Delinquency in 1961, a quite different approach was taken which was later adapted to a large extent by the Office of Economic Opportunity in its war against poverty. This new approach minimized the part that individual counseling might play and was aimed at "massive programs" designed to correct the major deficits in the social system that were closely associated with delinquency (in the case of the OJD programs) and poverty.

Analysis of 1960 census data, as already outlined in the foregoing section, revealed the important part which educational and vocational handicaps play in keeping poor people in poverty. Moreover, social science theory and community studies had pointed up the "powerlessness" and the exclusion of the poor from the so-called "community power structure." Largely as a result of these analyses and closely associated with the demands of leaders from poverty and minority groups, the antipoverty program focused on the following areas: job training (particularly for young people); enriched education (especially for preschool children through the Head Start program); community action and improvement in the "delivery system" of health, social, and legal services through such approaches as multipurpose neighborhood centers; involvement of poor people as employees, advisers, and policy-makers in poverty programs; and the employment of staff people from a wide range of backgrounds other than such traditional ones as social work.

Although the evidence is not all in because program evaluation is still in process, it appears that these antipoverty programs have made a considerable contribution to the slight reduction in the rate of poverty over the past five years. However, it will probably be impossible to ever sort out the various factors which contributed to this reduction and what part each played.

It would seem that the OEO program also made a number of other contributions. These include the opportunities that were provided to some of the poor for leadership, work experience in the human services fields, and involvement in the Head Start programs. It would appear that the latter program also made a significant contribution to increased public understanding and acceptance of the vital nature of preschool education, especially for disadvantaged children. The OEO program introduced, too, many new concepts into the thinking of professionals and community leaders. Although the reactions have been both positive and negative, to put it mildly, they have led to a ferment of reevaluation and new ideas in health, education, employment, and welfare fields.

There would seem to have been certain basic problems associated with the OEO programs, however. The most basic one is that they gave little cognizance to the fundamental importance of basic income support for poor people. This knotty problem was left up to the "old-line establishment" in the Department of Health, Education, and Welfare, whose functions include the administration of public assistance through grants-in-aid to the states. In most of the states the levels of public assistance are grossly inadequate both in terms of the size of the relief grants and in terms of restrictions on eligibility.

It is imperative that people have enough money to live on if they are to take advantage of such programs as vocational training, community involvement, remedial education, and all the rest. If people lack food, clothing, and shelter they are unable to turn their attention to other important, but less immediately relevant, concerns. Thus, guaranteed employment and an adequate financial assistance program for needy individuals and families are basic to all other antipoverty strategies.

The antipoverty program was set up with perhaps overly optimistic goals. It was claimed that this program would solve poverty within a few years. It is possible that such a goal is totally unrealistic, that one cannot easily solve a problem that has been in the making for many generations; however, the "war against poverty" was hardly an all-out offensive effort. It did not put money in the pockets of the poor. It had too little funding, and the programs were too short-lived. This lack of funding, and the short range of the projects, was closely associated with the diversion of funds to the Vietnam war. It also was associated with the reluctance of the taxpayers and, hence, Congress to appropriate a sufficient amount of money over a long enough period of time to finance the kinds of long-range projects that were needed. Along with this lack of sufficient funding went a shortage of administrative personnel to carry out the programs. Moreover, there would seem to have been too little time allowed and too little money for carefully designed administrative structures and fiscal controls.

Unrealistic methods were used in some features of the OEO programs. This particularly applies to the community action programs. Although there was lack of clarity in the administrative guidelines associated with these programs, their fundamental purpose, at least in some communities, was to bring about needed social changes through action programs which included "maximum feasible participation of the poor." These programs, deriving in large part from theory regarding community power structures and the exclusion of poor people from the "opportunity system," sought to increase the ability of the poor and minority-group people to participate as citizens in civic affairs, to make them feel a full sense of participation and acceptance in the society, and thus to enhance their sense of dignity and self-worth.

The value of maximum feasible participation is suggested by large bodies of social science and pragmatic evidence. It has helped people to assert themselves, and no one can question that the people's movements have been effective.

The debate rages around whether the "establishment" represented by legislative power should provide tax funds for attacks on itself (Marris and Rein, 1967; O'Donnell and Chilman, 1969). The government pays for all sorts of research for new knowledge. It has never consciously paid to educate for revolt against itself, although it has paid for new efforts that go counter to socioeconomic tradition, such as TVA, Medicare, and Medicaid.

Usually movements designed to change law, the social system, or any parts of it are financed by individual persons or organizations. Labor or professional organizations, for instance, do this often, and there have been poor people's groups in the past, as there are now. None of them was financed by the government, as is the community action program of the OEO.

Most importantly, in summary, the antipoverty programs administered by the Office of Economic Opportunity were almost too late, were too little, and were too short-lived. On the other hand, many of the basic concepts on which they were built (stepped-up job training, preschool projects, involvement of poor people in staffing and planning their own programs, and the development of multiservice neighborhood centers) would seem to remain sound with the major exception that they overlooked the crucial importance of adequate public assistance programs for unemployed or underemployed poor people. People who need money to live on, unless they have an adequate job, need money as a first priority.

The most effective OEO programs will remain and, as with Head Start —now operated by a new Office of Child Development in HEW—will move to operating agencies when all concerned agree that they should be transferred. These include the legal and neighborhood health services. OEO, after all, is not a Cabinet department but an agency in the President's office. It was designed to stimulate and bring about innovation and to get the establishment to change. These it did well. The coordinative function failed simply because one operating agency cannot coordinate its operating peers. True coordination needs power and should be above the chaos of operational competition.

Some OEO programs, such as multiservice centers, suffered from the fact that dozens of other agencies were also involved. Every agency, including OEO, was and still is competing for ownership of the neighborhood social welfare services and health delivery systems.

During this same period, efforts were being made to improve the Aid to Families with Dependent Children program as well as other public assistance programs. Many of the features of the public assistance programs, particularly AFDC, have been burdened with centuries-old punitive attitudes toward the poor. These attitudes obviously persist today in many segments of our society. They have been sharpened by the fact that the numbers of people receiving AFDC have been steadily increasing during the past decade and are continuing to increase at the present writing (early 1969). This increase has caused great public consternation, especially in view of the declining rates of poverty and the fact that we are experiencing times of high prosperity.

In 1968 about 4,500,000 children lived in families that were receiving AFDC payments. This number represented *less than half of the nation's children in families below the poverty line.* The assistance grant for children in most states left them deeply enmeshed in poverty. On the average, a family of four received an annual income of about $2,000 a year from the AFDC program: *only about one-half of a basic subsistence income.* Despite the clear evidence that the most serious deficit of the AFDC program is that it failed to provide anything like minimum financial support for needy children, the 1962 amendments to the Social Security Act (under which this program was established in 1935) put emphasis on improving casework services for poor people. Implementation of these amendments was left up to the states. At that time, it was thought that the AFDC rolls could be reduced by improving the quantity and quality of individual social services for assistance recipients. This concept was tied to the erroneous belief that families could resolve their financial problems through the improved adjustment of their individual members. By 1967 it was clear that the individualized casework approach had not made an impact on reducing the problem of economic dependency. In fact, AFDC case loads were rising rapidly. It was evident that although individual counseling may be effective in helping some poor people "make a better adjustment," they have to have something better to adjust to, such as readily available steady jobs with adequate wages, decent housing that they can afford, free facilities for good-quality care of children when mothers work, free or low-cost medical care to remedy physical disabilities, and the like. In short, individuals must have basic economic and other material needs met before they can turn their attention to other matters to which casework and the larger mental health programs generally address themselves, such as improving methods of child care and home-making practices, using community resources, resolving emotional problems, and the like. The seeming failure of the individual or group counseling approach to measurably alter the financial problems of dependent families played an important part in the development of the 1967 amendments to the Social Security Act, as will be discussed later.

While the intent of the AFDC is to strengthen family life and to maintain children economically, it has suffered from residual harsh community attitudes toward recipients, the absence of national standards, and the fact that each state essentially sets its own grant levels and administrative policies. Standards of support have been generally lower than an acceptable minimum level of "health and decency." Persons receiving aid were subject to public attitudes blaming them for their plight and subjecting them to an atmosphere of rejection and punishment for being poor.

Rejecting and punitive policies have included the following: extremely low and short-term grants; arbitrary withdrawal of assistance while families are still in need; denial of assistance if the father of the children is present in the home; methods of determining eligibility that have been slow and inquisitorial in nature; public assistance offices which are usually far from the homes of many applicants and involve long hours of waiting; public assistance rules and regulations that have often developed into such a complex maze that even the social workers—let alone the recipients and applicants—are at a loss to understand them; and, until recently, deduction of most or all of the earnings of a recipient from the assistance grant so that there was very little, if any, reward to getting and holding a job. Regulations such as these would seem to be designed for the failure, rather than success, of a program which is theoretically designed to help people escape from poverty. Incidentally, there is a widespread tendency on the part of the general public to blame social workers for the inhumanities and inequities of the public assistance programs in many states and localities. Fundamentally, the problem resides within the inhumane and inequitable provisions and financing of the system rather than in the people who administer it. Some staff personnel, as well as some recipients, may well be brutalized by this system, but the fault lies primarily in a citizenry that fails to support a generous and humane program.

The 1967 amendments to the Social Security Act attempted to eliminate some of the inequities in the public assistance system, but its major thrust was aimed at reducing the size of the AFDC case loads and the costs of this program. One of its major provisions was that all recipients over the age of sixteen, unless attending school, should be referred for training and employment if they were physically able to work or not required to remain at home because of the illness or incapacity of another member of the household. However, mothers of young children are not to be referred for training and employment unless necessary child-care arrangements can be made (The Welfare and Child Health Provisions of the Social Security Amendments of 1967, 1968). Unfortunately, adequate day-care facilities are virtually nonexistent in most parts of the country. There is no community in which they even begin to meet the needs of poor working mothers. Although federal aid is legislatively made available to states for development of day-care programs, the funding of this legislation is tragically inadequate.

The recent Social Security amendments further provided that AFDC recipients who found work would be permitted to retain more of their earnings. This is termed the work incentive program or, as some of the AFDC mothers have named it, "the work insensitive program." The great majority of mothers on AFDC have infant or preschool children. Although studies show that many prefer employment to public assistance, another group expresses a preference for staying home and caring for their own young children rather than placing them in child-care centers. Some point up that more advantaged women who are fortunate enough to have husbands who earn an adequate income to support the family have the right to choose whether or not they will enter the work force and leave the care of their children to other people. They also ask why they should get jobs which involve taking care of "rich people's children," as in domestic service, and pay someone else to take care of their own children when, in the long run, it would be just as economical for them to stay home and care for their own youngsters. These are cogent questions and complex issues. It would seem that one of the basic issues is whether poor people have an order of rights different from those of other more fortunate people. One suggested solution to this question has been that all mothers be paid a basic annual wage from tax funds for taking care of their children, since good child care in an economically secure home is very much in the public interest (Gil, 1969).

A particularly harsh feature of the 1967 amendments limits the federal sharing in costs of AFDC programs to the average monthly number of children under eighteen who received assistance in each state's AFDC program in the months of January through March, 1968. This is the so-called "AFDC freeze." It means, in effect, that the AFDC program in each state cannot receive federal support for a larger number of children than was the case in the winter of 1968. As of this writing, this so-called "freeze" has been eliminated by Congressional action, and the Supreme Court voided all state restrictions on residence.

Another feature of the amendments relates to inclusion of families in the AFDC program when an unemployed father is present in the home. The central features of this legislation provide that such families cannot receive aid unless it is demonstrated that the unemployed father has had "a substantial connection with the labor force." These provisions are particularly harsh in reference to very young fathers who have not had an opportunity to "form a substantial connection with the labor force." As pointed out near the beginning of this chapter, unemployment rates of low-income males, especially nonwhite males in poverty areas, are extremely high, primarily because steady, well-paying jobs are not available for people who lack educational and employment skills and who are handicapped by generations of poverty and discrimination. Provisions of this kind quite clearly tend to increase, rather than decrease, family breakdown.

At present, a number of proposals are being made to change the welfare system. There seems to be widespread agreement that steps must be taken to "straighten out the welfare mess." Quite naturally, there are different points of view as to what the nature of this "mess" is. Generally speaking, it appears that the nonpoor usually see the problem as being related to rising public assistance rolls and increasing tax costs. On the other hand, poor people are apt to view the problem as being largely one of low relief grants, punitive features in the legislation, and inhumane methods of administration. Various proposals are made, such as the negative income tax, guaranteed annual income, extended Social Security to cover the unemployed poor, and family allowances. Some of these appear to gain popularity because they are considered to be less expensive than the present system. It would seem that we have not faced up to the fact that there is no cheap way of solving the problem of poverty. No matter what system of public assistance is used, if it costs less than the present program, it cannot make any significant impact on the economic problems of the very poor. Moreover, no matter what name is given to public assistance and no matter how it is administered it will not be acceptable to people in need unless their fundamental economic requirements are met. Although poor people, quite rightly, object to being treated like second-class citizens because they need public assistance, more humane administrative methods will not reduce their basic problems or their basic objections unless the size of their grant or allowance or tax write-off is large enough to pay for their fundamental financial needs.

A number of changes are required for the alleviation of poverty in this country. Basic changes are needed in public attitudes, understanding, and willingness to invest in people who, through no fault of their own, have been left behind by the technological revolution. A positive approach is required that puts values on enhancing the potential of people rather than saving money. We must make larger, *long-term* investments in human beings: children, youth, fathers, and mothers. This includes adequate income support and a complex of health, education, vocational, social, and environmental services that are readily available, coordinated, and offered in such a way that poor people share in their planning and implementation. We need a flexibility and diversity of services aimed at strengthening families and individuals. We especially need more humane attitudes toward disadvantaged males and must include them in all service and public assistance programs.

A great increase in steady, well-paying jobs which disadvantaged people can hold is essential. It is particularly essential that there be an increase in the numbers of jobs available in the human service fields and a restructuring of these jobs so that they provide opportunities for career development, as well as opportunities for the employment of people who lack traditional technical or professional preparation in such fields as education, health, and the social services. It is important that jobs be developed and made available on a part-time as well as a full-time basis so that they may be held by mothers and young people in school. A number of these jobs might well be in such mental health-related fields as clinics, hospitals, Child Development Councils, schools, playgrounds, and the like.

Furthermore, it is important that we recognize that not everyone can obtain and hold employment in our modern society. At present, we accept the fact that persons who are handicapped by old age, severe physical disabilities, and extreme mental retardation cannot logically be expected to earn their own way through employment. We need also to accept the idea that society's interests might be better served by paying mothers of infants and young children to stay at home and raise these children rather than forcing them to go to work because of economic need. We need to accept the fact that some people are unable to work because of less obvious and more subtle problems such as those associated with serious emotional disturbance and mental illness.

It is important that we reexamine the work ethic of our society which originally arose out of the necessity that every able-bodied male be employed full-time so that enough goods could be produced to meet the needs of society. Now that machines have taken over much of the job of production this is no longer a necessity. This is another area in which social and economic changes are causing an upheaval in our value system. It is time that we reexamine our cultural patterns which hold that every family should be self-supporting and that, at least in the case of males, personal identity and self-respect are directly determined by occupational status.

Finally, we need to develop national, rather than local or state, programs directed toward reducing poverty and the many disadvantages which it imposes upon poor people. The states which can least afford to support and aid their poor people have the greatest numbers of the poor and need a greater share of national income to meet their problems. Furthermore, poor people move from one state to another in search of work or more adequate public assistance and related services. Therefore, national programs are needed which at the same time are highly flexible and diverse so that they may be adapted to the life styles and situations which obtain in different parts of the country.

HOW MUCH POVERTY FOR HOW MUCH LONGER?

How much longer will the people of this nation deny essential commitment to humanitarian principles? How much longer will they let more than 10,-000,000 children grow up in families where there is little to eat; where mothers are defeated and exhausted by too little of everything except children; where houses are crowded, infected with vermin, cold in winter, and stifling in summer; where fathers are humiliated by failure and rejection; where money is a small and sometime thing; where neighborhoods are dead-alive with violence, danger, exploitation, and the desperate search for a quick escape; where frightened and angry children go to crowded rundown schools to be taught by angry and frightened teachers how to pledge allegiance to the flag (with liberty and justice for all) and to read about an America they have never known; where, if one is black he finds that this automatically makes him inferior to *any* person with a white skin? And you get away from it all by looking at television or going to the movies, if you are lucky? There you find that there is a world of travel by plane and luxurious cars; a world of perfumes, furs, and private swimming pools; a world of pedigreed dogs who are fed only the finest meats; a world where men earn money "just by sitting at desks" and women spend their days cooking gourmet meals in spotless kitchens; a world where bad breath and stuffed-up noses are the most serious problems one can have.

The wonder is not that poor people have higher rates of emotional disturbance, school failure, poor health, unemployment, family breakdown, and crime than other people do. The wonder is that they survive as well as they do, that many do manage to "develop normally," get jobs, stay married, and fail to rise up in revolt against a society that has so much, shares so little, and condemns the poor for their "shiftless ways." The strengths, rather than the weaknesses, of so many of the poor are a tribute to them and the human urge to survive and aspire to a better world for their children, if not for themselves.

The stirring theme song for at least some of the poor and dispossessed of the 1960's has been: "We shall overcome—some day." Increasingly, the poor and dispossessed—and those others who are willing and able to *really* listen—are saying: "Not some day, but now." Such assertive action in behalf of one's own salvation is one of the important building blocks of good mental health. Are the more affluent citizens of our communities ready to truly support the assertions and the mental health of the poor— and thereby the mental health of *all* citizens?

SUMMARY

Eight major factors are closely associated with poverty: little education, the poverty environment, chronic unemployment, low income, life styles which are a product of impoverishment, poor physical and mental health, large families, and broken families. These factors interact in ways that keep poor families entrapped in an intergenerational cycle of poverty.

Clearly, poverty cannot be reduced or prevented unless there is a co-ordinated, simultaneous attack on removing or reducing these factors and their effects. This means that: free, high-quality education from preschool through vocational and graduate training must be available to all children and youth; the poverty environment must be radically and immediately improved through adequate housing, recreation, and other community services; vocational training, wages, and job opportunities in the public and private sectors of society must be guaranteed for those who are unemployed and underemployed, especially our youth; public assistance must be adequate to provide a decent standard of living and administered in ways that respect human dignity; high-quality, free physical and mental health and social services must be available to all those who cannot otherwise pay for them; parents and youth of all ethnic and socioeconomic backgrounds must be granted full and equal opportunities to participate in the planning and development of these and other community services. All of these programs could be coordinated through the neighborhood Child Development Councils and other advocate bodies recommended by the Commission. Advocacy functions could ensure that these programs and services are available to all children, youth, and their parents.

To effectively solve the problems of poverty, we must systematically reorder our impersonal and inadequate social and economic systems so they will meet human needs. If our communities are to achieve a mentally healthy climate, its citizens must look collectively at community problems and work together with professionals to use the knowledge we now have in order that new approaches can be developed to solve the problems that threaten the physical and mental well-being of every community member. We must act now on these data.

Children of Minority Groups: A Special Mental Health Risk

A note on the preparation of this chapter:

Very early in the Commission's study, it was recognized that the mental health problems of minority-group children are severe enough to warrant special consideration. Accordingly, a multi-ethnic, multi-professional committee of knowledgeable members was formed in mid-1967.

The Committee on Children of Minority Groups, as it has been known, had a maximum membership of thirteen plus liaison representation from the National Institute of Mental Health and the Division of Indian Health, both parts of the Public Health Service. This group has had a very deep interest in its task of promoting the mental health of the victimized children of minority groups. The Committee's report is an eloquent and valuable document.

In dealing with the issues of minority-group children in the Commission report, it was decided to handle these matters by securing the direct contribution of the members of this Committee. This chapter, therefore, is a product resulting from a very close working relationship among the Commission staff and members of the Committee on Children of Minority Groups. It has been reviewed by them. To the maximum extent possible, their suggestions have been utilized. This chapter, therefore, represents the views of the minorities involved, not the perception of their views by a person lacking group membership characteristics.

The mental health problems of minority-group children are so severe that they warrant immediate and drastic attention. Although this problem has been the basic concern of the Commission's Committee on Children of Minority Groups, it must be emphasized that we plead not only in behalf of these dispossessed children but for the future of our nation. A nation is only as strong as its people; its future lies in its young.

Poverty and racism have created a divisiveness which threatens our future and weakens our society and its citizens. There is, however, a new hope because there is a new spirit among the peoples of oppressed minorities. Each group is seeking—and even sometimes demanding—a recognition and acceptance of its unique cultural identity and right to equal opportunities. We believe this direction to be one which is conducive to good mental health.

We believe that mental health is the result of all factors—social, psychological, and biological—that permit a person to be free of crippling emotional states such as overwhelming fear, anger, envy, and racist projections. Such a person operates as a contributing member of his society and feels himself to be both effective and efficient. He is capable of strong and satisfying love relationships.

Presently, many minority-group children are denied the opportunities to achieve this ideal state of mental health. Only rarely does the child of an ethnic minority escape the damaging effects of racism. Often racism and poverty combine to cripple the minority-group child in body, mind, and spirit. The evidence presented below is testimony to the tremendous adverse effects which these two social factors—poverty and racism—have upon child development and child mental health.

THE PROBLEM OF RACISM

Racism is the number one public health problem facing America today. The conscious and unconscious attitudes of superiority which permit and demand that a majority oppress a minority are a clear and present danger to the mental health of all children and their parents. Traditionally, the criteria for defining public health problems are: (1) a problem that threatens a large number of people; (2) a problem that costs a large sum of money; (3) a problem that is impossible to treat on an individual and private basis; and (4) a problem that could cause chronic sustained disability.

The Commission's Committee on Children of Minority Groups believes that the racist attitude of Americans which causes and perpetuates tension is patently a most compelling health hazard. Its destructive effects severely cripple the growth and development of millions of our citizens, young and old alike. Yearly, it directly and indirectly causes more fatalities, disabilities, and economic loss than any other single factor.

Over the last two decades there has been a proliferation of scientific papers in the behavioral sciences attesting to damage to children, black and white, that can be directly traced to this endemic condition. Historically, minority groups of color have experienced the lash of racism. This is true whether we study the degradation of Indians, the subjugation of Mexican-Americans, the exploitation of the Puerto Ricans, the brutal relocation of the Japanese, the callous treatment of all Orientals, or the unresolved black question.

We must accept that the United States is not a white nation. The idealized image of the melting pot has, fortunately, never been realized. Our strength as a society rests in cultural pluralism. Biological evolution demonstrates the survival value inhering in a range of physical types within the species. So does a nation profit when the unique cultural skills, styles, and genius of diverse peoples are valued as societal assets.

The country is now experiencing an acute crisis. The legitimate demands of the alienated and emerging groups of this country, if unmet, constitute a threat to our continued existence as a nation, as well as our potential role in the international sphere. Social scientists now have the predictive ability to forecast that the Mexican-Americans in the Southwest, the impoverished Appalachian residents, the newly assertive Indians, and the isolated urban dwellers all have the same capacity for a violent resolution of our social crisis.

There are indications that the history of black people in the United States will be paralleled by other minority groups in America in the near future. Hope was generated by the 1954 and 1955 Supreme Court decisions.

During the late 1950's and early 1960's, hope was sustained while the blacks petitioned for economic viability through nonviolent means. However, the failure to correct social and economic inequities and injustices following the 1964 Civil Rights Act and other socioeconomic programs resulted in the mobilization of frustration and anger to the point of rebellion. Currently, the black population, filled with despair and ever aware of the failure of the actualization of bright promises, has become mindful of its need to unite in order to defend itself against the institution of repressive measures by the majority population. In a shorter order, the Mexican-American, the Puerto Rican, and the American Indian, without social intervention, may travel the same historical path.

The response to date by the mainstream culture has been not amelioration of grievances but punitive action. There have been few basic social or economic changes directed toward altering the value system of this society. There has been tragically little self-examination. The pathology of denial and lack of awareness has reached massive proportions. This indifference has robbed all Americans of the psychic energy so necessary for healthy functioning.

One of the realities of present-day America is that increasingly large segments of the minority population will be obliged to live in segregated communities, at least over the next couple of decades. In general, without massive intervention, this fact means that the majority of minority children born between now and the end of the century will be growing up in mentally unhealthy atmospheres rampant with substandard housing, inferior education, and poor health care.

The country must outgrow its legacy of racism. There must be massive outpourings of resources, both financial and human, if the problems are to be resolved. A minority child must grow up seeing himself and his life as having positive value. The white child must be equipped to live as a member of a multiracial world. These achievements will allow both children to grow up less handicapped by the effects of guilt, fear, anger, and anxiety.

The mutual distrust so prevalent in this country is leading to the polarization of Americans. The growth and viability of our society are dependent on everyone's achieving a full measure of growth and development. This is true no less of the majority whites than the minority group member. While the financial cost of eradicating racism in all walks of national life will obviously be immense, the result of making it possible for millions of wasted human beings to contribute to our national production and creativity, the development of millions of new consumers for our national product, the improvement of our commercial relations with problems of other nations, and the cut in the present enormous costs of inadequate welfare programs would seem to make it a relatively sound investment. The society can truly find new strength and integrity by an acceptance of all diversity.

MANIFESTATIONS OF RACISM AFFECTING THE MENTAL HEALTH OF MINORITY-GROUP CHILDREN

Racism now permeates the major institutions of our society. Racist policies and attitudes perpetuate poverty, crime, semiliteracy, and poor physical and mental health. While the consequences of racism affect us all, they pose a far more serious threat to the large numbers of children who are members of minority groups. It is these children who are most crippled in body and spirit, who are the targets of racist attitudes and practices which so threaten mental health.

Typically, we think of racist-type attitudes as being directed toward and affecting only those whose skin color differs from that of white America. While it is certainly far more difficult for people of color to escape from racist domination, such discrimination is by no means limited to non-whites. Phrases denouncing the poor as "immoral, lazy, and shiftless" defy all color bounds. These defamations apply to poor "white trash" as well, often with the expressed belief that such people, like the nonwhites, are biologically inferior.

The mainstream culture has yet to learn from its history that people can rise out of poverty to become contributing members of society only to plunge again into the depths of want and dependency when society withdraws the means for self-sufficiency. Appalachia has taught us nothing. The once independent mountaineer family is slowly disintegrating; its fate is now linked to those forces which determine the stability of the oppressed nonwhite. It, too, is falling victim to lack of economic opportunity plus a welfare system which perpetuates poverty and lowers self-esteem. The mainstream culture barricades itself against the weakness of its cultural and socioeconomic system by formulating racist rationalizations. Individuals —and even races—are held responsible for their own plight; inequality of opportunity is ignored. After generations of isolation and poverty, the oppressed themselves begin to doubt their own self-worth; a "self-fulfilling prophecy" arises from these doubts—one easily reinforced by the rationalizations and inequalities perpetuated by the majority.

Prejudicial Treatment of Minority-Group Youth by Social Institutions

The child growing up as a member of a minority group learns that his role in relationship to most social institutions differs from that of other children. He learns that members of his racial or ethnic group are likely to live in the least desirable section of town—the inner city, the ghetto, the barrio, the reservation, or the rural depressed areas. He discovers that hunger, poor health, and demoralizing housing are the lot of those who live in his neighborhood. The unemployment or underemployment of the adults around him does little to stimulate his interest in preparing for a career. Inadequate transportation and a paucity of recreational resources force him to find what entertainment he can in his home environment. In an overcrowded classroom, his teacher treats him in accordance with her stereotyped notions of his minority group. Not only his textbooks but television and the movies suggest to him that the good life is mostly white middle or upper class. Legal recourse, medical help, even adequate shopping facilities are not available in his neighborhood. Policemen become a visible manifestation of the enemy—the affluent world, the society that institutionalizes his degradation.

By the time he reaches adulthood, the minority-group youth realizes that he is inescapably branded by white racists as inferior because of a racial or ethnic inheritance from which he cannot escape. With the opportunity channels of the greater society closed against him, he feels more secure competing for whatever status positions are available within his isolated environment. Demoralized by the self-concept he sees mirrored in the eyes of society and debilitated by an unhealthy environment, he is not likely to escape from a cage of poverty and bigotry unless the social conditions which bludgeoned him into that cage are changed.

Maladaptive Life Patterns

To survive discrimination and poverty, many minority-group youths adopt a life pattern which in itself perpetuates the cycle of poverty. Motivation is stifled by a society which apparently prefers to support the poor with welfare payments which keep them at a level of bare subsistence rather than to allow minority groups an equal opportunity within the economic structure. The marginal activities of the ghetto, the reservation, the barrio, or the depressed rural sections are the only social settings in which many opportunities exist for enhancing self-esteem. Large families are at once a burden and a supportive group. Education may correlate with economic advancement, but the school institution tends to push out those children who cannot conform to the goals established by the school. Such life circumstances may be accepted in a pattern of ennui, hopelessness, and despair. A healthier adaptation may be rebellion.

Inadequate Mental Health Services

Although living in circumstances which continually threaten their mental health, for minority-group youth and the disadvantaged, mental health services may be virtually inaccessible. Clinics are often located at a distance from the poverty neighborhood. Service is preceded by a lengthy intake process and predicated on long-term treatment methods which may be inappropriate to the life style of the client. Mental health personnel are poorly equipped to understand the client's environment and feelings and may find communication beyond a superficial level to be impossible.

The disadvantaged are often reluctant to use what mental health services are available. Accustomed to the discomforts of ill health and unable to budget for medical care, the poor eschew preventive care and seek help only for emergencies. The poorly educated may not only ignore the first symptoms of mental illness but may hold unenlightened views of the nature of such illness.

Thus, our social arrangements to cope with mental health are, like other institutions in this society, less available to minority-group youth than to other youth.

PROBLEMS AND TRENDS RELATED TO THE MENTAL HEALTH OF MINORITY-GROUP CHILDREN AND YOUTH

Throughout the Commission's report there is overwhelming evidence of the relationship between poverty and minority-group status, particularly as related to Negroes, Puerto Ricans, Mexican-Americans, Indians, migrant workers, and white Appalachians. The facts and figures presented in other chapters show that unemployment, underemployment, and low wages are characteristic of large proportions of these groups and that among the multiple causes of poverty are racist policies and attitudes. The facts further show that education is still not the same vehicle to upward mobility for oppressed minorities as it is for the majority. Physical and mental health services continue to be dispensed on a discriminatory basis—if they are available at all to the poor.

As a consequence of these factors, millions of minority-group children suffer from untreated disorders. Millions are denied such basic human needs as adequate diets and housing, even where public assistance is granted. Further, many experience an unstable family life because of male unemployment and/or because public welfare measures, in some areas, encourage family breakdown. Many children must care for themselves because there are no adequate child-care facilities for mothers who *must* work.

We will not reiterate the facts and figures presented in other chapters but will attempt to convey the consequences of poverty and other factors upon the mental health of minority-group children.

DEMOGRAPHIC FACTORS

Age and Geographic Distribution

Tables 6 and 7 show the age and geographic distribution of the principal minority groups in the United States.

Table 6 shows that, in comparison to the white population, a larger percent of all minority populations is under fourteen years of age. The high percentage of youth among minority groups is significant in terms of the responsibilities which should be undertaken for the mental health of children.

Table 7 divides the United States into four regions and shows the distribution of principal minority groups in those regions. As shown, for each minority group included, more than half live within one region. Overall, Negroes make up the largest of these subgroups; they constitute about 11 percent of the nation's population.

Concentration in Urban Areas

Minority-group peoples are increasingly becoming an urban population. The majority of Puerto Ricans migrate from the island to New York City, the Orientals from their lands to Western cities. Of the more than 20,000,000 Negroes in the United States today, almost three-fourths are

Table 6.—Age Distribution of Principal Ethnic Groups in the United States, 1960

GROUP	14 YEARS AND UNDER	15 TO 19 YEARS	20 YEARS AND OVER	TOTAL
White	48,084,986	11,608,229	99,138,517	158,831,732
	30%	7%	63%	100%
Negro	7,085,970	1,496,991	10,590,715	19,173,676
	37%	8%	55%	100%
Indian	230,733	49,897	275,392	556,022
	41%	9%	50%	100%
Japanese	148,167	31,228	301,032	480,427
	31%	7%	62%	100%
Mexican-American[1]	1,449,629	306,979	1,708,391	3,464,999
	41.8%	8.8%	49.4%	100%
Puerto Rican	344,996	75,784	471,733	892,513
	38.6%	8.5%	52.9%	100%

[1] Data available only for white persons of Spanish surname in Arizona, California, Colorado, New Mexico, and Texas.

Sources: U.S. Department of Labor, Bureau of the Census, *Census of Population: 1960 United States Summary;* and Subject Reports on *Nonwhite Population by Race, Persons of Spanish Surname,* and *Puerto Ricans in the United States* (Washington, D.C.: Government Printing Office, 1963).

Table 7.—Regional Distribution of Principal Minority Groups in the United States, 1960

GROUP	NORTHEAST[1]	NORTH CENTRAL[2]	SOUTH[3]	WEST[4]	U.S.
Negro	3,082,499	3,446,037	11,311,607	1,085,488	18,925,631
	16%	18%	60%	6%	100%
Indian	26,356	98,631	127,568	271,036	523,591
	5%	19%	24%	52%	100%
Japanese	17,962	29,318	16,245	400,807	464,332
	4%	6%	4%	86%	100%
Mexican-American[5]			3,464,999		
Puerto Rican[6]					892,513
					100%

[1] Connecticut, Maine, Massachusetts, New Hanmpshire, New Jersey, New York, Pennsylvania, Rhode Island, Vermont.
[2] Illinois, Indiana, Iowa, Kansas, Michigan, Minnesota, Missouri, Nebraska, North Dakota, Ohio, South Dakota, Wisconsin.
[3] Alabama, Arkansas, Delaware, District of Columbia, Florida, Georgia, Kentucky, Louisiana, Maryland, Mississippi, North Carolina, Oklahoma, South Carolina, Tennessee, Texas, Virginia, West Virginia.
[4] Alaska, Arizona, California, Colorado, Hawaii, Idaho, Montana, Nevada, New Mexico, Oregon, Utah, Washington, Wyoming.
[5] Census data available only for white persons of Spanish surname in Arizona, California, Colorado, New Mexico, and Texas.
[6] Regional data not available for Puerto Ricans.

Sources: See Table 6.

concentrated in metropolitan areas. Mexican-Americans, who have traditionally tended to settle in the Southwest, are increasingly becoming an urban population. Only the white Appalachians and the American Indian continue to cling to the rural setting. About two-thirds of the Indians still live on reservations.

Displaced by mechanization of farms and other rural occupations, many minority-group families have looked to the city for a better way of life. Instead, most of them are met with the harsh realities of discrimination, lack of adequate housing, and little or no employment. Few training opportunities are open for the large numbers of poorly educated, semiskilled workers; however, full employment has been no guarantee of adequate wages for many of these families. The result for many has been confinement to the most depressed areas of our cities—a reality which has bred much bitterness and frustration.

While much of our research may be suspect because of middle-class biases, studies carried out in several large cities indicate that the very poor urban dweller may find little security or pleasure in his life, especially in public housing projects or other congested dwelling units. A sense of fear and mistrust is common, as are outbursts of violence. Many contacts are conflict-laden. In this environment, children have little chance to learn interpersonal skills or to develop a sense of trust in others (Chilman, 1966).

The physical environment of urban ghettos adds to the difficulties in child-rearing. Sanitation and garbage controls are often inadequate. Rat bites are not uncommon and are sometimes fatal to the young. Many ghetto residents complain of police harassment and of inadequate police and fire protection. The unequal distribution of legal services gives the poor a sense of hopelessness in attempting to rectify such complaints. Recreational facilities are also insufficient or lacking. Thus, at an early age the streets are used for recreational activities, and "street life" becomes one of the major environmental influences on the child's life. Unable to find employment, and often discouraged by the school experience, many minority-group youths join their peers on the streets, where existence is validated by "illegal" and antisocial activities.

The Rural Poor

Disadvantaged young people in rural areas fare no better than their urban brothers. The number of such children living in rural areas is difficult to determine. However, statistics show that 30 percent of all families receiving payments under the Aid to Dependent Families program in 1961 lived in rural areas.

Life is particularly difficult for Indians and migrant workers. Most reservations are underdeveloped areas characterized by semi-isolation, pervasive unemployment, and a myriad of problems related to social and community disorganization. Physical facilities are highly inadequate. By government criteria, 90 percent of Indian housing is substandard. Only one-third of the families have a safe water supply and waste disposal facilities. Their homes lack refrigeration, furniture, and adequate cooking space. Dirt floors add to the environmental hazards. At the present rate of construction, water and sanitation facilities will not be common for another fifteen or twenty years, and from thirty to forty years will be required to provide adequate housing for Indian populations.

The environment of children of migrant workers is similarly undesirable. Home is often a duck coop, an automobile, or a tent.

Education promises little hope for upward mobility for Indians and migrant children. It is estimated that 50,000 migrant children are traveling when they should normally be in school, and large numbers do not attend school at the beginning and end of school semesters. Many will continue to be in the fields rather than in school until they receive the same protection as other children under the Fair Labor Standards Act (Bennett, 1967). Education for many Indian children means little more than custodial care in boarding schools far from home and family.

Other disadvantaged rural youngsters face similar problems. Semiliteracy is still common in the South, in Appalachia, and in other rural areas populated by minority peoples. Because so few employment opportunities exist in these areas for disadvantaged youth, many migrate to cities. Few, however, are prepared to compete in the urban work setting. Low educational levels, inadequate work habits, and a lack of job skills combine with discrimination against young job-seekers and against minority-group or disadvantaged youth to limit opportunities for jobs and training at decent wages.

A Profile of Deprivation

The following profile of a Job Corps enrollee reveals a background characteristic of minority-group youth.

A further description of minority peoples and their problems should offer some insight into the factors which account for the profile of a Job Corps enrollee.

FAMILY PATTERNS

Among minority groups the family has been a principal contributing factor to the mental health of children despite the many difficulties imposed on family stability by poverty and discrimination. The strength and love of

Table 8.—PROFILE OF A JOB CORPS ENROLLEE

	MALE	FEMALE
DEMOGRAPHIC FACTORS		
Age	17.5	18.0
Race (percent Negro)	56.0	48.0
EDUCATION		
Years in school	8.8	9.8
Reading level (40% of Corpsmen in conservation centers read below third-grade level)	4.6	6.2
Math level	4.8	5.5
HOME RESIDENCE		
Rural	19%	5%
Small town, midcity	40%	35%
Metro (100,000+)	41%	60%
PREVIOUS BEHAVIOR		
No previous record	63%	82%
Minor antisocial behavior	27%	16%
One serious conviction	10%	2%
EMPLOYMENT		
Had full-time or part-time job prior to Job Corps	65%	50%
Of those reporting:		
• 60% said they made less than $1.25 per hour		
• Pre-Job Corps earnings reported to Social Security Administration averaged $639 per year, with 2.5 quarters worked		
INDUCTION STATUS		
Of those eligible for armed forces:		
• Failed test		47%
• Mental reasons		30%
• Physical reasons		17%
HEALTH		
Had never seen doctor or dentist		80%
FAMILY PATTERN		
Broken home		60%
Head of household unemployed		63%
Family on relief		39%
Substandard housing		60%
Asked to leave school		64%
Both parents had less than eighth-grade education		49%

SOURCE: Job Corps.

the Negro mother is virtually a legend in our culture. The positive influence of the Japanese family on its children is manifested in motivation toward education and economic success as well as in low rates of delinquency. Families of American Indian and Spanish heritage are reluctant to relinquish their children to institutions outside their ethnic communities.

Programs designed for minority-group children often fail because they are not compatible with the culture and patterns of social organization that prevail among these groups. A serious problem of ambivalence which approaches anomie can result when two value systems, those of the family and those of social programs, compete for the child's allegiance. Too often planners of health and welfare services have not taken into account such variables as the importance of extended family members, different child-rearing behaviors, etc.

Characteristic Patterns of Family Living Among Minority Groups

The minority-group families of America show many variations in life styles. Many—despite their ethnic origin—have become the disorganized, unstable families of the poor which have been described elsewhere in this report. Among these are many one-parent families, although as pointed out in Chapter IV, one-parent homes do not necessarily create problems in children.

Unemployment, more than any other single factor, threatens the stability of minority-group families. Within the ghetto, unemployment results in family breakups and generates a system of ruthless and ex-ploitative relationships. The plight of the Negro family is indirectly portrayed in Clark's (1965) presentation of the facts of life in the Harlem ghetto—the overcrowdedness, danger, disease, unemployment, crime, and drug addiction. His vivid description of the feelings of despair, escapism, defeat, and agony of slum dwellers conveys the ever persistent pathology which has become a common way of life. Spanish Harlem is similarly portrayed by Sexton (1965). Ralph Ellison (1966:11), appearing before the Senate Subcommittee on Executive Reorganization, summed up the Negro child's feeling of alienation thusly:

. . . these are American children, and Americans are taught to be restless. Our myths teach us this, our cartoons . . . the television cameras. He gets it from every avenue of life. . . .

So you see little Negro Batmen flying around Harlem just as you see little white Batmen flying around Sutton Place. It is in the blood. But while the white child who is taken with these fantasies has many opportunities for work-ing them into real life situations, too often the Negro child is unable to do so. This leads the Negro child who identifies with the heroes and outlaws of fantasy to feel frustrated and to feel that society has designated him to the outlaw, for he is treated as one. Thus his sense of being outside the law is not simply a matter of fantasy, it is a reality based on the incontrovertible fact of race. This makes for frustration and resentment. And it makes for something else, it makes for a very cynical and sometimes sharp perspective on the difference between our stated ideals and the way in which we actually live. The Negro slum child knows the difference between a dishonest policeman and an honest one because he can go around and see the numbers men paying off policemen. . . .

Now that so much money has been thrown into neighborhoods, supposedly, the papers tell us so, the slum child feels very cynically that it is being drained off, somehow, in graft. He doesn't know. He doesn't have the information. I don't even have it. All he knows is that this promised alleviation of his condition isn't taking place.

Given the existing situation, it is not difficult to understand why Negro parents often teach their children to mistrust white people. Mistrust is, for them, a means of self-preservation. The Negro child learns to be constantly vigilant and to never be surprised or disappointed by things that happen to him because of the actions of white people. This distrust makes it difficult to establish genuine communication between black and white people. The Negro withdraws, promotes distance, and never really allows white people access to his life compartment. In this way the situation perpetuates itself. Founded and unfounded hypersuspiciousness may be a relatively healthy adjustment for a Negro living in twentieth-century America, without which he is devastated and crippled .

But just as minority-group families are isolated from the mainstream, so are they becoming increasingly isolated from members of their own group. Unemployment, mobility, and exposure to public education and the mass media add to the factors causing strain among formerly cohesive families and groups. There is little in the majority culture to replace for these groups the stability which has been lost.

Nevertheless, most groups tend to consider traditional patterns as the ideal. The Indian, the Puerto Rican, the Mexican-American, the Japanese, and often the Negro place high value on personal relations within their own groups and on extended family ties. Mexican-Americans and Puerto Ricans tend to retain a strong patriarchal family, rigid sex roles, a belief that a mother's place is generally in the home, and a tradition of large families. Indians place great value on cooperation and sharing, values which often conflict with those of the larger society.

Rather than building upon the strengths which exist in each group, planners of services have tended to disregard—and sometimes even degrade —cultural differences. Children of minority groups are often derided by members of the majority culture because of their differing behavior and appearance. The result for many minority-group children is a loss of cultural identity and/or an ambivalence toward the life styles of their family or group. They become caught between two worlds, not quite belonging to either.

The poor among these groups have often been termed the "culturally deprived." The term itself is a residue of a racist society. Traditionally, the way the term has been used implies that being culturally deprived is a basic problem. Every national policy has been geared toward dealing with the problems faced by minorities because they do not have a homogeneous culture with the mainstream. In reality, these minority communities have cultures with value systems, mores, folkways, and life styles which are quite humane. Where these are weakened by the pressures of the dominant socioeconomic system, there is a tendency to lay the blame on the minority culture or, more typically, on the minority-group family.

We maintain that the best of parents cannot overcome the deficits and stresses which undermine the mental health of so many minority-group children—deficits in health and environment which stem from poverty; deficits in education which result from overcrowded, inadequate, and poorly staffed schools; stresses closely associated with the impact of prejudice, exploitation, failure, powerlessness, and insecurity. The impact of many of these deficits is related below.

The Mental Health Consequences of Poor Housing

Family income, in addition to discriminatory practices, makes the homes of many minority-group children particularly hazardous to well-being. We have already alluded to the poor housing and environments which are typical for many groups. The impact of these conditions on the mental health of children cannot be overemphasized.

In addition to endangering the child's physical health through risk of infectious disease, rat bites, and lead poisoning, poor home environments and overcrowding result in interrupted and insufficient sleep. This not only increases the child's vulnerability to infectious disease but diminishes his attention span for learning. Crowded conditions also result in over-stimulation since there is no insulation from either the sexual or argumentative actions of adults and older siblings. The relatively calm state of mind ordinarily observed in latency-age children is often replaced by a perpetual excitement with sex or violence among children from poverty families. This hinders the process of education and school adjustment and contributes to the impression that these children are unreachable (Solomon, 1968). Grootenboer (1962) also found a correlation between prolonged babyish behavior, resulting in poor social adjustment, and lack of privacy and overcrowded homes.

Crowded housing does not allow parents to meet the needs of the individual child. Overcrowding intensifies fatigue and irritability and contributes to erratic and irrational discipline. Such a home has little holding power for the child—it is not a place to which he can bring his friends. These conditions lead children to frequent the streets, where they are exposed to violence, seduction, alcohol, narcotics, and other hazards. Thus, the loss of parental control and adult supervision which occurs so early in the lives of many slum children must be laid partly at the door of their homes.

Crowded, unsanitary home conditions have further consequences for development. Rats and vermin have a specific emotional impact on children. Health workers in the inner city constantly see ghetto children who are plagued by nightmares of rats and insects crawling on them. These children are deprived of the normal course of child development in which nightmares and fears relating to bodily integrity gradually subside after the age of six. Such fears can be truly handicapping to the developing personality. Crowding also deprives adolescents of the privacy in which to "primp," at a life phase in which personal appearance is so important (Solomon, 1968).

Persons living in such housing move frequently, either to improve their lot or because of difficulties in paying the rent. This mobility has a deleterious effect on the child's school adjustment, sense of personal identity, peer group relations, and general trust in the environment.

Public housing expenditures have done little to alleviate these conditions for minority-group children.

EDUCATION

School Attendance

The educational institution touches on the life of virtually every American child, regardless of ethnic background or income. All but the most severely handicapped attend either public or private schools for at least the elementary years. Although this culture regards education as a means of improving social and economic status, the school's greatest failure has been in its inability to adequately educate youth from the lower socioeconomic groups, especially those of oppressed minority groups.

As noted in the last chapter, parental income is highly related to the school dropout rate and is particularly high where poverty is most concentrated—that is, among urban slum, rural, and nonwhite populations. Among some groups dropout rates are extremely high. For example, 60 percent of Indian children drop out of school between the eighth and twelfth grades (Ablon *et al.*, 1967). The dropout rate for Puerto Ricans in New York City is 70 percent.

The dropout figures are most disturbing when only eighteen- and nineteen-year-olds are considered. Of youths in this age group who are from low-income families and who are still living with their families, 31 percent are high school dropouts (Orshansky, 1965). This figure does not include those teen-age dropouts who have moved away from home or have already formed families of their own.

The disastrous occupational effects of dropping out of school were made apparent in a study of the first year's work experience of dropouts as compared to that of high school graduates. As compared to graduates, youths who drop out of school were shown to have much more difficulty in finding employment, lesser chances of progressing to skilled or semi-skilled employment, to have higher rates of unemployment after their first job, and to be far more likely to earn wages below the poverty line (David et al., 1961). Government figures show that this trend is typical throughout life. In 1967 between 48 and 75 percent (depending on the educational level) of those with less than a high school education were earning less than the national $7,579 median income of all family heads, whereas only 35 percent of high school and about 17 percent of college graduates fell below this annual median wage. The figures show that the lower the educational level, the greater the proportion of those below the poverty level (U.S. Bureau of the Census, 1967).

Family income is still largely a determinant of who will complete college. While the median educational attainment levels of the poor and Negroes are increasing, the percentage of whites and nonwhites with high school or college educations has remained stable over the past decade. Children of families at the bottom of the occupational hierarchy still have much less chance of moving into upper-level-income jobs. The chances of the white manual worker's son moving into an upper-level job are slightly more than half that of the Negro manual laborer's son. More disturbing is the finding that among Negro sons of white-collar fathers, 72.4 percent went into manual occupations, whereas only 23.4 percent of their white counterparts did so (Miller et al., 1967).

School Achievement of Minority and Low-Income Groups

Much has been written in recent years about the schools of the inner cities, the schools which serve children from slum areas. Many such schools are almost totally segregated in that the student population is comprised of one minority group. Certainly they are segregated in the sense that only low-income families are represented.

Although a wide range of achievment can be noted among individual children in such schools, a typical pattern of mean achievement for the student body as a whole is apparent. During a ten-month school year, poor students generally progress seven months in reading grade place-ment as measured by standardized reading tests. The deficit is cumula-tive. For tenth-graders, the mean reading grade placement score is generally at the seventh-grade level. Since much of secondary education depends on reading facility, the students are severely handicapped in all academic subject areas.

The failure of our schools to educate oppressed minority children in-dicates an inherent weakness in our educational system. For groups such as Indians and Spanish-speaking children, the failure of educators to recognize language and cultural differences and the tendency to impose the language and norms of white America are among the main factors which account for high dropout rates. But even among minorities whose language and values approximate those of the majority, the results are often similar. Ghetto schools, for example, are given less money per student than other urban schools; they provide the Negro child with the least competent teachers, the largest classes, and an unsuccessful curriculum. As a result, failure becomes cumulative. In the second grade, only 8 percent of all boys in ghetto schools are a full year or more behind the national average for their age group. However, five years later, 25 percent are behind; four years after that 39 percent are behind; and, by the twelfth grade, for those who have not dropped out, 57 percent are behind (Bagdikian, 1968).

The tendency for Negro school-age children to obtain below-average intelligence test scores has been reported for more than fifty years (see, e.g., Peterson, 1923; Schuey, 1958). Eighth-grade pupils in Central Harlem in recent years had a mean I.Q. of 87.7, whereas the average for New York City eighth-graders was 100.1 (Moynihan, 1965). A normative study of 1,800 Negro elementary school children in five Southern states yielded a mean I.Q. of 80.7 (Kennedy *et al.*, 1963). According to the most recent classification system accepted by the American Association of Mental Deficiency—which is used also by the U.S. Public Health Service—the average child in the latter study is "borderline retarded" (Heber, 1964). How much such inferior functioning can be attributed to health factors and home environment and how much to the inferior education and testing methods to which the Negro child is subjected has yet to be determined. What seems evident is that the Negro child is subjected to a host of factors which may be complexly interwoven and which make him, along with groups such as Puerto Ricans, Indians, and migrant workers, more disadvantaged than the average poor white child.

For the individual student, the failure to achieve in school depresses enthusiasm and motivation. His self-concept is impaired. The further he falls behind, the more overwhelmingly difficult classroom learning becomes until school achievement seems a hopeless goal. He may respond with attention-seeking behavior, by mentally withdrawing from the conflict, or by dropping out of school.

For the school as a whole, the effect is equally devastating. Generally teachers prefer to instruct the more able and conforming students. Consequently the ghetto school is regarded as an undesirable post and teachers seek transfers to less deprived neighborhoods. The general level of instruction, especially in academic classes, is geared to the learning ability of the majority of students in the class. Discipline becomes a major preoccupation of the teacher.

The School's Effect on the Mental Health of Low-Income and Minority-Group Children

The role of the teacher in a child's life is of vital importance. Not only is a year of the child's education in her hands, but she may also have a crucial effect on his mental health. Many teachers are neither educationally nor emotionally prepared for this responsibility. The behaviors learned by children living in a slum may be repugnant and even terrifying to the teacher. Some teachers become intolerant of ethnic differences after a frustrating year of struggling to teach effectively in a ghetto or barrio school. Others bring to the classroom a stereotyped preconception of what the black, brown, or red child is capable of achieving. Although the most competent and sensitive teachers are needed in schools serving primarily low-income and minority-group children, the salary schedule, the school facilities and equipment, the status, and other satisfactions to be derived from employment there do not attract many such teachers.

Guidance personnel employed by the school district are particularly concerned with the mental health of pupils. However, guidance services at the elementary level are generally extremely limited. Often the service is limited to one psychologist who serves several schools. Although secondary schools usually employ counselors, their case loads are heavy and they are assigned many noncounseling responsibilities. Through the counselor, school nurse, attendance officers, and administrators a working relationship is maintained with other agencies in the community concerned with mental health. Unfortunately, guidance and psychological services are seldom sufficient to ensure that the first symptoms of serious emotional disorders or mental illness will be diagnosed and that teachers will receive more than occasional assistance in creating a classroom climate which fosters mental health.

Grouping procedures employed by schools may also have a deleterious effect on the mental health of children. Despite the countless studies which have shown that student achievement is not enhanced in homogeneously grouped classes, many schools continue to use this procedure for assigning students to academic classes. Children quickly become aware of their placement in the hierarchy and label themselves and one another accordingly. Enrollment in the "slow" class not only tends to place a ceiling on the child's motivation but also limits his learning experiences.

The curricula in American schools are generally geared to middle-class white values and lack relevance for the minority-group child. The instructional program ignores the experiences and learnings gained from ghetto streets, the barrio, the reservation, or the farm. Instead, it is based on premises about the background experiences of and appropriate goals for middle-class children. Multiracial materials are now available in most subjects, and intercultural understandings are an objective in many courses of study. The number of indigenous aides employed in classrooms is rapidly increasing. Nevertheless, the real curriculum—that which is taught in the classroom—changes slowly, and the problems of racism are not a central concern in that curriculum.

The schools in urban areas, especially in urban slums, are often the oldest and least attractive structures in the school system. The classrooms are crowded, and grassy spaces in the schoolyard have been usurped by relocatable buildings. Often the campus is enclosed by a high fence to discourage vandalism and resembles a penal institution more than a school.

The rebellion of today's youth against ineffective educational programs may be but a juvenile desire to participate in the larger revolution. Nevertheless, "blow-out" seems preferable to dropout. If students feel that the schools can be responsive to the needs they voice and that an effort is being made to improve the relevancy of their education, perhaps fewer of them will leave school prematurely because of lack of interest.

Current Approaches to Improving Education for the "Disadvantaged"

State and federal aid have long been a major means of financial support for schools. However, only in recent years has any sizable effort been made to assist schools in serving low-income children. The Economic Opportunity Act and the Elementary and Secondary Education Act legislated preferential treatment for the "disadvantaged."

Economic Opportunity Act. Under the Office of Economic Opportunity, Head Start preschool programs were initiated across the nation. Eligibility is limited to the children of low-income families. Psychological, social work, and health services are at least theoretically provided for every classroom. The ratio of children to adults is reduced by using paraprofessional employees and volunteer workers.

Evaluation of Head Start revealed that the gains made by preschoolers were lost by the time the children had completed the primary grades. Consequently, a limited number of Follow Through pilot projects, funded by OEO but administered by the U.S. Office of Education, were launched during the 1967–68 school year at the kindergarten level. Follow Through continues the provision of special services and smaller class size through the primary grades. An important difference from Head Start is the requirement that the classroom enrollment be ethnically and economically integrated. Widely varied instructional programs are being tried in the pilot programs.

School participation in the Neighborhood Youth Corps and in Community Action Programs has also been beneficial. OEO's emphasis on parent and community involvement in CAP projects did much to open the doors of the school to the poverty community.

The Economic Opportunity Act also made funds available for the employment of paraprofessional aides and encouraged the recruitment of low-income community adults. A peripheral benefit derived from the employment of indigenous paraprofessionals in the classrooms has been an unusual on-the-job training for teachers. Many teachers questioned how helpful such aides could be and suggested that at least a high school education was necessary to be effective in the classroom. But teachers learned from the paraprofessionals. They learned that the aides, though poor, were not apathetic or resigned or unconcerned about their own children. They learned about the fears and hopes of the community. They observed the aides' interaction with students and pattern of responses. They marveled at the zest with which many of the paraprofessionals approached meaningful jobs and learning opportunities.

Disadvantaged students also benefited from the presence of indigenous aides. Not only did the students receive more individual attention, but they also observed a neighbor as part of the school staff. The teacher seemed less an outsider when teamed with a member of the community. The school and community environment began to overlap.

Elementary and Secondary Education Act. Title I of the Elementary and Secondary Education Act provides funds for school programs in low-income neighborhoods. The entitlements must be used in a defined poverty area for a limited number of children identified as educationally deprived. The ESEA project must provide services or experiences over and above those normally provided for the school district. Moreover, school districts are encouraged to saturate a target area with services rather than to spread a diluted program among all children in a district who could be considered in need of compensatory education.

The Office of Education has emphasized that the needs of preschool, kindergarten, and primary children should be given priority in planning compensatory education programs. The trend seems to be toward expending an increasing proportion of the available money at the early childhood level.

LAW ENFORCEMENT

Violence, crime, and police policy and practice have a strong effect on children growing up in minority-group communities. The nature of this effect and its relationship to mental health should be more closely examined.

The Kerner Commission aptly described the role of the police in the ghetto.

We have cited deep hostility between police and ghetto communities as a primary cause of the disorders surveyed by the Commission. In Newark, in Detroit, in Watts, in Harlem—in practically every city that has experienced racial disruption since the summer of 1964—abrasive relationships between police and Negroes and other minority groups have been a major source of grievance, tension and, ultimately, disorder.

In a fundamental sense, however, it is wrong to define the problem solely as hostility to police. In many ways the policeman only symbolizes much deeper problems.

The policeman in the ghetto is a symbol not only of law, but of the entire system of law enforcement and criminal justice. . . .

And yet, precisely because the policeman in the ghetto is a symbol—precisely because he symbolizes so much—it is of critical importance that the police and society take every possible step to allay grievances that flow from a sense of injustice and increased tension and turmoil (*Report of the National Advisory Commission on Civil Disorders,* 1968: 299–300).

Statistics show a higher crime rate for nonwhites than for whites. Such figures, however, do not portray the reasons for this higher incidence of crime—problems rooted in the poverty environment—in the high rates of unemployment, the pressure to turn to illegal activities, the greater likelihood of arrest, and so forth. Rather than attacking the underlying causes, society tends to react with such punitive measures as anti-riot legislation and more authority for the police. Enforcement seems to mean "containment" in many instances, yet most people are appalled by the implications of a containment policy. The black community has done considerable talking and writing about this policy. The American Indian does not need to talk about it; he lives with it, every day.

JUVENILE DELINQUENCY

A number of studies indicate that delinquency rates are higher among certain lower socioeconomic groups, especially those in socially disorganized areas (Conger and Miller, 1966). The question of whether or not delinquency should be equated with emotional disturbance in all cultural subgroups is still being debated. However, even if such behavior is "normal" among certain subgroups, the consequences of ensuing legal measures are not likely—by most present correctional means—to produce emotionally healthy results. For youth fifteen and over, placement is generally in jails, workhouses, reformatories, or prisons (U.S. Dept. of Health, Education, and Welfare, 1965).

The higher crime rates among some minority-group youths, as compared to middle-class youth, may well reflect biases in arrest records as well as law enforcement practices. Figures in recent years show a great increase in the nonwhite populations in all types of correctional institutions. Of all institutionalized children in 1960, 18 percent of white children, as compared to 40 percent of nonwhite children, were in correctional facilities, a fact which suggests that there may be vast inequities in the handling of behavior problems from children of different social and racial backgrounds (Rosen *et al.,* 1968). Thus, added to the handicaps of minority-group youths are the poor quality of care and rehabilitative services in these institutions, the impact of arrest records on future employment, and the paucity of opportunities for youths released from these institutions.

Our efforts to deal with delinquency have been highly ineffective. An effective preventive approach must deal directly with the cultural, social, and economic processes which give rise to delinquency.

COMMUNITY PARTICIPATION

This nation has always been a politically power-oriented country. Religious, ethnic, and racial groups have tended to become political factions which have sought control of their communities, individually and then though coalition with other self-interest groups at other political levels, and not necessarily along party lines.

Community control may express itself in many ways. For example, it may be necessary to actively train more Negro health personnel, particularly in the mental health fields. White psychiatrists and other white mental health professionals may be incapable of relating to the problems of the minority individual or masses. A community may deem it necessary to have black-controlled, black-staffed clinics.

Communities may demand the inclusion of Negro history or Swahili instruction in their public schools. This represents the struggle to find identity, self-esteem, group cohesiveness. State and local laws often bar such requests. If minority groups control their schools they may make these requests in more meaningful and forceful terms.

Community organization that provides for wholesome development of the minority culture's social system will offer children a good wholesome atmosphere in which to live. Some effects of disorganization in a community can be observed in the third- and fourth-generation Japanese-American. Formerly a strong identity within the Japanese-American group and a strong organization within their communities bound them together. However, the third and fourth generations do not possess this same cultural identity. Many were born in concentration camps and grew up later with the difficulty of finding out who they were. As a result, instability and delinquency are more prevalent in this group as compared to former generations, although their families are affluent, they attend the best schools, and they do not suffer the poverty and restrictions that their grandparents experienced.

One trend which may emerge from the black power movement and the war on poverty is increased community control of local institutions. Demands from minority-group neighborhoods for a voice in the policy-making of local schools illustrate this. Organizing the community for self-help programs is not sufficient. The dominant, strong, more affluent community must be responsive to the needs of the ghetto and must provide channels through which the ghetto resident can move from his own community. The mainstream culture must be organized in such a way that minority-group communities can relate to its various programs and institutions. If this cannot be achieved, the ghetto residents have little choice but to establish their own separate enterprises and institutions and operate them for the benefit of their own community.

HEALTH

A tragedy of our rich and technically advanced nation is that many children are constantly exposed to health hazards, receive limited health care, and have a curtailed life expectancy. Because of poor maternal health, inadequate prenatal care, and hazardous environmental conditions, almost twice as many nonwhite, as compared to white, babies die before their first birthday. Survival hazards in some groups are even higher. For example, one-third of Indian infants die between the first month and the first year of life, largely from *preventable* diseases.

The risk of disease continues throughout life for the Indian child, giving him an average life expectancy of only forty-three years. Typhoid, dysentery, diphtheria, hepatitis, tuberculosis, and other microbial infections often go untreated in this group. Middle-ear infections are so rampant in some Indian groups that on some reservations a quarter of the children have suffered permanent hearing damage. Trachoma, an infectious eye disease that often causes blindness, is almost nonexistent in this country— except on reservations. In one Apache group, a survey found that 61 percent of the children between the ages of five and eighteen were so affected (Farb, 1968).

Children of migrant workers also suffer a higher incidence of untreated disorders. Gastroenteritis is responsible for most deaths among these infants and children. The incidence of eye and ear infections, respiratory infections, caries, and oral and dental root infections is also high (Siegel, 1966).

Rural Negro children suffer even higher rates of undetected and untreated diseases than do their urban brothers.

Poor children in all groups receive little care. They are hospitalized less often but remain in the hospital longer.

Many of these poor children are stunted in growth and weakened in mind and body by malnutrition. Nutritional anemias are common, owing to economic insufficiencies and feeding habits and excessive milk intake. Many children seek gratification from the bottle rather than seeking a relationship with their mothers. They remain infantile and self-centered, fail to develop a trusting curiosity about the world, and do not reach out into the environment for satisfactions and challenges (Werkman *et al.,* 1964).

Children who are chronically sick and hungry may also come to question their own worth and the worth of their families. They may come to doubt any offer and to mistrust any favorable turn of events. As Dr. Robert Coles has noted, these children learn to be "tired, fearful, anxious, and suspicious" because they have experienced a kind of starvation in which "the body is slowly consuming itself." This bitter experience may breed potential recruits for riots in cities (U.S. Senate, *Hunger and Malnutrition in America,* 1967: 52–53). Federal food programs and public assistance measures have been inadequate to the challenge. In a land of abundance, children still suffer hunger. Many of these children belong to minority groups and are denied aid from federal food programs because of discriminatory practices.

Mental Health

The many complicating factors which hinder any definitive statement concerning the relationship between poverty or ethnic background and mental health are discussed elsewhere in this report.

However, the relationship which sometimes exists between poverty and mental disorders is shown in the incidence of mental retardation. Prematurity and complications of pregnancy—both higher among nonwhites—are correlated with all types of retardation. Large proportions of nonwhites are among the 75 to 80 percent of the retarded population that shows no obvious brain damage or organic defects. Many come from impoverished backgrounds. The causes of this seemingly inorganic retardation are linked to the poor diets and inadequate prenatal care for deprived mothers, and to malnutrition and the lack of stimulation for infants and toddlers.

A number of studies point to the high incidence of poor persons who are admitted to county and state and public mental hospitals. These studies, however, tell us nothing of incidence of emotional and mental disorders in the population but merely point to the relationship between inadequate preventive and outpatient services and low socioeconomic status.

Among some minority peoples, admission rates to state institutions exceed those of the general population. For example, Puerto Ricans in New York constitute about 9.1 percent of first admissions to state schools for the retarded, although their proportion of the state population is only 4 percent. No refined analysis has been made, but Fitzpatrick *et al.* (1968)

suggest that cultural, language, and class barriers may result in a diagnosis of retardation where it is nonexistent. They also question whether these differences might not account, in part, for the reported high incidence of schizophrenia among Puerto Ricans and for the large number of Puerto Rican children found in "special schools."

Ablon *et al.* (1967) raise this same question in relation to the low reported incidence of severe mental disorders among American Indians. Rates for alcoholism, neuroses, and social incapacity are high among Indians. Children's chances for successful social adjustment appear to be lowered through apathy, poor learning, and general withdrawal. However, mental breakdowns appear to occur infrequently, although severe mental disorders are known to increase with expanded detribalization and acculturation. It may be, however, that the low incidence of reported mental illness among Indian children is a function of our lack of knowledge of these people. As the authors point out, we once viewed Negroes as simple and happy people. We now know these stereotypes resulted from our ignorance. Persons involved in epidemiological studies have estimated that 20 percent of the Indian population is in need of some type of psychiatric care.

Although the data are inconclusive, reports in 1961 from 493 clinics representing 23 states indicated that nonwhite rates were higher than white rates for all age groups diagnosed as mentally deficient, for adults with brain syndromes and psychotic disorders, and for females with psychoneurotic disorders. In general, nonwhite rates were lower for personality and transient personality disorders in all age groups, for brain syndromes in children, and for psychoneuroses in males. The principal differences by color were the lower nonwhite rates in age groups three to eleven and eighteen to twenty. The nonwhite data came principally (70 percent) from Southern regions (Rosen *et al.*, 1964) but the trends have been noted by other investigators. The same differentials were noted in Monroe County, New York, where various types of facilities were surveyed (Gardner *et al.*, 1963), and in the study of a total clinic population in Maryland (Bahn, 1961). From all these studies it appears that nonwhites seen in clinics tend, more than whites, to be those with greatest impairment: e.g., psychotic disorders and brain syndromes. These findings indicate that nonwhites are referred for treatment and/or seek and receive treatment at a later date than whites.

Langner and his collaborators are currently engaged in a prevalence survey of children's psychiatric impairment and psychiatric disorders in Manhattan, New York City. Four hundred out of 1,000 randomly selected children aged six to eighteen have been given psychiatric interviews, ratings of impairment in various behavior settings, and psychometric scores and profiles developed on the basis of factor analysis of mothers' reports.

This data has been analyzed in relationship to treatment, familial practices and attitudes, and demographic variables such as sex, age, race, socio-economic status, etc.

Tentative figures for these 400 children show that 8 percent of the high-income, 12 percent of the middle-income, and 21 percent of the low-income group had "marked" impairment, or worse. However, almost no differences were found between low-income and high-income Negro children (18 percent vs. 19 percent). Little difference was noted between low-income (17 percent) and high-income (15 percent) Spanish-speaking children. About half as many high-income as low-income whites were considered "cases" (8 percent vs. 15 percent). High-income Spanish also showed a decrease as compared to low-income Spanish. However, 33 percent of high-income Negroes and only 21 percent of low-income Negroes were so considered. In most impairment areas, the high-income Negro child was found to be particularly unfortunate. For example, among all high-income groups, only Negroes showed any "marked" school impairment. (However, no mention is made of the quality of the schools which they attended as compared to other groups.) High-income Negro mothers were also found to have the most problems, e.g., body complaints, lack of un-derstanding of the child, general dissatisfaction, and poor self-image. In addition, marital discord was high among high-income Negroes.

Langner and his associates feel that real environmental stresses exist in high-income Negro families, leading to greater impairment rates. Such en-vironmental factors as prejudice and job discrimination—which in turn affect family cohesion and familial relationships—also prevent high-income Spanish-speaking children from obtaining a reduction in impairment com-mensurate with treatment.

Among the stresses on these families is inadequate income. More than 90 percent of the Negroes and Spanish-speaking groups in this study were excluded from "worldly goods." The fact that "high income" was cut at $6,500 in the Langner study—a sum below the $7,200 estimated for an "adequate health and decency budget" for an urban family of four—makes their exclusion even more apparent. Even college education fails to guarantee upward mobility for the Negroes in the study sample, as shown by the fact that the low-income group contains a higher proportion of college-educated fathers than the high-income group (Langner *et al.*, 1967).

Lack of income is, of course, one barrier to obtaining treatment. How-ever, there is a good deal of evidence indicating that poor children treated in public hospitals and public clinics do not receive the same treatment as their more affluent counterparts. Often, poor children are referred else-where. Rural youth are particularly deprived of mental health care, owing to lack of services in rural areas.

The poor child is usually referred to mental health agencies by the court or schools, both of which may reflect the ethnic and social class bias of middle-class professionals. Such referrals for children who are emotionally disturbed may be deferred longer, the lower the social class of the child (McDermott *et al.*, 1965). For the very poor, no referral may ever be made, despite the fact that the child's emotional disturbance is recognized.

There is also evidence of ethnocentric biases among professionals. As a result, treatment is less intense and prolonged. Data from one study indicated that when ethnic differences were accompanied by low socioeconomic status, the problems in treatment were compounded. A statistically significant relationship was found between increased ethnocentricity on the part of the therapist and lesser treatment received by the client. Therapists with low ethnocentricity more often treated ethnic minority patients in proportions comparable with their Caucasian clients (Yamamoto *et al.*, 1967). Langner *et al.* (1967) also found that therapeutic contacts were not "wasted" on Negro or Spanish-speaking children in Manhattan, or on any low-income group except whites. There were also differences in the type of therapeutic contact. Negroes were five times as likely to see a school counselor as whites, while few Spanish did. Negroes were also more likely to see a social worker. Whites, irrespective of income, were more likely to see a psychiatrist. Additional problems are created for Negroes in segregated mental institutions where workers care little for their patients (Coles, 1966). State-supported mental health clinics have also shown reluctance in accepting Indian referrals (Ablon *et al.*, 1967).

In addition to the fact that mental health services for minority-group and poor youth are insufficient in quantity and inadequate in quality, the delivery of services has been hampered by such obstacles as attitudinal barriers, administrative difficulties, lack of continuity in care, problems of emphasis, communication barriers, and transportation and time problems. The major problems are summarized below:

Maldistribution of mental health professionals. Few mental health services are readily available to children living in depressed areas, either urban or rural. Mental health facilities tend to be located elsewhere. Moreover, working in more affluent neighborhoods offers greater professional and financial rewards to the mental health professional. Often those professionals who do choose to serve the poor and minority groups are overwhelmed by the magnitude of the problems in minority communities and are frustrated by their inability to communicate within these subcultures.

Attitudinal barriers. Minority-group members and the very poor often view mental health services with distrust and misunderstanding. They may fear involuntary hospitalization or suspect that seeking services will brand them as insane. Often their experiences with welfare, law enforcement, and other agencies have been coercive and humiliating, and they anticipate the same kind of treatment from health agencies. Their perceptions of the nature of the illness and appropriate treatment may interfere with their acceptance of professional services.

However, the poor are becoming more sophisticated about mental illness. New approaches to working with the poor have also broken down some barriers. In some instances, self-help community programs have effected greater understanding among both the clients and the professionals.

Lack of coordination among agencies. Often a host of agencies and institutions are simultaneously providing services to a poor family. The welfare agency, the probation department, the school, the public health department, and others, all working separately, may impinge on the life of the family, each with its own requirements. Coordination among these services would not only improve the effectiveness of each in dealing with the family but would also eliminate unnecessary duplication. Administrative barriers between the various agencies and institutions frequently make communication difficult.

Lack of continuity in care. The client of one mental health agency or service often finds that movement from one community to another results in a break in service because of lack of coordination among agencies. A lack or inadequacy of facilities or the client's lack of skill in locating services may mean that treatment is discontinued. The client may be frustrated by time-consuming intake procedures. Supportive, therapeutic, and rehabilitative services may not be available in the home community for the patient leaving a state hospital. Consequently he feels deserted and may become increasingly incapable of functioning efficiently. Eventually, rehospitalization may be necessary.

Problems of emphasis and communication. Traditionally most of the mental health professionals have dealt primarily with intrapsychic problems. Minority-group and poor youth often have such serious difficulties in coping with their social relationships and their environment that these areas require prior treatment. The usual middle-class orientation of the mental health professional compounds his difficulty in communicating with the client regarding his perceptions of self and others. These circumstances argue for the employment of professionals who have had personal experience with life in the poverty community as a minority-group member.

Accessibility of services. Although the poor are most beset by lack of transportation, their communities are least apt to provide mental health services. For a mother dependent on public transportation to accompany a child to a mental health clinic outside her own community on a regular basis requires considerable stamina. If she is non-English-speaking and must depend on neighbors to care for other children in her absence, the difficulties in obtaining treatment may seem overwhelming.

Guidelines for the Provision of Mental Health Services to Minority-Group and Poor Youth

The mental health problems of the poor cannot be solved entirely by professional psychiatric means. Changes in the social, economic, political, legal, educational, and medical institutions of our society are required. The distrust, alienation, and hardships bred by poverty increase the incidence of mental illness in the United States. Nor can meaningful rehabilitation of the mentally ill be accomplished by a system of charities to be given or withheld by arbitrary selection.

For the following reasons, expanded and more efficient mental health services will have to be delivered to the minority populations in the immediate future:

a. a growing awareness of the need for an awareness of available services due largely to the influence of mass media;

b. an anticipated mobilization of anger and buried dissatisfaction by the masses of minority people;

c. increasing concentration of minority people into more crowded and substandard housing;

d. rapid widening of the technological gap plus the contemporaneous ineffectiveness and ennui-producing aspects of schools in minority communities.

The following principles of prevention and treatment stated by the Committee on Mental Health Services for the Disadvantaged of the Los Angeles Region Welfare Planning Council seem particularly pertinent (Mental Health Development Commission, 1967:15–19):

Physical well-being: The preservation of physical health is prerequisite for the prevention of mental disorders.

Psychological and social well-being: Such social conditions as the disruption of family life, poor housing, crowded living conditions, and unemployment are deleterious to mental health. Individuals must develop the skills necessary for social competence to compete for better jobs.

Continuity: Mental health services, including twenty-four-hour emergency service, short-term and long-term outpatient care, day-center care, and partial and full hospitalization, must be available to the poverty community.

Collaborative network: All voluntary and public helping agencies and community resources must collaborate effectively in service to the poverty community.

Accessibility: Mental health services should be conveniently located and oriented toward making the client feel welcome.

Consultation: Both direct and indirect services are needed. Often indirect services involve consultation with other non-mental health professionals and agencies.

Information/education: The socially disadvantaged have limited knowledge of mental health services. The mental health service must reach out to those in need of help and must provide mental health education for the community.

Training: The manpower shortage in the mental health field is particularly acute in disadvantaged areas. Training of mental health professionals and paraprofessionals to work within poverty communities is urgent.

SUMMARY

The mental health problems of our nation's minority-group children are intricately interwoven with socioeconomic factors. The high rate of poverty or near-poverty among minority peoples means that minority children are at high risk in areas of nutritional, physical, and psychological health. Racist attitudes and practices are reflected in employment and educational practices and differential opportunities in all areas of living. Among children, racism often contributes to impaired self-images, a high incidence of "educational retardation," alienation and isolation, and high rates of youth unemployment and underemployment.

Drastic changes are required in our human service institutions to ensure that equal opportunities and advantages are guaranteed all our nation's children. Many of the recommendations formulated by the committee on Children of Minority Groups in its original report (1968) to the Commission are included in the appropriate chapters of this report. Since the Committee identified racism as the number one public health problem, its original proposals on racism seem particularly relevant to this chapter.

RECOMMENDATIONS ON RACISM

Programs to eradicate racism should be initiated immediately because vast numbers of Americans appear ready to accept the fact, either from egalitarian or humanistic motives or from simple self-interest, that the dangerous and destructive mechanisms of racism must be abandoned. However, racism will yield only to the strongest, clearest, and most diverse campaigns of information and education. Therefore, this Committee makes the following recommendations:

1. That the President of the United States ask all levels of government to mobilize their resources to combat racism; that he address a joint session of Congress with the goal of educating them to the racial problem

and inspiring their support of programs aimed at alleviating ghetto conditions.

2. That specific efforts be made to preserve and sustain many of the features of minority populations. These strengths are needed to assure the advantages of cultural diversity and healthy psychological development.

3. That the existing power structures on national, state, and community levels be committed to effect real change in the attitudes and behavior of people in their sphere of influence through a program launched and led by the President and backed by a committee of governors.

4. That the President ascertain that each Cabinet department and independent federal agency is making every effort to eradicate racism.

5. That the President call for government action related to the Report of the National Advisory Commission on Civil Disorders; that members and staff of the commission who are acquainted with the methodology and findings meet regionally with various public and private groups to acquaint them with the scope of the report and its recommendations.

6. That the leadership for planning and implementing the campaign against racism come from the top of all sectors of American society including government, business, education, religion, medicine, the communication industry, and the arts; that a multiracial committee of nationally important leaders representing these sectors be immediately appointed to establish goals and policy.

7. That a National Foundation for the Social Sciences for the promoting and strengthening of these sciences, as proposed in S. 836—90th Congress, be created. It is further recommended that this foundation support not only basic research in the social sciences but that it also promote social science research, development, and pilot studies aimed at developing ways of coping with and of solving the major social problems of our society.

8. That the federal government not only develop adequate programs in the health, education, and welfare area but that it exercise surveillance of the effectiveness of these programs through the creating of a Council of Social Advisors to the President as proposed in S. 843—90th Congress.

9. That a new organization be established with adequate private and public support, to be called "The National Council Against Racism." The council would have both scientific and change-promoting functions. It would serve as:

a. a clearinghouse for valid and applicable data on effective racism-reducing programs and community organization efforts;

b. a clearinghouse for valid data on the psychosocial strengths and disabilities of various racial and ethnic groups in the United States (including "majority" groups) as well as data on programs that capitalize on these strengths and lessen the disabilities;

c. a research-promoting and idea-producing center;

d. an agency that directly sponsors a variety of appropriate pilot projects and action programs;

e. an organization energetically advocating the adoption of appropriate racism-reducing programs on federal, state, local, and private levels as well as providing consultation on the selection and implementation of such programs.

10. That the 1970 White House Conference on Children and Youth be devoted to examination of the problems of racism as they affect young children, thus mobilizing hundreds of national organizations associated with the Conference.

11. That mental health professionals be vocal in declaring that: The issue of universal human dignity is deeply interwoven in our international and domestic crisis. Furthermore, there are psychological contradictions inherent in the concept of a two-fronted war; that is, a war on poverty and an international war, presently typified in Vietnam. The bulk of our various national resources should be directed toward resolving the problem of racism and poverty.

12. That nonprejudicial attitudes, understanding, and the desire to make change be a prerequisite for public and private office and responsibility.

13. That the traditional networks of communications be drafted to provide exhaustive dissemination of whatever kinds of material are required to eradicate the misinformation, the conscious and unconscious hostility, and the false fears that are corrupting the minds and hearts of so many Americans.

14. That every effort be exerted to eliminate prejudice from communications media, including comic books, television, films, and textbooks.

15. That school boards include representation of minority groups within the community.

16. That the study of minority groups be a required part of the training of all teachers and school administrators.

17. That the study of the heritage and contributions of all ethnic groups in America be included in the early education of all children.

18. That the concept of the mental health team be broadened to include many other skills necessary to combat racism; this will require the development of such talent within the minority communities.

19. That each community assume responsibility for positive action in establishing and maintaining a society free from racism.

20. That housing integration efforts be directed at both cities and suburbs.

21. That innovative ways of implementing psychological change be explored by providing new methods of communication and interaction through which members of majority and minority groups affect a two-way

exchange of tolerance, understanding, and respect, and that new television channels and radio stations be licensed with the prior stipulation that they discharge their responsibilities in this sphere.

22. That the recommendations regarding press coverage of riots in the Report of the National Advisory Commission on Civil Disorders be applied to nonviolent events as well; that both sides of all controversies, confrontations, and other newsworthy material in race relations be carefully reported.

23. That prejudice in the individual be recognized as a psychological disability, damaging to the self and others and also limiting and reducing the quality and extent of the individual's interaction with his fellowmen.

24. That a nationwide campaign against racism be launched featuring such slogans as "Racism is the number one public health problem" and seeking to instill such understandings as the following:

a. America can no longer afford the material costs that stem directly from racism—the continuing physical decay of the inner cities; the rising bills for inadequate welfare payments; the property damage caused by riots and the subsequent programs of arson and looting; the loss of national income and taxes that could be produced by members of minorities if they had employment opportunities and equal access to capital; and the medical and mental hygiene cost to all public health services for repairing the human damage caused by ghetto life in the cities, on the reservations, or in the abandoned rural communities where automation has replaced human labor.

b. America can no longer afford the spiritual and psychological costs attendant to the atmosphere of violence and counterviolence, rebellion and retaliation. We can no longer afford the feelings of guilt, fear, anxiety, and the other crippling emotions that affect both sides in a national atmosphere of hostility and aggression evoked by racial tension.

c. America cannot afford the public image either at home or abroad of being a nation guilty of unfairness, intolerance, and disdain for human needs, contempt for human aspiration, and even blatant physical cruelty as shown on our television sets every summer and in the magazines and newspapers throughout the world. The sense of shame felt by Americans, particularly young Americans, as a result of being identified with such national and local action has become intolerable and is about to affect our national identity, our attitudes toward our laws and our leaders, and the very vigor of our national purpose and our will to maintain our national security.

d. America will be enriched as its people better appreciate the strengths and contributions of minority groups.

25. That long-range programs of research, experimentation, and eval-

uation be conducted to determine the most effective communication practices for eradicating racism; however, the urgency of the danger to the children of America inherent in racism requires that we launch a campaign against racism now rather than waiting for the results of such studies.

26. In a very real sense the mental health of minority children depends on the education and research findings of mental health specialists, educators, and administrators of welfare programs. Thus there is no more important institution in our society, relative to the mental health of minority children, than the Department of Health, Education, and Welfare. Though the practices of this department on the whole have been undeniably and immeasurably positive, the department must be evaluated critically in relationship to the mental health of the minority child.

For instance, despite the hundreds of qualified black physicians, sociologists, psychologists, social workers and nurses, this committee knows through the experience of its members only four blacks who have served the National Institute of Mental Health in a capacity of consultant, site visitor, study section member, or advisory councilor. We know of even less participation by qualified American Indians or Spanish-speaking Americans. Putatively, there are fewer than five intramural black professional staff members at NIMH. Insofar as "credentials" are held by dozens of blacks who are professors in "white" institutions of higher learning, all of them would qualify for any of these services.

The lack of participation by minority members at critical levels in the use of the public funds which most influence the research, education, and service of the mental health aspects of our society not only reflects racism but prevents the intellectual input from the minority community. Such circumstances, if connected, might help preclude serious social disruption in our country.

27. That agencies such as the NIMH, OEO, Children's Bureau, Bureau of Indian Affairs, Office of Education, and Labor Department discharge their responsibilities in planning and funding of services for children and youth of minority groups with a sense of urgency and daring. The vigorous recruitment for participation of professionals and nonprofessionals from the minorities must go beyond mere employment and consultation and must aim at high-level planning as well as direct delivery service systems which are compatible with the cultural values and life styles of the recipient. Programs for mental health, community action, manpower, and youth development unencumbered by myths about low-income and minority populations (e.g., cultural deprivation, time orientation, disorganized families) will assure that the minority communities will be strengthened in their capacity to solve their own social problems.

Such programs will fail if they are encumbered by administrative timidity, *a priori* prescriptions, and fear of "high-risk" program ventures.

28. That the emphases on changing the attitudes and behavior of minority persons be broadened to that of changing the attitudes and behavior of the white majority in the area of racism. New approaches to bring this about on a "wholesale" basis would need to be developed and the human and financial resources required be provided.

Emotionally Disturbed and Mentally Ill
Children and Youth

At least 1,400,000 of our youngsters under eighteen need immediate psychiatric care. This NIMH estimate is considered by that institute and most mental health professionals to be a conservative figure. There is no way of determining how many of these children and youth would have been spared their suffering if they had had available to them the broad range of preventive services and programs recommended in the previous chapters. No doubt the number would be less.

But of what benefit are conjecture and hindsight to the tragic reality of today? The needs of these children must be met. Their needs include all that we have considered in preventive services—a wholesome environment, good physical care, emotional support, education, and all the rest. In addition, these children often need services which are more specialized, intensive, and fitted to individual needs. At present, the majority are not getting this care, treatment, and services. Nor are there sufficient facilities and services for the millions of other children and youth whose problems, though less severe, require some kind of attention from mental health and other personnel.

DEFINITIONS OF MENTAL ILLNESS AND EMOTIONAL
DISTURBANCES

There is, as yet, no unanimity among mental health professionals regarding the definition of mental illness and serious emotional disturbances. Many different diagnostic categories and ways of viewing the problem exist. Similar problems have arisen in all emerging sciences, and psychiatry and clinical psychology are no exception. In fact, the study of emotional and mental disorders has proven to be exceptionally baffling and complex because of the very nature of man. The emphasis has, of necessity, been on relieving suffering more than on research to clarify theoretical problems. A full discussion of these matters will not be undertaken here. The American Psychiatric Association and other professional organizations are currently working toward more generally accepted and widely used systems of definition and diagnostic categories. However, a few of the current formulations will be presented in the following pages.

For example, some authorities suggest that when emotional and mental disorders are viewed in terms of their origins, five major categories can be distinguished: (1) faulty training and faulty life experiences; (2) surface conflicts between children and parents which arise from such adjustment tasks as relations among siblings, school, social, and sexual development; (3) deeper conflicts which become internalized within the self and create emotional conflicts within the child (these are the so-called neuroses); (4) difficulties associated with physical handicaps and disorders; (5) difficulties associated with severe mental disorders, such as the psychoses. It is estimated that 80 percent of emotional problems are related to the first two categories; 10 percent to the third category; and 10 percent to the fourth and fifth. Highly trained mental health and other specialists are required for handling the special problems of children in the last three categories; however, the other 80 percent of children with less severe problems can generally receive sufficient help from a variety of people who work with them, such as parents, teachers, public health and school nurses, child development specialists, social workers, paraprofessionals, etc.

One particularly promising approach is a system formulated by Dr. Dane Prugh for diagnosing, classifying, and treating emotional and mental disorders. Prugh ties this system primarily to the developmental stage of the child and the degree to which the child is handicapped or suffering from dysfunction. Mental health is viewed as being largely on a continuum, ranging from excellent to very poor psycho-social-physical functioning. His charts can be found in Appendix A of this chapter.

The Committee on Child Psychiatry of the Group for the Advancement of Psychiatry also proposes a classification system which is divided into the following main categories: healthy responses, reaction disorders, developmental deviations, psychoneurotic disorders, personality disorders, psychotic disorders, psychophysiologic disorders, brain syndromes, mental retardation, and other disorders.

This Committee has adopted three basic propositions: (1) there is a unity of mind and body and a close interrelatedness of psychological and physical processes; (2) diagnosis must be related to the developmental stage of the child; and (3) the child's behavior is deeply affected by his experiences in his family and the larger society. The Committee further stresses that a child's behavior is a product of many factors—physiological, psychological, and social—but concludes that, at the present, a classification system cannot take into account all of these factors in their great complexity and interaction (Group for the Advancement of Psychiatry, 1967).

Another approach, which might be termed social-psychological-educational, emphasizes that a child's behavioral difficulties are closely associated with gaps or deficits in his learning of social, behavioral, and academic skills. These deficiencies are a result of failures and problems in his environment: family, school, and neighborhood.

Yet another approach to the definition and description of emotional disturbance, not fully developed at present, may be called the ecological, or systems, analysis of the problem. The child is seen as defining a small social system of which he is an integral part and which includes his home, school, neighborhood, and larger community. The behavior patterns of the child in the context of requirements and expectations of a particular social system may lead to acceptance and support of the child or to his rejection, to his being defined as "disturbed" or "delinquent" or perhaps "mentally retarded." A child is identified as emotionally disturbed when there is too much discord in the system, when there is an intolerable discrepancy between the behavior of the child and the expectations of the normal socializing institutions. This concept is increasingly a part of most classification systems. When taken seriously, it leads to intervention that may include conventional psychotherapeutic procedures but would involve other strategies as well (Hobbs, 1966).

According to the Commission's Committee on Clinical Issues, the emotional and mental illness problems of preschool children may include:

1. Childhood psychoses which are the most serious forms of mental illness and which include such diagnostic categories as infantile autism and childhood schizophrenia.

2. Childhood neuroses which are characterized by such symptoms as extreme and unreasoning fears; continuing rituals carried out in a driven way; deep emotional depression; severe shyness and withdrawal from people and the environment; compulsive manipulation of parts of the self such as pulling of one's own hair, head-rubbing, unceasing masturbation, and the like.

3. Children with minimal brain dysfunction who demonstrate such problems as physical awkwardness, hyperactivity, and learning disorders.

4. A large group of disturbances which lie in the area of behavioral problems. "The latter category includes the dangerous child, the child whose tantrums, lying, and destructiveness set him apart from other children from a very early age."

5. Children with sexual deviations which lead to confusion over their sex identity and various forms of perversion and unusual sex interest. "Some boys, for example, show marked feminine interests from age two or even younger, along with compulsive patterns of sexual activity" (*Report of the Committee on Clinical Issues*, 1969).

To these might be added:

a. The failure-to-thrive syndrome, which is an important and serious condition found in some infants and young children. It manifests itself in the failure of some youngsters to grow and develop normally in the areas of physical, intellectual, and emotional development. This is becoming an increasingly widespread problem, the origins of which are not completely understood; however, it appears that at least some of these children are the victims of neglectful or unusually cruel parents (*Report of Task Force I, 1968*).

b. Children with physical or mental handicaps which are generally more disabling because of the associated emotional reactions of both parents and children.

THE NATURE AND SCOPE OF THE PROBLEM

The Commission has formulated the following definition of emotionally disturbed children: An emotionally disturbed child is one whose progressive personality development is interfered with or arrested by a variety of factors so that he shows impairment in the capacity expected of him for his age and endowment: (1) for reasonably accurate perception of the world around him; (2) for impulse control; (3) for satisfying and satisfactory relations with others; (4) for learning; or (5) any combination of these. The definition would seem to cover, in a general way, the major features of the various definitions which have been sketched previously. In reviewing various treatment approaches, Gioscia and associates (1968) conclude that regardless of varying diagnostic and theoretical systems, the basic methods of treatment tend to be fairly similar in actual work with disturbed children and youth (see also Chapter XI, "Research"). The goals of such treatment are generally tied to the five criteria of mental health presented above.

Incidence of Mental and Emotional Disorders

Estimates vary as to the number of mentally ill children and young people in this country. It is estimated that about .6 percent are psychotic and that another 2 to 3 percent are severely disturbed. It is further estimated that an additional 8 to 10 percent of our young people are afflicted with emotional problems (neuroses and the like) and are in need of specialized services. However, only about 5 to 7 percent of the children who need professional mental health care are getting it (Gioscia *et al.*, 1968; *Report of Task Force V*, 1968). According to the best available figures, only about 500,000 children are currently being served by mental health facilities—clinics, hospitals, private therapists. However, more than 10,000,000 young people under age twenty-five need knowledgeable help. As a nation, we do far better for our physically handicapped children than we do for those with emotional and mental handicaps. For example, it is estimated that 7,600,000 children are in need of services for the physically handicapped and that 5,600,000 receive such services (*Report of Task Force V*, 1968). It is clear that the present dearth of mental health services will become more acute in the immediate future.

Although mental health services have been greatly expanded over the past fifteen years or so, we are falling far short of our frequently announced national goals regarding a commitment to the children and youth of this nation. For instance, Eveoleen Rexford of the Boston University School of Medicine writes:

> Our national wishes and intentions to care adequately for emotionally disturbed children have been articulated repeatedly and with eloquence. For example, groups of citizens and government officials drew up the following statement at the 1930 White House Conference:
>
> The emotionally disturbed child has a right:
>   (1) to grow up in a world which does not set him apart, which looks at him not with scorn or pity or ridicule—but which welcomes him, exactly as it welcomes every child, which offers him identical privileges and identical responsibilities,
>   (2) to a life on which his handicap casts no shadow, but which is full day by day with those things which make it worthwhile, with comradeship, love, work, play, laughter, and tears—a life in which these things bring continually increasing growth, richness, release of energies, joy in achievement.
>
> There are in the United States: 2,500,000 children with well-marked behavior difficulties including the more serious mental and nervous disorders.
>
> Even as early as four years of age, it has been shown that more than 35 percent of the apparently normal children of self-sustaining families, average intelligence, have detectable behavior difficulties.
>
> A comprehensive program to prepare the emotionally handicapped child for life's work must include: early discovery and diagnosis which will determine the nature and extent of the handicap while it is in the incipient stages and when the greatest possible benefit may be secured from care and treatment.
>
> Protective legislation which will make a comprehensive program for the handicapped fully effective, safeguarding the interests of the handicapped as well as the employer.

Research which will determine the fundamental causes of mental and physical disabilities and discover the most effective methods of prevention and control of all handicaps.

National and central state agencies which will provide for the integration of national, state, and local educational, vocational, industrial, health, and welfare activities in a comprehensive plan on behalf of the handicapped child.

Have we really made headway during these 30 years, years during which we have attained the highest per capita income the United States and indeed the world has ever seen? We can note lamentably limited progress. What has been the cost to individual lives, what the waste to our nation of ignoring these recommendations? During 1967, the federal government appropriated $1.11 billion for cotton price support and one-twentieth that amount for child mental health services conceived in the broadest possible terms. What are our priorities? Do we indeed lavish care upon our children? What happens between the rousing statement of the child's bill of rights and the feeble, inadequate implementation of these goals?

Rexford comments further:

A curious factor has emerged about the basis for this support [support for this Commission]. Certain public figures have given such an endeavor their interest in "cutting down crime in the streets." . . . The extent and seriousness of youthful anti-social behavior are cogent reasons for wishing to plan more effectively and to ameliorate mental disturbances in the young; the possibility that the youthful delinquent becomes a serious adult criminal is often borne out. It takes one aback, however, to be told that protection of society *from* its children in this direct sense is the compelling motivation of many influential citizens for programming for emotionally sick children and youth and those at high risks (Rexford, 1969).

The failure of our nation to provide even minimally adequate services for the emotionally disturbed and mentally ill children and youth is related to many factors. One is the greater emphasis on providing programs for adults. For instance, special services needed for children have not been included in many Community Mental Health Center programs.

The failure of the great majority of states to include *any* plans for children in mental health programs presented to the U.S. Public Health Service (PHS) in 1963 led to the convening of a national conference that year on planning child psychiatric services within community mental health programs. However, the recent visit of a survey team to eight Comprehensive Mental Health Centers planned with and funded by the USPHS brought forth the distressing observation that only two had any kind of specific children's services and of these two instances, only one offered a satisfactory program. There were no plans in the other Centers to move ahead in providing appropriate children's services although these had been included in the original blueprints. . . . [Moreover,] Many child guidance clinics are currently the nuclei for mental health center programs, their staff serving adult patients, their activities for children steadily declining. Supposedly, this diversion from the children's program is temporary, but given staffing realities in many communities embarking upon a center program, it may not be unlikely that less service for children will be available within so-called comprehensive programs than was provided for children previously. It appears that wherever inpatient beds must be allocated to adult or child services, the latter rarely receive precedence. You may say that it is clearly more important to have the bed for the adult patient, but is that true? Is the adult's depressive and suicidal status so obviously more significant than that of a 10-year-old boy that no questions are raised about the decision? What of the suffering in the present? What of the import for the future? . . .

"Who speaks for the sick children?" is a question which might echo across the country these days as the planners, citizens, and government agents sit down together (Rexford, 1969).

Basically, there is a severe shortage of mental health programs of all kinds for people of all ages. However, children and young people are less well served than adults and seriously overlooked when we consider the size of the child population.

This appalling lack of services is extremely critical and shortsighted, especially in reference to children and young people. The experience of psychotherapists and other clinical personnel in the mental health field strongly indicates that the roots of mental illness and severe emotional problems usually extend far back into infancy and early childhood. In fact, many specialists in the field hold that the origins of most disturbances are found in a combination of the constitutional factors present in a child at birth, the effects of these factors on the feelings and attitudes of the child's parents or other caretakers, and the consequent interaction between the infant and the significant people in his environment in the first few months of his life (Lourie, 1967). Most clinicians agree that an extremely important time for intervening with both remedial and broadly defined preventive mental health services is during the mother's pregnancy and the very early years of infancy and childhood (*Report of the Committee on Clinical Issues,* 1969; see also Chapter VII).

Despite this general consensus, the present tendency in the provision of mental health services—to the extent that such services are available at all—is to identify children in need of professional help and refer them for help after they have reached the age of six or older and are found to present problems in school adjustment. There is considerable evidence, largely derived from clinical practice and theory and from related observation (Pavenstadt, 1965; Minuchin and Montalvo, 1967), that this is far too late for the most effective intervention in the child's basic adjustment. By the time the child has reached school age, his personality may have become highly disorganized or set in rigid patterns that are not easily changed.

This is not to imply that late treatment is of little use. Appropriate mental health service to children and youth of all ages may well be highly effective. The major point is that early intervention is usually the most helpful and may well prevent the cumulative compounding of the child's difficulties. The outcome of early intervention is even more favorable if followed by a wide range of supportive services to further aid and protect the child who is at mental health risk. Moreover, such continuing services are needed because early treatment is not an assurance that symptoms of disorder will not appear at a later date (*Report of the Committee on Clinical Issues,* 1969).

Part of any greatly expanded investment in programs for the mental health of children and youth should be focused specifically on treatment, research, and training in the field of services for mentally ill and emotionally disturbed children and youth. Particular, but not sole, emphasis should be placed on programs for those infants and young children who are in danger of developing severe disabilities. Every attempt should be made to coordinate programs and to eliminate the present fragmentation and overlapping of services.

Epidemiology

The exact number of emotionally disturbed and mentally ill children in this country is not known. There have been no national epidemiological studies of mental illness; but as formerly stated, it is generally estimated, on the basis of partial data, that .6 percent of our children and youth suffer from psychoses and another 2 to 3 percent from severe disorders. An additional 8 to 10 percent suffer from emotional disturbances. Among disadvantaged preschoolers, observation indicates that about one-third may suffer from emotional or mental disabilities.

As Dr. Rexford states:

As a nation we have not been able to look honestly at the scope of the problem of emotional disturbance in children and youth nor at the size and quality of the resources available to cope with these children. We have not developed the systematic surveys, the categories of conditions, the conceptual models, nor the adequate reporting and analyzing systems to know where we are.

However concerned we may be about the lacunae in our information regarding emotionally disturbed children identified by psychiatric facilities, the total situation may be far more serious. A large population of the children residing in correctional institutions, welfare homes, state schools, and foster homes undoubtedly suffer from emotional and behavioral disturbances. They may be labeled dependent, neglected, delinquent, or retarded and there is no way under present circumstances to include them in a comprehensive mental health survey. Each grouping of institutions has its own nomenclature and its own programming. There are those who believe that the reform schools and correctional institutions of the country are the sites of the same kind of neglect of mentally disturbed young individuals as the state hospital back wards were of adults (Rexford, 1969).

It should be borne in mind that for every child who has a severe mental health problem many more are affected—those who are in association with him in his neighborhood, in his school, and especially within his family. If only families are considered, one could estimate that at least three or four other people—parents and brothers and sisters—are intimately and deeply affected by a child's mental illness or serious emotional disorder.

It is likely that the prevalence and severity of emotional disorders will increase along with the increase in our child and youth population and the mounting stresses and demands of modern society. These stresses, as pointed out previously, presently affect young people of all socioeconomic backgrounds; however, poor children are additionally handicapped by the severe stresses of poverty.

At present, the precise extent to which poverty conditions cause higher rates of mental and emotional disturbance is unknown. This complex matter cannot be discussed in its entirety here; however, a few main points are in order. Although there appear to be higher rates of emotional and mental problems among people living in poverty, it is not entirely clear whether the conditions of poverty cause these higher rates or whether mentally ill people are more likely to drift into poverty. This theory of drift does not apply, of course, to children; however, it might well apply to older youth and to the parents of children who present emotional and mental disorders. Another school of thought attributes the apparently higher rate to the fact that there are fewer physical and mental health facilities which offer preventive and treatment services to the poor. In addition, rates are often based on admissions to public mental institutions which, because of costs and other factors, serve a disproportionate number of poor people. Then, too, it appears that psychiatrists and other mental health professionals are more likely to diagnose low-income persons as seriously disturbed than people from other income groups (Schneiderman, 1965; McDermott, 1965; Hollingshead and Redlich, 1958). The tendency is related not only to less understanding and acceptance of the poor but also to the fact that poverty evokes adaptive behaviors that might be labeled as emotional disturbance or mental illness in other, more affluent groups.

There is a growing recognition among mental health workers that the traits of fatalism, distrust, physical aggression, and alienation from society, so common among highly disadvantaged people, might be positive and helpful adaptations to the poverty situation. However, simply because poverty evokes these kinds of adjustments, it does not follow that these adaptations are positive in the broad sense in which we have defined mental health. Rather, these behaviors indicate that the poverty situation itself must be corrected and that, for poor people particularly, the environment is also the patient.

Efforts to help disadvantaged children and youth make a more healthy adjustment to life will not be effective unless their life situation is also changed. This does not mean that mental health services should not be made available to the poor. Rather, stresses in the environment should be relieved at the same time that high-quality mental health services are provided. Changing the environment will not, by itself, cure all the problems that poverty has caused within individuals.

Serious emotional and mental disorders are by no means limited to the poor. Being human is not easy for anyone. The processes of growing up are far from simple in our society. Probably all children and youth experience at least a few transitory emotional problems at some time in their development. These problems are related to the growth process itself and to the requirements that are placed on individuals to become members of a human society. The majority of our children, with the help of their parents and other social organizations, manage the strains of growth and socialization well enough so that, as adults, they function with a fair to excellent degree of adequacy, at least most of the time (see Chapters VII and VIII). However, as we have seen, a large number of children and youth fall victim to the miseries and handicaps that are associated with serious emotional and mental disabilities.

CAUSES OF POOR MENTAL HEALTH

The causation of mental illness and severe emotional disorders is a complex topic, and only a few highlights can be given here. At present, the causation of these disabilities is incompletely known and understood. There is general agreement among behavioral scientists and other mental health professionals that the causation of these problems is various and multiple and is related to the interaction of constitutional and biological factors; life experiences in growing up, especially in the family; and social and economic stresses and/or deficits in the larger environment. In the past decade, a shift in thinking has occurred within the mental health professions. There is less focus on psychological conflicts within the individual and increasing concentration on the social, familial, and cultural factors. Further, psychoanalytic theories over the past thirty years have placed increasing emphasis on developmental phases and crucial growth processes during infancy and childhood (Gioscia *et al.*, 1968; *Report of the Committee on Clinical Issues,* 1969).

Constitutional Factors

Constitutional factors present in the child at birth have considerable effect on his behavior and how he relates to people and things in his environment. These factors are related both to the child's genetic inheritance and to the physical health and life situation of his mother during her pregnancy. For example, a child may be born with a hunger drive that cannot be satisfied because of the physiological functioning of his body. Thus, he may develop a sense of distrust and dissatisfaction in his environment and fail to form the necessary dependent and close relationship with his parents. The parents in turn may become increasingly frustrated trying to meet the seemingly insatiable demands of this kind of a child.

Another example of the effect which constitutional factors may have on behavior is seen in the hypersensitive child who finds pain, rather than pleasure, in being touched. This turning away may eventually cause his parents to abandon their efforts to establish a relationship with him. This kind of situation is thought to be one of the factors related to causation in some cases of infantile autism or later neuroses.

Another case in point is the hyperactive child who receives overstimulation from his own body. This kind of child is extremely difficult to handle, and he finds it hard to relate satisfactorily to his own environment. In attempting to handle his own strong impulses, he may develop rigid controls over his feelings and activities and lose the important quality of flexibility of personality. Although hyperactivity is not always associated with brain damage, some children who are hyperactive suffer from brain damage. Such damage, in and of itself, may lead to rigid behavior patterns.

Babies differ in activity level at birth. Some are always active, and some tend to be quiet and passive. These tendencies have differential effects on the reactions of their fathers and mothers, depending on the kinds of behaviors valued by individual parents. Other constitutional differences account for the way some babies readily adjust to regular routines while others continue to be unpredictable. Moreover, some babies adapt easily and adjust readily to changes in their life situation, whereas others object strenuously to any shifts. There are also differences in human sensitivity to stimulation, in ability to concentrate, and in length of attention span. It is important that parents understand the constitutional characteristics of individual babies and learn to be sensitive and adaptative to them. It is obvious that parents will differ in their abilities to make these kinds of adjustments (see also Chapter VII, Section I).

It appears that a very small percentage of children are so biologically impaired at birth that even the most skilled and sensitive parents are unable to guide them into normal, healthy development. These children need a special sheltered environment, one more related to health and normal living than to illness. Long-term care must include vigorous treatment, rehabilitation, educational experiences, and other services (see Chapter I, Section II, Number 7, Page 38).

Autism

A small number of children with very severe behavior and learning disorders are diagnosed as "autistic." These children usually display bizarre, extremely withdrawn behavior and have severe learning difficulties, although they are not mentally retarded. It is probable that autism is not one disorder but a group of disorders, the causes of which are complex and very incompletely understood. Some clinicians believe the difficulty to be psychological in origin, whereas another group of investigators believe that genetic or congenital factors are predominant. Parents of autistic children are faced with tremendous emotional and physical stress in trying to care for and guide their handicapped youngsters. They must have help from the larger community so that they do not have to carry their heavy burdens alone (see also Chapter XI, "Research"). Parents also frequently need specialized mental health services for themselves and other family members because the presence of an autistic child in the family can lead to complex difficulties in the whole family interaction system, including problems of family communication, depressive and guilt reactions of parents and siblings, etc.

Brain Syndrome (Often Also Called "Minimal Brain Dysfunction" or "Brain Damage") (Clements, 1966)

The concept of brain dysfunction as a primary causative factor in learning and behavioral disorders among children has received increasing attention in the fields of medicine, psychology, education, and the language specialties over the past twenty years. The rise in the number of so-called "children with minimal brain dysfunction" may be explained in part by one or more of the following factors: (a) increased refinement in diagnostic techniques and skills over the last several years; (b) the growing need for a more exact classification of the learning and behavioral disorders of children; (c) an apparent increase in the number of children with neurological impairments which, unfortunately, is often related to improved medical services and the increasing ability of the medical profession to save the lives of babies with defects associated with genetic impairments, babies damaged by complications that develop during pregnancy, and those who were injured at birth; (d) a growing dissatisfaction on the part of many professionals who deal with children who feel that psychological and social explanations of children's behavior problems and learning difficulties are not always satisfactory (Clements, 1966).

Brain syndrome disorders are thought to be caused by impairment of the brain tissue which may be brought about by a variety of factors, including those already mentioned, and accidents, certain illnesses, disturbances in physical functioning, and serious deficiencies in nutrition. Although these disorders are relatively permanent, many children show a remarkable ability to compensate for them, to respond to special instruction, and to develop in a fairly normal fashion. The effect of these disorders is not always related to the severity and degree of brain damage. Outcomes in personality problems and learning disorders are related to the child's basic personality pattern, his current emotional conflicts, his level of development, the meaning of the disorder to the child and his parents, relationships within the family, and special services available in the community, particularly in the school.

These disorders may not become apparent until the child reaches school and may then show up in learning disabilities, such as difficulty in learning to read. Children with minimal brain damage often have normal or higher intelligence; however, they may be labeled as mentally retarded, primarily because their problems are incompletely understood and inappropriately handled within the family and/or by the school.

Personality and learning problems associated with minimal brain damage are frequently difficult to diagnose, partly because they are not manifested in any particular pattern of personality or learning disorder. Diagnosis generally depends upon careful observation of the child and a detailed history of the many factors in his development (Group for the Advancement of Psychiatry, 1967).

Reactions to Life Situations

A disrupting crisis in the child's life may bring about a strong emotional reaction which can cause a variety of emotional disorders. One of the most common reactions is a return to earlier levels of development. These precipitating crises may include severe illness or death in the family, and accident or serious illness suffered by the child, severe marital stress between the parents, the father's loss of his job, and the like. Although the birth of a new baby could hardly be called a crisis, it may well be perceived as such by the child. How well a child adapts to such events as these depends on many factors: his own constitutional and psychological strengths, the reactions of family members, and supports and services available in the community.

Family Behavior Patterns

There is growing recognition that a child's emotional disturbance is frequently, but not always, associated with the complex and intricate interpersonal relations within the family and the interactions that the family has with the larger social system. Some experts hold that difficulties within the family are not the basic *cause* of emotional disorders but that family problems arise initially out of the larger social and economic scene as well as from the biological and behavioral characteristics of the child.

The structures, history, organization, boundaries, relationships of the family as well as the family's place in the larger social unit of the community are regarded as critical aspects of emotional disorders. Thus, these experts advise that there can be no complete diagnosis unless there is a family diagnosis (difficult and complex as that may be), and there can be no lasting cure unless the cure takes place within the natural environment of the youngster (*Report of Task Force II,* 1969).

However, there is far from complete agreement on these points. Some specialists take the view that the causes of emotional and mental disorders are closely related to the attitudes, behavior situation, and functioning of family members, especially parents. They call for an intensive treatment focus on intrapsychic conflicts within individual family members and among these members.

Although these causal arguments await confirmation, there is clear evidence that lack of a close, dependable warm relationship between an infant and his mother or mother substitute is likely to have highly adverse effects on the physical and psychological development of the child. Also, as discussed in Chapter VII, children who are cruelly mistreated by their parents ("battered children") suffer serious personality, as well as physical, damage (*Report of the Committee on Clinical Issues,* 1969). Both marital conflict and family breakdown are also likely to have serious effects on the child's emotional health, as noted in Chapter IV.

In actuality, it is extremely difficult to arrive at clear understandings of the various causative factors in emotional and mental disorders, partly because causes and effects are so intricately interwoven with each other and partly because such a wide variety of social, economic, psychological, biological, and situational factors are likely to constitute interconnected roots of the problem (see Chapter XI, "Research").

Cultural Patterns

As pointed out in previous chapters, the cultural patterns or life styles of a family have a strong effect on how children are reared and how the

TABLE 9.—CHILD-REARING AND FAMILY LIFE PATTERNS REPORTED TO BE MORE
         CHARACTERISTIC OF FAMILIES OF CHILDREN WHO ARE EMOTIONALLY
         HEALTHY COMPARED WITH RELEVANT PATTERNS REPORTED TO BE MORE
         CHARACTERISTIC OF VERY POOR FAMILIES

EMOTIONALLY HEALTHY CHILDREN	POVERTY LIFE STYLES
1. Respect for child as individual whose behavior is caused by a multiple of factors. Acceptance of own role in events that occur.	1. Misbehavior regarded as such in terms of concrete pragmatic outcomes; reasons for behavior not considered. Projection of blame on others.
2. Commitment to slow development of child from infancy to maturity; stresses and pressures of each stage accepted by parent because of perceived worth of ultimate goal of raising "happy," successful son or daughter.	2. Lack of goal commitment and of belief in long-range success; a main object for parent and child is to "keep out of trouble"; orientation toward fatalism, impulse gratification, and sense of alienation.
3. Relative sense of competence in handling child's behavior.	3. Sense of powerlessness in handling children's behavior, as well as in other areas.
4. Discipline chiefly verbal, mild, reasonable, consistent, based on needs of child and family and of society; more emphasis on rewarding good behavior than on punishing bad behavior.	4. Discipline harsh, inconsistent, physical, makes use of ridicule; punishment based on whether child's behavior does or does not annoy parent.
5. Open, free, verbal communication between parent and child; control largely verbal.	5. Limited verbal communication; control largely physical.
6. Democratic rather than autocratic or laissez-faire methods of rearing, with both parents in equalitarian but not necessarily interchangeable roles. Companionship between parents and children.	6. Authoritarian rearing methods; mother chief child-care agent; father, when in home, mainly punitive figure. Little support and acceptance of child as an individual.
7. Parents view selves as generally competent adults and are generally satisfied with themselves and their situation.	7. Low parental self-esteem, sense of defeat.
8. Intimate, expressive, warm relationship between parent and child, allowing for gradually increasing independence. Sense of continuing parental responsibility.	8. Large families; more impulsive, narcissistic parent behavior. Orientation to "excitement." Abrupt, early yielding of independence.
9. Free verbal communication about sex, acceptance of child's sex needs, channeling of sex drive through "healthy" psychological defenses, acceptance of slow growth toward impulse control and sex satisfaction in marriage; sex education by both father and mother.	9. Repressive, punitive attitude about sex, sex questioning, and experimentation. Sex viewed as exploitative relationship.

TABLE 9.—(*Continued*)

EMOTIONALLY HEALTHY CHILDREN	POVERTY LIFE STYLES
10. Acceptance of child's drive for aggression but channeling it into socially approved outlets.	10. Alternating encouragement and restriction of aggression, primarily related to consequences of aggression for parents.
11. In favor of new experiences; flexible.	11. Distrust of new experiences. Constricted life, rigidity.
12. Happiness of parental marriage.	12. High rates of marital conflict and family breakdown.

SOURCE: Catherine S. Chilman, *Growing Up Poor,* U.S. Department of Health, Education, and Welfare (Washington, D.C.: Government Printing Office, 1966).

family conducts its life. Cultural patterns vary, depending upon the social group to which the family belongs. Life styles are generally formed in early childhood and are deeply affected by the individual's experience within his own family, even though each individual interprets these patterns in his own unique way. As noted in Chapter II, the cultural patterns generally found in each social class have their own particular deficits in reference to optional patterns of child-rearing. However, those life styles which are most prevalent among the very poor tend to be most harmful to the mental health of the child. Although adaptive to a life of poverty, these patterns interact with the many stresses of economic deprivation and tend to limit the growing child's opportunity for positive mental health.

Although research findings are, as yet, fragmentary and inconclusive, they point to the seriousness of the problem. An overview of related studies strongly suggests that very poor people, to a greater extent than others, often fail to adopt child-rearing and family life patterns which research indicates are associated with children judged to be mentally healthy in our society. These findings are summarized in Table 9. (Those studies which reveal factors conducive to positive mental health include the following investigations: Glidewell, 1961; Roff, 1949; Baldwin, 1948; Antonosky, 1959; Block, Patterson, Block, and Jackson, 1958; Law, 1954; Peterson, Becker, Hellmer, Shoemaker, and Quay, 1959; Watson, 1957; Radke, 1946; Porter, 1955; Thompson, 1962; Baldwin, Kalhorn, and Breese, 1945. Studies related to the child-rearing and family life patterns of the very poor include the following: O. Lewis, 1961; Myers and Roberts, 1959; McKinley, 1964; Handel and Rainwater, 1961; Davis and Havighurst, 1946; Rodman, 1959; Komarovsky, 1964; Herzog, 1963; Sewell and Haller, 1956; Bronfenbrenner, 1961; Clausen and Williams, 1963; H. Lewis, 1961; Miller and Riessman, 1961; Caldwell, 1964; Wortis, 1963.)

It should be noted that patterns of the kind listed on the right-hand side of Table 9 are not limited to very poor families, nor are they found universally among the very poor. Moreover, these patterns should not be considered as an indictment of low-income parents. They should be viewed as adaptations to the poverty situation and the social structure which tends to foster life styles that are related to fundamental psychological depression, poor impulse control, hostility, and/or surrender to overwhelming odds.

Social and Economic Stress

Continuing pressures imposed by the environment are seen as one set of factors that may play an important part in causing serious mental and emotional disorders. Individuals have varying ability to withstand environmental pressures, depending on their physical constitution, their previous life experiences, their present situation, and their anticipations and attitudes toward the future. Some children and young people are able to withstand considerable stress, while others have more limited strengths to cope with it. The severity and duration of stress also must be taken into consideration in terms of its effects. Along with those stresses imposed by economic deprivation are other pressures felt throughout most of our society—the explosive force of today's social and economic changes, life in the city, the terrifying threat of the nuclear age, conflicts between the races, air and water pollution, the population explosion, and the like. Individuals also experience their own particular stresses such as chronic illness or physical handicaps, continuing financial pressures, frequent moving, difficult employment situations, and so on.

PRESENT MENTAL HEALTH PROGRAMS

The critically severe shortage of mental health services for children and young people has already been noted. This shortage applies in all areas—diagnostic, treatment, consultative, and special education services. The services that do exist tend to be overcrowded, understaffed, and poorly coordinated with other mental health and mental health-related programs. Many of the deficiencies in our services were pointed out in Chapter I (see especially Section II), where a number of recommendations were made to improve these services.

We noted that in order to diagnose and treat emotional disturbance and mental illness in children, we need a coordinated network of services that includes the following elements: diagnostic, consultative, and treatment services available in outpatient clinics, residential centers, halfway houses, day and day-night services, emergency services, and supportive programs, including special programs in regular schools and mental health consultation to parents and teachers. No community has all of these services available for all who are in need; few communities have such programs even for a portion of the population; some communities have virtually no mental health programs. In those few communities where most of these services are available, the programs tend to be fragmented and lacking in provision for continuity of care for children and youth in different stages of their growth. Thus, the majority of young people who are in need get no services. A large group gets only diagnostic but no treatment assistance. In general, only a few—mostly the very rich— have all their needs attended in a coordinated way, and this is achieved mostly through access to costly private facilities and the care provided by private psychiatrists. The very poor, who need these services most, have least access to them. There are many reasons for this tragic state of affairs. For example, mentally ill and emotionally disturbed low-income children and youth are often seen as being untreatable by psychiatrists (Hollingshead and Redlich, 1958; Rudolph and Cumming, 1962; Gordon, 1965; Schneiderman, 1965). As noted in Chapter V, treatment is strongly related to social class, as is the length of treatment and the kind of diagnosis that is given to the person's illness. Lower-class people are less likely to be given intensive psychiatric treatment, more likely to be treated by inexperienced therapists, and more often labeled as psychotic or near-psychotic (Schneiderman, 1965; McDermott, 1965; Dunham, 1964; Hollingshead and Redlich, 1958). Lower-class individuals also have far higher rates of dropping out of treatment than do middle-class and upper-class persons (Baum, 1966; Cole, *et al.*, 1962; Rosenthal and Frank, 1958).

According to NIMH reports, about 473,000 children under eighteen years of age received some service in a psychiatric facility in the United States in 1966. Of these children, 84 percent were seen on an outpatient basis and 14 percent were hospitalized. As shown in Table 10, children accounted for about one-third of the total case load of outpatient psychiatric clinics. In contrast, persons under eighteen made up only 3 to 8 percent of the case loads of inpatient facilities.

The number of children under eighteen years of age receiving care in psychiatric clinics has almost doubled since 1959. This growth in the patient case load is only partly due to the increase in the child population in the United States. There is also a rising demand for and availability of these services. The number of patients under care during the last decade increased more rapidly than either the number of clinics or the professional man-hours available.

The adolescent group, aged ten to seventeen years, comprised two-thirds of the children served in clinics and, in fact, for boys was the largest patient group of any other comparable age span. Children aged five to nine years accounted for another third of the patients under age eighteen. Preschoolers accounted for only 6 percent of the clinic child population. Twice as many boys as girls were given service in clinics; however, the

Table 10.—NUMBER OF PSYCHIATRIC FACILITIES AND ESTIMATED NUMBER OF CHIL-
DREN UNDER EIGHTEEN YEARS OF AGE UNDER CARE DURING THE YEAR
IN EACH TYPE OF FACILITY, 1966

TYPE OF FACILITY	FACILITIES		TOTAL PATIENTS ALL AGES		CHILDREN UNDER 18 YEARS OF AGE		
	Number	Percent distri- bution	Estimated number	Percent distri- bution	Estimated number	Per- cent distri- bution	Percent of total patients in each type of facility
		(%)		(%)		(%)	(%)
Outpatient psychiatric clinics[1]	2,122	56	1,186,000	46	399,000	84	34
State and county mental hospitals	297	8	807,000	31	27,400	6	3
Private mental hospitals	175	5	105,000	4	8,400	2	8
General hospitals with psychiatric services	888	23	466,000	18	28,000	6	6
Psychiatric day-night units[2]	173	5	15,600	1	2,500	1	16
Residential treatment centers (not in state mental hospitals)[3]	149	4	—	—	8,000	2	—
Total	3,804	100	2,579,600	100	473,300	100	18

[1] Includes clinics of the Veterans Administration.
[2] Based on survey conducted in 1965 providing estimated number of children served in 1964. Includes day-night units of the Veterans Administration.
[3] Based on the average capacity or average number of residents reported for 92 facilities.
Source: *Directory of Facilities for Mentally Ill Children in the United States, 1967,* The National Association for Mental Health, Inc.
The Directory for Exceptional Children, F. Porter Sargent, Fifth Edition, 1965.
SOURCE: Beatrice M. Rosen, Morton Kramer, Richard W. Redick, and Shirley G. Willner, *Utilization of Psychiatric Facilities by Children,* NIMH, Mental Health Statistics, Series B, No. 1 (Washington, D.C.: Government Printing Office, 1968).

rates for boys aged eighteen to nineteen dropped sharply. This decrease is closely related to the discontinued contact with the schools and with the lack of major community programs which often serve as case-finding and referral agencies for young adults.

Almost 34 percent of the children who were terminated from clinic service received a diagnosis of transient situational personality disorder. Among children under five, brain syndromes and mental deficiencies accounted for almost half of the diagnosed cases. A large proportion of children received no diagnosis, a fact that reflects, to a large extent, the brief contact that many children have with the clinic.

The huge majority of children in state or county mental hospitals were over the age of ten, and more than half were between ages fifteen and seventeen. Again, boys outnumber girls two to one for first admissions to these hospitals and, once they are hospitalized, tend to remain longer in the institution. The major diagnoses for these hospitalized young people were schizophrenia and personality disorders (Rosen *et al.*, 1968).

As shown in Table 10, more than 27,000 children under age eighteen were in state and county mental hospitals in 1966. In most of these hospitals the usual practice is to place youngsters in wards with adult patients, frequently with those who are in an advanced stage of mental deterioration. These children and youth receive little, if any, therapeutic care, and no provision is made for the continuation of their education. An imprecisely determined number are left to "rot on the back wards," condemned to a hopeless life of continuing institutionalization. Another large group of young people who suffer from emotional disturbance or mental illness are labeled as being delinquent or mentally retarded and placed in institutions where they receive no treatment for their disabilities.

It is the conviction of this Commission that no child or young person should be placed in a mental hospital without a careful professional diagnosis and without preliminary attempts to help him through other forms of treatment on an outpatient basis in his own home or at least in his home community. If hospitalization proves inevitable, care should be provided in a special treatment unit for children or adolescents, as the case may be, in which provision is made for continuing therapy and educational and recreational needs.

Very little data are available on the number and characteristics of patients served in private psychiatric practice. One study showed that about 4 percent of private psychiatric patients are under age fifteen, indicating that very few children receive private psychiatric care. As of 1967, the relatively new Community Mental Health Centers were serving only 1,400 children under age eighteen—a number representing about 20 percent of the total patient case load. Two-thirds of the children served in these centers were boys; of those children under age twelve, boys outnumbered girls three to one (National Institute of Mental Health, 1968).

The present dearth of mental health services for children and youth in an average, but imaginary, community has been dramatically portrayed by Tarjan (1969):

The child population under 18 in the city is approximately 300,000. About 50,000 individuals, including 18,000 children, qualify as poor under the customary standards; most of these people live in one sizeable ghetto. Among the 110,000 children, there are some 7,500 who are emotionally disturbed, including 750 who are overtly or severely sick.

Approximately 20 children between the ages of five to 15 are diagnosed as autistic or schizophrenic. Three thousand children are diagnosed as mentally retarded with 500 falling into the moderately to more severely impaired categories. Almost no information is available on the prevalence of mental illness in the poverty population. It is very probable, however, that for most mental disorders the rates are higher than those found in the middle or upper socioeconomic classes. Even cursory review suggests, for example, that mild mental retardation as diagnosed by the school system, occurs 15 times as often in the city's minority population than in the residents of the suburbia-like areas.

All types of treatment resources are in short supply, even those that, to some measure, might substitute for psychiatric care. The city is served by a state mental hospital which cares for a population nearly three times as large as that of the city. The state hospital has no special programs for children, even though from the city alone nine children under 15 are in residence and a minimum of six are admitted yearly. There is neither a private psychiatric facility with a specialized program for children nor is there such a program in the two general hospitals which have a few psychiatric beds.

There are three psychiatric clinics but only one serves children, the others take only an occasional child for diagnosis. The three clinics see some 400 children under 18 per year. This may sound like a large number but it must be compared with the size of the emotionally disturbed child population of 7,500. We must also realize that only 100 of the 400 receive any treatment, others are seen, at best, for diagnosis. The clinic that gives some preference to children operates with a series of waiting lists: one for intake, one for diagnosis, and a hopelessly long one for treatment.

A Community Mental Health Center is about to open in temporary quarters. The people expect that the Center will pick up much of the slack in services for children, but the fact is that it will be overwhelmed by the needs of adults and therefore will postpone caring for children. A community facility for the mentally retarded is also under construction but it will be geographically located to serve the moderately to more severely retarded children of the middle classes and, for all practical purposes, will be unavailable to the citizens of the inner city where diagnosed mild retardation is most prevalent. It is also of importance to note that no special classes for emotionally disturbed children exist in the public school system and that the special program for the retarded reaches only two-thirds of the eligible educable and one-third of the trainable children.

It is obvious that the city cannot serve as a model for the delivery of community services and treatment. Yet, like most communities, it has one program relevant to childhood mental health which fills the city with pride. It is a private day school which cares for a few psychotic, severely emotionally disturbed, and neurologically handicapped children.

There is only one certified child psychiatrist in this city; he devotes most of his time to private practice and contributes only a few hours to one of the clinics. One child psychiatrist for 110,000 is near the national average. However, it would not be illogical to set a goal of one child psychiatrist for 15,000 children because in such a group one finds 1,000 who are emotionally disturbed, with 100 overtly sick. Parenthetically, we may note that there are some 20 general psychiatrists in the city but very few with interests in child psychiatry. The manpower situation is no better in such important fields as psychology, social work, or psychiatric nursing.

Care for Emotionally Disturbed and Mentally Ill Children Outside Their Own Homes

Intensive individual or group care outside the child's own home may be required for youngsters with severe emotional disorders and mental illness. The severity of their disorders presents extremely complex problems: those of deep emotional hunger, extreme overactivity, withdrawal from the outer world, high levels of aggression, violent uncontrolled behavior, bizarre and incomprehensible reaction patterns, and the like. These children need more than individual treatment. They need an all-embracing therapeutic environment and care which includes attention to their total development. For instance, they need individualized, highly skilled attention to their educational and recreational requirements. Their daily routine needs to be handled with psychological skill. These children need the help of highly trained mental health specialists who also serve as directors and consultants to a team of other professionals and nonprofessionals involved in delivering the wide range of services essential for their full care. Trained personnel should be readily available to conduct life-space interviews—that is, discussions with children of their difficulties at the moment they occur or at the moment the child feels ready to talk about them. In most cases, counseling services should also be made available to their parents.

When the child returns to his own home—often after a prolonged period of treatment—he should be followed up with therapeutic services which extend to other important people in his environment, such as his parents and his teachers. Because children have such a wide range of needs, and because intensive treatment is necessary for very sick youngsters, the costs of such care are high. For instance, the costs of residential treatment centers are generally estimated at between $10,000 and $18,000 a year. However, effective residential treatment at an early age may well save later costs—costs which extend beyond economic ones and which are cumulative in terms of the burdens that untreated, ill children are likely to impose upon themselves, their families, and their society.

At present, the small number of residential treatment centers and the cost to the individual family are factors which prohibit such treatment for the majority of children who are in need. The costs of such centers are so high that it appears that they cannot be extended and adequately financed unless federal aid is made available for this purpose (*Report of the Committee on Clinical Issues,* 1969).

Because there are not enough residential treatment and other specialized facilities, many children are placed in a number of inappropriate settings where their problems are likely to become more, rather than less, severe. These settings include mental hospitals which are designed for adults, institutions for the delinquent or the mentally retarded, and foster homes which are not designed to care for ill or disturbed children. Many ill, neglected children receive no treatment at all but rather roam the streets and the countryside, where they are a potential danger either to themselves or to others. Emotionally disturbed or mentally ill children from low-income and/or minority-group families are particularly likely to be misdiagnosed and placed in inappropriate facilities or neglected altogether.

In 1968 a survey revealed that 97 percent of the children in residential treatment were in private institutions. In 1966 there were a little more than 8,000 children in residential treatment centers; the number of seriously ill children under eighteen during that same year was estimated at 1,400,000.

There were 276 residential treatment institutions for emotionally disturbed children in this country in 1966. A number of states and territories had no such institutions. These included: Alabama, Arkansas, Georgia, Hawaii, Idaho, Mississippi, Nevada, Puerto Rico, South Carolina, Utah, and the Virgin Islands. The states with the largest number of such institutions are: California (38), Illinois (12), Massachusetts (27), Michigan (17), New York (24), and Wisconsin (14). A number of states, primarily those in the far West and in the Southeast, have only one such institution (Papenfort *et al.*, 1968).

Some existing residential centers offer good care. One example is the Hawthorne Cedar Knolls School, described in Appendix B of this chapter. As noted in this description, the Hawthorne Center provides total child care for the seriously disturbed in a structured milieu setting. Day care, group homes, and a halfway house serve as aftercare arrangements, providing a transitional phase between the institution and return to the community.

Other centers have weaknesses or deficiencies in their programs. This is particularly true of a number of institutions which offer care for emotionally disturbed or mentally ill children but which do not meet the standards set by such professional organizations as the American Association for Children's Residential Centers. The more conspicuous inadequacies, as described by some specialists, include the following:

In some institutional programs, well-trained staff members work with the children eight hours a day, five days a week; however, the children are cared for in the evenings and on weekends by personnel with the least training. Communication among the many professionals is often inadequate.

Many institutions for disturbed and retarded children provide diagnostic services only, with no place for children and their families to go to get help.

School is neglected or given secondary emphasis in many if not most residential treatment programs. Teachers are far down in the prestige hierarchy. They are often provided by public schools and are seldom the best teachers. They frequently remain on the fringe of the professional staff and seldom are central to it.

Very few institutional programs have adequately conceptualized and staffed liaison programs to work with the child's family, school, and community to speed his return home and to follow up so as to promote continuing progress and adjustment.

Once children are admitted to institutional programs they tend to remain for long periods of time, which may often be more a matter of custom than of the child's condition. A lengthy institutional stay is often associated with an inadequate liaison service.

Fully staffed residential treatment programs involving the traditional psychiatric team (psychiatrist, clinical psychologist, psychiatric social worker, psychiatric nurse, sundry kinds of therapists, teachers, aides) are expensive, as already indicated. Moreover, highly trained personnel required for such programs are now and will remain in short supply. These facts mean that we cannot meet requirements for residential care for all children needing it by building exclusively on the psychiatric team model. Such programs are essential but must be used selectively, with clear goals in mind and costs carefully considered.

Few residential treatment programs evaluate the outcome of their work in rigorously designed, well-controlled, scientifically objective studies.

These are harsh criticisms, but progress is not likely to be made until we take a hard look at current practice. This is not an indictment of any state or professional group. There are good residential treatment centers throughout the country, and under varied auspices, inspired by psychiatrists, teachers, social workers, and psychologists, at varying levels of cost. And there are many bad institutions that are underfinanced, understaffed, and poorly housed, whose devoted and overworked professional staffs know better than anyone how inadequate the places are and how much needs to be done. On the whole, we are doing a very poor job in supplying residential care for disturbed children.

There are times when a problem cannot be solved following accepted assumptions and procedures; such seems to be the case now in our efforts to extend traditional treatment models for the residential care of all emotionally disturbed and mentally ill children who need intensive specialized treatment. A not-too-sharp pencil can show what the problem is. Assume a most conservative estimate of the number of seriously disturbed children, say one-half of one percent of children under twenty. That means 450,000 seriously disturbed children in need of treatment. Assume that a psychiatric team is composed of one psychiatrist, one psychologist, two social workers, and three nurses—not to mention teachers, aides, etc. Give them a treatment load of 50 children in residence or intensive day care, a much heavier load than they can handle. This arrangement would require 9,000 child psychiatrists (six times the present number of child psychiatrists), 9,000 psychologists (more than the entire number of clinical psychologists), 18,000 social workers, and 27,000 psychiatric nurses. Assume further a per-day treatment cost of $40, which is on the low side. The annual cost of the program would be $6,570,000,000. Since traditional treatment programs tend to require about two years, this amount would need to be doubled to care for the children now estimated as being in need of help. Double the case load to reduce personnel requirements and the resulting figures are still staggering. The problem of residential and intensive day care for severely disturbed children simply cannot be solved the way we are trying to solve it.

Therefore, it is important to experiment with other approaches to care for disturbed children who, for one reason or another, cannot remain in their own homes. These approaches include other kinds of group care, such as those pioneered by Project Re-ED (see Appendix D of this chapter), day care such as that provided by the League School (see Appendix C at the end of this chapter), night-care programs, use of specialized foster homes, therapeutic nursery schools, and the like. In these programs very careful consideration should be given to expert diagnosis of the nature of the child's problems. Differentiation should be made between those youngsters with such severe disorders that highly intensive psychiatric and other forms of medical care are essential and those children who are likely to respond well to a more generalized approach. These various forms of treatment and care should be tried on an experimental basis and carefully evaluated with well-designed program research (see Chapter XI).

Included in such experimental approaches should be a more flexible use of mental health specialists who serve as consultants to other professionals, such as teachers and nurses, who are working directly with seriously disturbed children. Expanded use also should be made of paraprofessionals, that is, people without formal professional training who may do an excellent job in some aspects of group care for disturbed children, providing that such personnel receive appropriate in-service training, consultation, and supervision (see Chapters XI, XII, and the section in this chapter on services for adolescents and specialized programs in state hospitals).

Mental Health Services for Children in General

A number of problems are apparent in the provision of mental health services for children in general. In discussing those related to very young children, the *Report of the Committee on Clinical Issues* (1969) identifies three major difficulties:

1. There has been a tendency for many years to regard preschoolers as the primary psychological property of their parents; thus, treatment has been aimed at the parents, although clinical experience indicates that the child himself also often needs treatment before his problems become too rigidly imbedded in his personality.

2. There is a widespread lack of training and special professional skill developed for dealing with preschool children. The average child psychiatrist does not have specialized preparation for working with youngsters of this age.

3. There is a strongly held belief that preschool children should never be removed from their own homes. However, recent studies are indicating that children of this age may benefit from care in specialized foster homes, day-care centers, or residential centers if there are assurances that the child will receive a high quality of continuous care from parent substitutes.

While changes in the child's environment and the provision of supporting services such as day care and counseling to his parents may be extremely useful for many children, some youngsters need direct individualized psychotherapeutic help (Neubauer, 1967).

Services for Adolescents

Much of the treatment of the troubled teen-ager has fallen to clinics and private practitioners. The major unmet need for this group is that of vastly improved institutional care. An enormous number of teen-agers pass into and out of state institutions each year, and instead of being helped, the vast majority are the worse for the experience. This is true for the average state training school or state industrial or state farm for boys or girls; it is true, also, of the state hospitals in many areas.

The admission of teen-agers to the state hospitals has risen something like 150 percent in the last ten years. The number of youngsters in correctional institutions is also increasing, and few, if any, of these situations provide anything approaching adequate treatment or rehabilitation.

The usual picture is one of untrained people working without facilities attempting to deal with a wide variety of complex and seriously sick youngsters and producing results that are most easily measured by a recommitment rate that is often 30 to 50 percent and occasionally higher.

There is an urgent need for intensive skilled clinical and educational work with these many troubled youngsters and their parents. It is imperative that public attention be turned toward this shameful and correctable condition. State hospital programs for teen-agers are still seldom geared to the special needs of the adolescent population, as reflected in the tendency to place young people on adult wards without the benefits of the special recreation activities, education, supervision, and group experiences that teen-agers need. The result is, at best, a partial treatment program with many gaps left in what could be a major assist toward recovery from illness.

Although good institutional care is the most glaring lack in programs for teen-agers, mental health facilities in general are seriously deficient for this age group. Many child guidance clinics take youngsters only up to ages eleven or fourteen. For the older adolescent, there is not even the relatively commonplace clinic service, and outpatient care is only one of a whole series of necessary services. The nature of adolescence is such that to meet the upheavals and crises of this period of life, facilities are needed which will offer emergency service at any time. Backing this up must be a whole array of services beginning with a group-living halfway house. This might be a professionally run youth hostel, which has provisions for long-time residents who need an extended period in a protected and supervised state until they are ready for full community adjustment. At the same time, such a hostel would include facilities for transients, for youngsters under pressure who would leave home for a night or two or a week or two if they felt they must. It could provide a haven under socially approved auspices where they could also look for outside help and for relief from home pressures.

Protected work situations are necessary for many youngsters who need remedial education and on-the-job training to give them a sense of career and direction. For the more disturbed boys and girls, a day-care setup is recommended, where work training, school, recreational activities, therapy, group work, and in short, a total treatment program are all provided under one roof. To put it briefly, insofar as mental health care is concerned, as a society we fail our teen-agers at almost every level (*Report of the Committee on Clinical Issues*, 1969).

RECOMMENDED MENTAL HEALTH PROGRAMS*

Programs Based on Developmental Stages

As recommended in Chapter I, mental health programs should start before pregnancy with provisions for genetic counseling and family planning services. As increasing information becomes available regarding the relationship between genetic factors and mental retardation and physical handicaps, it is important that parents have access to skilled, sensitive counseling on this subject. Family planning should be available to all parents or prospective parents regardless of age or marital status, since an unwanted pregnancy presents a threat to the mental health of both the mother and her unborn child. Moreover, abortion services should be available at the request of the mother for the same reason.

As emphasized earlier, highest priority should be given to providing a wide range of physical health, mental health, and related services to expectant mothers and to infants and their parents. Current research on learning in infant life suggests that the kind of learning that goes on in the early months and years is probably more significant than anything the child learns during the rest of his life. There is rather substantial evidence that if severe deficits occur in early infant experiences, later therapy is likely to have only a partial effect. We do not yet know to what extent early deprivations can be undone later by therapy. We do know that such critical points in human life as pregnancy, childbirth, infancy, toddlerhood, preschool, and school entry represent optimal points of intervention both for ensuring good physical and mental health care and for working with families to help parents rear their children more successfully. This approach to families with very young children requires a large commitment on the part of the whole society, a willingness to invest in the development of infants and children and to regard their development as a very serious business (Gioscia *et al.,* 1968).

Our knowledge has brought us to the point where we can state with some certainty that it will be more economical—in terms of both financial and human resources—to organize services along the lines of the child's developmental stages and his needs at these different stages. To accomplish this goal, specialized personnel must be trained to deal with the character-

* In reference to most of the recommendations that follow, there is a lack of firm, research-based evidence as to the effectiveness of the various kinds of programs that are recommended. However, the need is so acute that it is not possible to delay action until all the needed research is completed. Basic and applied research must take place concomitantly with the launching and operation of a wide range of services (see Chapter XI).

istic problems of each period. Developmental knowledge must also be applied to the nature of agencies—their types and locations—and to practices and community relations wherever individuals are involved with children.

A Wide Range of Coordinated Preventive and Treatment Services

The establishment of services and training programs should include these goals: the treatment of every child as well as the family around the child wherever demonstrable emotional and mental disorders are found; an attempt to prevent these disorders by large-scale planning; and the reorganization of services in a way that will encourage the maximum flowering of each person's individual potential for self-realization and social contribution. In this planning, it is imperative that services be individualized and adapted to the needs of specific individuals (*Report of the Committee on Clinical Issues*, 1969).

A broad range of coordinated remedial mental health services must be provided for seriously disturbed, juvenile delinquent, mentally retarded, and otherwise handicapped children and their families. It is strongly urged that future services to the child be given according to the child's level of functioning rather than on the basis of diagnostic labeling. This will mean that children with many different diagnostic labels will be treated jointly under the same service program. Further, it is recommended that community-based facilities be developed so that children and youth can be kept as closely as possible within their normal, routine setting. For the more severe cases who must be removed from the normal setting, it is recommended that there be further development of residential treatment centers, special units in general and psychiatric hospitals, and separate caretaking provisions for children and adolescents in state hospitals.

Plans for care of the emotionally disturbed or mentally ill child should be based on: (a) the behavior stability of the child, (b) the strength and capacity of the family to support him, (c) the resources of the community. The disturbed child often needs a wide variety of services. It is essential that arrangements be made so that he may move easily from one service to another. Many emotionally and mentally disturbed children are excluded from services that they need either because a general service has made no provision for such children or because the cost of specialized services for these youngsters is beyond the means of the families involved.

A comprehensive mental health program for troubled youngsters should include:

1. *Informational-referral services* easily accessible and equipped to direct families to available services, resources, and facilities.

2. *Comprehensive developmental and psycho-educational assessment* of each child's special treatment and educational needs, as well as on-

going, periodic reevaluations to make certain the appropriate and adequate community treatment, training, and educational facilities are made available to meet the recommendations of the assessment service.

3. *Treatment* for the child and his family when indicated.

4. *Special education programs* which should be an integral part of the continuum of services to be provided.

5. *Rehabilitation services* to provide a planned and purposeful process of restoration, remediation, and psychosocial adjustment.

6. *Residential care* in facilities which offer milieu treatment and have adequate resources for medical care, psychological and psychiatric consultation, special education, and other support services.

7. *Transitional services* such as partial hospital care (as in day or night hospitals), halfway houses and hostels, and social rehabilitation programs.

8. *Relief services for the families* of children severely disturbed and mentally ill.

9. *Periodic assessment, evaluation, and follow-up* of the child (National Association for Mental Health, 1968. These are spelled out in detail in Chapter I, pp. 38–44).

Comprehensive continuous programs such as those outlined above might well be tied in with the functions and activities of the Child Development Councils recommended by this Commission and carried out in relation to community mental health programs.

Other recommendations emerged from a survey conducted by the American Association of Psychiatric Clinics for Children. The material was analyzed to assist the Commission in planning for mental health services for children. Some of the conclusions were summarized as follows:

1. Services which reach larger numbers of children at earlier ages or at earlier stages of disturbances are generally less expensive, more short-term, and achieve more favorable effect than those services which reach children later on when the children are more deeply disturbed.

2. The soundest progress in community organization for emotionally disturbed children and their families is achieved by developing services in "developmental succession," namely: preventive before diagnostic; diagnostic before outpatient treatment; outpatient treatment before hospital care, and so forth.

3. Communities with inadequate educational, preventive, diagnostic, and treatment resources are compelled to move children out of the community into institutions instead of reaching younger or less disturbed children more quickly and treating them with shorter, less expensive community and outpatient services.

4. In practice, it may be soundest to begin by making better use or

refocused use of existing resources than to establish and promote new services immediately. If a small community, for example, has a family service agency but no outpatient clinic, the addition of psychiatric services to the agency may be more economical than establishing a clinic itself.

5. No program can be soundly based which does not include careful diagnostic evaluation as the basis for any service or treatment planning. Such diagnostic evaluation means evaluation not only of the child and his problem but of the parent-child relationship, the parents, and the relationship of the family unit to the community and its resources.

6. When more specialized services are required, the transition for the child and his family should be as simple and as direct as good community organization and intra-agency cooperation can make it.

7. The multiple roles of the psychiatric clinicians and psychiatric services today have come not only from the many demands of various community services but have also come from contributions made by the many new directions in the field of medicine. For example, the contributions of psychopharmacology and genetics are having special present significance. Psychiatry is involved in the general present movement of medicine toward health preservation and the prevention of illness.

8. The child psychiatric clinician and the child psychiatric services today need to be aware of important class differences, value differences, and differences in beliefs regarding the role of the individual and the relationship between individual and group needs. Since we believe so fully in multiple causality, many different professional groups, using many different resources, have both an opportunity and an obligation to participate in helping troubled children and their families. However, it is precisely because the problems of an emotionally disturbed child are determined by a multiplicity of factors that the child psychiatric clinician and the child psychiatric services are useful in deciding which factor to be corrected is causal, and critical, and accessible to change. The unique contribution of the staff member of the child psychiatric service is his specialized clinical insight and his application of this to the methods of helping children (American Association of Psychiatric Clinics for Children, 1968).

Some mental health experts warn, however, that we should recognize that there is an extreme shortage of child psychiatrists in the country, not nearly enough to serve the function described above. Obviously, we must perfect new patterns of care that will use new kinds of personnel and extend the range of effectiveness of the child psychiatrist, a problem discussed further in Chapter XI.

Community Planning for Mental Health

When a community plans for psychiatric services for its children, it must be concerned with the quantity and quality of the health, educational, recreational, and welfare services which it provides for all its citizens. Services for emotionally ill children and their parents cannot be set up in a vacuum. They are related to, and affected by, other programs and services: both those concerned with children and those concerned with adults. All community services overlap and complement each other. They should be thought of as parts of a whole, not separate and unrelated programs.

Planning for comprehensive mental health programs should be coordinated with planning now going on in such areas as urban renewal and public housing, juvenile delinquency, the poverty program, and mental retardation. Great emphasis should be placed on the fact that mental health services for children are one segment of the total services in a comprehensive mental health program and that many and diverse facilities are component parts of this segment (American Psychiatric Association, 1964).

In planning such programs, states within a regional area, particularly those that are sparsely populated and have few facilities, may well coordinate the development of their programs on a regional basis.

In developing programs, certain fundamental principles of planning may be set forth: (1) emotionally disturbed children can be helped more effectively or adequately in communities that have a wide range of educational, preventive, diagnostic, and treatment facilities than in communities where there is a narrower range or a marked lack of such facilities; (2) services which reach children at early ages and at early stages of emotional disturbance are generally more effective, and therefore there should be a focus on treatment of young children and on early detection and treatment of emotional illness; (3) continuity of treatment for the individual child and his family should be a major consideration in organizing a program; (4) the order in which various facilities are initiated varies from one community to another. This depends basically on the services available, the degree of coordination among them, attitudes in the community (American Psychiatric Association, 1964).

Particular attention should be paid to the needs of low-income children and their families, whose problems are likely to be particularly diverse and acute and who are likely to especially lack needed services. In the past, the emotionally disturbed children from this group have tended to reach mental health clinics chiefly through referrals from juvenile courts and welfare agencies. Effective work with these children and their parents calls for a multiple approach and active cooperation with schools, juvenile courts, welfare agencies, child-care centers, public health nurses, neighborhood recreation workers, and the like.

Imaginative new methods may well be necessary for reaching and holding such families who tend to distrust middle-class professionals and the middle-class patterns of mental health services. These techniques include involving young people and parents in the planning and staffing of mental health facilities, using community outreach workers, involvement of parents and youth in neighborhood projects, and reaching parents through their participation in such programs as Head Start. At the same time, attention must be paid to the many adverse aspects of the poverty environment itself and the multiple reality problems that weigh so heavily on poor people, such as poor housing, lack of income, lack of community services, unemployment, rejection and discrimination and the like. Moreover, the cultural patterns of the very poor must be deeply understood and respected, in terms of both their cause and their effect on behavior.

In order to assure continuity of care for all children and young people, organizational arrangements should provide the following: (1) ready transfer of relevant information about patients from one facility to another, with the permission of the parents and with adequate protection of confidentiality so that information can be used to the best advantage and duplication of history-taking and services can be minimized or avoided; (2) sustained use of the same treatment personnel in different facilities to the maximum extent possible to avoid the disruptive effect of shunting the child from one stranger to another. For example, if a child who has begun treatment as an outpatient is seen later to have a more serious problem or if a family crisis intensifies the child's disturbance, hospitalization may become necessary. When the geographical location of a state or other hospital makes it possible, arrangements may be made, through cooperative planning, for the child's original therapist to continue in this role throughout hospitalization and during aftercare; (3) an unrestricted policy for the admission and transfer of children and families to various facilities through some arrangement for cooperatively determined clinical need. This unrestricted policy should be maintained without regard to ability to pay and with no residential requirements other than those imposed by whatever regionalization plan is in operation.

The mental health professional performs a wide range of functions. One of them is in his role as consultant. As a specialist, he uses his basic diagnostic and treatment skills in the important function of consultation with medical specialists, general physicians, nonmedical child-care personnel, and teachers. He works as a member of the diagnostic and treatment team. This team may include psychiatrists, pediatricians and other physicians, clinical psychologists, social workers, public health nurses, guidance counselors, teachers, speech therapists, neurologists, occupational therapists, and the like. He also has a role as consultant to the community in terms of community planning.

Care in State Hospitals: Specialized Programs

Inpatient programs in state hospitals can offer significant benefits on a long-term basis to chronically or very severely mentally ill children, those with severe brain damage, or others who require long-term care and treatment. This is often given in a "closed" setting with special provisions including staff precautions to prevent the child from harming himself or others.

These programs in state hospitals, separate from adult programs, have become more numerous in recent years as the special needs of children have been recognized. In the past they have been handicapped by a tendency of referring sources to use them as a means of acceding to community pressures by removing the disturbed—and disturbing—child from the community. The state hospital has unfortunately been used at times by communities to relieve parents, courts, and other agencies of problem children. Referral is still too often a matter of expediency rather than the result of clinical judgment or a decision intended to provide the treatment that is most appropriate for the well-being of the individual child.

Encouraging reports of new approaches to the care of children and adolescents in state hospitals are presented by the National Institute of Mental Health (1968). Since the start of the Institute's Hospital Improvement Grant Program (HIP) several years ago, nineteen state hospitals have chosen to develop new programs for children and adolescents as their first priority.

In one state hospital the new program for adolescents has forged together group psychotherapy, ward-patient government, patient discussions, a special therapeutic education school program, individual therapy, occupational therapy, and recreational therapy.

In addition to stimulating new combinations of treatment techniques, HIP has opened many new alliances between the state mental hospital and the community. In one new unit for adolescents, the year-end progress report notes that increased coordination with community agencies has occurred and several conferences have been held with county welfare boards, juvenile commissioners, religious welfare societies, and children's homes. This is an important achievement, since one of the major problems has been the isolation of the hospital from the community, with the result that children have become alienated from the community and lost to the channels leading back into it.

Still another hospital reports that one of the goals of its new project is to provide full school credit for work completed while the patient-student is hospitalized. The public school system within the area has cooperated excellently, the hospital notes, and has been perfectly willing to grant credit for work within the project and to accept the student in the regular school system upon his release from the hospital. The hospital is now working for full state accreditation of the project's educational program.

The Hospital Improvement Program has also contributed to speeding the use of a new educational and psychotherapeutic treatment pattern as the method of choice in childhood and adolescent disturbances. Under this pattern the formative procedures of education are applied to the growth potential of the child at the same time that psychotherapy is used. In the United States this fusion has been called educational therapy or psycho-education. In Europe it is known as orthopedagogy.

One hospital has inaugurated an "accredited therapeutic education" program that fuses therapy and education in a regime of physical education, recreation therapy, bibliotherapy, art therapy, and shop and occupational therapy with a staff at a one-to-one ratio with the children. The hospital reports "a very noticeable change in patient attitude, particularly on the part of the teenager, toward education." When first approached, the typical teen-age patient wanted no schoolwork. The hospital personnel believe this was because his difficulties had created problems in school for him, with the result that he had never had a successful educational experience. "We now find the students, without exception, very eager to go to school," the hospital reports, "and becoming rather perturbed when something happens which might either make them late or cause them to lose a day in school. Reports from ward personnel indicate that these individuals, since involvement in the school program, seem much better adjusted with a far better motivation and enthusiasm toward tackling problems, and much better able to conform to the give and take of ward living."

One hospital has established a program that seeks to provide vocational training and to enhance social functioning. Special facilities include a general shop area, welding, a print shop, and sewing, typing, and cooking areas. A chief vocational instructor, a social worker, a psychologist, a business education instructor, and a shop instructor work together as a unified staff.

Another innovation is the development of a project under which selected children live in a foster or boarding home and return to the hospital for a day-treatment program.

In yet another state hospital the director of research has demonstrated methods of providing secondary education for small, carefully screened groups of adolescents. The material came from the public schools and from selected correspondence courses. Films and texts on such life-adjustment matters as personal grooming, manners, and making friends were included, along with newspapers, magazines, and books which interest adolescents.

Vacations were scheduled to coincide with those in the nearby public schools, so that it would be possible for some students to spend these vacations with their families. Marked overall academic and psychological improvement was noted. Professional people from other states and Europe have visited the hospital to study the program.

The following recommendations regarding state hospital services for children and youth have been made by the American Psychiatric Association: (1) The state hospital programs should be seen as an appropriate resource in the general treatment plan for severely disturbed children. Depending on the needs of the state or regional area, the state hospital can provide moderate to long-term treatment, reeducation, and rehabilitation. It can also be developed to serve as a day facility, a week care unit, a night hospital, and even as a short-term crisis resource. All such uses of state hospital services should be integrated with other resources in the community. (2) The overall programs should involve the state hospital in explicit roles as to consultative and coordinating services so that it can gradually take its appropriate place in the total community program. (3) Responsibility for the child who is a patient in a state hospital should not be exclusively vested in the hospital but shared by the parents or a designated community agency. (4) Several factors which make for a change in attitude about rehabilitation and discharge should be encouraged. One is a change in staffing patterns with more well-qualified nurses, nursing assistants, child-care workers, counselors, and trained volunteers. Another is the growing practice of adequate diagnosis before admission, and a third is the increase in voluntary admissions. One may expect that in the near future the courts will no longer "commit" children to state hospitals because there is nothing else to do with them and that the state hospital will be used only when it is the treatment of choice. (5) The children's unit of the state hospital should have representation on planning councils along with representatives of social agencies and professional groups. Thus, the state hospital will play an active part in developing a comprehensive program.

Provision for aftercare is essential when a child leaves a hospital or residential treatment center. Aftercare measures should include continued psychotherapy when necessary, educational planning, recreational and vocational guidance, and specific welfare services to the child's family when appropriate. The child should not be sent home to face the same problems that originally gave rise to, or contributed to, his emotional illness. Aftercare should counteract the tendency of a family, neighborhood, or community to exclude the child, and it should help the family to create a healthier environment for him. If the family is not prepared to take the child back, then other placement should be arranged in the home community (American Psychiatric Association, 1964).

EMERGING TRENDS IN TREATMENT

In order to understand the new directions of treatment, it is necessary to review some of the problems inherent in the nature of therapy. Many emotionally and mentally ill children, even by the age of seven or eight, have chronic conditions that have existed for five years or longer. By this time, a good deal of psychological "scar tissue" may have formed. The illness may be entrenched and a part of the relationship life of that individual. Often the family has adapted to the child's condition. The entire pattern of illness may have a certain rigidity and stability. Such a situation is not easy to change.

The attempts to influence such conditions have therefore been rather slow-moving processes involving a good deal of highly expert professional time. Inevitably, this has generated a pressure to find shortcuts, rapid approaches, instant relief, or at least less expensive means of getting the job done. A time-honored means of approach has been to take the child out of an environment in which he is not doing well and put him in one in which he does adjust, or take the environment as it exists and change it. For example, if a child doesn't adjust or learn effectively in regular classes, the school can provide a special class for troubled youngsters where he *can* function. If the school, or the family, can't make such accommodations, it has been demonstrated that the professional can help them to do it by consultation, holding seminars, giving courses, and creating group meetings. For quite a few children, this combination is markedly helpful. Whatever the original source of their maladjustment, it is aggravated and abetted by the rejection and the sequestration they experience. And the relief and acceptance that follows from environmental manipulation of this sort often leads to a jump in performance that can be measured by I.Q. tests, by grades, and by general behavior. From the point of view of society, the improvement in the child's functioning has been material and worthwhile, and it becomes a matter of values and economics that decides which approach will be used.

The attempt to work with the child actively and directly has been similarly influenced by questions of expense and availability of skill. The most in tensive and expensive mode of approach to such treatment is child psychoanalysis. Many different forms of individual work with children have been developed since the original analytic model. These include a wide variety of psychotherapy methods which emphasize various possible tactics of approach. The names often describe their specific approach—rational psychotherapy, relationship therapy, reality therapy, existential therapy, nondirective therapy, directive therapy, relaxation therapy, paradigmatic models, etc. It is desirable that experimentation with new approaches continue as a means of reaching all children in need. The point is that so complex an entity as a malfunctioning child or adolescent is approachable on a wide variety of fronts: reassurance, direction, education, logic, personal warmth, sympathy, acceptance, reward, and, of course, punishment.

Pavlov's work on the "conditioned reflex" and the operant conditioning techniques developed by Skinner and others in this country have laid the foundation for another variety of treatment approaches. These include conditioning therapy, operant conditioning, behavior modification, and the like. The behavioral model, upon which these treatment approaches are based, presupposes that all behavior is learned and that it can be changed through planned relearning. Emphasis is placed on changing the behavior of the patient through teaching him more adaptive responses through the systematic manipulation of antecedents and consequences of undesired behavior. One of the assumptions of this approach is that if people behave differently they will have different experiences in their interaction with the environment and thus will begin to feel differently about themselves and others (Eysenck and Rachman, 1965; Skinner, 1953; Wolpe, 1958).

The attempt to increase the usefulness of scarce professional manpower has led in the direction of group therapy where one therapist sees several patients at a time. This has been extended and refined and is now a very important part of the treatment armamentarium. Nor is it merely a question of economy of time and personnel—there are profoundly important psychological events that are involved in being part of a group. Certain problems of children—for example, shyness, inhibition, difficulty in getting along with peers—can probably be more rapidly approached in group contexts than through any other means. Adolescents in particular lend themselves to group types of experience and often do very well with such measures. A number of variations of group therapy have also evolved, varying from group psychoanalysis to activity therapy of almost non-verbal character with grade-school children.

A development from group therapy is family therapy. Here the methods of working with a group are applied to the internal dynamics of the family, the child "patient," his siblings, and his parents all confront the therapist— and the problem—together and the work is directed toward altering the "ecology" of the child's human environment.

The extension of this form of treatment has resulted in exploring additional applications. Therapy groups composed of families where each group "member" is a couple, or an even larger family, have been undertaken. Group thinking has been turned to entire neighborhoods and, indeed, the logical extension of all this is "The community as patient." Therapeutic attempts with such "patients" are being made very seriously in some places.

Again, this is a field of practice with fresh new ideas and experimental methods, combining group therapeutic principles with approaches that deal with social forces.

There has been a recent emphasis on the role of social action, cultural, and community group programs to provide corrective emotional experiences. For the individual who has grown up in a disadvantaged environment and who has responded with apathy, hopelessness, poor self-image and/or alienation from the larger society, an opportunity is provided which can help him develop a new picture of his ability to be useful, active, and effective. These programs appear to have benefited some, and it is hoped that these efforts can help to reduce the level of problems created by racism and poor learning experiences. The emphasis is on using such influences as that of building on the still healthy components of an individual's makeup. However, the deprivations in early life can be so disabling that inevitably there are children and adolescents who cannot be reached by these newer approaches alone. They need assistance from a combination in which the more traditional treatment programs work collaboratively with these developing forces for creating social and community change.

As is inevitable, there are large numbers of "therapies" that are currently on the fringe of normal practice. Thus, treatment such as that based on enhancement of group therapy by all the participants being naked or by the use of agents such as LSD to achieve mystical group experience is being reported but its usefulness with children and youth has not yet been demonstrated.

Quite a different value may be set on the attempts to apply systems theory and communications theory to therapeutic processes. These approaches are currently under study and have all the uncertainties that attend any innovative technic; they involve reducing the therapeutic process to some form of model which can then be evaluated and worked with in "mechanical" terms. "Inputs," "feedbacks," "overloads," and other elements of cybernetic and system-analysis theory are called into play, interview data are translated into computer language and fed into computers, data retrieval systems are set up in agencies and information encoded, and many attempts are being made to adapt information theory, communication theory, and process analysis to therapeutic work on every level.

These approaches are tantalizing and suggestive. To date, they too have not yet proved their worth. However, their promise strongly indicates continued studies in this direction.

Attempts are also being made to wed our knowledge of neurophysiology and neurobiochemistry to our methods of treatment. The great advances in drug therapies for emotional illness that have evolved in the past two decades have left their impact on child therapy as well. For example, many residential treatment centers control the behavior of their more disruptive children as much by drugs as by psychological means; pediatricians are becoming more sophisticated in the use of amphetamines for the organically driven child, and the blending of drug medicine and psychological medicine is well underway in many areas.

Again, this is a major and fruitful field for research and bids fair to enrich both psychological theory and neurological knowledge. It has been disappointing to many that such major advances as the discovery of the centrencephalon, and the relation of the limbic system to emotions have not placed new tools into the hands of the mental health worker. But progress is rapid, and we may well hope for important new concepts and methods to arise in this area.

Psychoanalysis is also a major form of treatment and is primarily directed toward helping the patient free himself of deeply repressed unconscious conflicts which stand in the way of his full and effective rise as a person. In the case of the child, psychoanalytic treatment is aimed at resolving conflicts and repressions that stand in the way of his ability to grow and develop along relatively even, harmonious lines. This intensive mode of treatment is generally lengthy and expensive. Psychoanalysts have a major contribution to make, not only because of the treatment they provide to their necessarily limited number of patients, but also because they glean significant understandings and insights from their practice which are a valued resource in their work as consultants, teachers, and developers of fruitful hypotheses for further research (see also Chapter XII). Moreover, the more microcosmic, intensive investigations of individuals which are fundamental to the analyst's work provide many of the bases and techniques for therapeutic approaches to children and adults in general.

Restructuring the Environment

Other theoretical approaches to the prevention and/or reduction of emotional disorders and mental illness put emphasis on seeking underlying causation in the environment and conceptualizing needed related changes. This approach does not necessarily advocate the abandonment of treatment for individuals or groups of individuals but seeks to reduce the numbers of people who develop disorders which are at least partially associated with environmental stresses and deficits. Some of the related theoretical models follow:

1. *Epidemiological.* According to this approach, emotional and mental disorders are seen as being primarily related to stresses, deprivations, and pressures in the environment; thus, emphasis should be placed on locating and changing related problems in the environment rather than providing individual treatment (Laing and Laing, 1961; Kirchoff, 1967; Smelser, 1962). Underlying possible causes are sought in such factors

as poverty, racism, poor housing, inadequate education, unemployment, overcrowding, and the like.

2. *Social pathology.* If behavior is regarded as deviant by other people, this puts the individual into a labeled, deviant group and excludes him from society. The problem is seen as not being in the person but in his relation to the social situation. Examples may be found in racist attitudes and practices and in the ways in which our society generally regards and handles children who are labeled as mentally ill, mentally retarded, delinquent, welfare recipients, and the like. These discriminatory attitudes and practices call for social action to change related societal behaviors and attitudes rather than treatment which focuses on changes within the individual (Erickson, 1966 and 1967; Silverstein, 1969; Weinberg, 1967).

3. *Cultural pathology.* The cultural patterns of various groups are seen as playing a part in the origins and continuation of mental and emotional disorders. These patterns arise from social and economic situations; thus social action is required to treat the underlying situation. Involvement of people in planning and carrying out their own programs provides a new individual and group experience which may be effective in changing cultural values and attitudes, particularly if this action has an effect on the life situation of the people involved (Chilman, 1966; Rainwater and Yancey, 1967; Reissman, Cohen, and Pearl, 1964).

4. *Ethological.* Clues are derived from studies of animal behavior in reference to their interaction with the environment and planned manipulation of learning experiences. Implications are drawn for greater understanding of human learning and behavior and the possible consequences of planned environmental change. A great advantage of these studies is that the experiences of animals can be systematically manipulated and controlled, while this is not generally true in reference to human beings. Although question arises as to the extent to which it is possible to generalize from animals to human beings (Lorenz, 1966), findings from this field are provocative and provide rich theoretical sources for experimental action programs tied to research (see Chapter XI).

Some Prevalent Treatment Approaches

Prevalent treatment approaches, aside from those of psychotherapy and psychoanalysis, include:

1. Activity group therapy is now reemerging as a method of treatment along with other forms of group therapy. It is being applied, in a variety of forms, in working with older children, adolescents, and adults, as well as in group activity in therapeutic nursery schools.

2. Group therapy, in general, is being used in many ways, as in the case of interview group therapy for adolescents, group therapy for parents, couples' therapy, and the like.

3. Biological treatment through the use of drugs is now being seen as an adjunct of, and not a substitute for, psychotherapy and other related forms of individual and group treatment.

4. Treatment through the provision of "corrective relationships" with other people, such as mother substitutes and foster grandparents, has proven effective, especially for children and infants in hospitals, day-care centers, and day hospitals.

5. Filial therapy involves parents who are trained as therapists to work with their own children under the supervision of psychiatric personnel.

6. Home visits and treatment in the home have been found to be extremely helpful; however, they are also very expensive when conducted by highly trained mental health specialists. Such semiprofessionals as homemakers, tutors, and parent educators are proving to be a promising alternative, especially in instances in which the major problem is lack of appropriate stimulation and basic home care of the child.

7. Increasingly, outpatient care is regarded as being preferable to hospital care, when possible. Efforts to keep emotionally disturbed and mentally ill children and adolescents in the mainstream of society and in touch with their own families and neighborhoods are being made through a variety of approaches such as group day care, youth hostels, residential centers, day or night hospitals, special schools, increased use of mental health consultation to those who work with children and youth so that the young person can function better in his normal setting, and the like.

8. Environment therapy is a broad approach in which attention is focused more on the total social-psychological climate in which the person is living. For example, there is increasing recognition that all the people in a child's environment are important to his functioning and self-image. Attempts are made to provide a humane, psychologically sensitive, and supporting environment in such settings as the school, recreation programs, church-related activities, and so on.

9. Crisis therapy is focused on meeting the problems presented by people at the moment that a crisis arises. Twenty-four-hour services are recommended along with mobile crisis units (Gioscia *et al.*, 1968).

Some Special Projects

One approach to residential and day care for children who are moderately to severely disturbed is Project Re-ED, which is described in Appendix D of this chapter. Re-ED is designed to help children acquire competence in coping with realistic problems and to achieve joyous and purposeful living. Children and parents remain involved with each other, and there are programs for parents as well as children.

The schools are staffed primarily by teacher-counselors, carefully selected young people with specialized training at the master's degree level—considerably less than the least extensively trained mental health specialist. Selected teacher-counselors are used to provide liaison with the child's home, school, and community. Professionals serve as consultants in the program, thus extending their effectiveness by a substantial factor.

Careful follow-up research shows that the program is achieving results equal to traditional programs as reported in the research literature.

This approach is also stressed by L. Kohlberg (1968), who emphasizes that educational attainments are vital to the child's sense of competence and self-confidence. Kohlberg pleads for a "community mental health" or "Re-ED" approach to mental health services. The basic characteristic of such a design is an orientation to creating an environment in which children are able to develop and grow toward increasing social and educational skills and self-esteem. Children should not be segregated into special therapeutic environments which are radically different from those which they would normally encounter. Mental health services should be aimed at minimizing the amount of failure, rejection, and misery in a group of children (see also Chapter VII).

This same general philosophy underlies programs in several state hospitals. These tend to focus on the child's strengths, to establish an expectation for normal behavior and good work habits, and to encourage self-care and basic social adjustment. The use of child-care workers, student volunteers, and retired people, and the emphasis on small group activities throughout the total program, provides more intensive personal experiences and services for the child. The treatment goal is generally that of social recovery and return home as soon as possible (National Institute of Mental Health, 1968).

Partial hospitalization programs vary widely, as do the facilities offering them. At Los Angeles County General Hospital some adolescents spend their days attending school and therapy sessions at the hospital and go home at night. At other centers adolescents may go to school or to jobs in the community by day and sleep at the hospital. Many visit their homes on weekends and holidays, increasing their home stay as progress permits.

Considerable experimentation is being carried out with therapeutic nursery schools for preschool children. These youngsters may suffer problems ranging from mild behavior disturbance to severe autism and may require the therapeutic nursery setting in addition to individual therapy. At one center a three- to four-month nursery school experience for the child is supplemented by group therapy for the parents and by multiple family therapy for some of the families with severely disturbed children.

An NIMH-supported project in the predominantly low-income Negro area of Woodlawn in Chicago is designed to improve adjustment in first-grade youngsters. The program consists of weekly classroom meetings of children and their teachers, as well as consultation sessions with school administrators, teachers, and parents. One outstanding feature of the program is the active participation of the community. Neighborhood residents, including parents of the children, are members of the board of directors, which guides center policy and supports the educational effort. The success of school programs such as these depends on the key people in a child's life—parents, teachers, physicians, etc.—being involved in a concerted effort to provide a better environment for all children (National Institute of Mental Health, 1968).

Very little systematic research has been devoted to evaluating the effectiveness of the various treatment theories and methods which were briefly discussed in the foregoing section. This is also true of the program strategies which were recommended. Many more well-designed studies are needed, as will be discussed in Chapter XI.

INTERNATIONAL TRENDS

In many parts of the world there is an increasing interest in the problems of children and youth, a reawakened concern for the mentally retarded, the delinquent, and the disadvantaged. There is also a renewed interest in group care and protection of the family against the high economic costs of mental disorders and other illnesses. For example, broader social security coverage and/or mandatory health insurance programs are being established in a number of countries to cover the costs of mental illness.

Americans who visit these more progressive countries are impressed with the growing tendency toward experimentation with various approaches to the planning and delivery of services. In most countries of the world, child mental health services are an integral part of, or closely affiliated with, child health and welfare programs. These are usually seen as being more of a public than a private responsibility. Expenditure of tax monies for children's services is widely accepted. Greater responsibility and status are accorded the child-care staff, regardless of the amount of formal training, than is the case in this country. Many Europeans believe that the American concern with the costs of services for each individual reflects an outmoded viewpoint which has long ago been replaced in European countries with a combination of mandatory social security and sickness insurance benefits.

In many European countries there appears to be more concern with finding practical solutions to immediate problems and less preoccupation with abstract theories and concepts. For instance, there is considerable emphasis on the therapeutic meaning of work and on vocational training which can be of future use to adolescents. Industrial workshops are extensively staffed and supervised. Institutional training and work assignments are meaningful and relevant to the individual. They are not "make-work" programs.

In France and other Western European countries a new kind of professional known as an *educateur* is given considerable responsibility for residential and day-care programs for emotionally disturbed and other handicapped children. Some 2,000 *educateurs* are trained each year in special institutes which provide an intensive three-year course of training, including an internship. The training incorporates some of the understandings and skills of the psychologist, social worker, special educator, and recreational or occupational therapist. Psychiatrists, pediatricians, psychologists, social workers, classroom teachers, and other specialists are also involved in treatment programs, and the presence of the *educateur* trained in near-sufficient numbers, provides a stable, high-quality manpower base not now available in the United States. Competent observers report that residential programs for disturbed, retarded, and delinquent children in France are generally superior to those in the United States. A program for disturbed and delinquent children, based on the *educateur* or reeducation model, has been in successful operation in Montreal, Canada, for twenty years, under the direction of Mlle. Jeanne Guindon. The closest counterpart in the United States is the reeducation programs of Tennessee and North Carolina.

In sharp contrast with current United States practices are those social welfare-oriented and/or collectivist societies which have established central planning, state-directed coordination of services, and some control over manpower training and placement. These practices are buttressed by a strong tradition of comprehensive social security and sickness benefit insurance coverage. Examples might range from the more moderate programs of the Netherlands and the United Kingdom through the Scandinavian countries and Israel to the managed economies of the Communist lands of Eastern Europe.

Reports prepared by the 1968 U.S. Mission on Mental Health to the Soviet Union indicate that there is an elaborate array of child-caring services in Russia. These services include group care for infants, nursery schools, boarding schools, and invalid homes. Children are cared for days, evenings, or on a residential basis. After the mother delivers the child, the district children's clinic is immediately notified by the hospital. These clinics are the medical center of all services for children. There is one in every district, each serving approximately 15,000 children. These clinics also provide most of the medical and psychiatric services for kindergarten and school youngsters, including physical and psychological examinations.

The Soviet child is not lost in a welter of agencies. The district children's clinic is home base. This clinic has a number of staff specialists, including those in pediatrics, child psychiatry, and speech therapy. At age sixteen, the adolescent and his records are transferred from the child's clinic to a special clinic for adolescents. At age eighteen, his records are transferred to an adult service. Continuity of service to people of all ages is thus maintained.

Health-care services in the Soviet Union are closely related to basic goals which include the provision of a coordinated network of preventatively oriented, readily available, and geographically accessible mental health services, free of cost for all Soviet citizens. This is a reflection of the principle that health is a resource of the state, no less important than other natural resources. From this creed it follows that good health must be maintained and ill health prevented. In that sense, there is in the Soviet Union, unlike the United States, a clearly defined and explicit relationship between the structure of the government and the organization and delivery of health services.

The principle of continuity of care in the Soviet Union also includes provision for aftercare following discharge from a hospital or other child-care facility. Few if any American states have mandatory provisions requiring clinics to provide follow-up care to patients returning from state hospitals or residing in their service areas.

Although more data are needed to evaluate the impact of these programs, there is little doubt that child welfare is recognized as an important matter in state planning in Communist countries. Consistent with public health principles, emphasis is placed on those forms of prevention and treatment which can be applied rapidly, widely, and inexpensively. Many of these same trends also apply to programs in such countries as Israel, the United Kingdom, Denmark, Norway, and Sweden (David, 1969).

SUMMARY

Most of our emotionally disturbed or mentally ill children and young people do not receive the diagnoses, care, and treatment which they need. It is estimated that .6 percent are psychotic and that another 2 to 3 percent are severely disturbed. An additional 8 to 10 percent are in need of some kind of help from knowledgeable persons.

These children are crippled in their ability to learn, to relate to others, to see the real world as it is, or to adequately handle their impulses of anger, fear, and sex interest. They do not feel that they are a vital and effectual part of society. Predictions are that the number of mentally ill and emotionally disturbed children and youth will rise with the future increases in population and socioeconomic stresses expected in our rapidly growing technological society.

Even at present, there is no community in the United States which has all the facilities for the care, education, guidance, and treatment of such children. The few services which are available are poorly coordinated and are usually unavailable to poor and near-poor children. Many emotionally and mentally disturbed youngsters are poorly diagnosed and are institutionalized as being retarded or delinquent. Thousands are losing all possibility for partial or full recovery because they are forgotten and left to slowly deteriorate on the back wards of mental hospitals. Mental facilities and manpower are much more likely to be devoted to the needs of adults than to the needs of children and youth.

Research indicates that most children and adolescents with minor emotional and learning disturbances recover fully if they are given competent, understanding guidance and help. More seriously handicapped young people improve with appropriate treatment. While a few show no improvement despite the best professional efforts, they need humane care close to home, and their parents need help with their heavy responsibilities.

In order to appropriately care for these children and young people, a whole network of diagnostic, treatment, and care facilities must be available, including: a service information and referral center, physical and mental health clinics with special services for children and youth, mental health and special educational services in the schools, day-care and homemaker services with mental health consultation and supervision available, halfway houses for disturbed adolescents, residential treatment and other forms of group-care centers, special child and adolescent units in psychiatric hospitals, vocational rehabilitation and protected work situations, and family counseling services. Such services need to be closely coordinated and planned to provide sustained and continuing care for these children and their families.

To avoid many of these tragedies, services must be designed to reach parents at a very early stage—before conception of their first child, if possible. For example, genetic assessment and counseling should be provided in those instances in which there is reason to suspect that a biologically handicapped child may be born.

Specialized services for children with emotional and mental disorders should be planned and administered as part of a larger community program which is directed toward meeting the health, educational, recreational, housing, employment, social, and economic needs of all its citizens at all age levels. It is important that the different approaches to prevention and treatment of emotional disturbance and mental illness be carefully evaluated with well-formulated research.

DIMENSIONS OF PERSONALITY DEVELOPMENT
Physical, Psychological, Social
SCHEMATIC REPRESENTATION *

PERIOD	AGE	PSYCHOSOCIAL TASKS (Crises)	PSYCHOSEXUAL STAGES	RADIUS OF SIGNIFICANT RELATIONS	CENTRAL VALUE ORIENTATION	STAGES OF INTELLECTUAL DEVELOPMENT
	Birth					
INFANCY	3 mo.	Trust vs. Mistrust (I am what I am given)	Oral-Respiratory Sensory-Kinesthetic (Incorporative Modes)	Maternal Person	Hope	**Sensory-Motor** The infant moves from a neo-natal reflex level of complete self-world undifferentiation to a relatively coherent organization of sensory-motor actions. He learns that certain actions have specific effects upon the environment. Minimal symbolic activity is involved. Recognition of the constancy of external objects and primitive internal representation of the world begins.
	6 mo.					
	9 mo.					
	1 YR					
	18 mo.	Autonomy vs. Shame, Doubt (I am what I "will")	Anal-Urethral Muscular (Retentive-Eliminative Modes)	Parental Persons	Will	
	2 YR					
PRESCHOOL	3 YR					
	4 YR	Initiative vs. Guilt (I am what I imagine I can be)	Genital Locomotor (Oedipal) (Intrusive, Inclusive Modes)	Basic Family	Purpose	**Preoperational Thought** (Prelogical) The child makes his first relatively unorganized and fumbling attempts to come to grips with the new and strange world of symbols. Thinking tends to be egocentric and intuitive. Conclusions are based on what he feels or what he would like to believe.
	5 YR					
	6 YR			Neighborhood, School		

298

Thought

Conceptual organization takes on stability and coherence. The child begins to appear rational and well organized in his adaptations. The fairly stable and orderly conceptual framework is systematically brought to bear on the world of objects around him. Physical quantities, such as weight and volume, are now viewed as constant despite changes in shape and size.

Formal Operational Thought

The individual can now deal effectively not only with the reality before him but also with the world of the abstract, propositional statements, and the world of possibility ("as if"). Cognition is of the adult type. The adolescent uses deductive reasoning and has the ability to evaluate the logic and quality of his own thinking. His increased abstract powers provide him with the capacity to deal with laws and principles. Although egocentrism is still evident at times, important idealistic attitudes are developing in the late adolescent and young adult.

Stage	Age	Crisis	Period	Social Relations	Skill/Virtue
SCHOOL	8 YR	Inferiority (I am what I learn)			Skill
	9 YR		"Latency"		
	10 YR				
ADOLESCENCE	11 YR		Puberty	Peer In-Groups and Out-Groups	
	12 YR				
	13 YR	Identity vs. Identity Diffusion (I know who I am)	Early Adolescence	Adult Models of Leadership	
	14 YR				
	15 YR		Middle Adolescence		Fidelity
	16 YR				
	17 YR		Late Adolescence		
	18 YR				
EARLY ADULTHOOD		Intimacy vs. Isolation	Adulthood (Genitality)	Partners in Friendship, Sex Competition, Cooperation	Love
MIDDLE ADULTHOOD		Generativity vs. Self-Absorption or Stagnation	Maturity	Divided Labor and Shared Household	Care
LATE ADULTHOOD		Integrity vs. Despair, Disgust	Menopause Male Climacteric		
			Senescence	"Mankind" "My Kind"	Wisdom

* The writer wishes to acknowledge the help of Anthony Kisley, M.D. in the preparation of this chart.

PERIOD	AGE	PHYSICAL GROWTH	DEVELOPMENTAL STEPS (LINES)	DEVELOPMENTAL PROBLEMS
INFANCY	Birth	RAPID (SKELETAL)	"Normal Autism" (0-3 mo.)	Birth defects
			Anticipation of feeding	Feeding disorders: colic, regurgitation, vomiting, rumination, failure to thrive, marasmus, pylorospasm, feeding refusal, atopic exema
	3 mo.	Muscle constitutes 25% total body weight		
	6 mo.	Aeration maxillary and ethmoid sinuses	Symbiosis (4-18 mo.)	
			Stranger anxiety (6-10 mo.)	Extreme stranger anxiety
				Early infantile autism
	9 mo.	Eruption of deciduous central incisors (5-10 mo.)	Separation anxiety (8-24 mo.)	
	1 YR	Anterior fontanel closes (10-14 mo.)	Separation individuation (12-28 mo.)	Physiologic anorexia
				Sleep disturbances: resistance or response to over-stimulation
			Self-feeding	Extreme separation anxiety
		Eruption of deciduous first molars (11-18 mo.)	Oppositional behavior	Interactional psychotic disorder
			Messiness	Bronchial asthma
			Exploratory behavior	Pica
				Teeth grinding
		Increase in lymphoid tissue		Pseudo-retardation
	2 YR		Parallel play	Temper tantrums, negativism
			Pleasure in looking at or being looked at	Toilet training disturbances: constipation, diarrhea
			Beginning self-concept	Excessive feeding
PRESCHOOL	3 YR	SLOWER (SKELETAL)	Orderliness	Bedtime and toilet rituals
		Deciduous teeth calcified	Disgust	Speech disorders: delayed, elective mutism, stuttering
			Curiosity	Petit mal seizures
			Masturbation	Nightmares, night terrors
			Cooperative play	Extreme separation anxiety
			Fantasy play	Excessive thumb sucking
			Imaginary companions	Phobias and marked fears
	4 YR	RAPID (SKELETAL)		Developmental deviations: lags and accelerations in motor, sensory, and affective development
				Food rituals and fads
			Task completion	Sleepwalking
	5 YR		Rivalry with parents of same sex	School phobias
	6 YR	Eruption of permanent first molars (5½-7 yrs.)	Games and rules	Developmental deviations: lags and accelerations in cognitive functions, psychosexual, and integrative development
		Eruption of permanent central incisors (6-8 yrs.)	Problem-solving	Tics
			Achievement	Psychoneuroses
			Voluntary hygiene	Enuresis, soiling and excessive masturbation
		SLOWEST (SKELETAL)	Competes with partners	Schizophreniform psychotic disorder

Developmental chart (page rotated). Columns: Stage | Age | Physical Development | Social/Behavioral Development | Disorders

Stage	Age	Physical Development	Social/Behavioral Development	Disorders
SCHOOL AGE	7 YR	Frontal sinuses develop	Hobbies	Nail-biting
	8 YR	Cranial sutures ossified	Ritualistic play	Learning problems Psychophysiologic disorders
	9 YR	Uterus begins to grow	Rational attitudes about foods Companionship Invests in: community leaders, teachers, impersonal ideals	Personality disorders: compulsive, hysterical, anxious, overly dependent, oppositional, overly inhibited, overly independent, isolated and mistrustful personality, tension discharge disorders, sociosyntonic personality disorders, and sexual deviations Pre-delinquent patterns
	10 YR	Budding of nipples in girls		
	11 YR	Increased vascularity of penis and scrotum		
ADOLESCENCE	12 YR	Pubic hair appears in girls SPURT (SKELETAL) (Girls 1½ yrs. ahead)		Legal delinquency Anorexia nervosa Dysmenorrhea
	13 YR	Pubic hair appears in boys	"Revolt"	Sexual promiscuity Excessive masturbation
	14 YR	Rapid growth of testes and penis	Loosens tie to family Cliques	Pseudopsychotic regressions
	15 YR	Axillary hair starts	Responsible independence Work habits solidifying	Suicidal attempts
	16 YR	Down on upper lip appears Voice changes		Acute confusional state
	17 YR	Mature spermatozoa (11-17)	Heterosexual interests	
	18 YR	Acne in girls may appear Acne in boys may appear	Recreational activities Preparation for occupational choice Occupational commitment	Schizophrenic disorders (adult type)
EARLY ADULTHOOD		Cessation of skeletal growth Involution of lymphoid tissue Muscle constitutes 43% total body weight. Permanent teeth calcified Eruption of permanent third molars (17-30 yrs.)	Elaboration of recreational outlets Marriage readiness	Affective disorders: manic-depressive psychoses
MIDDLE ADULTHOOD			Parenthood readiness	Involutional reactions: depression, suicide
LATE ADULTHOOD				Senile disorders: chronic brain syndromes, etc.

301

PERIOD	AGE	ADAPTIVE MECHANISMS	EEG DEVELOPMENT	CNS MATURATION	DEVELOPMENTAL LANDMARKS
INFANCY	Birth		Neonate: Low amplitude and polyrhythmic 4-6 and 6-8 cycles per second appear	Brain weight: 350 grams Level of neural function: sub-cortical Transitory reflexes present (i.e.,moro,sucking,grasp,TNR)	Social smile (2 mo.) 180° visual pursuit (2 mo.)
	3 mo.	Incorporation			Reaches for objects (4 mo.) Rolls over (5 mo.)
	6 mo.	Imitation Denial Avoidance	Spontaneous K complexes appear (evidence of cortical response to stimulation)	Brain weight: 600 grams Brain stem in advanced or complete state of myelination Transitory reflexes disappear. Brain weight: 900 grams Cranial nerve myelination complete	Raking grasp (7 mo.)
	9 mo.				Crude purposeful release (9 mo.) Inferior pincer grasp (10 mo.) Walks unassisted (10-14 mo.) Words: 3-4 (13 mo.)
	1 YR	Regression			Builds tower of 2 cubes (15 mo.)
	18 mo.	Withdrawal Inhibition Displacement Projection	Subalpha 5-8 cycles per second become more evident Anterior fast activity disappears	Progressive integration of sub-cortical and cortical areas Babinski reflex extinguished Bowel and bladder nerves myelinated	Scribbles with crayon (18 mo.) Words: 10 (18 mo.) Builds tower of 5-6 cubes (21 mo.)
	2 YR	Undoing	Alpha development more dominant Irregularities in rhythms and distortions in waves give EEG "abnormal look." Sleep spindles may appear "spikelike." Drowsy record may show slowing paroxysms.Distorted sleep patterns can appear.	Brain weight: 1000 grams Spinal cord and cerebellum myelination complete	Uses 3 word sentences (30 mo.) Names 6 body parts (30 mo.) Uses appropriate personal pronouns, i.e., I, you, me (30 mo.) Rides tricycle (36 mo.) Copies circle (36 mo.) Matches 4 colors (36 mo.)
PRESCHOOL	3 YR	Suppression			Talks of self and others (42 mo.) Takes turns (42 mo.) Tandem walks (42 mo.)
	4 YR	Acting out in play and fantasy		Beginning single finger localization	Copies cross (48 mo.) Throws ball overhand (48 mo.) Copies square (54 mo.) Copies triangle (60 mo.) Ties knots in string
	5 YR	Repression	14+6 per second positive spikes start to appear. Transient disorganization of awake and sleep tracings is common.	Beginning right-left orientation Cerebrum myelination complete Level of neural function:cortical	
SCHOOL AGE	6 YR	Identification		Body image solidifying	Prints name Ties shoelaces Simple functional similarities Rides two-wheel bike Copies diamond Simple opposite analogies Names days of week
	7 YR	Isolation Pseudo-compulsions in thought, play Turning of emotions into the opposite Reaction formation Sublimation			
	8 YR			Cerebral dominance evident (laterality)	Repeats 5 digits forward Can define brave and nonsense

9 YR			Knows seasons of the year Able to rhyme
10 YR	Rationalization	Increase in alpha voltage and regularity	Brain weight: 1300-1400 grams (adult size)	Repeats 4 digits in reverse Understands: pity,grief,surprise Difficult functional similarities
11 YR				Knows where sun sets Can define nitrogen, microscope, shilling
12 YR	Intellectualization		(Growth in thickness of myelin sheaths continues for life)	Knows why oil floats on water Can divide 72 by 4 without pencil and paper
13 YR	Regressions			Abstract similarities
14 YR		14+6 per second positive spikes begin to disappear		Comprehends belfrey and espionage Knows meaning of C.O.D. Can repeat 6 digits forward and 5 digits in reverse
15 YR	Asceticism	Gradual evolution of stable adult patterns at all levels of consciousness		
16 YR				
17 YR				
18 YR				

ADOLESCENCE

303

B

JEWISH BOARD OF GUARDIANS
HAWTHORNE CEDAR KNOLLS SCHOOL

Brief Description

The Hawthorne Cedar Knolls School, a division of the Jewish Board of Guardians, is a residential treatment center in Westchester County, New York. It is located forty-five minutes from New York City on 228 acres of wooded land.

It serves a population of 200 boys and girls between the ages of eight and eighteen (150 boys and 50 girls). The majority of the children come from the New York metropolitan area, with a small number referred from various parts of the country.

The children present a wide range of emotional problems, including severe psychoneurosis, character disorder, borderline psychosis, and childhood schizophrenia, with behavior patterns ranging from impulsive, antisocial, sexual acting-out to bizarre, withdrawn, phobic symptoms. The median age of the children treated is sixteen years.

Sources of referral include schools, child guidance clinics, hospitals, the courts, departments of social service, private psychiatrists, voluntary social agencies, and parents.

All of the children fall within the range of normal intelligence or have indicated potential for normal intellectual functioning and achievement. The Hawthorne Cedar Knolls School is an open setting in which heavy reliance is placed on staff attitudes and a structured milieu to contain and treat the severely disordered child. It does not, however, accept children who are suicidal or homicidal risks and therefore in need of twenty-four-hour-a-day supervision.

In addition to its on-grounds residential program, Hawthorne carries a day-treatment case load of 15 Westchester County children and 15 New York City children. For the latter, who have had a period of care in residence, the day-treatment program represents a transitional phase between the institution and return to the community. Other forms of aftercare, providing a transitional experience, include such facilities as group homes (apartments housing up to seven children) and a halfway house in the City, which accommodates 27 young men between the ages of sixteen and twenty-one years.

The institution proper provides a total child-care and treatment program aimed at stabilizing the child's daily living experience. As far as possible, the program is geared to the needs of the individual child so that for some it will provide necessary limits and accountability for behavior while for others it will provide greater flexibility and super-symptom tolerance, all within a basic framework structured to permit a wide orbit of movement. It offers a regular but flexible routine which helps certain children to cope with reality demands with a minimum of personal struggle and without the crushing quality of regulations arbitrarily imposed by adults. The environment represents a synthesis of spontaneity and professional self-awareness, which allows for a natural emotional as well as trained and thoughtful response to the child, based on individual need, whether at the breakfast table in the cottage, on the ballfield, or in the classroom. The child's projections, distortions, and irrational impulses are acted out and acted upon in an atmosphere of adult sensitivity and response usually different in both tone and detail from his previous experience and thus expectations. Experiences may be modified to diminish anxiety or to increase anxiety, to test out newly acquired strengths, and to provide opportunities for new gratifications. The experiential aspects of the child's daily life are consistent with, parallel to, and interwoven with the clinical treatment process.

Major elements of the total program are (1) child care in the informal daily living situation; (2) education; (3) individual, group, and family therapy; and (4) recreation and play. All of these elements are encompassed within an integrated and planned milieu, which may be differentiated in terms of the individual child's special needs.

The school is divided into four *operational* units of 50 children each so that the unit staff has as complete a knowledge as possible of the children within the unit. A major *treatment* unit is the cottage or group-living situation, where a healing process takes place in the interaction with peers and adults. Because the process of corrective socialization and social change is rooted in the daily living experience, an effort has been made to provide sound professional management of this aspect of the child's treatment through the utilization of more sophisticated child-care staff trained in group and individual dynamics.

Overall, the school must function as a sensitive social instrument set up to respond to the aspirations and attitudes of its children and staff. While its culture is designed to project a particular life style, with its rules and limitations as well as opportunities, it is subject to the influences of the general community, the social conditions of its setting, and the unique interaction of its children and staff.

The institution operates a full-time, accredited academic school covering the elementary through the senior high school grades. Special curricula have been developed to motivate the child who has been a school failure, and opportunities for sublimation and symbolic fulfillment are utilized in the program. A primary goal is the rehabilitation of the child's ability to learn, and intensive remedial tutoring is provided as a method of repair. For those youngsters for whom formal education beyond high school is not planned, special vocational programs have been designed. Expectations are realistic and clearly defined for each child. Education is synonymous with "power," and while the child's illness is taken into account in the educational plan, the intent is to utilize the learning process itself as a method of emotional repair.

A fundamental tool in the care and treatment of the youngsters at the Hawthorne Cedar Knolls School is the design and structure of its various functional units—the cottage, the clinic, and the school; in other words, in the "psychogeography" of the institution itself. It represents a two-pronged effort to meet the generic needs of children and to deal effectively with the specific emotional disorders of individual children, avoiding replication of the pathological life style that brings the child to the institution in the first place. Through such opportunities for meaningful interaction with peers and adults and for a sound educational program with reasonable expectations, children are enabled to work through some of the problems that have denied and blunted their capacities for achieving some degree of success and satisfaction in their adaptation to life and society.

THE LEAGUE SCHOOL
FOR SERIOUSLY DISTURBED CHILDREN:
EDUCATION AS THERAPY FOR THE SERIOUSLY DISTURBED

BY DR. CARL FENICHEL*

In 1953 the League School for Seriously Disturbed Children challenged the ancient legend that the drastic surgery of separating a child from his family by hospitalization or placement in a residential center was the best and only solution for mentally ill children diagnosed as schizophrenic, autistic, or psychotic, and considered uneducable and untreatable. The League School offered a simple alternative: to take these children out of hiding and place them in a day-school program that would give them a chance to live and grow within their own family and community.

The League School began with the hypothesis that positive behavioral changes could be achieved by the use of special educational techniques in a therapeutic setting without individual psychotherapy. This hypothesis was based on the assumption that a properly planned and highly individualized program of special education with interdisciplinary participation could result in social and emotional growth as well as educational achievements for many mentally sick children.

The League School's emphasis on education and habilitation rather than on custody and segregation placed the school in the vanguard of an idea so compelling that it could not be ignored. Gradually, recognition and partial support came from government agencies on federal, state, and community levels. From the National Institute of Mental Health and the New York State Department of Mental Hygiene came grants for demonstration programs; from the New York City Community Mental Health Board came matching funds for a clinical staff;

* Founder and director of the League School, Brooklyn, New York.

and from the New York City Board of Education came increasing financial support for a large part of the school's teaching staff.

The League School found vast differences in behavior, communication, pathology, prognosis, and potential among all its children, despite a common psychiatric diagnosis. They ranged from the most passive and lethargic children to the most impulse-ridden and hyperactive; from those who were completely infantile and helpless to those who were self-managing and independent; from the most regressed and defective to some with relatively intact intellectual functioning. Often within the same child one found the coexistence and overlapping of features of childhood schizophrenia, infantile autism, retardation, and neurological dysfunctioning.

We soon realized that the psychiatric classifications had very little educational relevance and that what each child needs is his own personal prescription of special training and education based on a psychoeducational assessment of his unique patterns of behavior and levels of functioning. This means going beyond the medical and clinical work-ups and attempting to identify, analyze, and describe each child's specific skills and strengths, disabilities and deficits, lags and limitations in the many basic areas involved in the learning process, including sensory and perceptual intactness, neuro-motor development, spatial relations, body image, visual and auditory discrimination and retention, and ability to use symbols, understand language, and form concepts. The assessment also includes the many observable secondary symptoms of emotional and behavioral disturbances related to the primary disorders and defects. It then prescribes for the teacher specific remedial, training, and educational techniques and activities that attempt to reduce, correct, or remove these disabilities if possible, or to work around them and compensate for them if the disabilities are irremediable.

The major role of the school's psychiatrist, pediatric neurologist, psychologists, language therapists, and social workers is to pool their findings, skills, and understanding of each child and then, with the help of the special educational supervisors and curriculum resource specialists, to translate and make them available in functional and meaningful form for the daily program of the teacher.

The individual and group learning experiences of the child and his relationship with his teacher are the basic instruments of the League School program. The classroom curriculum, atmosphere, grouping, scheduling, regulations, and routines, and how they are handled by the teacher, all have implications and potential for positive learning and socializing experiences that can induce change, adjustment, and growth.

The educational and therapeutic value of the program will depend on how effectively the teacher employs individual tutoring and remediation based on an ongoing assessment of each child's learning and behavioral problems and deficits, and on how well she can integrate each child's individual skills, interests, and needs into the programming and group processes of the classroom. To be successful and meaningful, such a program requires a very small class size.

For those children who continue to function on a very low, defective level, emphasis is placed on impulse control and the development of self-help and socializing skills. Some of these children may eventually have to be institutionalized. Where academic achievements remain minimal, children are taught productive work habits and given prevocational and vocational training that will enable them to secure appropriate jobs within the community. The school educates and prepares as many children as possible for admission to appropriate public school classes—regular or special.

The League School has become the prototype of many day schools throughout the nation and abroad.

PROJECT RE-ED:

NEW WAYS OF HELPING EMOTIONALLY DISTURBED CHILDREN

BY NICHOLAS HOBBS*

The elliptic expression "Project Re-ED" refers to a project on the reeducation of emotionally disturbed children. It started as an eight-year cooperative effort of the states of Tennessee and North Carolina and Peabody College, made possible by a long-term NIMH pilot project grant. Two original Re-ED schools, Cumberland House Elementary School in Nashville and Wright School in Durham, remain in operation as permanent parts of the mental health programs of the participating states. Tennessee has opened three additional schools, including one for adolescents, and plans to convert its entire residential and day-care program for disturbed children to the Re-ED model. And schools are under development in other states.

At capacity each Re-ED school will serve 40 to 50 children, ages six to twelve (originally), in an around-the-clock reeducation effort that, coupled with intensive work with the child's parents, regular school, and community, seeks to return the child as quickly as possible to his normal life setting. Each school has a creative, challenging educational program, supplemented by primitive camping. The children are normal to superior in intelligence, but they have all been in serious trouble in school or have been unable to attend school. Labels such as emotionally disturbed, behavior problem, antisocial, withdrawn, schizoid, and schizophrenic appear in the children's records. The children are usually referred by psychiatric clinics.

Re-ED schools are staffed by teacher-counselors and liaison teachers, carefully selected young people with a background in teaching or other work demonstrating a meaningful commitment to children. We refer to them as "natural workers" to imply that we try through careful selection to capitalize on

* Director, The John F. Kennedy Center, George Peabody College for Teachers, and provost, Vanderbilt University, Nashville, Tennessee.

individual differences in ability to work with children, a product of an entire life history not likely to be modified much by professional training. Teacher-counselors actually receive nine months of graduate education leading to the Master of Arts degree. On the job they are backed up by consultants from pediatrics, psychiatry, psychology, education, and other fields, this backstop by high-level talent being essential to the success of the Re-ED idea and an important strategy in extending scarce mental health manpower.

From the start, Project Re-ED has been a reality-oriented operation. It was conceived in response to a still-present reality: that the nation can never provide adequate services for disturbed children by multiplying psychiatric treatment centers. There are not and will not be enough psychiatrists, psychologists, and other mental health specialists to staff them; costs are prohibitively high; and the model itself, as realized today in many respected institutions, often falls short of providing an optimum arrangement for restoring children to home, school, and community as quickly as possible. There will of course be a continuing need for medically oriented treatment centers, as well as for custodial care, but these two alternatives need no longer exhaust the range of the possible, nor provide the only models for helping children too disturbed to remain at home and in school.

The program that has evolved to help children in Re-ED schools is tuned to reality too. The central thrust of the effort is to help children here and now acquire competence in coping with realistic problems: how to read, how to play first base, how to approach school without fear, how to counter a dominating mother without recourse to asthma, how to take a stand against a bully, how to receive and how to give of one's possessions, how to know joy; in sum, how to be oneself fully, without guilt. Re-ED is further reality-bound in recognizing that children may live in a real world of less than adequate parents, of poor schools, of psychologically shabby neighborhoods, of communities that belie the word community, of territories unfit for human habitation. We believe that the most useful definition of an emotionally disturbed child is one that requires attention to both individual and social variables, with far more weight accorded the latter than is usual.

In Re-ED, then, we view the problem of the child called disturbed as a manifestation of the breakdown of an ecological system composed of child, family, neighborhood, school, and community. We frankly accept limited goals in our work. Our goal is not to cure a child or to prepare him to cope with all possible life roles but to restore to effective operation the small social system of which the child is an integral part. Cure seems to us a misleading concept. Effective living is intrinsically problematic. Our goal is to seek a point of adequacy where the probability of continued successful function somewhat outweighs the probability of failure. The Re-ED task is to get child, family, school, neighborhood, and community just above threshold in the requirement that each component makes of the other components. The Re-ED staff moves out of the system as soon as possible. Re-ED tries to avoid taking over indefinitely the responsibilities of the normal socializing agents of our society.

In Re-ED, goals and procedures are couched in the idiom of competence and self-fulfillment rather than of illness or pathology; intervention seeks the least practicable disruption of normal patterns of living. The strategy is to remove the child, in *space, time,* and *meaning,* the least possible distance from the people with whom he must learn to live, and who, in turn, must learn how to increase their contribution to his full development. On the *space* dimension, this means that Re-ED schools are located near the families they serve for ready access and communication. Both geography and policy make it possible for parents to visit easily. The children go home on weekends and vacations, so that the child and his parents and siblings can practice new learnings and test new resolves, so that the alienation so often a consequence of institutionalization can be avoided. And most children visit their regular schools periodically, to maintain their engagement with the institution that is second only to the family in responsibility for the socialization of children. On the *time* dimension, this means that Re-ED schools separate children from their families and regular schools for as short a period of time as possible to achieve the limited goals defined above. The average length of stay of a child in a Re-ED school is seven months. On the *meaning* dimension, Re-ED schools are designed with a high expectation of normal behavior, of zestful, purposeful, joyous living. Physical facilities are simple, open, homelike, uninstitutional. The daily program is planned to be so interesting, so engaging, so tuned to success, so instructive in group living, so self-fulfilling that the child is immediately caught up in behavior befitting a normal child. Human behavior is remarkably responsive to expectation. Re-ED goals are goals rich in metaphorical texture and evocative of the best that is in us all: children, parents, teacher-counselors, consultants alike. In the area of human behavior, prophecies tend to be self-fulfilling. No child can ever be more than what someone believes he can become.

It costs about $25 a day per child to operate a Re-ED school, a figure that compares favorably to the cost of traditional residential treatment centers. But a much more meaningful figure is the cost per child returned to home and school and community. Because of the comparatively short period of stay, this cost is about $5,000 per child.

A careful follow-up of children at discharge and 18 months after indicate a most satisfactory rate of improvement. The data show that Re-ED works.

Professional judgment is positive too. A "Panel of Visitors," composed of Eli M. Bower, Reginald S. Lourie, Charles R. Strother, and Robert L. Sutherland, followed the project from the beginning, visiting the schools and comparing observations. The panel concluded:

> That Project Re-ED represents a conceptually sound, economically feasible, and demonstrably effective approach to helping emotionally disturbed children, including the moderately disturbed and some seriously disturbed; that it does make available an important new source of mental health manpower and extends the effectiveness of highly trained and scarce mental health specialists; that it has developed concepts applicable to other educational and mental health programs for children; and that it has passed the crucial test of professional, public, and legislative scrutiny and acceptance. We therefore recommend the adoption of the Re-ED program as a primary resource for the help of emotionally disturbed children of the Nation.

Social-Psychological Aspects of Normal Growth and Development: Infants and Children

All the world loves a baby, so it is said. We as a society do not act that way. A newborn baby is a reaffirmation of the miracle of the creation of life. Most infants are near-perfect at birth and possess enormous potentialities for bringing deep joy to themselves and others. They come into the world with a great natural capacity for growth, for loving, for learning, for exploring and working. In them lies the hope of the future—for their families, their communities, the nation, and the world. Our infants and children can and must contribute so much to these larger societies. They therefore are the responsibility not only of their families but of these same societies. We as parents and citizens must firmly dedicate ourselves to the members of our new generation and to fostering their maximum growth and development into healthy children and young adults. We must dedicate ourselves further to creating a society devoted to families so that, in turn, these families may provide the best possible primary care for their young.

Tragically, large numbers of babies are warped and damaged in their growth, never to achieve the bright promise with which the majority of them are born. They are the victims of our society's indifference to the needs of children and of their parents.

Why do we let this happen? Compassion alone should prevent it. Enlightened self-interest should also demand that each newborn child be guaranteed his right to fulfill his innate promise. For those babies whose potentialities are stunted before they are born, we should be guided

313

by both compassion and self-interest to provide services and develop new knowledge so that such tragedies become rare exceptions.

Research reveals that most of a child's future growth and development is shaped by the events that occur from the time of his conception until he reaches the age of two. These very early years are of crucial importance and, for better or for worse, the foundation is laid—often irreversibly—for the individual's physical, emotional, social, and intellectual well-being.

Infancy and early childhood is the time during which the child is most flexible and will respond most quickly and easily to any needed remedial services. The Commission has placed special emphasis on recommendations related to the beginning and first years of life. Our proposals call for concerted medical, social, and educational services in such areas as: family planning, genetic research and counseling, prenatal care, high-quality intensive medical care, infant day care, homemaker services, parent counseling and education, income supports for poor families, and the like (see Chapter I, Section II). The need for such services will become more apparent in the discussion which follows.

Genetic Components

It is often difficult to differentiate genetic and environmental influences on human development. This is partly because the mother's health and nutritional status have a bearing on the development of her child from the moment of conception on through pregnancy. Great strides are now being made in genetic research. A few genetic factors have been isolated which show a correlation with certain psychological difficulties. These include at least one form of severe mental retardation and variations in the chromosomal structures which have been correlated to some maladaptive behavior. One widely publicized variation is that of the XYY chromosome aberration in males, which has been associated in some instances with acts of aggression and violence. Most scientists agree that not enough evidence is yet available to permit or require "genetic engineering," that is, the determination as to which people should be encouraged to reproduce and which people should be discouraged or even prevented from having children. For the present, the Commission urges that genetic counseling be available for those who are concerned about possible metabolic genetic disorders leading to mental retardation. Such counseling must be carried out with full recognition of the anxieties and fears that many parents may bring to such a counselor (see Chapter I, pp. 30–31).

Development During Pregnancy

A child's growth and development is affected by his prenatal, as well as his postnatal, environment. It is estimated that at least 250,000 babies are born each year with major and obvious defects. Others may have suffered damage in their development or at birth which may not be apparent until later. Some speech problems, some forms of mental retardation, epilepsy, reading handicaps, and various behavior problems may be related to brain injury during pregnancy or birth. It is widely believed that a number of mildly handicapped children, including many whose difficulties seem to be problems of social and psychological adjustment, actually suffered minor kinds of injuries to the central nervous system before they were born. Research indicates that the most critical period of brain development in the child is probably from the second week of pregnancy to about the eleventh week. The entire period of pregnancy is, however, a time in which damage may occur to the unborn baby. Among the factors that may cause this damage are: malnutrition of the mother, various virus infections such as German measles, infection by syphilis present in the mother, maternal diabetes, and a wide variety of drugs and toxic substances, including some present in tobacco. Moreover, there are higher rates of birth defects in the babies born to very young mothers, older women, women with chronic poor health, and women who bear too many closely spaced children. Furthermore, severe maternal emotional stress affects the biochemical equilibrium between the mother and an unborn baby. Research points to the close association between the mental and physical health of mothers before and during pregnancy and the physical and mental health of their children.

Statistics indicate that the infant death rate in the United States is higher than that in twelve other industrial nations. Despite our declining national rate, it is still 20.6 per 1,000 live births at the time of this writing (early 1969). There is a clear association between infant mortality and poor prenatal care. The infant death rate is five and one-half times higher for mothers who have received no prenatal care as for those who have. Inadequate prenatal care is not the total cause. Poor health and poor medical care prior to pregnancy, malnutrition, and poor environments are all added factors. Indeed, the total life situation of very poor people (who are also less likely to receive prenatal care) is more conducive to a high infant death rate. Obviously, a great many cases of infant death are avoidable. The Children's Bureau, in a recent analysis of the factors associated with high infant deaths, has indicated that this rate could be sharply reduced by the provision of a complex of intensive services in 56 key counties which contain most of the highly urbanized population in this country.

Babies who are born prematurely (with prematurity being defined as an infant with a very low birth weight) have relatively higher rates of mortality and serious handicaps such as brain damage, mental retardation, and blindness. Whether these problems are due entirely to prematurity is often difficult to determine, except in babies of extremely low birth weight. Causal judgments are complicated by the fact that prematurity is much more frequent among mothers who are not married, who have poor health, and who suffer from the handicaps of poverty. Premature babies need immediate and special assistance after birth. They often have difficulty in breathing and in eating and are much more susceptible to infections. Such babies are difficult to care for, and families usually cannot obtain the needed special guidance and supporting services.

The implications of the evidence given above are clear. It is extremely important to provide women the needed services and encouragement so that they can plan their pregnancies in terms of their overall physical condition, their age, the number of children they may already have, and the economic and social situation of the family. Fathers, or prospective fathers, should also be included in this planning and their physical and mental health taken into consideration. Presently, as we noted earlier, disadvantaged women have less access to family planning services. It is crucial that such services be made available, free of cost, to all people who cannot pay for this service. In addition, excellent medical care must be provided for *all* women from the early stages of pregnancy on through childbirth and postnatal aftercare. Other needed provisions, as recommended in Chapter I, include enriched diets for expectant mothers and provisions for prenatal and postnatal maternity leave with pay.

THE FIRST THREE MONTHS OF LIFE

The Need for Consistent, Affectionate Mothering

The newborn baby is totally dependent on those who care for him. Research shows that it is very important that he be cared for chiefly by one person. Ideally, that person should be his mother. If, for some reason, his mother is not able to give him the kind of care he needs, it is quite possible that he will thrive and develop well if a loving, competent mother substitute is provided and if that substitute is his main caretaker over a long period of time (*Report of Task Force I,* 1968). If he is cared for by a number of mother substitutes and does not have a continuing, close relationship with one "mother person," he is likely to develop later problems in his ability to relate to people.

A continuing, close relationship with one competent, loving person is important for many reasons. One reason is that, during the first year of life, a child needs to develop a sense of trust in his environment and in other people. This is essential to his basic sense of security about himself and the rest of the world. In effect, an infant learns to become a human being through his interaction with other human beings. He needs to know that he is loved and that he will be taken care of. His physical and intellectual as well as his social and emotional growth depends upon it.

Behavior Tendencies Present at Birth

The loving, consistent, and continuous care so essential to a child's sound development must also be highly individualized to fit each child's needs. There is a growing body of research indicating that individual babies are quite different from one another at birth. They vary in terms of activity, responsiveness, and sensitivity to the world around them. These differences appear to be consistent for a particular newborn child, and such behavior tendencies may persist into adulthood. It is not yet clearly determined which of these tendencies are inherited and which are more closely related to prenatal conditions and to factors at the time of childbirth, such as the length of labor, lack of oxygen, etc. (Escalona, 1968). It also appears that newborn babies differ in the ways in which they react to new experiences, the intensity with which they seek and react to experiences, their usual feeling mood, and their style of concentration (Thomas *et al.*, 1963). Obviously, the baby will receive better care if his parents are aware of, and sensitive to, his particular individual style and take cues from him as to how he may best be handled.

Special difficulties are likely to arise if the mother, or mother substitute, is insensitive to the special needs of her child or if she has quite different tendencies herself and cannot readily accept her particular kind of baby. These differences in individual infant style also suggest that if one person has major responsibility for the baby there is a better chance that his individuality will be better understood and handled. Research indicates that boys are more vulnerable than girls because of greater central nervous system inactivity. They may therefore require more maternal attention.

Need for Stimulating Experiences

The newborn infant needs more than good physical care and warm, individualized maternal love. He requires a variety of experiences which encourage his muscular and sensory exploration and development. At birth, his nervous system is not fully developed. It is important, for example, that he have light and a chance to see things in his environment so that his eyesight can develop. The baby is affected by stimuli from within his own body and by those provided by his environment. To varying degrees, babies reach out for experiences around them. It is critically important to their development that opportunities for proper sensory and motor experiences be available.

Physical discomfort and monotony in the environment reduce a baby's sense of contentment and his alert interest in learning. Hunger, fatigue, and physical ailments usually lead him to be less responsive and more backward in his behavior (Escalona, 1968).

A child's development is best brought about if he has alternating periods of excitement, quiet play, and times of peace and privacy. Although it is important that the young baby have many stimulating experiences, over-stimulation can adversely affect his development.

Hunt (1966) presents recommendations from his research regarding the needs of the newborn infant:

—proper and sanitary nutrition;
—clean clothing and repeated care for elimination;
—proper temperature and ventilation;
—opportunity to sleep;
—adequate medical care in cases of infections, nutritional disturbances, or other medical problems.

During his waking hours, the baby can profit from:

—being handled and rocked;
—having visual contact with a changing scene in which certain patterns like that of the human face appear and disappear repeatedly or having objects within view to look at;
—hearing a variety of different sounds in which, also, certain patterns like those of the human voice occur repeatedly.

Hunt also states that at this stage a baby further needs:

—consistent responses to his actions, at least most of the time; however, this consistency should be varied so that the baby learns new ways of getting what he wants;
—play with caretakers, because it is probably in play that the infant has the most natural opportunity to test himself and to grow and develop;
—an opportunity to hear speech and to get responses from others to his own attempts to talk.

It appears that the development of learned behavior is related closely to the child's level of biological growth, although present research is not conclusive. Apparently there are stages of growth at which different kinds of behaviors are most effectively learned and made an integrant part of the child's knowledge and skills. If such learning does not take place at the appropriate times, it may be less completely learned and may break down in times of stress (*Report of Task Force I,* 1968).

Moreover, the longer a baby or young child is exposed to inappropriate or harmful learning experiences, the more difficult it is to change any adverse effects on his development. For instance, a number of studies show that young children who are brought up in an impersonal institution appear to be apathetic and mentally retarded. If they are given personal attention and stimulating learning experiences, there can be dramatic changes in their behavior and their measured intelligence (Hunt, 1966). Until recently, it was generally thought that the apparent dullness and learning disabilities of many children of disadvantaged parents were an outcome of defective, inherited intelligence. Stimulated, in large part, by the work of Piaget (1952), a number of researchers in the past six or seven years have turned their attention to an intensive study of infant development and experimental procedures related to enhancing the intellectual and related capacities of babies through planned programs of stimulation (Richmond and Lipton, 1959; Caldwell and Richmond, 1964). Such studies show that infants usually seek out stimulation and seem to have an innate drive for competence. They have a need for novelty and complexity rather than monotonous repetition (Hebb, 1955).

The recognition that the growth of a child's intelligence is highly dependent upon his early experiences led to the development of the federally supported Head Start program, which was designed for children three years and over. It is now apparent that it might be far more effective to commence enrichment of the child's life at an earlier age, starting in the first few months of life.

Obviously, highly disadvantaged parents are less likely to have the energy to be able to provide the kind of stimulating environment that a baby needs. The strains and lack of resources imposed by the poverty environment tend to undermine parental ability to effectively meet the whole complex of a baby's needs—stimulation, excellent physical care, good nutrition, medical supervision, and competent, sensitive mothering.

We know that poor people do love their babies and have high hopes for their future, and that disadvantaged parents often care for their babies well. However, generations of poverty and its impact on health and vigor in many instances leads to apathy and conservation of energy for survival.

"Failure to Thrive"

Professionals in the human service fields have noted that some babies and children fail to grow and develop normally. The "failure to thrive syndrome" includes a complex of listlessness, dullness, withdrawal, and slow physical development. Such children are often small and puny. Although the causes have not been clearly established, there are clues from research and clinical practice which indicate that this failure may be associated with such conditions as emotional deprivation, lack of a stimulating environment, harsh and dominating child-rearing approaches, and malnutrition. A variety of genetic and environmental factors seems to be interactive, and thus the causes and symptoms of this syndrome may be different for each child.

The younger the child is, the more likely it will be that his physical problems may be manifested as behavior problems, or vice versa. Typical symptoms include failure to grow and gain weight, retarded development, occasional vomiting and/or diarrhea and other recurring physical illnesses, feeding difficulty, weakness, tiredness, and irritability. To arrive at a diagnosis of developmental problems, it is recommended that babies who fail to thrive be studied and observed by various specialists—such as pediatricians, psychologists, psychiatrists, and social workers—over a period of time and that, insofar as possible, these observations be made in the child's home setting.

Malnutrition

A great deal of publicity has been given recently to hunger and resulting malnutrition, especially among poverty groups in the United States. Experts in related scientific fields warn of overly simplistic one-factor interpretations. Although evidence from developing countries indicates that severe malnutrition, especially protein deficiency, in the early years of life has adverse effects on intellectual, physical, and personality development, the problem is not quite so clear-cut in this country, where such severe conditions are not as frequently found. Complex environmental factors in this country make it difficult to isolate the incidence and effects of malnutrition on the development of infants and very young children. However, there is evidence that malnutrition—together with illness and the many deprivations of poverty—plays a part in retarding development. Scientific experts emphasize that enriched diets, by themselves, are unlikely to bring the dramatic improvements in human growth and development that are now being claimed in some quarters (Dairy Council Digest, 1968).

The existence of poverty in both rural and urban areas of the United States, including 256 "hunger counties," was documented in a recent report (Hunger, U.S.A., 1968). The study pointed to evidence of retarded growth and possible lasting damage to mental capacity in children, resulting from malnutrition and other deprivations. Stine et al. (1967) studied height, weight, and other criteria of health and developmental status in 842 white and Negro children, approximately four years old, from Baltimore families which were described as "culturally deprived" and of a low-income level. Height and weight of these children were below standard values for this country and closer to values for malnourished children in developing countries. Percentile values for head circumference were all less than corresponding values for a "normal" population. A study by Woodruff (1966) indicates that conditioned malnutrition, or milder malnutrition associated with disease or stress—which is more common in the United States—has some of the same effects as the primary malnutrition found in children in developing countries. Woodruff comments that the management of conditioned malnutrition is far more complex than merely providing an adequate diet.

AGE THREE MONTHS TO ONE YEAR

Rapid Growth of Abilities

We have commented that a very young baby needs a chance to develop a sense of trust in his environment. He needs to have his dependency needs met. He needs pleasurable experience. He needs love and protection, and he needs recognition of his special individual characteristics. These same requirements are essential to his development between the age period of three months and one year. During this time span, however, the baby increasingly learns to differentiate himself from other people and from the physical environment. He learns more about his own body and the way it works. He learns more about the people in his life and the world around him. He also begins to adapt to a regular schedule of eating and sleeping. Most parents find this period of development far less stressful and far more delightful than the earlier time when the baby's needs were highly unpredictable and often highly intrusive into the needs of the parents. For instance, when the baby begins to sleep peacefully through the night, the whole character of family life takes a definite turn for the better.

Needs for New, But Not Too Many, Experiences

The first patterns of speech generally appear after age three months, and the normal baby delights in carrying on extended conversations with his parents in a strange and unknown language. He learns many new physical skills and develops more physical strength. His nerves and muscles develop so that he is able to impress himself and those about him with his new virtuosities. He learns to discriminate sounds and sights, tastes and smells. His need for more complicated toys and experiences increases. Yesterday's simple pleasures become a matter of indifference today. He learns to use his social ability to smile and laugh to win favors from adults, and he also learns the power of a piercing scream.

During this time it is important for him to have a wide range of experiences in seeing, hearing, touching, handling, and moving. However, it is quite possible to overstimulate him. For instance, in some disadvantaged homes the confusion and high noise level of the environment may cause him to become irritable or nonresponsive. Conversely, many such homes lack the diversity and kinds of stimulating experiences that promote a child's intellectual and physical growth. Stimulation not developmentally or individually adapted to the child also occurs frequently in more advantaged families. A number of parents have been impressed with the messages in the mass media concerning the importance of a rich environment for their children. Achievement-oriented, ambitious parents may well overdo the stimulus regime. Besides stimulation, babies need periods of quiet, rest, and privacy.

As he grows a little older, a baby needs to start learning that he cannot always have exactly what he wants exactly when he wants it. The ability to withstand some frustration and to accept some controls is important for his later development and for his adjustment to his family and his larger social world. His growing drive for independence also should be respected, and he needs to be encouraged, but not pushed, to do things for himself.

During this time it is still difficult to diagnose the problems that a child may have or the causes of these problems. Professionals are far too prone to advise anxious parents that the child will simply outgrow some observed difficulties. A number of signs may suggest problems, such as: disturbances in physical functioning related to sleeping, eating, and digestion; excessive crying; repetitive unhappy moods; fearful and withdrawn behavior; persistent tension and irritability; nonresponsiveness (*Report of Task Force I*, 1968).

There are critical deficiencies in services for infants under the age of one. The growth of such programs as the maternal and child health clinics, however, has provided a greater service emphasis on this stage of child development.

THE CHILD ONE TO THREE YEARS

A Neglected Age Period

Children between the ages of one to five often are not reached by the services they need from the medical, dental, and mental health professions. Service deficits for this age group are even greater than for infants. Developmental and related deficits often go unnoticed until the child reaches school at the age of five or six. At such a late date, our research studies show, it may be extremely difficult, if not impossible, to reverse the damage that may have already occurred. As preschool programs are developed further, the child may come to professional attention by the time he is three or four, but the age period for one to three still tends to be critically neglected (*Report of Task Force I*, 1968). Good physical care, adequate nutrition, medical attention, immunization against contagious diseases, and identification and correction of physical handicaps all continue to be important during this age period.

Some Behavior Characteristics of This Stage

Between the ages of one and three the youngster develops an increasing sense of self and some concept of his sex identity and the identity of other people. By the time he is three, he is likely also to have some awareness of racial identity. His drive for independence increases and becomes particularly strong. Probably every parent has experienced the drive of the two-year-old for independence and self-determination or, as the experts call it, autonomy. This is the age during which the word "no" seems to be the standard response to any request made of the child and "me do" and "mine" become regular features of the vocabulary.

Learning Self-Control

Children seem to vary in their drives for aggression and passivity, independence and dependence. These variations are probably related to reaction tendencies present at birth and to the way in which the child has been nurtured. The young child's drive for autonomy is one that should be respected and encouraged. However, he should learn controls over his own drives and a respect for the feelings and rights of other people. This kind of self-control takes a long time to develop, and it is important to recognize that it is a gradual process which is difficult for the youngster—one which is more difficult for some children than for others. A child is best able to learn these controls and still achieve healthy social and emotional development if he is given steady, supporting love combined with firm, mild, consistent discipline. An inconsistent approach leads him to test every situation in order to find out how far he can go in doing what he wishes. Inconsistency, combined with harsh, physical punishment, tends to adversely affect his development. Such parental behavior may lead the child to become overly aggressive, violent, and quarrelsome or to repress such aggressive hostile feelings and become fearful and withdrawn. On the other hand, general permissiveness with few, if any, restraints tends to result in a child's being socially unacceptable and unable to discipline himself. Development seems to be most enhanced by kindly, consistent discipline adapted to the child's age, his individuality, and the situation. This helps a youngster to develop freely within known and predictable limits so that he can grow toward a sense of satisfaction in himself and his life, with an accompanying ability to handle the real world of both limitations and opportunities.

Adventures and Explorations

As the child moves from his first to his third year, he has a growing need for social relationships with other children as well as with adults. It is important for him to experience relationships with people at various age levels rather than only with adults or children of his own age. When he plays with his own age group he tends to engage in what has been called parallel play. In other words, he plays alongside other children, often imitating what they do but not generally engaging in cooperative play. Play of all kinds helps a child develop. He learns from playing with many kinds of toys and has a growing need for more and more complex, but not too complex, playthings.

This is the time, too, in which his ability to talk is growing and in which his curiosity is aroused about the many things in his environment. Here, again, every person who has cared for an active two- or three-year-old is well acquainted with the youngster's drive to explore and to find out what he can do and how things work. His need for protection is likely to increase during this time because his energies and enthusiasms far outrun his knowledge and judgment. Accident rates for this age span tend to be high, and it takes an active and knowledgeable adult to protect the child from the many complexities of today's complicated home and neighborhood.

A youngster needs to experience many successes and relatively few failures as he strives to acquire new skills. He needs to learn how to channel his aggressive feelings and divert them from acts of physical violence to verbal expressions or substitute harmless play activities. He also needs to learn how to express his sex-related curiosity in relatively indirect ways, such as talking about them, playing with water and clay, and the like.

A child's interest in sex is likely to be clear and open at this time. Parents and other adults are frequently disturbed by the child's obvious interests. These interests should not be denied or punished. Rather, the child should be helped to satisfy his curiosity through having his questions answered, having an opportunity to observe animals, and being gently guided toward socially desirable behavior, such as keeping his clothes on in public. It is obvious that the attitudes of parents and other caretaking adults about their own sexuality and sex life strongly affect how well they will be able to handle the child's growing sex identity and interests.

Intellectual Development

The intellectual capacities of the one- to three-year-old child are in a sensitive and rapid stage of development. It has already been remarked that the child should have many kinds of learning experiences and opportunities to develop and test his skills. The teaching style of the parent evidently has a significant effect on the growth of the child's learning capacity. For instance, children who have normal or higher I.Q.'s tend to have parents who give the child emotional support and gentle guidance when he is attempting to master a new task. A loving, nonauthoritarian approach combined with interested involvement appears to be helpful. The child is helped if his parents talk to him about how a task might be performed, give him clear directions that he can understand and follow, and point out the basic principles that are involved—such as in matching colors, forms, and the like (Hess and Shipman, 1965). It has been found that middle-class parents who have had similar experiences in their childhood are more likely to use such teaching styles than are lower-class parents. In fact, the tendency of better-educated parents to talk to their children in ways that include basic principles and concepts is related to the fact that they are more likely to have children who achieve well in school (Bernstein, 1961; John and Golstein, 1964).

It has been claimed by some that lower-lower-class parents do not talk to their children. This is an inaccurate statement of what generally happens. It is more likely that these parents do talk quite a bit to their children. They are more likely to deal in action words related to the immediate situation. This tendency is associated, of course, with the parent's own early experience, present situation, and lack of advanced education.

AGES THREE TO FIVE

Increasing Independence and Activity

The three- to five-year-old follows the same general growth and development trends as those noted for the younger child. Beyond the age of three, however, the child's social experiences increase. He generally takes great pleasure in the company of children his own age. His drive for independence grows. He still tends to depend on his parents for love and protection, but these needs are not quite so great, partly because he has learned more and more about how to take care of himself. Moreover, if his needs to be dependent have been met earlier, he has a foundation of self-security and self-esteem on which to build so that he has the courage and confidence to venture forth into the world on his own.

Children of this age tend to be highly creative and imaginative. Of course, this trait varies from individual to individual and is found in differing forms and degrees of expression. Through imaginary play, young children begin to sort out the differences between what they both fear and wish and what is real. They also practice for life's future roles. Little girls busily occupy themselves being small mothers, and little boys play at being cowboys, Superman, and other "heroic" figures. Creativity is also expressed through a barrage of questions, a flurry of mudpies, drawing of pictures, and so on. It is important that children be given many outlets for their urges to create, to experiment, to imagine, and to learn.

The modern home is often hard-pressed to accommodate such exploratory drives of the young child. The difficulties are usually even greater in the overcrowded and constricted homes of poor people, and often compounded by the lack of yards and playgrounds. As indicated earlier, disadvantaged parents often lose control over their children by the time they are four years old, since they become involved in the street communities of children and adolescents. Thus these youngsters, lacking other opportunities for experimental play, seek the excitement and dangers of the streets. In general, many homes and neighborhoods lack the facilities for providing children with the rich, but safe, experiences which they require for maximum growth and well-being. To meet this need, the Commission believes that the development of preschool programs, supervised playgrounds, and other recreational facilities should be an important part of the network of services recommended for our nation's children (see Chapter I, Section II).

Growth Toward Greater Self-Control

During the three- to five-year age span, children should gain increasing control over their impulses and show more and more ability to work in cooperation with others. The same principles of firm, mild, consistent discipline, combined with loving care, apply here as, indeed, they apply to children at older ages. Parents and teachers can also help children develop constructive ways of handling their impulsive feelings. These ways include talking about feelings rather than acting them out. This occurs most effectively when play, engagement in creative activities, and development of a wide range of skills and interests are facilitated.

Establishing Identity as a Boy or a Girl

The three- to five-year-old child has an increased awareness of sexuality and of his or her own identification as a male or female. A number of varying theories and opinions attempt to explain the growth of sexual identity during this period, which is often referred to as the Oedipal stage of development. This topic is far too specialized and complex for an adequate discussion here. However, it is generally agreed that it is important for the little boy to have a close, companionable relationship with his father and to learn more and more about the masculine role. It is also important that he feel that it is a good thing to be a boy and that both his father and mother approve of his masculinity. Basically the same thing can be said about a little girl in relation to her mother and father. While some claim that the absence of a father from the home inevitably has serious adverse consequences for the developing child at this stage of his growth, we have noted there is a lack of evidence that an intact marriage is universally of such critical importance as has been widely assumed (see Chapter IV). A conflict-ridden marriage, for instance, may be more damaging to a child than the divorce or separation of parents. If there is no father in the home, little children of both sexes may find help from other men who are present in the neighborhood, the school, and/or the family. Program planners should make every attempt to engage more boys and men to work with little children in such settings as the preschool and the playground. It is time that we abandoned the prevalent assumption that the care of children should be delegated solely to women.

Recent Emphasis on Intellectual Development of Young Children

At various times in our country's history we have placed differential stresses on the social, intellectual, emotional, physical, and moral development of children. This has led to the tendency to consider one or another of these factors as being central and all-important in the development of programs and policies. As we have stressed so often in this report, however, all of these aspects of development are crucial to a child's well-being, and a broad conceptualization of positive mental health includes each of these in interaction with one another. It is on this basis that we must develop and carry out programs which are aimed, in a coordinated way, at enhancing the potential of children and youth.

The intellectual development of children has received special emphasis in recent times, partly because of the accumulation of evidence pointing to its critical importance to success throughout life and to the significance of early learning experiences. For example, in an analysis of many studies of child development, Bloom (1964) presents impressive evidence which indicates that, on the average, 50 percent of the development of the measured intelligence of seventeen-year-olds apparently takes place between zero and four years and another 30 percent takes place between the ages of four and eight years. The word "apparently" is used advisedly here. Although space does not permit a technical discussion of this topic, question can be raised about the method used in Bloom's study. His conclusions are drawn from statistical manipulations of the results from a number of studies, and there is some uncertainty as to whether these manipulations are completely satisfactory. For instance, the results show a relatively low correlation between measured intelligence at the ages of three and adulthood, and it is highly questionable whether adult intelligence can be predicted from scores obtained by children before the age of six (Bayley, 1940; Honzik, MacFarlane, and Allen, 1948). In addition, there may be considerable variability among children. Some are known to be genetically late developers. For instance, some individuals have been found to vary in their measured intelligence by as much as 50 points during their school years. Only 15 percent of the children in the Bayley study were found to maintain as little as 10 points variation in measured intelligence during their growth from childhood through adolescence. No studies have been made of changes and variations in the measured intelligence of disadvantaged children over a long period of time. Bloom's conclusions are based largely on studies involving middle-class children. Moreover, *measured* intelligence may appear to remain fairly stable because children generally remain in the same kind of social and educational environment until they are grown. We do not yet know what difference planned enriched educational experiences for older, as well as younger, children might make in affecting measured intelligence and educational achievement.

All Aspects of Development Are Important

Although the question has been raised as to whether there has been a recent overemphasis on the intellectual development of young children and on the exact ways in which intellectual capacity can be determined in early childhood, this is not intended to denigrate either the importance of this development or the need for a wealth of learning experiences during the first five years of life. The main point is that these early years are tremendously significant for all aspects of a child's development—his physical health, emotional health, and social adjustment, as well as his intellectual growth. All of these factors must be considered together in providing the child excellent and coordinated care and guidance. Neglect of any one of these critical aspects of a child's development may cause life-long problems. If the youngster has a sound foundation to his life, he has a far better chance for healthy functioning in the future as he grows from childhood to adolescence to youth and to maturity. Attention to these various aspects of the young child's life implies that he should have: continuing, high-quality medical and dental care, good nutrition, competent parenting, a wealth of intellectually enriching experiences, diversified opportunities for active and quiet play, a time of rest and privacy, a safe and healthy physical environment, and specialized professional attention to serious physical or emotional problems if they should appear. He also needs to be understood and treated as a unique individual with his own particular style of growing, learning, and behaving.

Consideration must also be given to the fact that boys and girls, on the average, tend to be quite different in their patterns of growth and development. On the average, boys are more vulnerable to physical and emotional stress than are girls. They tend also to be slower in their development of fine physical coordination, as in learning to talk and dress themselves, handling small objects with skill, and the like. Conversely, most boys are superior in the development of large muscles and usually have a greater need for vigorous play that requires the use of these muscles. In planning programs for young children and in seeking to understand and guide them, we need to pay far more attention to these sex differences.

Possible Symptoms of Mental Health Problems

Some young children may have special problems in growth and development. There may be signs that specialized physical and/or mental health services are needed, at least for careful diagnosis. Such children may exhibit one or more of such symptoms as extreme shyness; appearance of being listless or tired much of the time; lack of interest in the environment; frequent whining and/or crying; being easily upset and frightened despite reassurances; poor appetite and/or feeding difficulties; inability to speak distinctly or understand spoken words, with few or no signs of improvement by age three or older; frequent falling and lack of physical dexterity; general and continuing irritability; inability to play with other children without frequent and extensive quarreling, by age three or so; frequent and severe temper tantrums; insistence on a set routine for many aspects of life; nightmares; sleepwalking; marked fears and phobias; extreme risk-taking behavior; excessive thumb-sucking or masturbation; lack of sex curiosity; markedly slow learning of simple skills; lack of interest in learning; strong dependency on parents with few or no signs of increasing independence; head-banging; serious sleep disturbances; strong and determined resistance to reasonable controls; running away, by age three or more; cruelty to animals and people; extreme destructiveness; frequent diarrhea or vomiting that has no apparent physical cause; poor weight gain or growth; and "failure to thrive" (adapted from Prugh, 1968).

Many, if not all, children show a number of these behavior symptoms to a moderate degree, or briefly, at different stages in their growth. The question of whether any behavior signifies a serious problem generally revolves around the continuity and severity of the symptoms. Their seriousness and meaning can be determined only by medical and psychological experts in the professions concerned with early childhood. Since the symptoms described above, as well as other less common ones, may indicate serious but correctable (or reducible) difficulties that can have long-term consequences if they are not identified and treated, it is exceedingly important that diagnostic and remedial services be available to children when these problems first appear (see Chapter I, Section II).

Importance of the Middle Years

The midstage of childhood is that period which reaches from age six to preadolescence. It usually ends at about age ten for girls and age twelve for boys. It is frequently referred to as the golden age of childhood because during this period most children have attained a considerable amount of independence and physical and psychological stability. This is generally a relatively harmonious time of slow, steady growth and development in which the child has an opportunity to build up and further establish physical and emotional resources which he will need later, especially during the preadolescent and adolescent growth spurt which is made even more difficult by the many stresses of our society.

Although the first five years of life are generally considered to be the most important to the child's total development, the midstage of a child's growth is also crucial from many points of view. The child of this age is still in a relatively early period of development and is still highly impressionable. Services designed to correct physical, emotional, social, and intellectual difficulties are likely to be more successful at this time than if they are provided later. Schooling, of course, is particularly important during this age period, and learning problems should be treated as soon as they appear. These problems, if not diagnosed and treated, may be cumulative and progressively more handicapping. This same basic principle applies to other aspects of the child's well-being: his physical and mental health and his social adjustment. Failure to help him, as he needs it, in these critical areas may well lead to a compounding of problems which mount in their severity and adverse effects. Moreover, earlier efforts to ensure maximum physical and mental health are likely to have little long-range pay-off unless they are continued in a way adapted to the needs of his developmental stage.

The midstage of childhood is frequently overlooked by researchers and specialists in child development, partly because serious difficulties are usually not as obvious as in infancy, early childhood, and adolescence. However, during this period the child is building on the foundation which he acquired earlier. He needs to accomplish a number of "developmental tasks" if he is to be effectively prepared for both his adolescence and later life. As time goes on, he will probably become more and more his unique individual self, not only because increasing differentiation is a basic aspect of human development but because our society, at least in part, cherishes individuality. We, however, as parents, teachers, recreational leaders, and the like, often do not actually want to pay the price of developing the child's real individuality. Highly individual children raise awkward questions, defy social conventions, and are often noisy and disruptive. Therefore, individualism is often simultaneously encouraged and discouraged. Too often, there is a great deal of pressure on the child to conform merely for the sake of peace and appearance. This may rob him of such qualities as creativity, a zest for living, an openness to new ideas and experiences, and a sense of his own integrity as a person.

Increasing Contact with the Community

The majority of youngsters are affected most deeply by their experiences in their own families. As they reach the age of five or six, however, they are influenced more and more by the society around them. Children at the midstage of development are somewhat like small commuters who travel back and forth between their own families and the way stations of neighborhood, school, church or temple, and the various child-serving organizations and facilities. The older a child grows, the more wide-ranging are his commuter activities and the less frequently does he return to the home station of the family. Many other people assume significance as models of what it is like to be a human being. He is affected by his friends, the older children and adults in his neighborhood, his schoolmates and his teachers, his religious leaders, club directors, doctors, and other significant people. His attitudes about himself and the world around him are shaped by these people and experiences. Quite naturally, the quality of these experiences and the nature of other people make an enormous difference in his attitudes, as do the experiences of members of his family and the attitudes which they have toward themselves and which other people have toward them.

One vital aspect of a child's growth at midstage is the development of his sense of being a part of his community. He needs to feel an identification with this community, and he needs to acquire large amounts of knowledge and large numbers of skills so that he can become an effective member of it. In earlier chapters we pointed out that there is a crisis in community life in many parts of the United States. Groups and individuals are pitted against one another. Many people are questioning the values and goals of our society, and some are in active rebellion against these values and goals. Individuals and families are often isolated from each other. The distrust and isolation among the various social classes and ethnic groups is reaching acute proportions. It is questionable whether communities can survive if their members do not have a deep sense of belonging to them and if their members do not become involved in determining and supporting the community's values. Communities are built upon common consent, communication, and common knowledge of their members. Just as communities need people for survival, so do people need communities (Inkeles, 1968).

Thus, it is in the interest of our society to cherish and foster the loyalty and competence of its members, including its children and youth. On the other side of the coin, it is in the interest of individuals to develop a sense of belongingness and a capacity for effectiveness in their communities.

Some experts in the field of human behavior have seen society as being, more or less, an enemy of individual fulfillment. Such experts generally attempt to help individuals find ways to develop their own capacities and satisfactions more or less in spite of the requirements and limitations imposed by society. Such a strategy may have been and may be necessary under an autocratic form of government. It should not be necessary or desirable in a democracy. These comments may seem rather far afield, but they have deep and serious meaning for children growing up in our society. Children cannot identify with our society or believe in it unless they have positive experiences in their day-to-day living. They cannot believe in, or commit themselves to, a society which proclaims such ideals as "liberty and justice for all" if they find that they and their families experience mostly restriction and injustices. If our society permits children to go hungry and their parents to go unemployed, ignores treating their sicknesses or handicaps, rejects them, allows them to live in crowded and unsanitary housing in disorganized neighborhoods, gives them no help when they are failing in school or forces them to attend segregated schools, and arrests them for behavior which is rooted in emotional or social problems, can they be expected to react other than with alienation and cynicism on hearing such pronouncements as "our nation stands for the right of each individual to life, liberty, and the pursuit of happiness"? Children can develop a deep and real sense of community commitment only if they and their parents find that the community has real commitments to them as individuals, and that their needs and actions can influence the community.

The Drive for Mastery and Independence

Children in this middle age of development have other and more specific needs. Erikson (1959) has referred to this period of child development as "the age of mastery." Most children during this stage have a great drive to learn and perfect many different kinds of skills—physical, social, and intellectual (Biber, 1968). Their world is constantly expanding, and if the child is in good physical and emotional health, he tends to be eager to participate actively in his environment. He often flits rapidly from one interest to another. He practices new skills with great avidity. If all is going well, he will grow steadily in his capacity to perform increasingly complex tasks. As he reaches the age of nine or so, social groups will probably become more and more important to him. Membership in "secret clubs," demands for independence and privacy, and participation in adventurous group exploits are commonplace. However, growth does not go forward in a straight line. The young commuter is likely to waver back and forth between dependence and independence, between mastery and failure, between the courage to adventure and the fear that he can't measure up to the expectations of the outer world. This is a time in which he needs help with his drive for mastery, comfort for his fears and failures, and encouragement and guidance to try again. He needs the experience of doing things on his own. However, he also needs to be protected from the many dangers of our complicated world. This is a time in which accidents are likely to be the highest cause of injury or death.

The problem of giving the growing child enough, but not too much, protection is particularly difficult when the physical environment does not provide safeguards such as protected recreation areas, traffic control, law enforcement, neighborhood zoning and services, and the availability of concerned adults who can appropriately guide the child. Special difficulties are likely to arise for those children who live in disorganized neighborhoods, and for those whose mothers are employed outside the home in after-school hours.

Special consideration must also be given to the child's ability to get along with other people as well as his competence in handling his own drives and feelings. Overly rigid adult controls are likely to lead either to open rebellion or to unhappy withdrawal into the self. Few or no controls may well lead to extremes of selfish, impulsive, and antisocial behavior. Reasonable controls, which are discussed with the child and which are set with kindness and consistency, allow him a chance for needed free expression within definite limits. If the child is not able to act in consideration of others, as well as himself, he is likely to be treated with rejection or exclusion as he encounters the larger social world. Part of the growing child's task is to learn how to be a member of social groups without surrendering to the group his own identity, interests, and beliefs. This, of course, is a life-long task. The growing child is merely exploring various ways to deal with such complex problems. Pressures for him to "adjust and belong" may short-circuit this search for both belonging to society and maintaining his own integrity as a person (*Report of Task Force II*, 1969).

Each child approaches these various tasks of mastery in his own individual way and will achieve mastery in different areas with different degrees of success, partly because of the treatment he receives at home and in the larger society. It is extremely important that the child have experiences which will enhance his self-confidence, self-image, and overall mental health so that he can attain the needed sense of mastery and independence.

Intellectual Development

If the child is developing as he should, his intellectual ability will be expanding rapidly. As he reaches the age of ten or eleven, he should show an increasing ability to handle basic ideas and principles, rather than simple arrays of facts (Biber, 1968). He should be able to see cause-and-effect relationships more and more and have an increasing sense of time and place and his relationship to it. His vocabulary should be growing at a rapid rate, and his knowledge of words should become increasingly complex and related to basic concepts.

The child's school experience plays an important role in all aspects of his intellectual growth. However, the family also plays a critical role. The child's intellectual development is highly dependent on the support parents give to the school and to the child as a student, and also upon the kinds of stimulation and understanding provided in the home. Parental attitudes toward learning, the kinds of vocabulary used in the home, the intellectual interests of the parents, and the breadth of enriching life experience available to the family all play an important part in developing the child's intellect. As noted in Chapter IV, long-term poverty and/or discrimination tends to produce family life styles that are not strongly supportive of educational achievement. Moreover, the school system tends to provide an inferior brand of education to these children who need special help with their learning.

The Development of Competence

Another way of looking at the child's drive for mastery is to consider it as being related to his need for the development of competence. Competence might be defined as the capacity to effectively perform one's role* for the enhancement of the self and for the well-being of the self and society. Smith (1968), following White (1959), proposes that competence is essentially based on self-esteem and self-respect. These feelings lead to attitudes of hope which enable one to take initiative in actively coping with the environment in an independent fashion. This formulation is somewhat like that of Erikson (1959), who theorizes that trust, confidence, initiative, industry, autonomy, and hope are basic to sound human functioning and are the positive side of such negative attitudes as those of self-doubt, passivity, dependence, fatalism, and despair. It can be seen that children at midstage, if they are developing in the desired directions, are building on experiences largely acquired in their own families and on an earlier sense of trust and confidence which is so crucial to self-esteem and self-respect. As they move out into society, they need further adult support so that they can continue to develop their competence to cope with the larger world. If they come from disorganized, unhappy, or neglectful

---

* Role is a somewhat complex concept. It might be defined simply by saying that it is the part one plays in one's various functions in life as, for instance, a family member, an employee, a student, etc. Each role has its values and expected behaviors which have been developed, over time, out of the needs and functions of society.

homes in which their self-esteem and self-respect are not adequately promoted, they will need a great deal of extra help and understanding from adults at school and elsewhere in the community.

It is held by some that competence is synonymous with positive mental health. While it would seem to be an extremely important quality and closely related to the well-being of the individual and the society in which he lives, it would appear that, in actuality, life would be quite barren if competence were the chief goal. One might say that this is an instrumental concept which relates to coping with external reality and to achieving well in such endeavors as work and community participation. An expressive side to the personality is also necessary, since it is closely associated with warm, enduring person-to-person relationships and with a sense of individual identity (*Report of Task Force II*, 1969).

The Capacity to Give and Receive Love

The expressive function might be more simply and appropriately defined as the capacity to give and receive love. Large bodies of research attest to the tremendous importance of warm, supporting parental love to the sound development of children. Love might be equated with the life force and generous, positive feelings and behaviors in relation to other people. These qualities are greatly needed in all parts of society, not just in the home. However much a truism, this has been seriously overlooked, especially in recent years, with the concurrent emphases on productivity, achievement, and vocational success. Warm, positive, loving attitudes are desperately needed to offset the forces of hostility, separatism, and violence which beset our society. The capacity to give and receive love is essential in all the human service fields. It also has an important place in the community and all employment settings. Current widespread attitudes of alienation and despair may well be related to our present overemphasis on achievement and deemphasis on positive, close human relationships. If children are to develop into healthy, happy human beings who have a commitment to society as well as to themselves, it would seem essential for them to have many fulfilling and strengthening human relationships which are inspired by affection as well as by respect and training for competent self-mastery. Such relationships need to be provided within all the social institutions which deal with children and youth. They should not be limited to the family alone.

Individual and Sex Identity

Youngsters at midstage may seem to have relatively few sex interests. According to some theories of human behavior, they are in the so-called latency period, when other interests, such as those we have described, override sexual concerns. However, it seems likely that children of this age have acquired greater sophistication in dealing with adults than they had when they were younger, and that they have learned to mask many of their interests. Although their sex interests and drives will become stronger and more obvious as they reach adolescence, these drives are by no means forgotten during the middle years. This is especially true as youngsters move toward preadolescence. It becomes increasingly important to them to firmly establish their identity as being either boys or girls and to have this identity accepted by their associates. This desire to confirm one's masculinity or femininity generally leads to confining much of one's social life to the same-sex group. In effect, boys learn how to be boys and girls to be girls from absorbing information, skills, and acceptance from members of their own sex.

In our society there seems to be more demand on boys to prove their sexual identity than on girls. Toughness, courage, strength, and athletic prowess become a must for boys. These pressures for proving one's masculinity account, in part, for the studied disdain and separateness which boys of this age usually show toward girls. Beneath the masculine swagger and careful disinterest often lie quite opposite feelings. These feelings are frequently expressed in such commonly observed activities as teasing and chasing girls, taunting them for their feminine weaknesses, showing off masculine prowess, and so forth.

Girls, although keenly aware of boys, hide their feelings of uncertainty about their own feminine charms by overt rejection of the male sex. Society generally pushes them in the direction of receptivity rather than open aggression. Their giggling responses to the boys and their complaints of being pursued are part of their growing interest in the fascinating "battle between the sexes." In fact, some recent studies have shown that both boys and girls of this age group generally have a keen interest in the opposite sex and entertain "secret crushes" for a special "other" (Broderick, 1969).

During this time, most children are gathering considerable amounts of information about sex. They frequently gain this knowledge from one another, and, unfortunately, it is often based on confused and faulty information. Some experts say that, ideally, children should be able to receive sound sex education from their parents and that they should feel free to discuss sex-related matters openly with their parents as a natural part of everyday life. Such easy interchange usually does not occur, partly because parents lack the needed information and, more importantly, because of their own confused and guilty feelings on the subjects. Other experts point out that parents may not be ideal as *the* agents for sex education during middle childhood and adolescence, partly for the reasons given above and partly because of the close emotional ties between parent and child. To a considerable extent, a child's developing sexuality is associated with his developing emancipation from his family. If he is to grow into an emotionally and sexually mature adult, able to fuse sexual and psychological love in a man-woman relationship, he needs to separate both his sexual self and his psychological self from his parents. Thus, it appears that schools, religious organizations, and other child-serving agencies should share, with parents, the education of youngsters in matters related to sex as well as other aspects of the child's developing self.

Some fathers and mothers seem to push their children into sexual precocity for which they are not yet ready. The parents may do this somewhat unknowingly in response to the surrounding culture—particularly in some middle-class and upper-class neighborhoods. Thus, dances and other such social activities may be staged for youngsters who are only ten or eleven years old, complete with all the trappings of "sub-deb" clothes, corsages, and the like. This premature pushing of social functions goes way beyond the level of most boy-girl interests at this age. When youngsters are prodded into behaviors for which they are not yet developmentally ready, they may react with feelings of embarrassed inferiority, resentment, and confusion about their social and personal competence. Some of the current enthusiasm of youth for highly informal manners, clothes, and hair styles may be related to early resentments at being pushed into overly elaborate social situations.

Some Differences Between Boys and Girls

Differences in the ways that boys and girls develop generally become more marked as children get older. Some of these developmental and behavior differences seem to be inborn; however, others apparently are a product of our cultural expectations regarding masculinity and femininity. On the average, girls develop more rapidly than boys in verbal skills. These superior skills are a great asset to girls in their educational achievement. Girls tend to do better in elementary school and in high school than boys. They generally receive better grades, fewer of them fail, and fewer of them drop out of high school before graduation. Even in the lower grades, boys tend to do better than girls in mathematics and science, but, on the average, this superiority is not enough of an asset to bring about equal educational achievements.

The tendency for boys to experience greater difficulties in school is probably related to the fact that the majority of teachers are women, especially in the elementary school. This makes it difficult for boys to see school as being an appropriate masculine activity. Moreover, most women teachers find the active aggressive behavior of boys more difficult to accept than that of girls. Generally speaking, boys tend to be more aggressive and physically active than girls. These tendencies seem to be partly innate and partly a result of family life experiences and cultural pressures (Kagan and Moss, 1962). The greater tendency of girls to be more passive and dependent than boys is also related to inborn tendencies, family experiences, and cultural expectations.

More boys than girls of elementary school age are brought to mental health clinics because of emotional problems. Boys, on the average, also show a greater need for remedial reading; higher delinquency rates; and a higher vulnerability to physical disease and psychological stress.

A greater understanding of the social and psychological differences between the sexes on the part of parents, teachers, and other people who work with children might well reduce the higher tendency of boys to have learning and behavioral difficulties.

Better Programs Needed for Boys: School and Recreation

In addition to understanding on the part of adults, there is a need for changes in school and other community programs. Experimental approaches are called for which include not only the addition of more men to the faculties of elementary schools but, also, changes in the school curriculum, teaching methods, and regulations which often put a premium on passive obedience in grading systems. Most of our elementary schools tend to be more feminine than masculine in nature. Emphasis is frequently placed on such qualities as neatness, orderliness, conformity, being quiet, and the like. Such requirements are generally easier for girls to follow.

Boys are likely to experience considerable rejection and lack of understanding, not only at school but in the home, where feminine values espoused by mothers tend to be dominant, especially as cities prevent the active work and exploration which exist in the expanding frontiers or rural areas. Thus boys, harried by their inner drives for activity and aggression, pressured by the larger culture of the masculine world to prove their maleness, are thwarted in many settings by the feminine barriers that block their entrance to the male society. In addition, their self-esteem is undermined by conflicting and impossible demands that they act manly but live by feminine standards.

Recreational and youth-serving organizations also need to plan their programs more appropriately for boys. These agencies often overlook the needs of young boys or provide female leaders for their programs. Many more well-qualified men and older boys are needed to provide leadership and recreational opportunities in all of our neighborhoods. The need is particularly acute in disadvantaged communities, where the hazards are exceptionally high for male children who lack safe and rewarding opportunities for self-expression and growth through healthy play.

Some Rewards of Camping

Camping experiences are highly desirable for both boys and girls, but perhaps more so for boys. A well-run camp, staffed by leaders who have a deep liking and understanding of children, can yield exceptionally high dividends in both physical and mental health. Camping can provide a number of rewarding opportunities. It gives the child a chance to live away from home with his peers and to relate to leaders who are different from, and perhaps more youth-oriented than, his parents. It allows him to experience the freedom and challenge of the out-of-doors. It provides a setting in which the child can learn new skills for coping with a more natural environment and develop a greater understanding of, and appreciation for, the natural world. All of these can be important gains for children, especially for impoverished youngsters. While we cannot discuss the complex subject of camping, it should be emphasized that camping, per se, does not necessarily provide a good experience. Like other programs, its promise lies chiefly in the quality and training of the individuals who serve on the staff (see Chapter I, pp. 88–90).

Growth Through Play

Play is an essential part of childhood and the basic learning modality of the preschool child, an activity in which children may learn many things which may be as important as those they learn in school. Through play a child may learn a host of physical, social, and intellectual skills. Play provides opportunities for the child to acquire moral principles related to such values as justice, honesty, and sharing. Play also allows the child to develop his capacities for planning and organization and to express his great need for creativity and imagination. The child develops, in large part, through play —from infancy on. The opportunities which our society provides children for healthy recreation experiences is of vast importance in promoting their total development. Presently, these opportunities are particularly needed for children in poverty or near-poverty neighborhoods.

Development of Moral Character

The study of the development of moral character has been largely neglected by behavioral scientists for almost forty years. It has recently received renewed research attention. There is also an obvious and prevalent public concern about the so-called breakdown in values among many people in our society.

Moral behavior might be defined as behavior which conforms to those standards which a society establishes as being good or right and for which the group administers disapproval or punishment if transgressions occur (Maccoby, 1968). The definition of moral behavior and enforcement of it provides a structure which allows a society to function. Ideally, moral behavior controls the individual's desires for self-centered satisfaction of his own pleasures and needs, which can be followed only at the expense of the needs of others. Every society has to have moral codes if it is to endure, although these vary from society to society. Some rules, however, are common to most societies, such as those of honesty, respect for the property of others, responsibility to others, and control over hostility, aggression, and the sex drive.

Moral principles are also somewhat similar, in definition, to the conscience. The foundations of conscience are laid early in life, mostly within the family, and are built upon as the child and young person grows. A number of factors are closely associated with the development of moral strength, particularly those related to the child's gradual development toward control of sex and aggression.

Moral development takes place slowly. As the child grows, he should show increasing capacity for moral judgment, He should be able to move from a simple recital of rules to a gradual, but increasing, understanding of such abstract moral principles as honesty and justice. Most young children tend to be very rigid and specific about rules, such as those involved in playing games or proper school behavior. Over time, they usually gain a broadened understanding of moral principles. They should move beyond obeying rules simply to avoid trouble or to win approval from others to incorporating moral principles which they can and do act on because they understand and believe in them. This process of moral development appears to be partly a process of normal growth and development; however, it is also importantly associated with the child's experiences. Quite clearly, a number of adults have not had the experiences which would enable them to move beyond the early stage of moral growth. Consequently, they tend to act opportunistically and are not motivated by basic moral principles which they have absorbed and made their own.

Moral character does not seem to be developed through the didactic teaching of moral principles. It is more closely associated with the following: democratic, affectionate child-rearing methods; mild, reasonable, consistent discipline; the developing capacity of the child to grasp concepts and principles; models set by parents and adults in their own behavior; and the discussion and clarification of moral values with the child along with explanations of the serious consequences that are likely to occur as a result of "immoral" behavior (Kohlberg, 1964; Hoffman, 1963; Maccoby, 1968). There are also indications that the development of moral strength is associated with healthy ego development, a strong sense of self-respect, good intellectual capacity, and life situations which are conducive to "moral behavior." Moral behavior is a reciprocal learning in which the child reflects the moral behavior of society's agencies and its mediators toward him.

Learning Opportunities Essential

It should be clear that the qualities we described above—growing independence, mastery, social adaptation, community commitment, competence, capacity to give and receive love, and moral development—are intimately related to the child's experiences in the home, school, and community, and that they are also dependent upon and intertwined with all aspects of his physical, emotional, and intellectual health. If children at midstage are to grow and develop in these desired directions, they must acquire related basic attitudes and skills. In order to acquire these skills and attitudes, the right learning conditions must be made available to them.

For example, in order for a child to learn effectively he, as an individual, must *want* to learn. He must believe he is able to learn. He must find that learning is rewarding, and he must have access to the opportunity to learn. Since children are still deeply rooted in their families during their elementary school years, it is important for the school and other institutions to involve parents in this learning process of their sons and daughters. In order to stimulate a person's desire to learn, the person has to feel involved as an individual. This is true for both the child and his parents. Each must feel that learning is relevant to improving life for the child. It is important, for instance, that children and parents feel that school is related to their family life and the life of their neighborhood. Yet, particularly for disadvantaged people, school may seem like a quite separate world, one which excludes parents and has no relationship to the day-by-day realities or future expectations of the impoverished child. Current trends such as decentralization of urban schools and involvement of parents as school employees and school advisers are based on a recognition that school programs need to be much more closely related to the lives of children and parents if effective learning is to take place.

It is not only important that a child wish to learn, but he must also *believe that he is able to learn.* He needs to feel competence as a person and learner. His sense of competence, as noted, is closely related to his sense of self-esteem, and his belief in himself is closely associated to his parents' belief in him and in themselves. A sense of power to control one's own life and to cope with the environment is fundamental to a sense of self-esteem. This seems especially true for males, from whom the culture requires such traits as independence, achievement, and self-direction. If parents and children feel powerless vis-à-vis the school and other systems of society, their self-esteem will be seriously threatened and they may lose faith in their ability to become an effective part of the larger society.

Lack of self-esteem and a disbelief in oneself as a learner and doer are likely to bring about feelings of anxiety, attitudes of fatalism, alienation from society, and the setting of low or unrealistically high aspirations for oneself. Thus, if children are to acquire the knowledge and skills that are imperative for their own and society's functioning, they must have a sense of power and participation in the various parts of society, including its educational system. As already mentioned, children at midstage have a great drive for mastery, self-direction, and acquisition of many skills. They need support for these drives from their parents and from such social institutions as health, welfare, education, and recreation agencies. The child and his parents must have a sense of real participation in these agencies rather than seeing themselves as being helpless and passive recipients of programs imposed by other aloof and powerful persons.

If a child is to learn these lessons which are so necessary to society, he must be able to see and experience that *learning has a pay-off for him*. He must experience more success than failure in this learning and find that it is related to coping more successfully with his environment. Children have a natural urge to explore, to adventure, and to be actively involved with the people and things around them. If these drives cannot be expressed through rewarding and related experiences available to the child through organized society, he will turn to the pleasures, excitements, and rewards of a disorganized society. This often happens to the child of the urban slum, who finds that his disorganized neighborhood offers far more pleasure, excitement, and rewards for learning than does organized society with its frequently rejecting, unrelated, and incomprehensible approaches and programs. The disadvantaged child all too often finds more advantages in acquiring commitments and skills related to the deviant life of the disorganized community than in attempting to compete in the life of organized society which offers so few rewards and opportunities for him and for those around him.

In summary, if all our young citizens are to be "socialized" to effectively adapt to goals and needs of organized society, we must find ways to enhance their desire to learn social goals and skills, their belief in their ability to learn, and their recognition and experience that learning does have a pay-off. This implies that all the social systems which reach children and their families—such as the school, church or temple, and health, recreation, and welfare organizations—need to provide ways for all individuals to participate with greater equality. It also implies that these systems must be organized to recognize the integrity and potentiality of all individuals—children and parents—and to ensure that they obtain both immediate and future economic, political, and social rewards for acquired learning and skills.

It is for such reasons as these that the Commission emphasizes the participation of children, youth, and parents in the planning and direction of neighborhood Child Development Councils and local Child Development Authorities.

Some Symptoms of Emotional Problems

The behavior characteristics of children at the midstage of development are sometimes indicative of later adult difficulties. This is particularly true of aggressive and antisocial behavior. Although behavior problems of this kind may be predictive of later maladjustment, the exact nature of the behavior may not be the same when the child becomes an adult (*Report of Task Force II,* 1969). The more frequent and more severe these symptoms are in childhood, the more predictive they are of future difficulties.

On the other hand, children who show shy, withdrawn behavior do not necessarily have emotional problems in their later years; however, poor social relationships with other children do tend to be predictive of some later forms of emotional and mental health problems.

Contrary to general opinion, difficulties in academic achievement, by themselves, may not be directly related to poor mental health or poor emotional adjustment in adult life.

Whether or not certain kinds of behavior are symptoms of emotional maladjustment is a complex matter. Different behaviors have different kinds of meaning, depending on the sex of the child and the social class to which he belongs. For example, aggressive, defiant behavior on the part of lower-class boys is more likely to be related to life styles of poverty neighborhoods than to emotional problems within the child (*Report of Task Force II,* 1969).

Other behaviors which may be indicative of problems in emotional adjustment at this age include: sleepwalking, extreme dislike and fear of school, nervous mannerisms, poor control over toilet functions, nail-biting, learning difficulties in school, inability to form relationships with people, lack of clarity as to what is real and what is imaginary, excessive masturbation, persistent thumb-sucking, extreme fearfulness and dependency, temper tantrums, defiant and persistent refusal to accept discipline, cruelty to animals and/or other children, marked overactivity, frequent stealing, destructiveness, recurrent diarrhea, vomiting or headaches, persistent feelings of fatigue, markedly effeminate behavior in boys, and masculine behavior in girls (adapted from Prugh, 1968).

Many of these behavior symptoms commonly occur from time to time among normal children. The chief question is how frequently they occur and how severe they are. It is important that children who display such symptoms over a period of time be referred, with their families, to mental health personnel for careful evaluation and diagnosis and that treatment be provided if the need is indicated. Since most children of this age are in school, teachers and other school personnel can play a critical role in identification, referral, and cooperation in treatment plans for such youngsters.

SOME SPECIAL SUBGROUPS OF CHILDREN IN TROUBLE

The Abused Child

A number of children show the symptoms of having been cruelly mistreated and abused. Nationwide child abuse cases total 2,000 to 3,000 children injured each month and one or two killed each day, according to the estimates of two associates with the University of Colorado School of Medicine.

Dr. C. Henry Kemp and Dr. Ray E. Helfer say the number of children under five years of age killed by parents each year is higher than the number of those who die from disease. Although statistics make it appear that the cases of child abuse are increasing, the figures are actually more reflective of state laws enacted in the early 1960's requiring reports of child abuse (New York Times, October 10, 1968).

Parents who abuse their children are found to come from a wide variety of educational, socioeconomic, racial, and ethnic backgrounds. Ninety percent of these families have serious social problems, unhappy marriages, and financial difficulties. Many appear to be in a state of continual anger. The only stimulation needed for the direct and violent expression of this state is some normal difficulty in bringing up children. Other abusing parents clearly reject a certain child and feel that he is a real and constant threat to them. Many of these parents have a long history of emotional instability. Their childhood was often marked by deprivation of nurturance, parental concern, and emotional warmth.

Serious child abuse is not one act, or even many, but rather a basic condition about which the involved parents rarely seek help. Such parents typically withhold information about themselves and their families, and seem not to be concerned or guilty about the child's poor condition.

Attempts to help these parents have proven to be extremely difficult. It seems unlikely without the major effort of social agencies that their behavior can be significantly improved.

Children who are cruelly mistreated by their parents are likely to develop a great deal of hostility toward the world in general and may become violent and deeply disturbed adults. It may be necessary to remove children from such homes permanently, although early diagnosis and early psychiatric and casework treatment may be helpful in some of these families. Such services are extremely inadequate in most parts of the country (*Report of Task Force I,* 1968).

Childhood Neglect

Childhood neglect may occur in minor degrees in many families. Severe childhood neglect includes gross parental inattention to the needs of their children, abandonment, starvation, and/or unusual isolation of the child from the family and the community. Studies of neglectful parents and neglected children are practically nonexistent; however, social workers, physicians, and others concerned with child welfare report that this is a problem of widespread and national importance.

Parents who neglect their children come from many walks of life. Middle-class parents may find ways of hiding rather subtle neglect of their children, but the results of such neglect may show up in the poor development of the child. Parents who severely neglect their youngsters have been found to have a variety of personality problems—psychosis, high impulsivity, and so on. In some ways, many of them resemble abusive parents, except that usually they do not show such aggressive and cruel behavior. A large percentage of neglecting mothers show behavior patterns that indicate a sense of discouragement, depression, frustration, and surrender to unsatisfying life circumstances. These attitudes may stem from very poor social and financial conditions, chronic physical health problems, or personality difficulties. Many of these mothers seem to feel that "nothing is worth doing" and that they are completely inadequate to cope with their situation or problem. They may be suffering from heavy burdens of child care and isolation from any form of help. If supporting services are given, such as counseling, day-care services, or homemaker aid, these mothers may be able to learn to take care of their children fairly well. Without help they tend to become depressed, disorganized, and inadequate.

Children suffering from the most severe forms of neglect show a failure to thrive as described earlier in this chapter. Usually with warm attention and good child care they show marked improvement. Clearly failure to thrive is a condition which calls for continuing medical supervision and treatment and supportive services (*Report of Task Force I,* 1968).

Children in Foster Care

More than 200,000 children in this country are in foster care. The effectiveness of such care is questionable. A number of recent studies show that about half of the children in foster homes do not grow up satisfactorily (Murphy, 1964; Gil, 1964; De Fries *et al.,* 1965). Moreover, child welfare services are often not available at the time children and families need them. A number of children have been placed in foster homes at least several years after it first became known that the situation in the child's own home was obviously very bad. Most child welfare agencies do not have, or do not use, such preventive services as homemaker and day-care facilities. There is also evidence that a large proportion of abused children belong to families who were known to social agencies for a considerable period of time before their children were removed from the home. It has been found that no action is taken in most cases until the situation is extremely severe (Jenkins and Sauber, 1966).

Social agencies have failed to develop clear guidelines as to when children should be separated from their families. This decision is often more dependent on the availability of foster homes than on the needs of the child and the family situation. Although foster home placement is generally regarded as a temporary measure, this is often not the actual case. For two-thirds to three-fourths of the children in foster care, there is no specific plan as to whether and under what circumstances they can return home (Maas and Engler, 1959; Jeter, 1963). Many children never return home but are placed from foster home to foster home. The major reasons for this situation are the severe shortage of foster homes and the fact that foster parents often find that they do not receive needed help to work with the children and therefore cannot continue to keep the children they have accepted. Children in foster homes have great difficulty in establishing their sense of identity and in forming relationships with their various foster parents. It is assumed that the social worker will be a stable adult in their lives, but the inadequate staffing, poor training of workers in helping foster families, and large turnover in social work staff makes this most unlikely.

Although foster home care is regarded as temporary until the child's own family can improve, child welfare agencies typically provide almost no service to the child's family.

Foster care is expensive. It is estimated that it costs about $8,000 a year per child. For this same amount, many other kinds of services could be provided which might keep the child with his own family, such as day care and other supportive services. It is important that child welfare agencies have a broader range of available supporting services and that they plan for children in partnership with the children's families. Parents should not be forced to keep a child when this is beyond their capabilities. Conversely, a child should not be removed from his own home as a punitive measure or a judgment that the family is nonconformist. The most important decisions should revolve around the questions of whether the child's needs are being met and what kinds of services might be planned with the family to improve the situation when difficulties occur.

A number of improvements are needed in children's welfare services.

For example, better methods are needed to diagnose the causes of children's problems. Services such as homemakers, day care, and overnight care also should be available. Moreover, payments for the care of children should be made to relatives who may have much to offer the child but cannot afford to take him without payment. These payments would reverse the present trend of thought, that is, that relatives should not receive payments from social agencies for child care.

In addition, group-care programs in small group settings are needed, especially for preadolescents and adolescents. These programs should be flexible and combine work and recreation experiences, as well as further opportunities for the young person's education.

Housing projects could accommodate day-care centers within them which offer flexible programs for part-time and full-time care. Insofar as possible, children should be kept in the mainstream of their own society, rather than being shunted off to separate institutions. Where it is certain that a child cannot ever return to his own home because of the severe problems of his parents, planning should be made for his permanent care, including the possibility of legal adoption (*Report of Task Force II,* 1969).

PROGRAMS AND SERVICES FOR THE PARENTS

The Complex Job of Parenthood

We have discussed some of the severe problems faced by children when their parents are unable to meet even their most basic and elementary needs. These parents, although not large in number, are particularly handicapped by a variety of conditions that are usually related to deficiencies from their own childhood experiences as reflected in their own personality or life situation. For some of these parents the major source of difficulty may lie in the characteristics of a particular child rather than primarily in themselves. Whatever the difficulty, the simple fact is that this group of parents cannot provide adequate care for all or some of their children. It is important that their inability and the needs of their children be understood and accepted. There must be greater public investment in alternative care arrangements for youngsters who need to be cared for away from their own homes.

The great majority of parents can provide positive growth and developmental experiences for their children if the community shares this opportunity and responsibility with them by providing the wide variety of coordinating services which have been recommended in previous chapters.

In this chapter we have pointed out in greater detail how complex and demanding is the job of parenthood. It requires of the parent almost superhuman capacities to meet the many diverse needs of the child, from the moment of the child's conception onward. We have shown how parents need to be sensitive to the individual tendencies of each of their children;

how they are called upon to minister to the child's needs for first-rate physical care and protection; intellectual growth and development; understanding and guidance of his emotional drives; training in social skills; support of his activities in the neighborhood, school, and community; and adaptation to his differing developmental stages. As if all this were not enough, most parents have at least two or three children—all in different stages of growth and all different in their individual traits.

Obviously, the demands on parents are tremendous. Eager as nearly all parents are to do an excellent job of child-rearing, they cannot deny their own human needs—physical, psychological, and social. Nor can they put aside the totality of their own life experience that has made them what they are and molded their behavior as parents. Furthermore, fathers and mothers cannot cope single-handedly with the many handicaps that the social and economic systems may impose upon them and their children. If parents are to be effective in the tremendously important task of child-rearing, they need the supporting cooperation of other systems outside the home. Some of the programs and services which should be provided by these systems will be discussed here as they apply particularly to parents.

Can Parent Education Help?

Programs in parent education are being recommended increasingly throughout the country and have been strongly supported by many of the advisers to the Commission. There are a number of reasons for recommending such education, including the following:

1. There is increasing knowledge about children and factors associated with their healthy growth and development. This knowledge should benefit parents in the task of child-rearing.

2. The rapid changes in society to which the child is exposed in the larger community threaten to create a gap between parents and children. It is important to try to help parents keep abreast of such changes, particularly as they apply to changes in the schools and newer methods of education. A greater understanding of school programs is especially needed for those parents who have had little education themselves and for whom the gap between school and home is apt to be especially great.

3. Logically, it appears that there is much to recommend in parent education programs addressed to such areas as: consumer education, homemaking education, nutrition education, sex education, health education, and the like.

Despite the fact that there is much logic to the recommendation that education for parents be greatly expanded, other factors should be taken into consideration. For instance, a recent review (Chilman, 1969) of all parent education projects over the past twenty-five years or more, including currently ongoing ones, reveals that very few have been objectively evaluated. When such evaluation is applied, the findings almost universally indicate that parent education programs typically reach only about 5 percent of the parents to whom they are addressed. The attendance even of this small group is sporadic. There is scanty evidence to suggest that these parent education programs have any measurable impact on parental attitudes and behavior. Although it appears that these groups are attended more frequently and more enthusiastically if the programs include parent activities and free discussion rather than simply a lecture or a film, even the former type of program seems to meet with small measurable success. This is true even when transportation and child care are provided, neighborhood parents are involved in reaching out to other parents, refreshments are offered, and meetings are held in places familiar and acceptable to the parents. Although it is quite possible that parent education programs may have important, but hitherto unmeasured, positive effects on some parents, the evidence seems quite conclusive that parent education per se is not particularly useful as a major approach to reaching parents and improving their child-rearing behaviors.

Broader Forms of Parent Participation Indicated

The Commission believes that parent education would be most effective if it involved parents as participants, not only in the planning and carrying out of parent education but in other ways, such as through their employment in human service programs, through their involvement in action for social change around issues that seem important to them, and through their active involvement in the development and administration of such programs. It is probable that parents, even more than young people, need to feel that they have a significant voice in the affairs of their communities. Their adult status should place them in responsible, participating roles rather than in passive, dependent ones. It is time that professionals in the human services agencies adopted the basic principle of working in full partnership *with* parents rather than independently devising programs and services *for* parents and their children (U.S. Dept. of Health, Education, and Welfare, 1968).

Parent education programs probably would be even more effective if they were part of a whole range of services which the parents themselves see as being needed and helpful. These include health services, employment training and placement, economic assistance as needed, legal aid, homemaker services, aid with housing problems, and so forth. Basic to the successes of any program directed toward the child-rearing behavior of parents is the recognition that the survival needs of a family must be met before parents are free to consider the less immediate needs of their children and themselves. For example, one could hardly expect parents to be concerned about the child's intellectual development if the family does not have enough to eat and does not have a home in which to live.

A recent trend in helping very young disadvantaged children has been in the area of home tutoring. While the experimental projects vary somewhat, the basic idea is to reach infants and/or very young children in their own homes and provide intellectually and physically stimulating programs for them so as to enhance their "cognitive" development. In most instances, attempts are made to involve mothers in this process. Evidence indicates that attempts to so involve these parents are variously successful, depending on the life situation of the mothers and their own social and psychological characteristics. Such efforts would be far more successful if programs of this sort were combined with a wider range of services designed to meet the many needs of *all* family members.

Some studies show that the majority of parents are not interested in learning about child growth and development in general but are immediately concerned with the specific problems of their own children. They tend to view the physician as being the major source of help for both infants and preschool children, whereas the teacher is viewed in this role for older children. It is evident there is an important counseling role for teachers, doctors, and nurses. Since there is such a shortage in these professions, it is recommended that aides be trained to work with these professionals in the role of counseling with parents as well as in other capacities (see Chapter XII on mental health manpower). Parental counseling must be addressed to the particular needs that parents bring, but it is important that the total life situation, the family constellation, the cultural pattern, and the developmental stage of each individual parent be considered. Especially in the case of people who are poor or members of minority groups, the counselor must recognize that the parent is likely to bring with him attitudes of fear, anger, and distress engendered by a long history of past rejection and discrimination.

One function of the Local Neighborhood Councils recommended by the Commission would be the provision of at least emergency counseling and the development of counseling and other services for parents where such services do not exist.

It is quite evident that the majority of parents in this country have learned a great deal over the years through reading about child development and family relations, seeing films related to the topic, and other such materials. As remarked in Chapter III, most of these educational materials are addressed to middle-class parents. They are unrelated to the life situation, cultural pattern, and reading levels of less educated and less affluent fathers and mothers. It is recommended that pamphlets, posters, and films be developed in cooperation with low-income parents and that these be made widely available in neighborhood Child Development Councils and other appropriate places.

A number of experimental approaches are indicated, such as:

1. The provision of mental health consultant programs to schools which include mental health services to both parents and children. These should be aimed primarily at early prevention of behavior disorders. Mental health consultation should also be available to school personnel. This consultation might include the training of teachers for interviewing parents more effectively and making more visits to the families of children.

2. A family counseling service located in the school and linked to other community resources and pupil personnel services. This family counselor would have the responsibility of offering an interview to all parents of children in the school at least once a year in order to gain an understanding of parental goals and concerns and to offer further family services. Particular emphasis would be placed on reaching parents whose children are at the kindergarten and first-grade level. Family counselors might be specially selected people who do not have professional training but who are provided in-service supervision and training by teaching and mental health personnel.

3. Parent cooperatives of many sorts might be experimentally developed and financed, especially in low-income areas. This might include parent cooperatives to purchase their own health, legal, educational, or counseling services.

4. Improvement is called for in reference to delivery of services to rural areas. Mobile services, manned by a team in the fields of physical and mental health, represent one useful approach. Every effort should be made to coordinate the delivery of mobile service, to avoid duplication and fragmentation. Particularly in rural areas, it is recommended that service programs be coordinated, as relevant, with the activities of the Department of Agriculture in both the food programs and extension services.

5. Programs that serve parents as well as children should be set up very closely to or actually within public schools. Many school buildings are not used after school hours or during the summer. Additional use should be made of these facilities. Moreover, it would be desirable to form as close a link as possible between school and the family and to render services closely coordinated with the school to all family members. Such a procedure would help in creating positive attitudes on the part of parents toward the educational system and would strengthen the educational programs for many children whose learning problems are related to family difficulties. Such programs might well be coordinated by the Child Development Authorities and Councils.

There is no one service or service strategy that will meet the needs of all individuals and families. A wide range of services and methodologies is needed. Families have a wide diversity of problems and needs. They are ready, willing, and able to use different kinds of services. Their choice will depend, in part, on what they are like as individual human beings, their different cultural patterns, personality characteristics, levels of information, life experiences, and current situation. Individuals and families should have *freedom* to choose what seems to them to be most useful. Their choices should be based upon information about and participative experience with a variety of services (U.S. Dept. of Health, Education, and Welfare, 1968).

SUMMARY

The healthy development of children is related to many interwoven factors: biological, social, emotional, and intellectual. Research shows that a child's development is greatly affected by the physical and mental health of his parents—especially his mother's nutritional and emotional state in the nine months or so preceding his birth. He is also influenced by the spacing and number of children in the family into which he is born and his family's social and economic situation.

The first few months and years of a child's life are of critical importance and profoundly affect all aspects of his total development. Thus high-quality prenatal, natal, and postnatal care are imperative to unimpaired development.

The quality of parental or substitute parental care is of fundamental importance. Warm, loving, continuous care by a parenting person on whom an infant or child can depend and whom he can trust to be sensitive and responsive to his needs is essential. Ideally, this person is his mother. Society has a responsibility and a vested interest in each infant's care. Research shows that proper attention to the baby's needs for loving attention, first-rate physical care, good food and housing, and a wealth of learning experiences is essential to development of his full potential.

Continued services to assure the physical and mental health of infants and very young children must be continued for preschoolers and older youngsters. This means that we, as a society, must be continuously concerned about the growing child's total well-being—and the well-being of his parents, who are his primary supports.

The normal, healthy growth of children is, indeed, a miracle. Their capacity for growth from helpless dependence toward ever-increasing skill, competence, self-direction, and capacity to relate to others requires constant attention and help from parents and trained persons and a concerned society and its agencies.

Social-Psychological Aspects of Normal Growth and Development: Adolescents and Youth

PREADOLESCENCE

Children do not suddenly burst into adolescence. They grow into it gradually, after a long preadolescent period. Preadolescence begins for the average girl at about age ten and for the typical boy at around twelve For girls, this period is marked by rapid growth, which occurs before the onset of menstruation. However, the growth spurt in boys takes place after puberty arrives. For both boys and girls, the preadolescent period brings a characteristic increase in activity and probably in energy. Play tends to be vigorous and appetites large. The emotional disturbances related to the physical and psychological changes during this period may lead to such behavior as excessive sloppiness in habits and dress and even a lack of concern about personal cleanliness, as well as negativism, stubbornness, unruliness, disobedience, and other behaviors which adults find irritating. The child often becomes highly sensitive and seems to overreact to even minor criticism.

A common difficulty experienced by children during this period stems from the fact that they mature at different rates and yet are treated as if they were all at the same stage of development. The girl, particularly, is likely to have troubles, since most girls mature earlier than boys and are far ahead of the boys of their own age in sexual maturity, interests, etc. Early- and late-maturing children obviously require different attitudes and experiences. The late-maturing children may feel inferior or uneasy among those whom they regard as their more "hip" peers.

These differences in growth and development, plus the mounting

353

social, biological, and emotional pressures of this period, account for much of the behavior upheaval that is well known in junior high schools. Parents, club leaders, teachers, and other involved adults may further enhance these problems by treating the child as if he were at a certain calendar age rather than a particular developmental age. For instance, prohibiting dating until the child has reached the age of fourteen may be entirely inappropriate for the girl who matures at age eleven or twelve. Youth activities and school programs planned on the basis of developmental stages rather than on specific chronological ages would probably help significantly in ministering to the different individual needs of young people at this stage of development. School counselors should also be specially prepared to work with this age group on an individualized basis.

ADOLESCENCE

Adolescence as an Opportunity

Adolescence is not only a biological or physiological given but also a psychological and social opportunity. Adolescence is not a fixed number of years but rather a possibility for an experience of psychological and social growth which *may or may not* occur after puberty. If real development in terms of emotional, ethical, and intellectual aspects is to continue beyond childhood, there must be continuing support and acceptance of adolescent growth from the family, the school, and other agencies of the larger society. Without this kind of support the development of an adolescent may be foreclosed or distorted with results that may show themselves not only in the obvious forms of personality problems or deviant behavior but in a curtailment of human potentialities for self-fulfillment, independence, psychological maturity, and creativity. Only a minority of young Americans are given the opportunities for real adolescence, and many, for one reason or another, are not supported in their efforts to move ahead to a more complex, more responsible, and more self-directing adulthood (*Report of Task Force III, 1968*).

During adolescence, ideally, the young person undergoes considerable restructuring in terms of psychological changes within himself, changes in his relationships with other people, and changes in his value system. He needs the opportunity and freedom to gain broader experiences, to test himself in many ways, to raise questions and seek answers to them. He also needs guidance, protection, understanding, and some controls as he struggles for growth into adulthood. This is a period that has become notorious as a time of upheaval, confusion, and trouble for all concerned: for the adolescent himself; for parents and other family members; for the school; and for society in general. It is a time in which the young person experiences alternating joy and misery, energy and lethargy, idealism and cynicism, and feelings of independence and dependence.

Each adolescent, as in his earlier years, behaves in his own unique way—a way that has been strongly affected by his many experiences in his home, school, and society. His behavior is also affected by the present situation in which he and his family are living and by the cultural patterns of the people around him, including their expectancies of what an adolescent should be like.

Some Differing Theories About Adolescence

The nature of adolescence has given rise to a number of different theories. For example, psychoanalytic theory holds that during adolescence unresolved earlier problems—both conscious and unconscious—are reworked by the individual and, in a sense, he recapitulates the essential elements of his life experiences up to that point, especially those of his relationships with his parents (Josselyn, 1968).

Others take a somewhat more modified point of view but agree that one of the central tasks of adolescence is for the individual to gain increasing emancipation from his own family and grow toward his separate identity as an individual. For instance, according to Erikson (1959), adolescence entails the integration of emerging intellectual abilities and potentials into actual lived life; the integration within the self of new values, ethics, and purposes; and the developed capacity to live with one's own sexual, aggressive, and other instinctual drives. Adolescence involves a movement away from the simple mirrorlike view of the self which developed in childhood to a new, more self-directed, and individual sense of the self. It also involves a heightened drive toward independence and further development of the capacity to relate and involve oneself with others in close, give-and-take relationships.

Although the general picture of adolescence is one of overt stress and difficulty, at least several intensive studies raise questions about this assumption. In a 1957–58 survey of 3,000 adolescents between the ages of fourteen and sixteen, Douvan and Adelson (1966) found that the majority of young people whom they interviewed seemed to be going through adolescence with at least a superficial calm. These teen-agers tended to show "an avoidance of inner and outer conflict, a premature determination of their identity, a constriction of their individuality and values, and a general unwillingness to take psychic risks." These findings suggest that a large number of adolescents in our society tend to side-step the growth struggles which potentially lead to their full development as individuals.

Another recent study of normal adolescents was carried out by Dr.

Daniel Offer, associate director of the Institute for Psychosomatic and Psychiatric Research and Training in Chicago (Kramer, 1969). This four-year research project, directed toward middle-class, suburban high school boys, revealed that the majority were generally accepting of themselves, their homes, their schools, and their society. In general, they expressed positive feelings toward their parents and the parents had similar attitudes toward their sons. Most of these boys were coping well with school requirements, and delinquent behavior was rare. They had conservative, conventional attitudes toward sex, and most were oriented more toward sports and friends of the same sex than toward dating and girl friends.

The researchers conclude that the relatively secure earlier years experienced by these boys provided a basis for a generally smooth adolescence in which the boys showed a basic trust in their parents, confidence in themselves, and hopeful attitudes toward their future.

Other less intensive studies carried out by surveys and written questionnaires often show that the great majority of adolescents seem to be well satisfied with themselves and with society. These findings may reflect the desire of adolescents to portray themselves in a good light, both to survey directors and to themselves. These findings may also indicate that a great many young people prefer conformity to the pains of individualistic growth. Such conformity is encouraged by many segments in our society. For instance, it appears that the majority of parents, teachers, leaders of youth organizations, and employers emphasize obedience and deference rather than self-expression. It is quite clear that many are concerned about overconformity and believe that our society does not sufficiently promote or sanction individuality so that adolescents might nonconform without criticism. Some of the rebellion of students—blacks, young people, and other minority youth groups, including middle- and upper-class white youngsters—may be partly a response to pressures for conformity. Some young people from all economic levels, white or nonwhite, show rebellion through delinquent or disorganized behavior. However, many of the disadvantaged or highly advantaged youth who rebel do so not only because they are responding to adolescent turmoil or pressures for conformity but also because they are distressed about moral issues. Some seek changes in various aspects of the social order, as will be noted later. Another large group of youth apparently keep their rebellious feelings mostly to themselves or repress them so deeply that they are generally unaware of them. The need to be well thought of and to conform is a general one among most adolescents, especially in the middle class.

Some hold that adolescence tends to be a time of greater difficulty than childhood, partly because older youngsters are simply able to get into more serious difficulty. During adolescence, the range of operations is wider, pregnancy becomes possible, physical strength increases, and youths are exposed to a greater range of temptations. In addition, society is less forgiving of the older child who behaves in nonconformist ways, and parents are more deeply disturbed when their older children show symptoms of not preparing adequately for the adult tasks of marriage and eventual employment.

Central Tasks of Adolescence

Regardless of what theoretical approach one takes on adolescence, there is rather general agreement that at this time life presents the young person in American society with certain central tasks. Douvan and Adelson (1966) stress the fact that adolescent tasks are quite different for boys than for girls. The boy's major concerns and psychological growth are focused on and expressed in the areas of achievement, self-direction, authority, and control over the sex impulses. The girl's key concerns revolve around friendship, dating, popularity, and the understanding of interpersonal relationships. A boy finds his identity largely through the development of his own competence and independence in handling such tasks as work and achievement. A girl is more likely to find her identity through close attachments and intimacy with other people. In our culture the need to marry and find acceptance in love exerts such pressure on the young girl that she hardly has the time and energy to invest herself in the discovery of her own individuality until she has gained some measure of security in a stable love relationship.

In Chapter II we pointed out that the very nature of our society today presents adolescents and youth with both particular problems and special opportunities. All of our young people are faced with swift and radical social changes, with pressures for educational and vocational achievement, with demands for great strength and competence, and with being members of a very large youth population. A great many young men are faced with being drafted for a war in which they may not believe, and many adolescents feel a sense of helplessness in connection with the H-bomb threat. Separation and hostility between the races presents another excruciating issue. Young people are likely to be highly stimulated and confused by the unrealistic and highly commercialized messages from the mass media, by shifts in values, by the temptations for impulsive behavior that surround them on all sides, by the current "now" philosophy, which reflects the many uncertainties of our world. The majority have far more money to spend than was true for an earlier generation, and they are courted by the many businesses and industries that cater to the "youth market." They live in a sexually stimulating environment in which modern contraceptives make sex "safe" but frequently forbidden to the young.

Many have a prolonged period of dependency after they have become physically mature. The average of biological maturation has been gradually dropping so that it is now about age twelve for girls and fourteen for boys. Yet many young people are not in a position to marry and support themselves until they have finished long years of advanced education.

Two Stages of Adolescence

There is considerable agreement that adolescence is divided into two stages, although there is no clearly marked division between the two. In early adolescence the young person is largely preoccupied with the issues of emancipation, independence, and freedom from the family. In later adolescence there is a growing concern with questions about the future, and a further development of a sense of social role and personal purpose. This gradual shift away from preoccupation with family issues toward an expanding interest in the wider world is by no means automatic or guaranteed by the passage of time. This growth is unlikely to occur unless both society and the family recognize and support its importance and validity to the young person.

Two major issues arise in late adolescence. One revolves around finding one's place in the wider world and the other around developing a capacity for intimacy, including psychophysical intimacy with the opposite sex. Thus, occupational choice and marital choice are both crucial issues to the older adolescent. The choices are related not only to individual development but to what is actually available to the young person in the society in which he lives. For the advantaged youth, the central problem will be the difficult, but luxurious, question of choosing widely between many available opportunities. However, the disadvantaged young person may have only two choices: to accept social rejection and educational or occupational failure in a pattern of fatalism and passivity or to lash out violently against the society which condemns him to inferiority, deprivation, and humiliation (*Report of Task Force III,* 1968).

Adult Attitudes Toward Youth

Adults hold confused and conflicting attitudes toward youth. Many express hostility, suspicion, and rejection of the young. Although these attitudes seem to be age-old, they are probably more extreme now because of the nature of our society and the sheer magnitude of our youth population. It is probable that these adult attitudes include envy and fear, both of youthful vitality and of the competition posed by young people. In addition, some older people may mistakenly see in youth their own hidden and repressed wishes for sexual and aggressive adventures. Moreover, parents and other middle-aged adults are plagued by their own particular anxieties, such as advancing age, their employment, and their place in the community. Parents also have worries about the safety and normal growth of their sons and daughters. Conflicting demands are made on young people by the older generation. They are expected to behave in a grown-up manner, yet they are often prevented from showing independence and taking on real responsibilities. Legally they are considered adult at different points in time for different purposes, and these legal definitions are not consistent from state to state. For example, in most states young people can get an automobile license and leave school at age sixteen, yet they are prohibited from engaging in many kinds of employment. Boys may be drafted at eighteen, but in some places they are not allowed to vote until they are twenty-one. Even the legal age for marriage varies, from age fourteen for girls in some states to age twenty-one for both boys and girls in others.

There is a tendency in our nation to deplore the ways of youth and at the same time to worship and glamorize youthfulness. Among the middle class in particular, some parents seem to push their children into a premature adolescence and overindulge them with material possessions yet are unwilling or unable to entertain young people in their homes. The attitudes of parents, the nature and size of many of today's homes, and the drive of youth to separate themselves from their parents are all factors which have led large numbers of adolescents today to find their own gathering places, far from the guidance and supervision of adults. This situation, together with the automobile, presents obvious hazards, especially for young adolescents.

Strivings for Independence

The striving for independence from one's own family is a crucial prelude to becoming a separate adult. This striving may be manifested in open rebellion, rejection of parental standards, and criticism of parents. Or the emancipation process may take the form of quiet withdrawal, secrecy, and an insistence on privacy. The latter is more likely to be a feminine tactic, partly because the culture disapproves of open aggression on the part of girls. Typically, adolescents both want and fear independence. They still have deep emotional ties to their family and yearn for the love and protection of earlier childhood. This is one reason why they seemingly resent being given actual independence and tend to push the limits further and further for proof that their parents still care enough about them to take a disciplinary stand. This ambivalence about independence also plays a part in the irritating, provocative behavior in which young people often indulge, basically as a bid for parental attention.

Boys, especially, are often unable to communicate their inner conflicts by talking about them to other people, especially their parents. The sensitivities of youngsters at this age are apt to be so extreme that they take on outer defenses of bravado, boredom, or "playing it cool." Risk-taking behavior is common, partly to prove one's own strength and to mask an inner sense of weakness.

Most young people are extremely sensitive to criticism. Their feelings are intense, and their self-esteem is frequently low. Especially among younger adolescents, inner struggles require so much energy and attention that the youngster may seem to be focused only upon himself.

Social Development

The majority of adolescents have a drive to conform to their own age group in such matters as dress, manners, appearance, and speech. Wanting to "do what everybody else does" probably results mainly from inner feelings of inferiority and anxiety about one's own adequacy. For most adolescents, the so-called peer group assumes an increasing importance, usually more so for boys than for girls. Girls are more likely to identify with a few very close friends and, in effect, practice their social and emotional skills with their own sex before they muster sufficient confidence and courage to develop a close love relationship with a boy.

"Crushes" are common at this period. The "crush" often involves elements of hero worship and may seem to be sexual, at least in part. The young person, unknowingly, is using these attachments partly to outgrow his dependence on his own parents. These intense attachments usually fade with the passage of time, but from them stems the eventual ability to form a deep relationship with a member of the opposite sex.

Hero worship is common at this age and is related to the youngster's search for an ideal self. He is trying many different ways of being an adult and has dreams of glory about his own heroic role in the future. It is important that he have adults available whom he can worship and who are allied with the basic goals of organized, rather than deviant, society. Community leaders, teachers, employers, religious counselors, and youth leaders may be the objects of hero worship. If such people, through their own fallibilities or lack of understanding, exploit this worship or fail to accept adult responsibility for it, the young person may be seriously dis-illusioned.

Communities must provide more opportunities for adolescents to find satisfying, safe outlets for their social, emotional, and recreational needs. Presently, adequate recreational facilities and centers are the exception rather than the rule. The lack is particularly serious in low-income neigh-borhoods but also a frequent problem in more affluent communities. Such centers need to be related to the particular interests of young people and must include their participation in planning and administration. This participation requires an adherence to democratic principles. Adults must provide guidance but avoid authoritarian methods. Later in this chapter we will present some suggested guidelines for youth participation.

Sex Development and Behavior

The heightened sexuality during adolescence is strongly, but not completely, influenced by physiological changes. In girls this sexuality is frequently repressed and expresses itself chiefly in romantic dreams of love. For the boy, the sex drive tends to be much more explicitly biological and direct. There seem to be prevalent attitudes and expectations which reinforce the boy's tendency to regard sex as largely a biological, impersonal matter. Girls are frequently taught to fear and protect themselves against boys. Boys are often regarded as being unprincipled young savages who are bent on ruthless exploitation of females. These expectations and attitudes in our society seem to create and perpetuate difficulties between the sexes in the interpersonal realm and to particularly undermine the boy's sense of personal worth.

The earlier maturation of girls adds to the difficulties between the sexes, as does the fact that adolescent girls are more likely to have greater social skills and do better academically. These kinds of differences between the sexes during adolescence add to problems in heterosexual relationships, particularly when boys are taught that they should be superior to girls and protect them as the weaker sex. Our tendency to promote strictly age-graded activities, to compare boys invidiously to girls, and to offer boys and girls differential sex education and counseling would seem to undermine opportunities for promoting qualities that are important in marriage, such as the capacity for free and open communication, fusing of feelings of love and sexuality, shared interests, and interdependence.

The So-Called Sex Revolution

There are sweeping claims today that we are in the midst of a sex revolution. However, changes related to sex roles and sex behavior are more a matter of evolution. These changes go back to the late nineteenth century in the United States and the period of growing industrialization which brought with it increasing economic, social, and political equality for women. The development of modern contraceptives has contributed to woman's quest for equality and has given further impetus to the search for new values that are more closely related to our technological, urban society. Although there are many indications that values related to sex behavior seem to be undergoing a radical change, related research indicates that these changes are not as revolutionary as they might seem. Recent studies carried out by Reiss (1969) indicate that the proportions of males and females engaging in premarital sex relations have actually increased very little over the past twenty-five years or so. The main changes are in more open discussion about sex and higher rates of premarital petting. It seems that the major revolution in terms of the sex behavior of women was launched in the 1920's. There apparently has been relatively little change over the years in the sex behavior of men, except as they have had to adjust to the new concepts which women have of themselves in their relationships with men and the larger society.

Some observers of the current scene comment that many of the current trends are healthy, since Americans have long been too secretive and uninformed about matters relating to sex. They also comment that the present open discussions represent greater honesty about actual feelings and behavior. In the past, sex was very much a matter of separate moralities. There was one set of standards for public pronouncements and another for private behavior. These same commentators also observe that many of today's young people (mostly middle- and upper-class youth) are developing a new and healthier morality: one that supports personal commitment and responsibility between sex partners, both within and outside of marriage, rather than mutual exploitation and an exclusively physical relationship (Kirkendal and Libby, 1969).

Anxiety About Physical Development

Most adolescents of both sexes are anxious about their physical development and appearance. This anxiety may manifest itself in compulsive cleanliness, long hours spent before the mirror, a fixation on clothes, and the like. This anxiety may reverse itself by an apparent sloppiness and self-neglect which may be a gesture of despair about one's attractiveness or an expression of revolt against parental overemphasis on "keeping up appearances." These adolescent anxieties are exploited by commercial interests which make large claims about the magic road to love and popularity via the right pill or soap.

Intellectual Development

Intellectual capacity generally expands rapidly during adolescence with the growing ability to handle abstract concepts and new ways of conceptualizing time and space and one's relationship to it.

It is in adolescence that the intellect "cuts loose" from the concrete events of daily life and becomes a powerful force, for better or worse, in the governance of daily behavior. In this process (which at its best is an extension of rationality and at its worst a flight into unreality), the adolescent normally vacillates between romantic, highly intellectualized theory building and impulsive daily behavior which may bear little relationship to his high ideals and theories (*Report of Task Force III*, 1968).

The newfound ability to develop theories and to imagine a world that does not exist is one of the factors that leads adolescents to indulge in elaborate daydreams. As the young person imagines the world as it might be, he may develop resentment of the world as it is. His ability to dream of a radically different future makes it possible for him to build a world of the imagination that may serve not merely as a goal and ideal but as a means of escape from the trials of the present. He tends to try out in his imagination the kinds of things he might be and do before he actually engages in action. As he grows a bit older, he should be able to accept more easily the gap which is bound to exist between ideal images and the actualities of real life.

Moral Values

The redevelopment of moral values, which should occur during the adolescent period, is partly related to the increased ability to reason abstractly. Moreover, the young person must re-form values and make them his own rather than accepting them blindly from his parents, as he once did. This is part of his emancipation process from his family. It is also part of the need to develop broader and more flexible moral concepts, rather than simply reordering childhood rules of behavior. He is likely to become aware of the often large differences between what other people tell him to do and what they actually do themselves—and no one is more likely to be the object of bitter criticism in this regard than his parents. He needs to realize that his mother and father are not superhuman idols (as he probably saw them in childhood) but are human beings with human strengths and weaknesses.

As the adolescent seeks a new morality he can make his own, he also tends to closely examine the actual practices of society. Highly principled youth, in particular, may develop a sense of outrage over the gulf between social ideals and actual social practices (Silverstein, Rosenberg, and Weingarten, 1967). This examination of moral values is a particular characteristic of the present because rapid social change has given rise to a general value upheaval in our society.

A major moral concern of adolescents revolves around the control of sexual and aggressive impulses. The sexually maturing adolescent must learn to control these impulses but still be able to freely express verbally his desires for sexual pleasure, love, and intimacy. Equally important, adolescence brings with it new drives and abilities for violence, drives which are made more disturbing both to the adolescent and to the adult world because of the young person's increased strength. In an attempt to control and yet accept his impulses, the adolescent may swing dramatically and rapidly from one behavior to another. For instance, he may shift from being very active sexually to a period of denial of sex. Rage, fury, and violence may be replaced suddenly by peaceableness, self-restraint, and saintlike gentleness. These shifts should not be seen as perverse and unreasonable adolescent behavior. Rather, they should be regarded as one normal aspect of development in which impulsive action and excessive self-control swing back and forth in ever-narrowing cycles which, ideally, lead to the slow development of the young person's ability to acquire flexible and realistic controls over himself rather than being dependent on the controls imposed by his parents and other adults (*Report of Task Force III,* 1968).

As the young person develops these kinds of controls, it is important that he also acquire the ability to release his feelings without guilt or anxiety. Because uncontrolled aggression and sexuality cause highly visible social problems, they command immediate social attention. However, if the young person is forced to overcontrol both his anger and his sexuality, this may lead to an adult life marked by quiet desperation and poor capacity for human relationships.

There is considerable evidence that adolescents who live in families in which the style is democratic rather than authoritarian are more likely to be able to control their behavior without becoming overly inhibited and constricted. For example, the interview survey of Douvan and Adelson (1966) found that young people from democratic families tend to be "unusually self-reliant, poised, and effective. They are free to criticize and disagree with parents, but have generally warm companionship with them." In authoritarian families, adolescents are found to be obedient on the surface but beneath this façade they show strong feelings of rebelliousness and impulsivity. Unlike the more principled first group, authoritarian-reared youth ". . . tend to have an externalized morality, to define morals as what one can get away with." In democratic families, the interviewers found that parents allowed the young person a fair degree of independence, included him in important decisions affecting his own behavior, and tended to use verbal, rather than physical, discipline. On the other hand, authoritarian parents set rules without consulting the children, allowed little independence, and tended to use physical techniques for enforcing discipline.

Trends for Today's Youth

Today's youth are highly diverse and represent many groups with different major concerns, such as white and black radicals, student activists, the dropouts from society (the alienated), the social activists, and those in the conformist majority. Although only small groups of young people are actively engaged in rebelling against our present society, the questions which they raise and the attitudes which they espouse may well have an extensive influence on both current and future generations. In historical perspective the youth communes, "the hippies and flower children," are not a new phenomenon. A number of European countries have experienced strikingly similar movements among youth. Our current student unrest is a common phenomenon on other continents.

Today's dissident youth tend to identify with members of their own age group rather than with their elders, a particular social class, or an organizational structure. They often form alliances among themselves, frequently in opposition to sanctioned authority and in protest against traditional forms of social organization. They view the concepts and values of earlier generations as being outworn and unrelated to the current scene. Never has this age-old tendency of youth seemed as strong and widespread as at the present, when the communication media transmit the spread of dissident international youth movements.

One adhesive force among many of our youth is their continual awareness of the world in which they live. Emphasis is placed on open discussion of issues. Many demonstrations by student, and other, groups can be explained as an expression of anger at the failure of the adult world to honestly recognize an issue and be willing to discuss it. The awareness and acceptance of the pace of social change by these more activist youth is related to their distrust of leaders and their view that today's problems may not be answered by yesterday's wisdom. They see the world as a global village and react to events in other countries as keenly as they do to events in their own. They are moving toward an international, rather than a national, point of view. They have been born into a technological society and accept it as a matter of course. They do not resist the conveniences of this society but are opposed to the nonhumane aspects of the environment—the depersonalization, commercialism, and devaluation of human relationships.

Another tendency, somewhat in conflict with the alliance of youth, is the central value our dissident young people place on personal development, part of which is an emphasis on openness to all new experiences and interactions. They feel that their "true identity" is in constant flux and that they have an obligation to continue to grow to meet the many changes in the current world scene. Being psychologically free and able to interact with anyone, in any situation, no matter how alien the other person or situation may be, is an ideal goal. Face-to-face human relationships are treasured. These values stand in contrast to the "game-playing" and achievement-oriented manipulation of others which is so much the life style of Americans who want to move up on the social and economic scale.

As a part of the bid for psychological freedom, nonconformist adolescents and youth today strive to move away from the puritan tradition of the Protestant ethic. To express one's self without inhibition is a primary goal, particularly if one can do so creatively. The desire to be able to enjoy life colors many of their actions. In this era of affluence, many of the young choose work for its quality and enjoyment rather than for purely practical reasons. With the advent of the "pill," sexual relationships are chosen for their meaningfulness; exploitative relationships, sexual or otherwise, are disapproved. To be able to enjoy sex without fear or guilt is a concomitant of the capacity to "be one's self."

These trends in the attitudes of youth are encouraging. What may appear to be real innovations in the style of young people in today's world may prove to be necessary conditions for existence in the world of tomorrow. The trend toward identification with international, rather than national, social class, or family membership; the continual flexibility and capability of personal growth; and the movement away from violence and toward the humanization of our world's society may prove to be attitudes that could well mean the difference in quality of life in the twenty-first century and, indeed, could well mean the difference between life or destruction for the human species (*Report of Task Force III,* 1968).

Gaining a New Sense of Community

Today's revolutionary changes are difficult for both young people and their elders. In general, vast social and economic upheavals have brought about a loosening of the bonds of community in our society. "Between rich and poor, black and white, the pre-industrial and the modernized world are appearing ominous gulfs, reflecting an absence of common experience, common interests, common values, and of the sense of sharing of common human fate. A similar failure of community is affecting the relations between young people and the adult world. This is the meaning of the much belabored 'generation gap' " (Smith, 1969). This failure of community and decline of authority has left the individual without the usual supports and guidelines. The resulting confusion is particularly difficult for young people, especially for those who are the most sensitive and who most value basic moral principles. The associated sense of aloneness may lead the individual to become involved in violent or outrageous acts as a way to make him feel that he actually exists and that he is part of a "passionate fellowship in crisis" (Smith, 1969). It is important that adults in a position of authority resist the temptation to rely on punitive and authoritarian attitudes in dealing with youthful rebellion. By a wider sharing of power, by the development of approaches that allow greater cooperation in coping with common tasks, by rational and open discussion of the issues, by showing a readiness to change in reasonable directions, it may be possible for the two generations to arrive at a greater sense of community, with norms and goals which are more adapted to the present situation.

Student Activists

Many have called this "the generation of protest." Actually, only small minorities have been actively committed to political or social change, even at those colleges and universities where student protests have been most publicized. In general, the rule is student apathy or indifference, and the exception is student activism or protest. Although the activists make up only a small percentage of the student group, they exert a great influence on the vast majority of other young people. They, together with the alienated youth, are a major force which is helping to shape the character of this generation. The nature and meaning of most student dissent is grossly misunderstood, not only by the general public but by many college administrators. For example, it is widely thought that student activists are "misfits" who are in some way rebelling against parental authority. In fact, activists are drawn from among the most academically talented, idealistic, and committed of today's college students. They generally come from politically active and liberal families whose values they are implementing, rather than rebelling against (Flacks, 1967; Smith, 1969). Unlike the alienated, activists are strongly committed to traditional American ideals of justice, equality, and democracy as well as faith in human nature and the effectiveness of human action. It is unfortunate that administrators, law makers, and the general public so often fail to appreciate the nature and promise of today's student political involvement and that they seek to limit the activists' involvement in crucial national and international problems. Activists, frustrated by the deafness and restrictiveness of those to whom they address themselves, are tending toward more and more desperate efforts to draw attention to their causes. An attitude of opposition to student political and societal involvement does not help them become responsible members of a democratic society.

High schools and colleges should encourage students to become knowledgeable about and actively involved in local community issues. Youth should be viewed as helpers in the sense of the domestic peace corps.

It is imperative that schools defend the right of free speech in general, not the particular right of some partisan group with a vested interest in one position. Whenever possible, student publications should be self-governing and, when feasible, financially independent. They should be limited in their freedom of expression only by the laws that govern the press in the United States. High schools, colleges, and universities ought to encourage this "generation of protest" by meeting with and listening to students who present demands, grievances, and concerns (*Report of Task Force III,* 1968).

Alienated Youth

A small group of our more affluent young people feel that our present society is so corrupt and pointless that they must withdraw from it. These young people reject the materialism and other dominant values of middle-class America. They see middle-class family life as essentially pointless and repressive to humanistic interests and objectives. They tend to live rather secluded lives in their own communities where financial interests are of secondary importance and poverty, although at times uncomfortable, is seen as socially and spiritually ennobling. These young people see their elders as essentially unfulfilled, as having denied their human potential by "selling out" to economic and social security. Alienated youth feel that they cannot develop their own individuality if they participate in a society of this kind. They find much hypocrisy about them and believe that schools and colleges do not prepare them for the present and future realities of modern life.

There is some evidence that this withdrawal from the major society into "hippie retreatist colonies" may cause lasting damage to the individual development of some young people. However, it is likely that, in time, many an alienated youth will be successful in finding his own identity and many will return to the larger community. Our challenge for the present is to create a society in which our young people feel they can belong without a loss of personal and moral integrity (*Report of Task Force III,* 1968).

Working with, Rather than Against, Adolescents and Youth

There are a number of mistaken assumptions which society often makes in handling young people. These assumptions include the following:

1. The first commonly held but misleading assumption is that "clamping down" on and isolation of the young from society are necessary and beneficial disciplinary procedures.

2. A second incorrect assumption is based on the idea that there is a single or major cause of any behavior or social problem, such as delinquency, school dropouts, and the like.

3. Another misleading and almost fatal assumption is "youth are not old enough to know what is good for them, nor mature enough to participate in the planning and operation of their own development and education."

4. Adults generally assume that they know better than young people what youth needs (*Report of Task Force VI,* 1968).

Because society has changed so enormously in the past ten years or so, young people who have grown up in it are likely to understand many aspects of the current scene better than their elders do. Moreover, young people have great resources of energy, vitality, imagination, and flexibility to bring to our communities. They have a drive to find a significant place for themselves in society, to commit themselves to important undertakings, and to test their competencies in a wide range of experiences related to their future careers as employees, heads of families, and community members. It is important that young people be given the chance to work in partnership with adults in many kinds of enterprises.

For example, young people should participate in planning their own educational experiences in elementary schools, high schools, and colleges. Moreover, they might well serve in voluntary or employee positions, either part-time or full-time, in the human service fields of physical and mental health, recreation, welfare, and education. For instance, high school youth could serve as tutors, playground leaders, and classroom aides in elementary schools. They should be given a part in planning community service projects and in carrying them out. A number of experiments along these, and related, lines have been carried out in various parts of the country with reportedly good results (*Report of Task Force VI,* 1968). Of particular relevance to the mental health field is the use of college students as volunteers in state mental hospitals. Several thousand college students participate each year in various activities in local mental hospitals, such as individual tutoring, occupational therapy projects, and programs designed to teach long-term hospitalized patients how to live and act in the community.

Human service programs which involve youth in various aide and professional activities probably will be more effective if the following guidelines are adopted:

1. Participation of young people in the planning and program evaluation process.

2. Preparation for human service work, either volunteer or paid, through brief orientation sessions followed by on-the-job training and competent supervision which is democratic in nature and allows for free discussion and questioning.

3. Involvement of young people in the determination of standards of work and any limitations of behavior, speech, dress, and the like.

4. Clear job descriptions with provisions for the young person to try out a variety of work activities.

5. Open, free communication between adults and youth.

6. Willingness on the part of adults and youth alike to experiment with

new approaches with a readiness to tie these experimentations to already existing knowledge and to frequent objective examination of their effectiveness.

7. Understanding on the part of participating adults of young people, as individuals, and of the underlying dynamics of adolescence and youth as stages in development. Of equal importance is the adults' understanding and full acceptance of youth from a diversity of social and economic backgrounds.*

Experiences in the human service fields, whether voluntary or paid, potentially offer many advantages to those youth whose interests, aptitudes, and values attract them to such programs. Appropriate participative experiences for selected youth in the human service fields, if skillfully handled by administrators and regular staff people, can help young people acquire a greater sense of their own significance, give them a chance to test themselves in activities related to their own future functions in work, family, and the community, provide an opportunity for them to carry responsibility and achieve further independence, and create an outlet for their idealism and desire to give. Such experiences also potentially provide youth with a wider range of adult models with whom they may wish to identify and from whom they may derive new knowledge and aspirations. Such positive outcomes, of course, depend on the quality and behavior of the adult models.

The Child Development Councils and Authorities recommended by the Commission should serve to help youth take advantage of the wealth of opportunities that are present for volunteer or paid experience in the human service field. We already have evidence of youth response in such programs as the Peace Corps, Vista, domestic and overseas youth service programs conducted by church-related groups, and college student ghetto tutoring projects.

National Council of State Committees for Children and Youth

The National Council of State Committees for Children and Youth has had a long, continued interest in promoting the involvement and participation of the young and in 1963 established a standing committee to promote the concept of youth participation (Clendenen et al., 1968).† Patterns of state youth partnership vary in structure and method. From questionnaires

* These suggested guidelines have grown out of related theory, observation, and experience. They are yet to be validated through research directed toward an assessment of youth participation programs.

† The names of the various state committees vary. Therefore, in this report the term "state council of youth" has been used to cover all.

completed by the various state committees, the National Council was able to identify several suggested principles of adult youth partnership. They include:

1. Grant young people responsibility and allow for the learning experience of mistakes and failures.
2. Keep adult-youth communications open at all times.
3. Make sure participation is meaningful to youth.
4. Assure regional, socioeconomic, and ethnic membership.
5. Besides orientation materials and sessions for new youth members, include in the format opportunities for discussions of the happenings in meetings, both for clarification and as a sounding board for youths' reactions.

Past members of youth councils who evaluated their experience on state committees agreed that the most successful involvement of youth in community activities was that in which the councils were connected with the mayor's office or similar civic offices. Past members' evaluations pointed out the error of involving youth without really giving them a voice or influence. Participation must be real; it must be meaningful and *capable of having a meaningful impact on youths' lives*.

The National Service Secretariat (1968) has published a directory of service organizations to identify agencies in which young people may serve in various areas. The National Service Secretariat, whose purpose is to conduct research and provide information and consultation on matters related to youth service, restricted this directory to agencies which could be expected to meet the criteria for a national service program if and when one comes into effect.* Basically, this means that the organizations must offer young people opportunities to perform needed tasks contributing to the welfare of others; be able to communicate across racial, social, and economic barriers; aid in developing the individual's sense of self-worth and civic pride; and provide opportunities for youth to get involved and to learn while serving.

Many organized youth activities such as the National State Committees, to date, have been rather weak ad hoc bodies, which are not always broadly representative. The Students for a Democratic Society and other student groups, such as the black youth organizations, have been organized by youth themselves and appear to generate a greater feeling of meaningful involvement. While these youth-organized movements represent only a minority of youth, such groups do have an impact on the total youth population.

* These criteria are not to be understood as necessarily implying endorsement of the national service concept by the agencies in the directory.

Participation of Youth in the Political Process

The Commission believes that youth should be granted the opportunity to actively participate in the political processes which govern their lives in so many ways. Serious consideration should be given to lowering the voting age to eighteen years *(Report of Task Force III,* 1968). Today's young people are in general far more knowledgeable about the issues that face our nation than was true of earlier generations. Not only do they mature earlier and have higher average levels of education, but they also frequently have a clearer understanding of current and emerging issues. Their readiness to participate was reflected in the 1968 Presidential campaign. All these are cogent arguments for extending the right to vote to this younger group who show a rightful concern about having a more effective voice in the public policies and legislation which affect their lives so deeply.

SOME SPECIAL PROBLEMS

Emotional Disturbances and Mental Health Problems of Adolescents

As noted in Chapter I, there is a rise in emotional and mental health problems during adolescence. The emotional upheavals often associated with adolescence may lead to such wide swings in behavior that it is frequently difficult to know whether the young person requires psychological treatment. No one would wish to begin psychotherapy with young men or women whose painful struggles are moving them closer to an understanding of themselves or of their relationship with the outer world. But for other individuals, hard to distinguish from their fellows, the general confusions of adolescence mask a diffusion and despair not characteristic of a developmental phase but indicative of emotional disorder. Expert diagnosis may be necessary to know whether or not the young person is seriously disturbed.

It is a mistake to assume that the upset young person will necessarily "just grow out of his difficulties." There is no symptom of the disturbed adolescent that does not in one way or another fit into the category of normal adolescence. It is the degree, the crippling, and the unchangeableness of the symptoms that should be the criteria for evaluating whether the individual's behavior is that of a normal adolescent or an indicator that something, at least potentially, is going awry (Josselyn, 1968).

Most, if not all, adolescents suffer from passing feelings of depression. Psychotherapy is indicated if depression is the dominant and continuing mood. Too persistent concern over body functioning, with a wide range of poorly defined symptoms and a general feeling of exhaustion, also suggests that the individual may need help from a therapist. However, such symptoms are not always psychological. It is important that early symptoms of real illness be diagnosed and treated. Perhaps the physical conditions that are most frequently overlooked are diseases such as infectious mononucleosis.

Some adolescents react in an opposite way to their anxieties about their bodies and clearly neglect ther physical needs. When physical care is neglected to an extreme degree, it indicates that there is probably an underlying serious psychological disturbance (Josselyn, 1968).

Daydreaming may also be a symptom of disturbance if fantasies are dominating the life of the young person and preventing him from coping with the outer world.

It appears that schizophrenia in the adolescent is much less frequent than was formerly believed. Improvements in the treatment of schizophrenia have led to indications that many adolescents were previously misdiagnosed as schizophrenic. There is need for much further study of this question. At present, one can only suggest that there is a psychosis of adolescence that should not be confused with schizophrenia. The adolescent with such a psychosis has been overwhelmed by the multiple demands made upon him, and as in any psychotic breakdown, he lives in an unreal and disorganized world. However, when he recovers he does not retain schizoid characteristics. He is like a machine that has functioned well until a belt slips off a wheel; when the belt is replaced or put in proper position, the machine functions as well as it ever did (Josselyn, 1968).

Suicide in the Adolescent and Youth Population

The death rate by means of suicide rises among our young during adolescence. The national rate for the total population is a little higher than one percent a year; for the adolescent and youth population it is about one-half of one percent. Although this rate has risen somewhat since a low point in 1954, it is still much lower than it was in the early part of this century and considerably lower than it was during the peak Depression years. Suicide risk is directly related to advancing age. It is nonexistent under age five, virtually nonexistent at five to nine years of age, rare between the ages of ten and fourteen, increases in frequency about seven- to eight-fold at ages fifteen to nineteen, and more than doubles again in frequency in the twenty-to-twenty-four-year age group (U.S. Dept. of Health, Education, and Welfare, 1966). Although the rate increases alarmingly during late adolescence and early youth, the overall rate for these years remains below one percent. The rate for males is triple that for females, and, generally speaking, the rates for nonwhites are lower than those for whites, although rates for nonwhite males seem to be increasing recently.

The reasons for suicide are, as yet, little understood. The rates are about the same for all socioeconomic levels, so it appears to have no direct association with amount of income. It appears that suicide rates are higher for college students than for other young people of the same age. For instance, at some colleges the rate is as high as 2 percent or more. For several years, suicide has been surpassed only by accidents as the leading cause of death among the college population. Various reports suggest there may be an increase in the *number* of college students who commit suicide, although there is no evidence showing an increase in the *rate* of college suicide (Pennington, 1968). There is no clear evidence that academic pressures are related to this higher suicide rate among college students. Conflict within the young person's family, loss of a parent or rejection by a parent, and isolation from friends all seem to be related to suicide. Extension of suicide prevention centers and improvement of college mental health counseling services are strongly recommended as a means of reducing this problem (*Report of Task Force VI,* 1968).

"Overt or covert references to a desire to commit suicide, are expressions of continued hopelessness in regard to life, should always be taken seriously and are an indication of the need for expert psychotherapy" (Josselyn, 1968).

Juvenile Delinquency*

The increase in our youth population has also brought about an increase in the numbers of juvenile delinquents over the past ten years or so. Whether or not the prevalence of delinquency in the population has actually increased is not definitely known, because delinquency rates are partly determined by police and court practices. Despite this lack of clarity, it is apparent that delinquency and crime are very serious problems, both for our society and to the young people involved.

Delinquency rates rise markedly from age eleven onward and are five times higher among boys than girls. Among boys, the rate doubles between the ages of eleven and twelve and more than triples between the ages of twelve and seventeen. The arrest rate for first offenders is highest for boys who are fourteen years old. In large cities, delinquency rates are much higher in poverty areas, although this is not necessarily the case in smaller cities and rural neighborhoods. It seems that crime, among all age groups, is exceedingly high in our city slums. In Chicago, for instance, one very low-income inner-city ghetto neighborhood had 25 times as many serious crimes against persons per 100,000 residents than did a far more privileged

---

* This subject is too large and specialized to be adequately covered in this report; other special commissions have prepared reports and recommendations on this subject. Here, we will merely sketch some of the emotional factors that seem to be associated with juvenile delinquency.

area. (*Report of National Advisory Committee on Civil Disorders,* 1968).

Further evidence of the seriousness of delinquency is revealed by the following facts. It is estimated that 11 percent of all children in the United States will reach the juvenile court by the time they are nineteen years old. In 1965, persons eighteen or younger accounted for 24 percent of all persons charged with forcible rape, 52 percent of those charged with burglary, 45 percent of larceny charges, and 61 percent of those charged with auto theft. At some time during their lives, 90 percent of all urban Negro males will be arrested for something more serious than auto theft (*Report of Task Force V,* 1968).

There are a large number of factors that play into delinquent behavior, including the adverse effects of poverty and the poverty environment, the general pressures and upheavals of today's society, the strains associated with migration from rural areas or other countries to large urban areas, the repressive and punitive behaviors of people in authority, the blocking of the opportunity system for disadvantaged young people, and high rates of youth unemployment.

There are other delinquency-related factors that might be termed primarily psychological. For example, there are some indications that boys who belong to delinquent groups are more likely to have social and emotional problems than other boys of the same social and economic background. Various studies have shown several psychological differences between delinquents and nondelinquents. For example, boys in delinquent groups are more likely to have far higher aspirations for success than their life situation would warrant. They tend to show a great concern for their status, which flows primarily from their feelings of inferiority and inadequacy. They frequently show very poor social and interpersonal skills and tend to be highly anxious, extremely self-centered, and lacking in the ability to assert themselves as people. Contrary to general impressions about the group spirit of delinquent gangs, it has been found that the members of such gangs have little warmth, loyalty, or trust in one another. They react with a show of bravado to cover inner feelings of dependency. Moreover, they have an orientation toward violence and hostility which leads to many fights within the group. These young people frequently come from homes in which they received little consistent love, parental support, or steady discipline. Many of these homes lacked a father. In cases where the father was present, he tended to be hostile and authoritarian (Short, 1966).

Most specialists in the field of delinquency believe that there is a wide range of individual psychological differences among delinquents. Such specialists hold strong convictions on the need for individual diagnosis, followed by any necessary care and treatment planned on the basis of the diagnosis. In somewhat similar fashion the psychological causes for delinquent behavior vary enormously and interact with the individual's stage of development, social and economic background, life experience, and present situation. Delinquency is only a symptom of a host of deficits or errors in the individual's life. In the case of a few children and adolescents, these may prove to be constitutional. What is more certain is that deficiencies in families, neighborhoods, health and recreation agencies, schools, police and court systems, employment opportunities, and the like all contribute to the problem of crime and delinquency.

Polier (1968) has commented that today's delinquents are "yesterday's neglected children on whose behalf the community has failed to act." While it is clear that many delinquents need remedial services rather than punishment, most are dealt with harshly. Youngsters from disadvantaged minority groups and poverty neighborhoods, particularly, are committed more often to correctional institutions than to treatment facilities. Moreover, it is well known that disadvantaged youngsters are often treated with brutality and suspicion by the police and are far more likely than more advantaged children to be arrested either on the grounds of suspicion or for minor infractions of the law. When a young person is defined as being delinquent by society, he is far more likely to act in aggressive and antisocial ways. When his arrest record blocks his future employment in legitimate activities, and his confinement results in refinement of the art of crime rather than rehabilitation, it is quite likely that today's delinquent will become tomorrow's adult criminal.

According to recent testimony before the Senate Subcommittee on Employment, Manpower, and Poverty, some 100,000 children in 1965 were incarcerated in adult prisons. Of the 833,507 juveniles taken into custody that year only 2.9 percent were referred to a welfare agency. One-third of the juvenile courts in the nation have no probation officer or caseworker available to them. Eighty-three percent have no regular access to any psychiatric or psychological assistance for the treatment of offenders.

According to the same subcommittee report, a recent survey of thirteen states revealed that training schools were grossly overcrowded, a problem that was being met by premature discharge which resulted, in turn, in a high rate of repeat commitments. The annual total operating costs of all state training schools in 1965 totaled $144,600,000. Most schools were still operating only custodial programs. Despite the lack of success with institutional programs, state and local governments—without federal grants—plan a 42 percent increase in training school capacity by 1975 (U.S. Senate, 1967).

A recent survey of 233 state and local agencies revealed that training schools were being used for various purposes other than those for which they were intended, e.g., as maternity facilities, detention facilities, custodial care for the mentally retarded and/or children with severe psychiatric problems, etc.

This survey revealed that only 12 percent of agencies handling juvenile delinquents had any psychological or psychiatric services available to their probation departments. Where such were available, waiting lists were long. Diagnostic rather than treatment services were generally provided. Foster care and group homes—although seemingly successful probation alternatives—were limited. Group homes were offered by 10 percent of the agencies but cared for only 322 children. There were 4,967 children living in foster care through the auspices of 42 percent of the agencies; however, more than one-half of these children were living in three California counties. Although halfway houses were not evaluated, public opposition to these facilities was noted ("Correction in the United States," 1967).

All types of institutions showed a sharp increase in nonwhite population between 1950 and 1960—a rise of 76 percent in training schools and 92 percent in other types of correctional institutions. Jails, workhouses, reformatories, and prisons reported approximately 35 percent nonwhite adolescent populations (U.S. Dept. of Health, Education, and Welfare, 1965). Of all institutionalized children in 1960, 18 percent of white children as compared to 40 percent of nonwhites were in correctional facilities. This suggests that there are vast inequities in the handling of behavior problems of children from different social and racial backgrounds (Rosen *et al.*, 1968).

The increase in delinquency—particularly among the poor, and especially among the ghetto population—makes imperative a preventive approach. The inability of most correctional institutions to truly rehabilitate delinquents calls for a greater effort to use means which have a greater potential for effectiveness. Noninstitutional community-based programs which encourage youth participation are one such example, especially programs which include training in social competence. Job-training programs also offer potential. However, any such programs must be more than crash efforts which offer hope to disadvantaged youth only to breed further discouragement because funds and manpower are either insufficient or are withdrawn after a short period. Nor can we expect reasonable gains from job-training programs that train for nonexistent jobs (*Report of Task Force VI,* 1968).

At present, prevention and treatment programs are poorly funded, lack coordination, reach only a few, fail to provide individual diagnosis, and lack relationships to the specific problems presented by different individuals (*Report of Task Force V,* 1968).

We must deal directly with the cultural, social, psychological, and economic processes which interact in their effect on the individual and give rise to delinquency. For these purposes, the conventional individual casework and psychotherapeutic approaches are inadequate by themselves (U.S. Senate, 1967). Further, psychiatric intervention, by itself, appears to be ineffective with habitual delinquents. Reviewing the data on delinquency, as related to psychiatric treatment through court-connected child guidance clinics, Rodman and Grams (1967) concluded that efficacious treatment is dependent upon effective diagnosis, upon the placement operation, and upon the treatment programs which are designed for each *type* of delinquent.

It has been demonstrated that the treatment and rehabilitation needs of many children who exhibit delinquent behavior are not different from the needs of children with emotional disorders who are not delinquent. In these terms juvenile delinquency does not describe a child. It is rather a legal and social term.

Use of Drugs

The exact extent of drug use is unknown, partly because of the legal prohibitions against their sale for other than medical purposes. However, surveys on several college campuses indicate that about 20 percent of students have used marijuana at least once and between 2 and 10 percent have tried LSD at least once. Keniston (1967) estimates that about 5 percent of the total student population on college campuses are using drugs. Kifner (1968) reports that drug usage among high school students is becoming extremely widespread.

There is currently widespread public concern regarding the use of drugs. This concern is heightened by lack of sufficient information and by prejudicial attitudes as well as the association of drug use with illegal activities. There is no doubt that this is a grave problem especially among our youth.

It is possible here to present only a few highlights on the subject. In the first place, it is important to recognize that there are many different kinds of drugs and not all of them are highly dangerous or physically addictive. Drugs include the following major categories: narcotics, sedatives, tranquilizers, stimulants, and hallucinogens.

The narcotics include opium, morphine, and heroin, which can produce physical and psychological dependency as well as addiction. These narcotics tend to dull fear, tension, and anxiety. The addict is usually lethargic and indifferent to his environment. Sedatives, which are depressive, have many medical uses, and most are safe and efficient under medical supervision. Phenobarbitol is one exception to this case. This drug can lead to both physical and psychological dependency, and its abuse is more dangerous than alcohol or narcotics abuse. It can lead to intoxication which is much like that produced by alcohol (Smith, Kline and French Laboratories, 1967).

Tranquilizers counteract tensions and anxieties. Although their abuse can lead to physical and psychological dependency, their use has not become "a street problem." The stimulants (amphetamines) do not seem to produce physical dependency but can create psychological dependency in some people. The abusers of these drugs tend to be talkative, restless, and highly excitable.

The hallucinogens, which include marijuana and LSD, produce a sense of euphoria and dreaminess. They do not lead to physical dependency, but psychological dependency on them can lead to lethargy, self-neglect, and little constructive activity. The usual effect of these drugs is to loosen inhibitions, but this does not generally lead to action. LSD affects the central nervous system and produces changes in mood and behavior, but psychological dependency on it appears to be rare. Devotees generally use this drug when it is available but do not develop a serious craving for it. The use of LSD can have serious effects for some people. It has been known to lead to psychoses and both homicidal and suicidal urges. The findings are inconclusive and conflicting as to whether it has genetic effects on the next generation as has been claimed (Smith, Kline and French Laboratories, 1967). Apparently there has been a decline in LSD use since the discovery that it may produce psychoses and possibly chromosomal breaks.

Many people use drugs today with no adverse effects or addiction. Many people use them secretly, others openly. A number of college students use them socially as other people use alcohol (Student Committee on Mental Health of Princeton University, 1967). Some people use drugs in an experimental mood or to meet the pressures of a specific situation. Some of these people, in time, become increasingly adapted to them, and an unknown proportion become addicted (Alskne, Lieberman, and Brill, 1967).

The causes of drug use are multiple and vary according to the drugs, the individual using them, and the situation. Among adolescent users, a number of possible factors are suggested: the psychological strains of adolescence, the adolescent's desire for rebellion, experience, and membership in peer groups, and the alienation of some of today's youth (Alskne, Lieberman, and Brill, 1967).

Those more likely to become addicts may have long-standing psychological problems which include poor interpersonal relationships, early childhood deprivation or overprotection, and fear of the responsibilities of adult life.

Drug addiction probably occurs equally at all socioeconomic levels; however, more affluent individuals are better able to hide it. For low-income groups the pressures of poverty, discrimination, the slum situation, and the culture of disorganized neighborhoods all play a part in creating addictions. This is shown by the fact that the epidemic areas in New York City, where drug use is extremely high, are relatively concentrated settlements of disadvantaged minority groups, mainly Negroes and Puerto Ricans. These areas are marked by poverty, unemployment, disorganized family life, dense population, and highly crowded housing (*Report of Task Force VI*, 1968).

In their study of drug-using youth gangs, Chein, Gerard, and Lee (1964) found that there was less street warfare among those who used drugs.

Drug users were marked by a deep sense of the futility of life. In almost all families of addicts there was a great deal of conflict within the home and lack of warmth between parents and children. The mother in these families was usually the dominant member, and the father had little relationship with either the mother or the children. The few drug users from more stable families were more likely to make frequent efforts to break the habit. Although many delinquent youth used drugs, this use did not cause delinquent behavior except in terms of the need to find money to support the habit.

Despite a Supreme Court ruling (*Robinson* vs. *California,* 370 U.S. 660, 1962) to the effect that criminal punishment for addicts constitutes cruel and unusual punishment, punitive approaches still prevail and proper treatment has been developed only in a few areas. Thus, the punitive atmosphere which the young person experiences in the slums is continually repeated by the larger society. While proper treatment may occur in a few cases, more often youthful addicts are removed and confined, without treatment, to various kinds of penal institutions, only to be released later to the environment which produced their problems in the first place (*Report of Task Force VI,* 1968).

Several preventive approaches to drug use have been suggested, including education about drug use and its dangers, enhanced opportunities for low-income youth, and group and individual counseling. The importance of the educational approach to curbing drug abuse has been particularly emphasized by Dr. Helen Nowlis, director of a drug education project of the National Association of Student Personnel Administrators.

Approaches to treatment include not only controlled detoxification but also psychiatric evaluation and therapy and continued medical supervision and counseling. Community services are needed to help the ex-drug user from slipping back into former patterns and to resist the pressures of his drug-using friends.

A variety of treatment approaches are being used, including Narcotics Anonymous, a volunteer group modeled after Alcoholics Anonymous, and Synanon, a private organization which runs a group of residences for addicts throughout the country which are managed by ex-addicts.

Various drugs are being used which appear to aid the individual in conquering his addiction. These drugs are used in combination with individual and group therapy, remedial education, vocational training, and job placement (Smith, Kline and French Laboratories, 1967).

SUMMARY

Adolescence is not only a time in which physical maturity advances rapidly but also a social and psychological opportunity for significant growth into mature individuality. A comparatively smooth adolescent stage is tied to early and continuous friendly relations and open communication with parents, a sense of positive self-esteem that has developed over the years, and the use of democratic, rather than authoritarian, child-rearing patterns by parents. A relatively calm adolescence is more frequently found among middle- to upper-class youngsters.

On the other hand, many youngsters from poverty backgrounds are likely to have quite a different adolescent experience, handicapped as many are by a complex of depriving and adverse experiences in their past and in their present and by their meager hope for a markedly better future.

It is quite clear that the individual adolescent brings to this stage his entire life history and his own unique biological traits. The young person does not become a different individual simply because he is adolescent, although he may express himself in somewhat different ways at this period as he progresses toward becoming a full adult.

Adolescence is a different process for boys and girls. For boys, there is particular pressure for achievement in sports and the larger world of occupations and advanced education. For girls, the major pressure is for becoming a lovable and marriageable young woman.

Adolescence in our culture seems to be divided into two stages that merge into each other. In early adolescence, the young person is primarily concerned with winning independence from his deep involvement in his family. At a later stage, the average adolescent is more involved in establishing his own place in adult society in terms of his readiness for love, intimacy, and marriage, his employment and career, and his status in the community.

During adolescence these two-way urges become more acute with childhood clearly in the past and adulthood looming on the horizon. In today's society the adolescent has a particularly difficult role to play. His growth, of necessity, is uneven. He is physically mature long before society is ready to give him adult roles; he is intellectually adept long before he has had enough education and training to prepare himself for these roles; he is idealistically motivated long before he is able, through growth and experience, to evolve the principles on which he can realistically and flexibly build his adult life. He is ready for significant participation in society while adults are still demanding that he be a passive, dependent onlooker of a scene that affects him deeply and which is changing too profoundly and rapidly for his adult mentors to understand and manage. These sets of conflicts within and between the generations frequently create an explosive situation.

It is extremely important that adults support the growth of adolescents and youth toward mature individuality and that they provide the services which are essential to this growth: education, employment, physical and mental health, counseling, and recreation. Moreover, these services should include a comprehensive approach to helping the young person prepare more effectively for marriage, work, and parenthood.

Adults must be willing to share power and position with young people. This willingness to share should increase as the young person grows from early adolescence on toward adulthood.

Unless adolescents and youth are allowed to actively participate in the building of a new society, we will witness, in all likelihood, an increase in current trends of youthful protest and violence and/or, conversely, a "tuning out" or turning away from a society which has become too rigidified, too selfish, and too sterile to meet the young person's needs.

Education and the Mental Health of Children and Youth*

THE SCHOOL AS A SOCIAL SYSTEM

Schools as Partners in Mental Health

There is a close association between the child's mental health and his education. Schools have a tremendous potential for enhancing the mental health of all the children who attend them, preventing the development of serious emotional disorders, and improving the condition of those children who are already suffering from such difficulties.

This function is in line with the Commission's philosophy that the mental health of all children is of concern to the community, and that the promotion of positive mental health through education, etc., is just as important as the treatment of specific emotional and mental disorders.

This is not to say that the school is solely responsible for the mental health of all children. Rather, the school is one of many institutions in the community that has this responsibility and opportunity, which it shares with families, physical and mental health services, religious organizations, social service agencies, and youth organizations. At present, one of the problems encountered by the schools is that these various child- and youth-serving systems are uncoordinated and separated one from the other. The

---

* This chapter is limited to a brief presentation of some basic mental health concepts as they might be related to the schools. The reader is also referred to other chapters in this report, especially Chapters IV–VIII and X. No attempt has been made to provide a thorough discussion of the very large field of education itself.

school has tended to develop a host of special services of its own, often without awareness of the other resources in the community.

At present, there are great needs for a better meshing of school and other community programs, for more understanding and trust between the various child- and youth-serving professions, and for a greater involvement of the parents and young people themselves in the whole process of planning and carrying out programs designed to enhance the overall healthy growth and development of young people. One of the functions of the Child Development Council recommended by the Commission might well be the promotion and coordination of child-serving activities that take place within the school and other community agencies.

The Past Multipurpose Tradition of Schools

Traditionally, our schools have been charged with multiple responsibilities for "the whole child." This sense of total responsibility is a result of the school's own tradition and of community expectations, especially the expectations of parents.

This tradition of trying to be all things to all children evolved in rural America and was intensified by the many waves of immigration to this country. The children of these immigrants benefited in important ways through the central responsibility that many schools assumed for them. Although the schools have been subjected to barrages of criticism from all sides, they have, by and large, done a magnificent job over the years in serving many children and youth. It is through the public schools that the huge majority of our children have moved upward to better jobs, enhanced the use of their leisure time, become more informed community participants, and so forth. Education remains the major passport for upward movement to higher occupational and income levels.

However, it is no longer realistic to expect schools to be *the* major child-rearing institution. The task has become too difficult and complex because of the knowledge explosion in all fields and the complexities of today's society, and because other child-caring specialties and systems have developed.

Schools: A Major Target of Criticism

There is a tendency for communities to expect the impossible of schools. Adults approach schools with a very complex set of attitudes and emotions. It appears that we, as adults, both love and hate our schools. Nearly all our citizens have had some childhood experience with the educational system. They bring memories of past triumphs and defeats, past joys and memories, to their present attitudes and expectations. Added to this is the fact that most adults are also parents, and thus school also becomes an object of their hopes and fears for their children. Few parents are able to accept the fact that their children may have problems which largely originate either in the children themselves or within the family. It is common to project children's difficulties onto the school. However, no school, just as no parent, can supply magical solutions to the arduous tasks of growth and development from childhood to maturity. Nevertheless, schools have always been a target of mixed community attitudes of respect and devotion on the one hand and scorn and hostile criticism on the other.

Everyone knows that the schools are in particularly grave difficulty today. There is nothing unique and special about the schools' situation. All our social institutions are in a state of upheaval. All are being criticized and show signs of disorganization. All are burdened with a sense of failure and a loss of morale. This is true of such institutions as the family, the church, and the systems of social welfare, health, employment, communication, housing, transportation, recreation, public safety, and the many levels and departments of government.

Schools Reflect General Social Upheaval

The problems encountered by our systems are fundamentally most related to the vast technological changes that are shaking the very foundations of our society. These changes are so disturbing to the life patterns of all our people that we tend to respond with attacks on such various institutions and the people who run them, rather than recognizing and facing the fundamental problems and the necessity of finding creative, flexible, humane ways of solving the basic issues that confront us. The tendency to scapegoat a particular person or institution, to advocate simplistic solutions, to call for punitive action, is a normal human response to the anxieties bred by crisis. Normal though this response may be, it will only increase our problems in all areas, including those of the schools.

The schools have become the scapegoat, then, for the problems they reflect but do not necessarily create. The schools have become the target for angry protests from all points of the ideological compass and from all sectors of society, ranging from the very old to the young, from the very wealthy to the very poor, from white racists to black power advocates, from inner-city residents to the privileged exurbanites.

These attacks spring, in part, from the stresses engendered by social changes and the impact of these stresses on the mental health of us all. Such attacks also erode the mental health of the people who are responsible for the schools: administrators and teachers alike. This erosion of the psychological well-being of school personnel cannot help but have adverse effects on the children, adolescents, and youth who attend these schools. One aspect of the school and its role in contributing to the mental health of children is the development and maintenance of a healthy environment—both in terms of obvious factors, such as physical safety, and in terms of less obvious ones, such as the nature of the psychological and social principles and practices that guide the school in its dealings with teachers, children, and parents.

The School System and Its Impact on Mental Health

A psychological-social environment which promotes mental health depends upon many factors. These include a school system administered in a democratic way, rather than in an authoritarian or loosely permissive one. Such factors also include a school system which provides teachers with a sense of economic and psychological security, a sense of significance and participation, a sense of challenge and opportunity, and a sense of competence and success. All of these conditions are important in establishing an environment in which teachers can teach and children can learn. The same factors are important ingredients of the kind of teaching which stimulates and promotes the child's mental health and his success as a learner. Teachers cannot employ approaches of this kind, establish a positive mental health climate in the schoolroom, and promote the healthy growth and development of each individual child unless they work in a climate that both promotes the mental health of teachers and allows for sound teaching practices. Moreover, children and youth are not likely to respond to the efforts of a single teacher unless the whole school environment supports the child's sense of significance and individual worth.

The schools cannot establish a democratic environment which promotes mental health unless they are given community support to operate in this way. The schools cannot maintain real democracy when they are pushed in other directions or when they are under extreme pressure to produce impossible results. It is quite obvious that the schools have been under almost impossible and frequently unrealistic pressures in the past twenty years or so.

Current Pressures on the Schools

Pressures on the schools include the following:

1. A huge rise in school population associated with the post-World War II baby boom and increasing school attendance of all, or nearly all, our children and adolescents.

2. Pressures on schools to escalate the achievement levels of the entire child, adolescent, and youth population. These pressures have been a

matter of public policy, especially since 1958, and have also resulted from the rising aspirations of parents and of the young people themselves for higher and higher levels of academic achievement and education beyond high school.

3. Pressures associated with the rural-urban migration which brought with it huge numbers of people from isolated areas who had suffered the severe adversities of poverty and discrimination for many generations (see Chapters IV and V).

4. Pressures associated with the 1954 Supreme Court decision which called for integration in the schools. By now it is apparent that real integration has not occurred and that racism in society is reflected in the schools in such a way as to deny most minority-group children the high-quality education they so desperately need and which they and their parents so increasingly and rightfully demand.

5. The explosion in knowledge and in new kinds of educational techniques which have put tremendous demands on the schools and on teachers for increasing their expertise both in subject matter content and in the understanding and evaluation of new educational methods.

6. Tremendous rises in the cost of education which are associated with the larger numbers of children in schools, the greater numbers going on to high school and advanced education, the mounting costs of buildings, supplies, and teachers' salaries, and the public's rising expectations for high-quality education. These higher costs have been particularly difficult for city schools to bear, since the major financial burden for education is still assumed by localities and cities which have been steadily losing their more affluent residents to the surrounding suburbs. It is, of course, in the metropolitan areas that high-quality education is most critically needed because it is in the cities that the most educationally disadvantaged children dwell.

7. Although the supply of teachers has increased in recent years, there are still severe teacher shortages in many parts of the country. It has been particularly difficult to find teachers with the skill, ability, and willingness to work in the inner-city schools where they are so critically needed.

8. The schools are faced with a new and different child and youth population. These are the postwar young people who have grown up in the automation age. They have suffered the stresses of this age, and most have benefited from its advantages. They bring to schools a new set of strengths and weaknesses that teachers who belong to a different generation have difficulty in understanding (see Chapter II).

9. The schools are faced with the shifts and confusion in values that afflict the rest of society. They are faced with the problems of increasing drug use, more open sex behavior, and rising numbers of delinquents

among their students. Although it is unreasonable for the community to expect the schools to be able to handle all ranges of deviant behavior, many schools feel a responsibility in this regard, and the community frequently demands that the schools "do something about the situation."

Under these multiple pressures it would seem that the schools have done amazingly well in many ways. Perhaps the impressive thing is that they have done as well as they have rather than that they show signs of strains. The schools need community support and understanding if they are to deal effectively with these pressures and with the associated challenges, responsibilities, and opportunities, and make the changes required in our rapidly changing society with its very diverse student populations.

Open Schools in Open Communities

The schools need the support and cooperation of parents, the child-serving institutions, and all sectors of the larger society. Conversely, the schools need to open themselves up to parents, the larger community, and the other human service organizations.

Part of the current crisis in the schools is a crisis in participative democracy. This crisis is one of the roots of both student and parent protests. In this sense, the current conflict and unrest is hopeful. It represents pressure for a democracy that will exist in daily life, rather than a selective democracy that is a reality for some but exists for others only in textbooks and political campaigns.

Real democracy, as was stated, is fundamental to mental health, at least as the Commission has defined mental health in our society. A democracy is real only if it ensures every young person the opportunities and services which will provide him the chance to develop his full potential—physically, socially, psychologically, emotionally—within a democratic framework. This means, among other things, that the schools must be openly receptive to the greater participation of their students and the community. Conversely, it means that school personnel and students must be given a far greater opportunity to participate in community life as a legitimate, living part of the educational function and process.

If children and youth are to have more real contact with adult society and participate in an open school which relates actively to the community, a climate must be fostered to promote experimental approaches. The Commission suggests that new approaches include giving children and young people a chance to participate in the planning and administration of the work of the school (see Chapters VIII and X). It also recommends that schools greatly expand present programs which provide opportunities for children and youth to visit a host of community enterprises; that work-study programs be enlarged (see Chapter I, Section II-E); and that many more adults be encouraged to be actively involved in the work of the school in both salaried and volunteer capacities, such as teachers, tutors, and recreation leaders. In almost every community there are many adults who have special knowledge, abilities, and interests which can enrich the lives of children. These adults could be involved in the life of the school in far more imaginative ways, especially if flexible approaches are adopted which ask for only part-time or occasional participation of men and women who may have busy lives of their own. It is of crucial importance to the mental health of children that these approaches include ways to achieve the active participation of parents from all socioeconomic levels and backgrounds. The closed system of the schools has too frequently excluded parents from any real involvement with the educational enterprise (see Chapter VII, pp. 348–352).

The current trend toward maintaining an open community school after school hours and during the summers should be encouraged and supported. Schools that offer a wide range of recreational and educational programs to adults as well as to children provide a potential means for enhancing the human resources of the larger community. If schools are seen by parents as being related to their own needs as well as to the needs of their children there is a greater likelihood that fathers and mothers will participate more wholeheartedly and knowledgeably in the education of their children. Increased communication between home and school can yield many important benefits, the greatest perhaps being that it can help the child feel that school and home are closely related, that he is not asked to make painful choices between loyalties to teachers and loyalties to parents.

The Child Development Council recommended by the Commission can be an important expediter of helping the school and the community find better ways to relate to each other and helping children, youth, and parents participate in a wide variety of ways in the programs of the school and other facets of community life.

Opening up the Adult World to Children and Youth

For too long now, we have clung to history and tradition and considered the school as a separate society responsible for all aspects of child care. This view of the school has been reinforced by our tendency to seal off children, adolescents, and youth into worlds separate from those of adults. We frequently have taken the irrational and overly protective attitude that children and adolescents are radically different from adults, that they should be shielded from the dangers and pleasures of the adult world, that their (falsely presumed) childish innocence should be preserved. It is obvious, too, that many adults do not want to be burdened with the strains of closely relating to children and dealing with their strong emotions, their high energy levels, and their drive for exploration, mastery, and self-determination. Many adults would rather provide *for* children, as, for example, through the schools, than interact closely *with* them. However, this sealing of children into separate societies leads to a discontinuity in the growth experience, a lack of integration of the many parts of the world into which the child comes into contact, twisted perceptions of reality, and a learned incapacity to relate to adults. The only effective way to prepare children and youth for adult society is to give them increasing opportunities to have contact with it, to share in many aspects of community life, and to have a more open, realistic learning experience in school.

Opening up the Curriculum

More realistic and appropriate preparation for adult life as worker, citizen, and family member must include an opening up of the curriculum of the schools so that it deals more realistically and honestly with many phases of contemporary child and adult life. Teachers should have a larger role in curriculum development, specifically in relation to the particular children and young people they are teaching, rather than being forced to accept curriculum materials that are determined by the school system as a whole (*Report of Task Force II*, 1969). Some schools are pioneering in bringing students into the curriculum-building process. Studies are being related to the actual lives of the children through current events as reported on television and in the daily newspapers, classroom and community activities undertaken by the students, and the like.

Opening up the curriculum so that it truly engages the interests and experiences of children and youth means that more open communication must exist in the schools. There must be greater provision for children and young people to express themselves openly through increased freedom in speech, in writing, in play, and in other forms of expression such as music, drama, and art. If teachers are required to keep rigid control over the speech and other forms of behavior of children and young people, it is likely that most youngsters will continue to view school as boring, repressive, and unrelated to the important things they are thinking and wanting to learn.

Teachers as Whole, Participative Adults

Opening up the school also includes a more open way of selecting, training, supporting, and encouraging teachers to be fully effective adults who participate freely in the life of the school and community. Just as we tend to seal off children and young people in the separate community of the school, so we tend to seal off teachers from being whole persons. This practice has adverse effects on their teaching and on the kind of model they present to children of what it is like to be an adult. In order to promote the functioning of teachers as effective, whole adults, a number of approaches are suggested:

1. As already mentioned, it is imperative that schools be democratically administered and that teachers operate in a climate in which they participate as full-fledged citizens with clearly defined rights and clearly defined responsibilities.

2. At present, many teachers are trained for their professions largely through lectures and classroom drills. Through this experience they tend to teach in the same constricted way in which they have been taught. Much more emphasis should be placed on a breadth of experiences for student teachers in working with many kinds of children and youth in many kinds of classrooms and, also, in becoming involved in the community. These experiences should be closely related to seminars in which there is full opportunity for free discussion of their learning, their reactions, and their observations *(Report of Task Force II, 1969)*.

3. It is important that greater recognition be given to the fact that teachers are human beings with their own stages of development, their own life situation, their own orders of interests, feelings, and attitudes. Thus, in both teacher training and the supervision of teachers on the job, more attention should be paid to their need for social and psychological support for the difficult tasks they are undertaking. This is not to imply that schools of education or supervisory personnel in schools should engage in providing therapy for teachers. Personal counseling and therapy are another matter; however, such personal counseling should be made readily available to teachers if they should wish it, at little or no cost, since the mental health of teachers is so importantly related to the mental health of the children with whom they work.

4. Teachers should be regarded as full-fledged professionals working in partnership with other professionals, such as the mental health specialists. There is a tendency to downgrade teachers as being less competent and knowledgeable than specialized mental health personnel. It should be recognized that teachers have their own particular specialization. Potentially, they have a great deal to offer in terms of their own observations and experiences with children in joint consultation with such specialists as psychiatrists, psychologists, social workers, guidance counselors, school nurses, and the like. Each of these professionals plays a particular role. The child's needs will be best met through joint consultation and joint planning based on mutual respect between the different members of the professional team.

5. The work of different teachers should be made far more flexible.

Within a school faculty each teacher has special interests and strengths. Some teachers are particularly adept at curriculum-building, some at working with individual children, some at conducting discussions, some at teaching particular subjects. Teachers should be encouraged to play different roles at different times, and experimentation along these lines should be carried out and combined with evaluation of the results in which the teachers and children participate *(Report of Task Force II,* 1969).

6. The practice of using many kinds of aides in the classroom and other parts of the school should be encouraged. Children, adolescents, youth, parents, and others who are interested in the schools can participate in a host of ways to enrich school programs and free the teacher for specialized educational roles.

The School Administrator

The principal and administrative staff in the past have not been chosen from the curriculum and subject-oriented teachers but primarily from among those who could control children. All studies done on schools indicate the need for using educators as administrators.

Men and Women in the Schools

Over the years, most of the schools have become largely feminine enterprises. The reasons for this situation are economic, historical, and cultural. Traditionally, women teachers have been willing to work for less pay than men teachers. Thus the schools, especially the elementary schools, have become largely feminine institutions. This has been far more typical in the United States than in other industrial nations and has been considered a problem, particularly in relation to the education of boys, for more than fifty years *(Report of Task Force II,* 1969).

There is abundant evidence that this feminization of the schools has had particularly adverse effects on boys. We have already noted that many more boys of elementary school age are brought to mental health clinics than are girls; that they show a greater need for remedial reading; and, as compared to girls, a greater probability of failing in all grades of the elementary school and of dropping out before finishing high school. There are clues from research that this situation does not have to exist and that the psychological climate of the school can be an important factor in reducing the emotional and academic problems of boys (see also Chapter VII).

Commission members recommend that every effort be made to increase the number of males in the teaching profession. "Increases in salaries are not enough to attract and hold men in teaching. With greater part in responsible decision making, with the organization of responsible power in teacher groups for goal-directed behavior, teacher morale could be sufficiently enhanced to offset the imbalance in the sex ratio of the faculty of our public schools" (*Report of Task Force II*, 1969).

Education: Addressed to the Intellect Alone?

There is considerable confusion about the role of the schools in meeting the needs of each child. Some experts proclaim that the school is specifically and exclusively an educational institution, that its job is to impart knowledge and information, develop learning skills, and prepare children for further education and eventual employment. Subject matter is emphasized, and teacher preparation is seen in terms of making teachers academic specialists in their particular knowledge field. This emphasis has been particularly popular in the past ten years or so. Some of the proponents argue that the mental health component of this approach is to increase the child's competence as a learner. This increase in competence gives him a greater sense of mastery, power, and self-confidence which positively affects his mental health (Bower, 1960). The school may recognize that other problems exist for children but see their role as being specifically in the intellectual-rational realm. The proponents of this approach proclaim that concern for emotional and social problems of students are the function of the mental health personnel and other specialists and not of the classroom teacher.

On the other hand, there are also many experts who emphasize that education cannot be effectively carried out when it is addressed only to the rational, intellectual side of the child. Integrated learning which is lasting and usable to the child must be addressed to his emotional and social needs as well as to his intellectual and rational ones. Also, if learning is to promote creativity, flexibility, resourcefulness, and individuality, it must be carried out in such a way that the child has access to the rich world of his feelings and total life experience. Furthermore, it is impossible to overlook the fact that the child brings his whole life to school with him. This deeply affects his abilities, interests, and motivations, which play so large a part in his effective learning. It is not really possible to overlook all aspects of the child's physical, emotional, and social background and functioning if one truly wants the child to be able to learn to his maximum capacity—to learn not only for the present or for the taking of tests but for permanent, integrated learning that will have meaning to him in his future life. One way of conceptualizing this approach of combining the emotional and the intellectual aspects of the child's life is presented by Biber in the *Report of Task Force II* (1969):

Range and depth of sensitivity to world around

Differentiated, discriminating perception as basis for action and interaction.

Attitude that there is an open, varied world all around which invites penetration; experience to be probed and unravelled; human interchange across wide range of emotion.

Openness to receive and react, etc.

Cognitive power and intellectual mastery of the symbolic systems of word and number

Search for relationships among discrete elements of experience.

Re-organization of perceptual meanings to larger order concepts and generic meanings.

Conceptual mastery of experiential elements.

Competence in the logos of our society, etc.

Synthesis—integrating across cognitive and affective domains

Outcome of learning experience which takes symbolic expressive form.

Transformation of some part of child's encounter with the outer world that reflects and utilizes the forces—the cumulated meanings, feelings, wishes, conflicts—of his inner life of impulse and affect.

Integration of diverse stimuli, general intimacy with non-rational processes as basic to creativity.

Differentiated interaction with people

Availability of variety of modes of communication, verbal and non-verbal.

Use of interchange with people as source for understanding commonness of human feelings and conflicts as well as mode of emotional refreshment.

Experience with peers for joint productivity and building codes of interpersonal relationship.

Relating to adults, selecting, as part identification figures.

Adaptation to requirements of social situations

Acceptance of denial for sake of alternate fulfillment.

Adherence to rules and regulations as protection of learning.

Internalization of regulating codes.

Recovery from frustration or failure.

Mergence of individual drive with group purposes.

Self-understanding

Depth and range of acquaintance with self.

Reality of expectations and aspirations.

Identity as an individual.

Moral judgment

The School Is Not a Mental Health Institution, But It Does Have a Mental Health Role

The above comments and conceptualizations do not mean that the school is a therapeutic institution. The function of the school is not to treat emotional and mental problems any more than it is to treat physical ones, but it does have a role in understanding these problems, taking them into account in methods of teaching, styles of relating to the child, ways of discipline, and expectancies for the youngster, and in the development of a curriculum tailored to the student's interests and abilities. Although the school is not a therapeutic institution, its ways of working with individual children may well have either positive or negative therapeutic effects depending on the skill and sensitivity of teachers and depending on the availability of needed helping resources.

Besides taking the characteristics of the individual child into account, the school has a role in being alert to possibly serious problems that he may present, in seeking consultation for these problems, in working in partnership with treatment specialists and parents, and in referring children and their parents to specialized services, as these services seem indicated.

A sensitive teacher can make a difference in the life of a child. One such teacher commented on what was learned about a child by reviewing the cumulative records of the school and by the biography that one youngster wrote when he was in the eighth grade. According to teachers' comments about this boy, there was almost unanimous agreement that he was a serious problem, a poor learner, and an all-around undesirable student. There was one exception to these reports. The fifth-grade teacher wrote, "Billy is really an unhappy, neglected child. At first, he was a serious behavior problem in my classroom. As I came to know him better and realized how much he needed success and kindliness, I found that his behavior problems disappeared and that he made good progress in his school work." Billy wrote in his biography: "I have always hated school. All of my teachers were down on me and thought I was dumb. The one thing I wanted to do was not have to go to school at all—except for the fifth grade. I had a good teacher then who liked me. School was fun and I learned a lot in that grade."

Individual Growth and Development and the School

In Chapters VII and VIII we traced some of the outstanding social and psychological features of individual growth and development from infancy through young adulthood. The research findings and concepts that were detailed in these chapters have been applied by many schools and should apply to educational practice in general.

Chapter VII dealt with the importance of the early years of life to all aspects of development, including intellectual development. We recommended that much more attention be given to children from infancy through age three. The Child Development Council and the child advocate system recommended by the Commission could play a particularly critical role in this respect. The Head Start preschool program, although not designed for very young children, was devised largely because of the growing recognition that the early years of life are of basic importance to the child's adjustment to the school situation. Evaluation of the results of Head Start are somewhat confusing and fail to give clear-cut answers to indicate that an enriched preschool experience makes a significant difference in the child's readiness and ability to learn in school. However, some controlled studies indicate that regular kindergarten and first grade are not designed for these children. The demands made upon children in these traditional schools may have adverse effects or negate gains made in Head Start.

Problems both in the research design and in the great diversity of Head Start programs may account, to a great extent, for the lack of straight-forward proof that this program had a beneficial effect on the total group of children who attended it. (See also Chapter XI on research.) This should not suggest that such programs be abandoned. It suggests rather that they should be strengthened and extended, that further careful evaluation should be applied to different kinds of programs serving different kinds of children, and that special enriching education should be continued at least through the elementary school years. It would be fallacious, indeed, to assume that a few months or years of early enriched education alone could make up for the many disabilities and handicaps of poverty and racism. Unless we find ways to greatly strengthen the educational and other supportive services for such children, a large proportion will be condemned to school failures, followed by later problems in employment, community membership, and family life.

In general, we may find that high-quality preschool programs have a measurable, positive effect on all or nearly all children, not merely those who have been educationally handicapped in their earliest years. Further experimentation and evaluation in this field is important. However, it seems premature to assume, at this point, that *every* child will benefit from a preschool experience. Attention should be given both to the quality of the experience and to the characteristics of individual children and their families. For example, some very young children are particularly sensitive and easily overwhelmed by group experiences and may not benefit from such programs. Also, some parents especially enjoy their preschool children and are particularly competent in providing many enriching experiences for them in their own homes.

As the child moves through school, teachers and other members of the school staff should continue to be aware of the individual characteristics of each child as well as the special aspects of children at different developmental stages. However, since each child goes through each stage in his own unique way, it is important that simplistic assumptions not be made that a child behaves in a certain way because he is a certain age. A more dynamic view of behavior is called for, one which recognizes the many complexities of interacting forces within the child or young person and his relationship with others and the total environment.

Poor Kids in Poor Schools

The severe problems of children whose lives have been damaged by poverty and/or discrimination have been presented in considerable detail in Chapters IV and V. We have shown how the situations of poverty and racism have undermined the capacities of families and children to deal effectively with the social systems of the more affluent, white society. It is well known that such children tend to come to school with many physical, mental, and emotional handicaps that lessen their ability to adjust and learn in the usual school environment. The problems of these children are greatly escalated by the pressures encountered by most of the schools they attend. However, it has been found that the problems of inner-city schools and of the children who attend them are not unique; they are merely extreme examples of the problems encountered by most schools and by many children and youth at all levels of society (*Report of Task Force II*, 1969). In general, our schools need to be upgraded. New approaches are required if we are to develop better educational methods adapted to today's young people and today's society.

There is a danger of stereotyping children from poverty and/or minority-group backgrounds and of assuming that they will be poor learners and present behavior problems. This kind of assumption tends to become a self-fulfilling prophecy.

Solutions have not been found to meet the needs of many of these youngsters. Many of the suggestions given earlier in this chapter would seem to be particularly relevant to inner-city schools and their children. Moreover, just as it has been found that disadvantaged youths who are being trained for jobs need a multiple of supporting services before effective training and job placement can take place, so it would appear that children of poverty would be in particular need of supporting services beyond those which the school alone can supply. (See also Chapter X.)

Low-income families are frequently blamed for not providing the physical care, emotional support, and intellectual enrichment that youngsters need in order to profit from the school experience. However, families that are harassed by the crisis of poverty can hardly be expected to provide ideal care for their youngsters. These families need a whole range of supports: income, health care, day care, homemaker, housing, and other services so that they can create a more adequate home for their children. The child advocate system recommended by the Commission can be a strong force in mobilizing and ensuring these services for children.

Many schools are adopting a number of experimental approaches to working more effectively with youngsters of poverty backgrounds. For example, some behavioral scientists are finding that they can achieve remarkable results in helping extremely difficult children control their diffuse aggression and associated inability to learn by planning a series of rewards for specific pieces of desired behavior and by overlooking destructive behavior. These experimenters report that the children not only behave and learn better but seem to be far happier than they were before they could control their aggression. But however useful one approach appears, there cannot and will not be a simple, one-factor, easy solution to these difficulties. It is strongly recommended that evaluation be built into these experiments together with flexible, open-minded attitudes.

Temporary Disturbances in Children and Adolescents

It is important that school personnel be aware of the temporary but frequently disturbing upsets in the lives of their young students. As we have pointed out earlier, it is estimated that 10 to 12 percent of children in elementary school are suffering from psychoses or serious emotional disorders. Beyond this group are those 20 percent or more who experience temporary upsets. (Actually, this group is probably far larger than has been generally recognized.) These upsets may relate to family crises, to critical periods of growth in the child, or to problems that the child may have experienced in his neighborhood or school. If communication is open between teachers and students and if schools have ready contact with families, there is much greater likelihood that teachers and other personnel will have a deeper awareness of the difficulties that children are facing and that they will make allowances for these stressful periods.

Some critical periods in the child's life are likely to arise with the entry into the first grade, the shift from elementary school to junior high school, and movement into high school. It is extremely important that the child's early experiences in school be good ones. His attitudes toward himself as a learner and toward the school as a place for learning are being significantly shaped at this time. The shift from home to school requires great inner resources on the part of the child. It means he must give up some of his early dependence on his parents, face the world away from the protection of home, test himself with his peers, and encounter a strange environment filled with the terror of the unknown. Warm, supporting teachers who are sensitive to the child's reactions can make a great difference in helping the youngster bridge the perilous gap between home and school. Close relationships between the teachers and parents are also particularly desirable during these transition years.

During the junior high years, developmental differences in children are particularly great. It is recommended that schools be more flexible in their classroom and activity grouping of children so that they not be put into rigid and age-specific categories. This kind of flexibility is probably most important during the junior high years when there are such differing levels among youngsters in social and physical maturity.

Children with Emotional and Mental Disorders

Although the school is not a therapeutic institution, it can and should do much more than is currently done for disturbed children. According to the *Report of Task Force II* (1969), teachers should be exposed to various degrees of disturbed behavior within the classroom during their training years. This should include an emphasis on new techniques of remediation. Later during their career years, teachers should have realistic mental health consultation available. Realism in this sense means mental health consultants who themselves understand the world of education and the problems of the school system. This recommendation assumes concurrent changes and increased collaboration among education and mental health systems at national, state, and local levels. Collaborative consultation would also reduce the unnecessary polarization of therapy and education which now exists in the schools.

Preparing teachers to deal with a variety of individuality in children as well as with different degrees of disturbance would render less necessary the placement of children in special classes for the emotionally disturbed. The Task Force wishes to register unequivocal disapproval of the present custodial nature of many special classes for emotionally disturbed children, while it recognizes the necessity for special classes for children with particular handicaps. Where special classes for emotionally disturbed children are actually classes for psychotic children, the true purpose of these classes should be kept in mind; euphemisms such as "educationally handicapped" obscure the nature of these classes and make it more difficult to think clearly about their value.

The essential failure of special classes for emotionally disturbed children to reduce "the size of the problem" added to the increased tendency to commit children to state mental hospitals for lack of any other alternative and the disadvantages of commitment to detention centers cause us to recommend the establishment of day care and residential centers for the severely emotionally disturbed. We conceive of day care and residential centers as intermediary structures in the community, standing between hospitals and schools. Such centers would be based on flexible admission and discharge arrangements so that children could stay for brief or long periods of time, for day or total care, and would not find their return into the community hampered by elaborate administrative procedures. The Re-ED Project serves as a good model for such intermediary residential and day care centers. It would be desirable if such centers were more closely identified with educational and public health agencies than with courts or hospitals. This recommendation reflects our concern with the adverse effects of excluding children from the mainstream of the life of the school (*Report of Task Force II*, 1969).

Mental Health Services in the Schools

Specialized services related to the mental health of children have been established in many of our nation's schools. The exact nature of these services varies from community to community, state to state. They reflect the growing body of knowledge related to the many factors that affect a child's school adjustment and ability to learn. They also reflect the concern of the school that specialized services be quickly available, as needed, in the school setting and that these services be closely coordinated with other parts of the educational enterprise, such as teacher methods, attitudes, and behavior; curriculum development; school administrative policies and practices, and the like.

These services frequently include staff specialists such as guidance counselors, school psychologists, school social workers, psychiatric consultants, school physicians and nurses, remedial speech and reading specialists, etc. Ideally, such staff members operate as a team and work closely with one another, other members of the school staff, parents, and children. A problem often encountered in this area is that of inadequate coordination of services, duplication of effort, and misunderstandings between the various professional groups. Also, professionals frequently have too rigid a view of their own particular specialized roles and functions. A broader, more flexible way of working is preferred, one which is based on the concepts of child development approach.

This approach is basic to the work of all mental health specialists concerned with the schools. A mental health service related to the school needs to include people who are capable of bridging the gap between the community and the school, bringing together the child and the curriculum, consulting on the learning and behavior of children with other school personnel, communicating and translating mental health concepts to the teacher, working with the teacher so that he can function in his classroom more effectively, and working with parents on a variety of child-rearing problems. Knowledge of ways of performing these functions does not need to be the particular specialty of any one professional group. They can be performed or shared by all, depending on the person's individual skill, experience, and training.

Schools should carefully appraise their present approach to the development and use of specialized mental health services. As indicated earlier in this chapter, many of today's communities have a wide range of specialized services for children and youth. These services should be coordinated with those of the school. Duplication and separation between the school and other community services should be avoided. It is often argued that community agencies outside of the school fail to understand educational issues and thus their treatment suggestions for children cannot be applied well to the school setting. However, professionals from these other organizations are not likely to learn how their services to children and families can be coordinated with those of the school unless a free and open communication system is established between school and other agency personnel. There is no good reason why all child- and youth-serving professionals should not be given an opportunity to develop deeper understandings about today's educational system, just as there is no good reason why teachers and other school personnel should not be given an opportunity to learn more about the work of community agencies in mental health-related fields.

Our children would also benefit if more attention were paid to the common core of knowledge in the human service fields—medicine, education, psychology, social work, religion, and recreation.

Students preparing for these various fields might well be trained together in such courses as human growth and development, community organization, principles of mental health, and the like. In-service training and institutes for working professionals could also be conducted across the various professional disciplines. Sharing of common training experiences might well promote closer cooperation among the professionals who serve children and youth. After all, the overall well-being of our young people is, or should be, *the* major focus of professional activity. With this common concern and commitment, the various professions should be spurred to adopt the flexibility and openness of approach that is necessary if we are to improve the quality of the human services which are so essential to our young.

SOME SPECIAL CONSIDERATIONS

Mental Health Content in the School Curriculum

Expert opinion ranges on many sides of the question as to whether or not there should be mental health content in the curriculum, one which might also include family life and sex education. Programs of this sort were quite popular during the 1940's and 1950's but were frequently discontinued after 1958, when public policy and opinion swung strongly toward emphasizing academic content in the schools and deemphasizing the so-called "soft life adjustment classes." It seems entirely appropriate to introduce into the curriculum of elementary and secondary schools new theories and knowledge from the social and behavioral sciences which are, indeed, closely related to concepts of mental health and society. There is considerable disagreement about the extent to which such content should be personalized in terms of dealing with the specific problems of individual children. It is probably more appropriate to present this material in a more generalized fashion and to avoid a discussion of specific problems raised by specific students. This is an area in which it is important for teachers to be clear about their roles as educators rather than therapists. However, in teaching such courses, teachers should be alert to individual problems of children and young people. Teachers should also be aware of the importance of seeking mental health consultation and/or referring the young people for special mental health services. When these matters are opened up for discussion and a positive school climate in which human and social problems are realistically accepted is established, young people may find themselves readier for specialized help than they might otherwise be. In general, most students are likely to feel that these subjects are closely related to the real issues that they are facing in their daily lives. That is, they are likely to feel this way if the teacher has such traits and skills as the psychological warmth, openness, and knowledgeability that are requisite to the teaching of this subject and, indeed, to the teaching of all subjects.

Although some experts have great enthusiasm for the teaching of courses of this kind, it should be pointed out that there is no research evidence which indicates that these courses have a measurable impact on the values and behaviors of young people. Feelings and attitudes toward such matters as dating, courtship, mate selection, marriage, and sexual behavior are complex and are deeply rooted in the total life experience of the young person. Related behaviors do not yield readily to change through educational approaches. This is not to deny that these courses may have positive effects; however, it suggests that in this instance, as in others, one cannot expect education alone to markedly affect the whole complex of factors that underlie human behavioral outcomes.

It is important that the shortcomings of relying solely on education be understood. Too often the community expects the schools to "do something" about such problems as drugs, delinquency, and sex behavior. While the school has a role in educating students on such matters as drug use, legal restraints on behavior, and the various aspects of sex behavior, it cannot be expected to "control the problem" alone.

School and the Teaching of Values

As pointed out in Chapter VII, the moral development of the child is of great importance and has recently received renewed attention from researchers in the behavioral sciences. For a variety of reasons, the public schools have tended to avoid the issue of teaching moral values. This practice is, no doubt, closely related to the separation of church and state in this country. It is also associated with the position held by social scientists that values are deeply rooted in the total life experience of the individual and are related to his particular ethnic, national, social class, and religious background. Therefore, the school should avoid "interfering" in such matters. Such a value-free, objective position is a tradition that has been extolled as the scientifically correct one for serious scholars. Furthermore, there has been a reaction against the earlier tendencies of teachers to take a judgmental position toward the behavior of children and youth and to try to impose their own moral beliefs upon them.

Although it is entirely inappropriate for teachers to espouse a particular set of values which they ask their students to assume, it *is* appropriate for the schools to encourage children and young people to freely discuss moral principles and values. These are matters which deeply concern the adolescent. Through open discussion, young people can gain a better appreciation and understanding of the diversity of values among their peers and also examine their own principles more critically.

Although many would disagree, it would seem appropriate for teachers to share their moral principles with their students if they make it clear that these *are* their personal values and that the students are not obligated in any way to accept them. One of the reasons for this suggestion is that teachers provide students with images of what it is like to be an adult. If the student perceives the teacher as having no basic moral values and principles which are of importance to him and upon which he builds his life, the student may conclude that this is a desirable style of adult living. However, if teachers do share their own values with their students and declare that these are their own and are not to be copied uncritically by others, such declarations may not be sufficient. It is also crucial that teachers not communicate in any fashion that they believe there are deficiencies in the moral beliefs of their various students and their families. Such criticism may tend to force the youngster into conflicting loyalties between home and school. This kind of conflict creates highly undesirable discontinuities within the child or young person between his life in the school and his life in his home.

All in all, it is suggested that more attention be given in teacher training to a consideration of the principles and dynamics of moral development in children and youth and to an examination of the moral beliefs held by the teacher or student teacher himself. Perhaps one of the problems in today's society is that too strong an emphasis has been placed on a detached, value-free position rather than an appropriate emphasis on the centrality of integrated moral principles as an important component in the life of all human beings.

SUMMARY

The schools possess an enormous potential for affecting the mental health of our children and youth. They can be an effective agent in the prevention of emotional and mental disorders and the promotion of the young person's healthy growth and development, through effective education and meaningful curricula and through remedial services provided in cooperation with other community agencies.

The school, like all our social institutions, is showing alarming signs of strain. Everyone, or almost everyone, criticizes the schools at the same time that they expect almost miraculous feats from them. Upheavals in the schools are fundamentally related to social stresses in our society.

These stresses include such factors as: the enormous growth in our child and youth population; the rising demands that schools successfully educate all youngsters at higher and higher levels of competence; the problems of the inner city engendered by poverty, racism, massive population shifts, and the loss of an adequate tax base; the shortage of highly qualified teachers; the critical link between educational achievement and occupational success; current shifts and confusion about values; and deficits in needed human services of all kinds.

In general, schools need to open up their doors to the community—and the community should open its doors to the schools. Children and youth stand to gain from such a process. Their education should be deeply and immediately related to life and all its opportunities to learn about the realities of living in today's society. School is meant to prepare youngsters for adult life. Such preparation is bound to be distorted and inadequate if it is conducted in a closed social system. Opening up the school to the larger society also means opening up the curriculum to the issues of living in today's world. It requires changes in the expectancies and attitudes we have toward teachers and other school personnel to accord them the rights and freedom we give other professional adults. It calls for greater flexibility and experimentation in school practices and for expanding the work opportunities for men in the field of education.

Democratic procedures are closely associated with the mental health of the schools and of those persons associated with them. The total environment of the school deeply affects the child's mental health in all its aspects: physical, social, emotional, and intellectual.

Our school system must devote specific attention to children with particular problems, including those related to emotional and mental disorders. To the maximum extent possible, these children should be kept in the mainstream of the school's life, not shunted off to special schools or classes. To help meet this problem, greater support should be given to providing teachers and parents consultation from mental health specialists.

Employment: Problems and Issues Related to the Mental Health of Children and Youth

Work and Mental Health

The mental health of our children and youth is closely associated with the preparation that home, school, and community gives them for a smooth entry into the world of work. The gradual growth and development of children from infancy through adolescence is primarily directed toward becoming a competent, healthy adult who is able to cope effectively with reality and to find satisfaction and challenge in living and working, either in the home or on the job. In our society, work has long been considered a central feature of every adult's life. Although the relevance of this tradition in a postindustrial society is now being questioned, occupational achievement and success are still necessary for the great majority of people, not only as a means of family care and support but for a sense of status and significance.

It is of particular importance to a man's sense of identity, although this is also becoming increasingly true for many women, especially after their children become older.

Despite the centrality of work to most adults, we do little in our society to prepare children and adolescents for their future occupational roles. This is related to changes in society which have moved occupations out of farms, homes, and neighborhoods and into factories, large business firms, professional offices, and the like.

Until the latter part of the nineteenth century, most American children grew up in homes which were close to the occupational lives of their parents and, indeed, often went to work themselves at an early age. Especially as business and industry grew larger, more mechanized, and more impersonal, children and youth were frequently exploited as employees. In a move to protect them from this exploitation and to give them a better chance for more years of education, child labor and compulsory education laws were passed. While these have yet to be extended to all children, especially those of migrant workers, such laws were important gains for most children. However, we may have gone too far in protecting children and keeping them away from the dangers of overexposure to work.

We have tended, in this country, to create separate age-specific societies for our young at school, in religious and recreational groups, and in the neighborhood. This practice has probably been enhanced by growing recognition during the past century that children are not just miniature adults. They have particular capacities, needs, and interests related to each developmental stage, and it is important that the special nature of these be recognized. It is equally important to recognize the fact that children are not radically different from adults, that they are young people in the process of slowly growing toward adulthood. This growth process should be continuous and related to their future status. We, however, have created discontinuity by our overinsistence on cutting them off from the many aspects of adult society, including the occupational sphere.

The Need for a Developmental Theory of Work

The mere fact of working, more than the type of work involved, has an impact on the development of the early adolescent or preadolescent (Engel *et al.*, 1967). But work, as we noted, is no longer an expected role for children in our society. However, many view work as salutary for children, and particularly for youth, as long as it does not take the form of child abuse. Work is viewed as beneficial in terms of developing the adolescent's sense of self-respect, accomplishment and competency, the management of time, and sense of responsibility to outside authority, and as valuable in developing an overall appropriate understanding of and orientation toward work.

However, there have been few studies that have investigated the psychological implications of early work experience, and we have yet to scientifically determine the effects. Generally, those interested in the vocational behavior of children have studied such preemployment variables as occupational preference, aspiration, and expectation, and recently there has been some investigation into the developmental aspects of the process of occupation selection (Holland, 1964). However, there have been few conceptual tools produced which are appropriate to the study of working children. Studies of adults have focused primarily on worker productivity and satisfaction, the relationship of personality characteristics to occupational group membership, or the relationship of specific occupational groups to the larger social structure. These approaches are inapplicable to the study of working children, primarily because the variety of jobs open to children is severely constricted, and occupational group membership below the age of fourteen lacks stability.

One study, in attempting to evaluate the work experiences of young Caucasian boys aged eight to fourteen, developed five variables that when grouped together represented an individual boy's work style (Engel *et al.*, 1967). These included the degree to which work provided a means of living out a sense of identity for the youngster, the degree to which the boy attempted to control the conditions of his work, the degree to which he expressed an interest in future vocational activities, the span of time covered in the boy's consideration of his future, and his investment in adult relationships which would not exist if he were not working. Surprisingly few of the subjects had an occupational orientation, and they did not appear to have considered how their work could have implications for their future vocation. However, in general, when these boys thought about their future, they did so in terms of vocational activities, even though their reasoning was grossly inaccurate or lacked conviction. Little is known about the basis of occupational preferences in early adolescence. Plans for careers formulated in the eighth or ninth grade are only moderately useful in predicting occupational activities or career plans a year or two after high school.

This concept of work style, that is, the manner in which children behave at work, should aid in our understanding of the developmental processes of vocational behavior in childhood and promote an understanding of the choice of an adult occupation as a mode of personality expression. Such research is needed on the relationship of the growing-up process to vocational behavior in childhood and to eventual occupational selection and satisfaction. This is particularly needed, since the choice of a specific occupation is so overdetermined by life circumstances, luck, opportunity, and unpredictable setbacks.

Another study conducted in Boston of a representative sample of working boys of all races below the age of fourteen found that an astonishingly high number—73 percent—of these boys stated that they had worked at one time for strangers for pay (Engel *et al.*, 1968). At the time of the questionnaire, 47 percent claimed to be working, indicating that child work may be more prevalent than expected. These boys worked before and after school hours. This study showed that race had no significant relationship to child work, but that socioeconomic level did. The highest proportion of working boys was found to be in the lower-middle and upper-lower levels, rather than in the more affluent upper-middle or the poorest lower-lower class. If child work was a matter entirely of economic necessity, those in the lowest level would have had the highest proportion of workers. However, other factors, such as the availability of jobs and attitudes toward work, may override the need for money. In this study, the model age for beginning work was about ten, regardless of social class. This study therefore indicates that whereas whether a boy works may be primarily determined by social class, the age of starting work may be developmentally determined. It further pointed out the fact that child work is not a random phenomenon and that boys who work between the ages of nine and fourteen differ in a number of ways from their peers.

There is a need to know more about the mental health correlates of early work experiences, as combination work-school programs are increasingly being posed as part of the solution to our youth unemployment-job preparation problem. In both adult and youth working situations there is a need to look into ways in which employment contributes to mental as well as physical health. The nation is moving in the direction of viewing the goals and functions of the work experience as more than an avoidance of poverty, insecurity, and illness. We are looking at ways to progressively advance worker well-being in keeping with the continuously rising aspirations and expectations throughout our society. Experiences in the work force have differing and complex effects on the individual's various roles—as a school attendant, a family member, a social participant, or a political and community decision-maker. The quality of employment has a major effect on the quality of the individual's life in general and subsequently on his children's attitudes and opportunities for satisfying work situations.

Although the meaning of work to an adolescent is undoubtedly influenced by the meaning of work to those in the parental role, we do not know fully what the function of the parent is in preparing children for work—whether through education, training, or as role models. In the Boston study of working boys previously cited (Engel et al., 1968), there was no relationship between child work and mother's employment. Nor did being the child of foster parents account for any differences. However, there was a significant relationship between father absence and child work. Further refinement of this relationship is needed; however, it does indicate that the absence of a father may have a strong bearing on whether or not a boy works before the age of fourteen. Research on the complex interrelationships among the characteristics of the individual, his family and environment, and his job, as well as the attitude toward work that is passed to the child, needs to be expanded. Planning designed to improve the mental health of youth must encompass their experience in, and preparation for, the world of work and its relationship to the developmental process. The act of working does have an impact on the identity formation of the child, and we must find ways to enhance this process.

Some Directions for Change

The Commission is not suggesting that children and young adolescents should enter the regular labor market. However, more thought should be given to how they may be exposed, more realistically and thoroughly, to the many ways in which people in today's society earn a living. This exposure to the modern work world should become increasingly broad and intensive as the youngster grows older. It should include attention to the masculine and feminine roles required for family life and homemaking as well as occupations outside the home.

New ways must be found to integrate work as a natural part of a child's life, along with education and play. This effort should begin early in the school years, starting at the preschool level. Children should be encouraged to participate in the normal, ongoing work of school, home, neighborhood, recreational, and religious settings. Opportunities for work experiences should be broadened and intensified as the child grows older.

Such an approach would be a radical one for this country at this point in time, but it is well worth considering. It has much to recommend it from a mental health point of view as being one of a number of approaches to helping children and youth grow more competently, comfortably, and knowledgeably into adulthood.

Preparation for work, choice of a vocation, obtaining employment, and vocational development represent central tasks for most of our youth, both male and female. Most young people would be greatly benefited by preventive programs designed to facilitate their growth and development and enhance their full potential as workers as well as members of families and communities. There are some groups, however, who need remedial programs to help them resolve immediate unemployment or underemployment problems.

Since the threat of unemployment and underemployment is the more immediate and critical one for about one-fourth or more of the nation's youth, some examination of this issue is in order.

Prevalence of Problems

Although the United States requires a larger proportion of its children to remain in school for a longer period of time than does any other nation, our youth unemployment rate is the highest of any industrialized country (*Manpower Report of the President,* 1968). The reasons for this are incompletely understood. Very probably they are closely related to the nature of our occupational structure, our public policies, the size of our youth population, and the ways in which we fail to prepare many of our young people for successful employment.

The Unemployment Rate

Despite new education, training, and job programs for youth, the high unemployment rate among our young people persists (see Figure 7). The rates are high for youth in all income groups, but particularly for those in low-income nonwhite families.

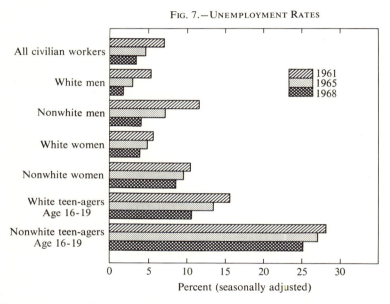

FIG. 7.—UNEMPLOYMENT RATES

Percent (seasonally adjusted)

The growth in the number of jobs available plus recently established youth training programs have been compensating factors in keeping youth unemployment rates from rising even higher at a time when so many young people are currently entering the labor market. As Figure 8 (see page 411) indicates, more than half of the total labor force increase between 1961 and 1968 was made up of young workers.

Rapid population growth among all teen-agers in this decade will continue into the 1970's before declining. In the total sixteen-to-twenty-four-year-old range, it is estimated that there will be almost 19,000,000 in the labor force by 1970 and more than 22,000,000 by 1980. This represents almost a 49 percent increase in the youth of this age in the labor force during the 1960 to 1970 decade, and more than a 19 percent increase in the 1970 to 1980 span. It thus appears that an already acute problem will be further magnified.

FIG. 8.—MORE THAN HALF OF THE LABOR FORCE INCREASE
BETWEEN 1961 AND 1968 WAS MADE UP
OF YOUNG WORKERS . . .

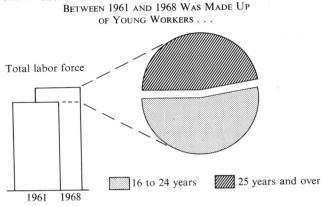

Total labor force

16 to 24 years   25 years and over

1961   1968

THEREFORE, THE PROPORTION OF THE LABOR FORCE
UNDER 25 YEARS OF AGE ROSE SIGNIFICANTLY

1961   1968

The Subemployment and Hidden Unemployment Rates

The subemployment rate reveals other kinds of employment problems related to the underutilization of manpower. Subemployment affects major groups of workers: those employed below their actual or potential skill level; persons outside the labor force who desire or need work; full-time year-round workers with inadequate earnings, and employed persons who are relegated to short work weeks for reasons beyond their control. Youth tend to fall into the last two categories, that is, to be underemployed or working at a job which does not pay an adequate wage.

Hidden unemployment particularly affects the jobless rate in poverty areas, where many individuals are not included in the usual rates of unemployment. They are not counted as being in the labor force because they are not registered as looking for work nor have they worked at regular steady jobs. Such persons—many of them young people—lack the knowledge and confidence to seek work through the usual channels. The "hidden" unemployment rate greatly increases the estimate of those not working. In large metropolitan centers actual rates of those not working have been judged to be as high as 30 or 40 percent.

Causes of the Problem

Youth unemployment is associated with a number of factors. A leading cause is the increasing complexity of business and industry and associated demands for employees who have high levels of business, professional, or technical skills. During the next decade, these kinds of work requirements will increase (*Manpower Report of the President,* 1969). Major job increases will occur in a wide range of services and white-collar occupations. The long, sharp decline in jobs in farm work will continue, and the smallest amount of job growth will be in laboring and semiskilled work. Routine, repetitive, low-paid jobs are being eliminated in business and industry with the increase in mechanization.

Because of the rapidity of technological change, those who have learned only one set of skills may be faced with obsolescence within a decade. A premium is placed on the worker's ability to learn new patterns and adjust readily to changing circumstances. The apparent contradiction of jobs which go begging while job seekers are idle is already a fundamental aspect of the employment situation in most large cities. Programs which seek to train youth for employment must achieve a balance between meeting the immediate needs of the labor market and developing the individual so that he can readily adapt to changing conditions.

Employment Problems of Special Groups

It would be difficult enough to meet these challenges if all young people had similar training needs and employment potentials. The task becomes more formidable when an attempt is made to meet the particular needs of special groups.

Impoverished youth. The very poor have a particularly difficult time in getting good jobs that have a future. Poverty, low educational attainment, and limited employment history are circular in their effect, as shown in Chapter IV. Children who are reared in poverty suffer its many deficits and are handicapped in job-seeking both because of their individual lack of necessary knowledge and skills and because of prejudical attitudes of employers. Barred from the larger society, many such children turn to their immediate neighborhood for a sense of identity and belongingness. Rainwater (1966) has proposed that the lower-lower-class male is so shut off from the mainstream of society that he is threatened with total loss of his sense of being a person. Since existence is impossible under these circumstances, he is forced, to preserve his own sense of identity, to consider the major society as being unreal. Having nothing to offer as proof of his identity other than himself as a person, he tends to place a high premium on such qualities as "lots of heart" and the daily excitement that can be gleaned from a life "on the streets."

For the urban slum youth, the lure of such a life may become a fixed pattern—one which will shut him off from developing attitudes and behaviors necessary for employment success. For these youth, "hustling" can represent the same thing that work does to those young people who have been brought into the regular occupational system. Both provide money, recreation, food, and companionship with the opposite sex. In fact, "hustling" can give the individual a sense of satisfaction and competency that he may not receive from the kind of legitimate work that is open to him.

In many cases, slum youth may have been encouraged in school to be "realistic" and aspire to or accept the very types of low-income, low-prestige jobs from which they hope to escape. They may accept occupational goals far below their desires, and perhaps well below their potentials, and in some cases, settle for a life of marginal employment. For the ghetto youth, this choice is not made voluntarily in the context of numerous choices available to him. It is forced upon him, and the consequences have harsh, corrosive effects on his self-esteem and on his future and that of his family.

Young people from poverty environments are as often fired for inappropriate work attitudes as for poor work performance. One study revealed that those fired for poor work attitudes disliked run-of-the-mill competition, were indifferent to such things as improvement in physical working conditions, a promotion-on-merit atmosphere, a sense of group belongingness, and congenial fellow workers. These workers were found to have self-defeating patterns of excessive drinking, quarreling, and absenteeism. Such patterns were associated with hostile attitudes toward their parents and resentment of dependence or domination by family members. The investigators noted that these workers appeared to reenact in the working situation the patterns they presented in their early life—an attitude of being short-changed at home and on the job (*Report of Task Force VI, 1968*).

Since motivation for regular employment in business and industry is often not seen as being relevant to the life situation of the very poor, the disadvantaged young person is apt to encounter influences in his home, peer group, and neighborhood that are adverse to his seeking and holding a job in the larger society. Failure to receive support from these groups can result in conflicting attitudes and confused feelings that impair the strenuous efforts he must make to adjust occupationally. For example, disadvantaged youth who enter trainee programs sometimes fail to receive encouragement from their peers or family. An unemployed father or an older unemployed sibling may view the trainee's employment as a threat to his own status and self-esteem. Trainees have been known to request working hours at night so that their family or peer group will not know they are working and consequently downgrade their employment.

Members of minority groups. A high proportion of impoverished youth face additional employment problems because they are members of minority groups. For instance, the New York Puerto Rican population has a high proportion of unemployed teen-agers whose acute job problems are compounded by lack of language facility as well as poor education and discrimination. A sample survey in the Bronx in the spring of 1966 revealed that for Puerto Ricans in the four-to-nineteen age group the unemployment rate was 24 percent, while that for the twenty-to-twenty-four age group was 19 percent. Comparable figures for Negroes in the Bronx at this same time were 10 and 16 percent, respectively (*Manpower Report of the President,* 1968).

The Mexican-Americans in the Southwest are also handicapped in the search for better jobs by their low educational attainment and language problems. In general, Mexican-Americans have relatively little education but their income positions are remarkably better than their levels of educational attainment would seem to warrant. It has been suggested that Mexican-Americans face less discrimination in the labor market than do Negroes, which may explain their comparatively high income position. Generally speaking, the unemployment rate of Mexican-Americans is higher than that of whites, but lower than rates for American Indians or Negroes.

Little is known about the employment situation of Indian teen-agers, but data for adults indicate that Indians on reservations are among the most disadvantaged minorities in our country. There is only scanty information about those who leave the reservation. Fragmentary information indicates that some occupational upgrading is taking place. Fewer Indians are working at farm jobs and more at skilled and semiskilled jobs (*Manpower Report of the President,* 1968). Compared with the labor force generally, however, these advances are minimal.

Although the unemployment rate for white teen-agers has recently dropped as employment opportunities have increased, the rate for nonwhite teen-agers has remained high and has dropped very little from 1961 to 1968. In 1968 one out of every four nonwhite teen-agers was unemployed, a proportion almost two and one-half times that for white teen-agers. Nonwhite teen-age girls have the highest unemployment level for any population group (*Handbook of Labor Statistics,* 1968).

While it is common knowledge that there is a positive association between education and income, few serious studies have been made of this relationship among members of disadvantaged minority groups. For these groups, education is not such a crucial factor in solving employment problems. Additional education is not necessarily converted into proportionately higher earnings at the rate experienced by whites. Those Negroes, Mexican-Americans, and other minority group members who have educational levels similar to those of whites do not earn similar amounts of money or hold similar jobs. Less than half of the difference between white and nonwhite income can be explained by differences in educational attainment (Fogel, 1965). Some of this difference can be explained by the lower quality of education frequently provided for minority-group members. A great need for these groups, however, is on-the-job training. A nationwide study showed that more than 80 percent of the difference between white-black incomes could be explained by differences in occupational experience. Negroes receive much less of the type of training that includes actual work experience (Thurow, 1968). In addition, when job-hunting, a white high school graduate has a three-to-one chance over a white high school dropout, whereas a Negro high school graduate has barely any edge at all over a Negro who failed to finish high school (*Federal Programs Assisting Children and Youth,* 1968).

Cultural differences in work attitudes are also a factor in the employment of some minority-group members whose values tend not to be congruent with those of the dominant society. For example, a prevalent attitude among American Indians is that work is valuable only when it is necessary either to protect or to provide for their social group. A job means the ability to buy or do some desired thing, and when enough money has accumulated for this objective, they often quit working. Many Mexican-Americans have somewhat similar attitudes. Work is good only because it provides money for the essentials and the pleasures of life, and it is to be valued along with other equally important things such as family, friends, enjoyment of life, and a cultivation of one's personal interests (Joint Commission on Correctional Manpower and Training, 1967). The Anglo-American's attitude is generally very different. A man's job is his most important function—his social status, standard of living, and prestige all depend upon the job.

School dropouts. Most of the young people who drop out of school come from poverty backgrounds and are handicapped by the many deficits that such a background is likely to impose. A disproportionate number are further handicapped by racial discrimination. Thus, the employment problems of dropouts are frequently compounded by prejudice, by their lack of familiarity with the language commonly used in the work world, by attitudes toward work which conflict with those of the larger society, as well as by their lack of the required education and skill training.

In the metropolitan North and West, black students are three times as likely as white students to drop out of school by the age of sixteen or seventeen. In these areas, 20 percent of the eligible black population is not enrolled in school, in contrast to 6 percent of the eligible white population (Coleman *et al.,* 1966). The national Indian dropout rate from the eighth to the twelfth grade is unusually high—around 60 percent (Ablon *et al.,* 1967). The percentage of dropouts among Mexican-Americans is also extremely high (Office of Education, 1968).

Comparative data on white and nonwhite youth show that in October, 1966, the dropout rate among youth sixteen to twenty-one years of age was 42 percent for white boys, 29 percent for white girls, 61 percent for nonwhite boys, and 44 percent for nonwhite girls (*Federal Programs Assisting Children and Youth,* 1968).

Those who drop out generally have a history of grade and subject failure, which often has begun early in elementary school. When they weary of experiencing repeated failure, they leave school, only to repeat the same pattern in their working life experiences. From a mental health point of view, leaving school may be a realistic adaptive measure (Engel, 1969).* When the family situation is bad and the school is not something with which the youngster can identify, leaving school may be a sound move in terms of what some behavioral scientists call the "search for an alternate identity."

However, the dropout may bring an attitude of failure with him, which adds to his employment handicaps. The National Education Association indicates that unless Herculean efforts are made to help this group finish high school, more than one-third of the young people who pass into the labor market annually will be school dropouts. One-third of these dropouts will have had the overwhelming handicap of less than eight years of formal education (NEA Research Division, 1967). Two in three will not have completed more than grade ten. Thus, most will drop out before they become exposed to occupational and vocational information as it is now generally offered in the schools.

The nonwhite high school dropout is at the bottom of the job market today. The highest unemployment rate is for all nonwhite dropout girls— more than 33 percent of the 1965–66 dropouts were seeking work in 1967 (*Federal Programs Assisting Children and Youth,* 1968).

In the great majority of cases, lack of mental ability is not the major cause of failure to finish school (Schreiber, 1962). Being forced to go to work from economic necessity is probably not the major factor in dropping out either, although school records show that many students give this as a reason (*Report of Task Force VI,* 1968). Rather, a number of conditions interact and add to the dropout problem. In general these include a broad educational disability which results in an indifferent, discouraged, or anxious attitude as well as a dislike of the school experience combined with low-income life styles, rejection by school personnel and classmates, adverse emotional factors, and inferior schools.

* Engel, M. Personal communication with Joint Commission on Mental Health of Children, March 5, 1969.

Delinquent youth. The interrelationship of dropping out of school, delinquent behavior, and subsequent limitations on employment opportunities is well known. Traditionally, employers have relied on schools to produce eligible personnel, and when the school closes the door on the dropout or delinquent, so does the employer. The delinquent youth who drops out of school is at a crossroads. Either he must be assisted in developing a work identity and occupation which are congruent with the dominant culture or he may develop an alternate identity which competes with employment or which does not value legitimate work. The life style and quick pay-offs of this alternate identity can provide the youth with a sense of security, with social participation, and with a feeling of status that would normally be provided through the worker-provider role (Rainwater, 1966). In some cases, by the time a delinquent drops out of school, this anti-work identity is well developed. The situation was recently summed up by Julius Hobson, a Negro activist and former head of CORE for the Washington, D.C., area, in these vivid terms:

There's a psychological thing there—a man who's living on his wits, sleeping 'til ten in the morning, on the hustle on the streets or the pool rooms—he figures a guy working eight hours a day for eighty bucks a week just isn't smart. If you just get a guy like that a job and turn him loose, you're wasting your time—he won't last a week. After 30, maybe 25, a man living on his wits reaches a point where he just won't hold a regular job. You've got to catch them young (*Report of Task Force VI,* 1968).

According to recent studies, the rate of delinquency among dropouts may be as much as ten times higher than among children who stay in school (Schreiber, 1963). As pointed out in Chapter VIII, there are many kinds of youngsters who are classified as being delinquent and there are many interacting causes of delinquency. No one kind of treatment or rehabilitation program is appropriate for all these young people. Work training and work placement are indicated for some delinquents, but the kind of training and/or placement depends upon the characteristics and needs of the individual.

Rural youth. The problems of our rural areas are reflected in the plight of our rural youth. Although all boys who enter farming come from farm backgrounds, only a small percentage of those born on farms can expect to become farmers. Farms are becoming fewer in number, more mechanized, and larger in size, and the number of farm boys greatly exceeds the supply of available agricultural jobs. Therefore, at the present time and in the foreseeable future, the majority of rural youth who enter the labor force must do so in nonfarm occupations (*Manpower Report of the President,* 1967).

Studies indicate that those who were raised on farms are much less likely to be successful at nonfarm occupations (Burchinal *et al.,* 1962). In general, studies show that growing up in an agricultural community often imposes a handicap in the competition for more remunerative and higher-status non-farm jobs (Burchinal *et al.,* 1962; Beale *et al.,* 1964).

Generally speaking, boys who plan to farm have much lower levels of educational aspiration than those who plan other careers. If a boy decides to farm, the decision is often made before he enters the tenth grade. Thus, he shows less interest in broad occupational information and is generally unaware of the objective requirements of today's larger world of work (Haller, 1966). Because fewer teen-age youth will have the opportunity to become farmers, it is necessary to plan programs which will develop the knowledge, skills, opportunities, and aspirations necessary for them to perform adequately in other jobs.

One of the most disadvantaged groups is the 300,000 or so children of migrant workers who follow the crops each year. They work in fields alongside their parents and may be on the road five, six, or more months a year. In some communities they are barred from the school. Their opportunities for adequate education and skill training, particularly as jobs in agriculture continue to decline, are at the barest minimum.

Blue-collar youth. There are few studies on young blue-collar workers. From what is known, there appears to be little difference between the young and the older blue-collar workers. A number of studies have shown that the fully employed and "stable" workingmen view employment chiefly in economic survival terms. Legitimate work is not expected to be a source of personal satisfaction. The reasons for this orientation are highly complex; some are obviously tied to the fact that the jobs available to the blue-collar worker have little status in our society. These jobs are merely time-serving occupations which fail to engender the worker's pride in being trained or employed in a highly respected occupation that affords a sense of individual competence and significance.

Unlike their elders, young blue-collar workers tend to take the union for granted; although they understand its function, they do not appear to have the same personal relationship to it as do the older men who helped to bring the union into existence. With both young and older workers, satisfaction appears to be found outside of working hours, not particularly on the job, and promotions from the rank are generally limited—a condition which is accepted. The young blue-collar workers are likely to be relatively affluent, and job security rather than interesting work is usually seen as the advantage of higher education.

Although there does not appear to be a difference in working-class attitudes based on age, there may be one based on race. One study in Akron, Ohio, showed that the black workers were more nearly attuned to many of the issues which affect the college-educated young. These blacks understood the antiwar protestors, the hippies, the activist college youth, and the generation gap, whereas the young white workers understood none of these.

It has been suggested that working-class white youth may be experiencing a growing rift between themselves and others as they cling to traditional values in a society that has become less traditional or at least less willing to cling to traditional values (Simon, 1969).

The mentally and physically disabled. For the young who are physically handicapped, mentally retarded, or have a history of mental or emotional disorders, a job may be a necessary condition for rehabilitation. Although figures are not available on youth alone, physical and mental impairments limit the work activity of perhaps 16,000,000 Americans seventeen years of age and over, not counting those handicapped by alcoholism (*Manpower Report of the President,* 1969). Disabling conditions are especially prevalent among the poor. Chronic disabilities increase with age, but within each age group these proportions increase dramatically as family income goes down (*Manpower Report of the President,* 1967).

Psychological problems, which may accompany physical handicaps, often render individuals unemployable. However, the ability to secure and hold a job can be a major factor in promoting the emotional stability of such persons. The stigma attached to former mental patients makes it especially difficult for them to get employment. Three-fourths of all former mental patients feel that they have to hide the fact of hospitalization in their search for jobs (Posner, 1969).* The adolescent who has had psychiatric treatment is at an even greater disadvantage than the adult. Since such youth have had little time to build an adequate work experience record, it is of extreme importance that they gain a better than average work skill.

Although mentally retarded persons have often proved to be loyal and reliable employees, few can use regular vocational services in the community. Since defeat is a common experience for retarded adolescents, programs that strengthen and preserve self-esteem in the preschool and school periods are of extreme importance and tend to increase their employability more than later remediation programs (Rusalem *et al.,* 1967).

Does Everyone Have to Work?

As suggested in Chapter IV, it would seem to be important to reexamine the so-called Protestant work ethic which has prevailed in our society and which has been closely associated with an economy which is geared to industrial development and production. Now that our economy has reached what some term the "postindustrial stage," in which we have highly mechanized production and no longer need as many workers employed full-time, it is appropriate to reassess our value systems related to work and

---

* Posner, B. (Deputy Executive Secretary, President's Committee on Employment of the Handicapped). Personal communication with Joint Commission on Mental Health of Children, March 28, 1969.

leisure. Question must be raised about the "full employment" ideal, the identification of every male in terms of his occupational status, the emphasis on work achievement, and the identification of women and children in terms of the occupation and income of the father of the family. We must find other criteria by which to accord approval, status, and significance to individuals so that a person can be unemployed and still retain his self-respect. Volunteer activities, hobbies, leisure occupations, and the like need to be accorded greater value. These comments particularly apply to the "marginally employable" for whom full-time productive work is a great effort and for whom modern business and industry often have very little use. Many in our society who suffer from serious emotional, mental, and physical handicaps may fall into this group. Along with greater recognition of their worth as individuals, whether or not they are productively employed, must go public provisions for their economic support as a matter of right rather than of grudging charity. These points should not be interpreted as a disclaimer of the responsibility of a person to support himself and his family if possible.

Studies of other societies suggest that productive, paid employment is not essential to the well-being and self-respect of individuals if the values of the culture do not demand this kind of activity. Such values grow out of survival necessities imposed by demanding environments rather than innate human needs to be productively employed.

These comments do not imply that human beings have little or no need for activity. It appears that most do have a drive for self-expression and self-development through being and doing. This suggests that we must pay more attention, in our society, to providing many kinds of opportunities for recreation and education for the individual throughout his life-span. The trend in this direction is already apparent; it should be encouraged for people of all socioeconomic and age levels.

It is impossible to predict the outcomes of these trends with great clarity and exactitude. Changing values about work and leisure are but one aspect of many current value upheavals associated with the changing nature of our economy. Flexibility, willingness to experiment, readiness to accept a diversity of life styles for many types of individuals, and assessment of the outcomes of shifts in programs and policies would seem to be the appropriate approach in the work-leisure spheres as well as in other aspects of our complex society.

EMPLOYMENT AND COLLEGE YOUTH

Enrollment in institutions of higher education among college-age youth increased about 80 percent during the 1960's, an increase more than double the rise in the youth population. Altogether, more than 40 percent of young high school graduates are going to college today, and proportionally more college students are working. For many college students the continuation of their schooling is dependent upon having a job. (This is also true of many high school students, and proportionally more of them are also working.) The increase in the number of college students who work may be due to several factors, such as the rise in college expenses, the creation of part-time jobs through government programs, and better economic conditions which have created more jobs for these young people.

The proportion of college students who marry while in school has remained substantially stable since 1960 (U.S. Bureau of the Census, 1967–68). In 1966 about 12 percent of college students were married, and nearly six out of ten of these were in school full-time. In 1968 a considerably higher proportion of married college men were employed than was the case for their single counterparts; the proportion of employed, married women students was, however, only slightly higher than for single ones.

There is no evidence that working either hinders or enhances the scholastic performance of students (Bernert, 1958). We know very little about students who work—whether they are exceptionally capable, exceptionally bright, or average, or how the working experience may affect their mental health.

There are a few programs for college youth which provide for education and employment, alternately arranged, on a full-time basis. The Antioch College plan is the classic example. In very recent years, some large employers have initiated arrangements with a number of colleges in a co-operative education situation. Ford and Lockheed, for example, have co-op programs in which undergraduates alternate trimesters of college with trimesters of work for the participating company. The object, of course, is to interest the students in working for that company full-time after graduation. Personnel men appear to be enthusiastic about this program, indicating that these employees *"fit in better than anyone."* (Rukeyser, 1969; italics in original.)

At present there is a ready market for college graduates. Negro college graduates are in particular demand but in short supply. The vast majority of upper-middle-class vocational positions are occupied by college-trained persons, and the number of these positions has been increasing rapidly. There are indications that this is changing. Those who have analyzed the supply and demand of college graduates have indicated that we are beginning to enter a period in which there may be some shortages of trained personnel in specific fields, but, generally, there may well be a surplus of educated persons (Havighurst and Neugarten, 1962; Folger and Nam, 1964). By 1975 there will be a much larger supply of people available for these jobs, owing to the World War II baby boom. By this same date, despite possible shortages in certain higher-level occupations, a larger share of the nation's jobs will be available only to persons holding a college degree. Either college graduation or advanced graduate work will be required in more than 14 percent of all positions, as compared to 12 percent in 1966 (Rosenthal and Hedges, 1968).

Young college graduates and college dropouts increasingly tend to seek work which they consider to be significant and personally satisfying. Many are not satisfied with the vocational roles which society expects them to fill and tend to look for positions in which they will have the opportunity to work for social change. These young people primarily constitute that portion of youth which was described in Chapter VIII as the activists and idealists. Though this is a relatively small group, it is a highly influential one.

These young people feel that they can work for social change and still earn a living in employment that suits their particular skills and temperament. A pamphlet entitled "Vocations for Social Change" expresses this viewpoint:

What's really going to change America is the fact that more and more members of this much maligned "younger generation" are not interested in wasting their lives doing jobs that are useless, pernicious, or boring, just because they pay well. . . . Some want to work actively for social change, or to help people in some real and concrete way; many more are simply holding out for a job where they can live like human beings and accomplish ANYTHING that's real and concrete (Kleinberger, 1968).

This trend is reflected in a college survey published by *Fortune* magazine in January, 1969. The following statement was chosen by 42 percent of the survey sample: "I'm not really concerned with the practical benefits of college. I suppose I take them for granted. College for me seems something more intangible, perhaps the opportunity to change things rather than make out well within the existing system." Those who agreed with this social change statement were mostly students in the arts and humanities, and only one-quarter of this group came from blue-collar families. The majority, however, took a more conventional approach and agreed with this statement: "For me, college is mainly a practical matter. With a college education I can earn more money, have a more interesting career, and enjoy a better position in society." One-third of the practical-minded students who chose this formulation came from blue-collar families, and the majority of them were enrolled in business, engineering, or science-oriented courses.

Generally speaking, those who work with college youth feel that the number of young people who subscribe to the social change and personal fulfillment credo is growing. Improved salaries and advancement opportunities, therefore, may not be enough to attract the youth who have the freshness of outlook which industry seeks. Increasingly, many young college graduates are evaluating potential jobs on the basis of the challenge, the creativeness, and the usefulness that work can offer to them as individuals.

CURRENT ATTEMPTS TO SOLVE YOUTH EMPLOYMENT PROBLEMS

Efforts to meet the vast and varied occupational needs of our many kinds of young people have been far too limited. The more forward-looking projects that do exist are mainly of recent origin and were largely started under the impetus of federal aid programs. Among the major efforts are those initiated by the Vocational Education Acts and amendments of 1963 and 1968, the Economic Opportunity Act, the Manpower Development and Training Act, the summer work programs of the President's Council on Youth Opportunity, and such military programs as Project 100,000 or Project Transition. In addition, other types of programs have an employment and training component which may involve youth, such as those of the Model Cities. Private industry has also developed a number of programs, and voluntary agencies have been increasingly involved in modifying or expanding their traditional approaches to vocational development.

Programs for the Disadvantaged

The chief emphasis of most programs has been on low-income youth, members of minority groups, school dropouts, delinquents, or those young people who have a combination of these and other handicaps.

Although the earlier projects revealed an awareness that large numbers of disadvantaged youth needed medical, legal, family, and mental health assistance, it was assumed that many of these problems would be dispelled by the salutary effects of a genuine work experience. In actual operation it was found that such problems were too pressing and too troublesome to permit many young people to solve their multiple problems through employment or job training alone. Consequently, to increase success rates, it was necessary to buttress these programs with medical, dental, legal, financial, family, mental health, and ameliorative services. In addition to skill training, medical treatment, and efforts to increase motivation and emotional stability, most of these programs included education and training in such behaviors as promptness, politeness, good speech, and good grooming.

In brief, there are two large components to the work-training approach—vocational preparation and supportive services. Vocational preparation includes components aimed at developing positive employment motivation and work-related habits, interpersonal skills, basic educational achievement, peripheral knowledge related to jobs, and occupational skills. Supportive services generally include counseling, testing, guidance, and other services necessary for appraisal and adjustment.

Staff members of virtually all work programs have accepted the responsibility for locating and developing jobs as well as for training and assisting youth as individuals. When broadly conceived, job location and development include concern with labor market conditions and trends, public and private occupational structures, and business and union policies and practices. More immediately, job development includes locating existing employment for individuals, persuading employers to create jobs for them, and encouraging employers to redefine job qualifications in order to increase opportunities. (See also a later section on public policy and employment opportunities.)

Since failure in the job interview is common to those youth below age twenty-one, the "vestibule" program has been developed as an additional component. This program attempts to prepare young people to meet a prospective employer in an existing work situation or community agency, thus affording him an opportunity to evaluate the individual on the job and help him to adjust to the work situation.

The most critical phase in work placement occurs 15 to 30 days after assignment, when the individual finds adjustment to the work environment most difficult. It is generally conceded that follow-up supportive services are essential during the first few months on the job in order to promote the individual's successful adjustment. Principal emphasis is on counseling, continuation of occupational and remedial education, and provision for legal and other services.

In addition to these broad vocational programs for the disadvantaged, there are a number of programs more limited in scope. For example, there are bilingual employment services, including testing in Spanish, and a trend toward teaching English in schools as a second language as an effort toward upgrading the employability of Spanish-speaking Americans.

School Work Programs

There are various programs aimed primarily at preventing young people from dropping out of school. One of the most successful has been authorized by the Vocational Education Act of 1963, in which students work part-time in employment and go to school part-time. The purpose is to offer realistic work experience combined with formal education in order to simultaneously develop knowledge, more skill, and appropriate work attitudes. In the view of the Advisory Council on Vocational Education, this part-time cooperative plan is the best program in vocational education (*General Report of the Advisory Council on Vocational Education,* 1968). This program is also popular with students. It consistently yields high placement records, high employment stability, and high job satisfaction. Due to the large number of students that apply and the inadequate number of programs, only the best students are selected to participate, a probable factor in its success.

The program has rarely been used in junior colleges, even though it would appear to be an excellent method at this level of instruction.

Summer work programs are also used to help youth stay in school. These programs range from summer jobs for college students to jobs for disadvantaged youth. The President's Council on Youth Opportunity has been particularly concerned with the latter group. This council announced that in the summer of 1968 there were more opportunities to work, learn, and play than in any previous summer, but that there were also more youth to be served. Under the council's program, 832,000 specifically identifiable poor youth were employed during the summer of 1968 (about 5 percent of unemployed youth). This employment was believed to be one factor in lowering the unemployment rate in the twenty largest metropolitan areas in the country. Such employment includes direct federal jobs and work opportunities in business provided in the fifty largest cities by the National Alliance of Businessmen (The President's Council on Youth Opportunity, n.d.). It is clear that more funds are needed for such programs if the unemployment problems of young people are to be dealt with effectively.

In all these and other programs for the disadvantaged, relatively little consideration has been given to the problems of those who may be the most difficult to prepare for employment: the delinquents, the mentally retarded, and the emotionally disturbed. Delinquents have been included in general programs for the disadvantaged, and employers who have been involved in planning such programs have relaxed some of their stringent policies against hiring youth with probation and parole records.

For the mentally retarded, vocational rehabilitation services have made particular gains recently in developing cooperative vocational rehabilitation school programs designed to assist the retarded young person to move from school to work. Such programs have reduced the school dropout rate of retarded youngsters and have provided a technique for enabling at least some of these young people to gain a work skill.

Change in Basic Vocational Training

In addition to the development of many educational-vocational programs for youth with special problems, basic changes are taking place in the vocational training of all young people. There is increasing recognition that vocational education must be redirected from training in a few selected occupational categories to preparing all groups in the community for their place in the work world. The Vocational Education Act of 1963 calls for redirection and reorganization of many aspects of the nation's vocational education programs, including areas of training emphasis, teacher education, school construction, and stepped-up program research. This act established a new definition of vocational education which specifically incorporated basic and general education as a prerequisite for adequate vocational preparation. It provided that vocational education be available to all persons in all communities and that it support unified rather than separate training programs in selected occupational categories.

Special Needs of Delinquent Youth

The effectiveness of the correctional system in the vocational rehabilitation of adjudicated delinquents is a specific area in which we urgently need more research-based knowledge. The placing of adolescents with adults, overcrowding, and the amount and extent of diagnosis, treatment, and adequate work training are all part of this complex area. In such institutions, however, realistic and effective vocational training is crucial.

Special employment problems of youth who are arrested as delinquent, or suspected of delinquent behavior, are created by present practices concerning arrest records and bonding. A large number of young people who are arrested each year and brought before a court are found to be not guilty. However, discrimination in employment is based on the record of arrests rather than on a conviction. It has been increasingly recognized that conviction may not rest on guilt but may depend on the circumstances of the arrest, the availability of legal aid, whether or not bail can be afforded, and poverty and/or minority-group membership. In addition, the type of the arrest record and the type of offense committed may not be as important in obtaining employment as the mere fact of having been arrested. A youngster's denial of an arrest record is normally grounds for dismissal in all types of employment once the falsification is discovered, regardless of the outcome of the arrest and his performance on the job.

If court proceedings indicate that the youth is not guilty, job disqualification on the basis of the arrest is a misuse of judicial machinery. Misuse of the arrest record creates the proverbial "self-fulfilling prophecy" (Sparer, 1966). Denying youth job opportunities does, in fact, promote the likelihood of criminality. These outcomes are especially unjust and unfortunate in that prejudice against low-income and/or minority-group youth may play a large part in the initial arrest.

At the present time, juvenile, youthful offender, and wayward minor records may be viewed by prospective employers through a "waiver" of confidentiality signed by the applicant. Young people who have run afoul of the law, therefore, may be perpetually stigmatized as a result. Juvenile, youthful offender, and wayward minor records should not be disclosed to anyone except other courts, the probation department, and institutions in which youths are placed.

Assistance in obtaining bonding also raises problems, as bonds are increasingly being required by employers in jobs involving property responsibility. An arrest record usually bars an applicant from obtaining a bond from a private underwriter. Frequently arrest records of Negroes are regarded as more serious than the same record for whites. If this barrier to employment is to be overcome, "high-risk" bonding programs must be implemented. There has been some experimental bonding in this area, and this experience needs to be built upon (*Manpower Report of the President*, 1967).

Special Needs of Handicapped Youth

The professionals who work with handicapped children and youth need to become more aware of training for employment as one aspect of the total treatment or rehabilitation process. It must be recognized that there are a number of children and youth who are so handicapped that they will never be able to function on a job. However, for many others some form of work may serve as an aid toward independence and improved mental health.

NEEDED PROGRAMS AND APPROACHES

It is evident that many of today's young people have employment problems which range from mild to severe. Those most critically affected are young people of poverty backgrounds, members of oppressed minority groups, rural youth, school dropouts, youngsters with a court record, and those with physical, emotional, and mental handicaps. Another group experiencing problems is those college students who are seeking social significance and personal fulfillment through their careers.

These employment problems arise from two major sources: (a) the characteristics of these young people as individuals and (b) the nature of the economy and its associated occupations.

If we are to reduce the occupational problems of young people, two chief strategies are needed: those designed to prepare individuals for work and those directed toward making the economic and employment systems more adaptive to individual differences and special needs.

Broadened Approaches to Individuals

Programs addressed to individual change call for a number of approaches. These should be based on a deeper understanding of human growth and development and the many factors which interact to affect human behavior. Just as the child brings his total life experience and unique characteristics to school, so he also approaches employment as a total person, affected by all that has happened to him in the past, by his present situation, and by his hopes and fears in relation to the future. Just as we have tended to divide up the child's world in specialized, uncoordinated services addressed separately to his physical, social, emotional, and educational needs, so we have tended to view his vocational needs as separate from the rest of his life. Thus, attempts to help him vocationally have been too cut off, conceptually and programmatically, from his total life situation.

Clearly a broader conceptual base is needed for vocational education and guidance. Current trends in this field are encouraging, as noted at the end of the preceding section. Recent changes in vocational education legislation and policy are directed toward a closer coordination between academic education and vocational education, reaching all community members with vocational education, and the support of general vocational education rather than narrow training for occupational specialties. This broader concept of vocational education should be extended further to include a deeper and more realistic recognition of the individual as a whole person whose occupational life is but one facet of his total life history and situation.

Both preventive and remedial approaches to the youngster's future work roles must be based on these kinds of understandings as well as on sound knowledge of the nature and requirements of occupations in the present and the near future. Preventive programs should start with the young child and provide him appropriate experience with the work world as one aspect of the adult society.

Along with pioneering ways in which children can have more direct and indirect experience with the world of work, it is important to recognize that all supportive programs which we have discussed in earlier chapters have a bearing on the occupational as well as other aspects of the child's future. These programs include those which are addressed to his physical, social, emotional, recreational, and educational needs. As we have remarked so frequently, a child's mental health depends upon all of these services. Furthermore, occupational success not only is based, in part, on the young person's mental health but also, in turn, affects it. Services addressed to the prevention of occupational problems are, in large part, the same services that are generally supportive of the child's healthy growth and development.

More specific to occupational preparation, a wide variety of experimental approaches should be undertaken which are directed toward increasing the child's experience and understanding of work as it relates to himself and his future occupation.

Only a sketch can be given here of the ways in which more work experience and knowledge might be provided for children and adolescents.

Work Experience in School

It is suggested that experimental programs be undertaken which provide for a wide participation of children in the ongoing work activities of the school with such experiences starting at the preschool level and going on through high school and college. Generally unexplored areas include those which are related to serving as teaching assistants, assisting in the lunchroom and on the playground, helping in the school office, assisting in school construction and maintenance of building and grounds, work with audiovisual aides and the library, and the like.

In somewhat similar fashion, work experiences could be provided for children and adolescents in such facilities as hospitals, clinics, playgrounds, camps, social service and related programs, youth-serving organizations, child-care centers, and the like.

In all such programs, it is important to take into account the age and developmental stage of the child, individual differences, prevention of exploitation, coordination of work with educational experiences, adequate work supervision, appropriate work hours, and training of supervisory personnel so that the work will be a sound developmental experience.

These kinds of work programs have much to recommend them not only in terms of providing growth experiences for the young person but in terms of reducing critical personnel shortages in human service and related fields. In these programs, it is important to provide sex-appropriate activities and competent supervision by males as well as by females. It is particularly important that realistic and sound work experiences be provided for boys, not only because of their future work roles but because so many boys in our society lack a number of male models with whom they can identify and from whom they can learn masculine roles.

It is obviously impractical to attempt to teach children and young people all they need to know about occupations through providing direct work experiences. The world of occupations is too complex for such an undertaking, and youngsters are not ready to participate in all possible occupational fields. Thus, indirect means of occupational education and counseling are also important. These might include a greater emphasis on field visits to work settings and on including in the school program working adults who can share their occupational experiences with children and adolescents. Parents should be involved in these work experience programs as much as possible so that they can gain a greater sense of participating in their children's educational and vocational development.

Vocational education and counseling are also important parts of the school program, as we have indicated. Schools also need to be more closely linked to the employment services than is usually the case.

Remedial Services

In the earlier sections of this chapter we described various kinds of occupational problems which handicap our young. Solving the problems of these young people is far from easy, for reasons ranging from behavioral patterns and attitudes to physical, emotional, or mental handicaps, as noted. Moreover, the nature of today's economy and occupations make employment in the private sector a dubious matter for some of our young people who have numerous educational, vocational, and psychosocial deficits.

As already indicated, many of these youngsters need a whole battery of coordinated services if we are to prepare them for work and stable employment. Besides these services, attention must be paid to such practical problems as transportation, the proximity of the job to the young person's home, child-care facilities for young working mothers, and the like.

Besides these kinds of considerations, careful attention must be paid to factors associated with various jobs, such as the level of wages, the hours of work, the chance for career development, Social Security coverage, and the like.

Job Development

A review of programs aimed at training the educationally vocationally disadvantaged has revealed that the presence of a job which is available to the person who is being trained is just as important as, if not more important than, job training, remedial education, and the provision of other services. Special attention must be paid to young people who live in areas of overall poverty where employment opportunities are simply not available. Training is of no avail unless employment opportunities can be brought to the region, or unless provisions are made for helping the person go where the jobs are and supporting him while he is making an adjustment to the new location. Studies also indicate that, especially for disadvantaged youth, job placement needs to precede job training. The young person who has grown up in poverty and suffered its many rejections and humiliations tends to be wary of promises of future success. His willingness and readiness to learn is apt to follow the actual experience of having a job and earning money.

The development of enough jobs for the disadvantaged and the otherwise handicapped probably will require the further expansion of jobs under public auspices. Intensive study of the job market and the characteristics of the severely disadvantaged unemployed or underemployed sector of the population strongly suggests that private business and industry is and will be unable to offer full employment at adequate wages to all of these people. It is apparent that there must be an increase in jobs under public auspices, not only to provide employment for those who otherwise would not be able to find adequate work, but also to fill large gaps in our public services and the lack of employees to perform necessary work, especially in the human service fields (Sheppard, 1969).

Further expansion of work opportunities in public human services could play a significant part in expanding many of the programs recommended in this report. Using children and youth as aides to professional personnel in these programs would not only allow them to participate in the world of work but would provide a needed source of manpower in the human service occupations.

SUMMARY

Work satisfaction, security, and success play important roles in the mental health of our children and youth. Work continues to be a central part in a man's—and increasingly a woman's—sense of personal identity, significance, and status. To most Americans, it is the major source of individual and family income, a particularly critical matter in our consumer-oriented society, and thus a critical factor to the individual's mental health.

Careful planning is needed if we are to solve the problems of work satisfaction in a technological society and of employment for each individual to earn a living for himself and his family. We need to look at the facts of employment as they affect our youth. Our youth unemployment rate is the highest of any industrialized nation even though our young people stay in school longer than youth in these other countries. A large proportion of our young people are underemployed in low-paying, non-rewarding jobs that offer little future. Working-class youth find little personal satisfaction in their generally routine jobs in large organizations: work is merely a means to an end—economic security. Many of our youth, however, do not view economic security as a primary goal. Almost half of our college-trained youth are dissatisfied with the junior executive jobs in business and industry which they find open to them. They are seeking employment that is personally satisfying, creative, and directed toward social goals.

Work, like play and education, should be an integral part of the child's life, increasing in range and complexity as he grows older. Work experience should be tied to the child's developmental level and special interests and abilities. We need to experiment with new, flexible ways to find a means of involving children and youth in the work of the schools, neighborhoods, and ever-widening communities, and, at the same time, protect them from exploitation. Such an approach would be a radical one in this country, but it has much to recommend it from a mental health viewpoint. One mechanism for such an approach can be found through the Child Development Councils and child advocate systems recommended in this report.

Many of our attitudes toward work are outmoded. We must come to accept the fact that some people, through no fault of their own, cannot earn a "living wage" through employment and that they have a right nevertheless to dignity, respect, and adequate public assistance. However, many unemployed and underemployed persons possess the capacities to become productive members of society. We need only to capitalize on their potential. In all fields of human service—medical, social, educational, recreational—we are woefully short of services and personnel. Greatly expanded services are needed, as shown in other chapters of this report. Many people need the jobs that such expanded services would offer.

CHAPTER

XI

Research

INTRODUCTION

One task of the Commission was to use our existing knowledge about how we might enhance the development and mental health of our children and youth. This we have attempted to do. Yet, we were continually faced with the painful awareness of all that we do not know. Much of the complex process of human growth and development remains an elusive mystery. Only slowly are we beginning to make inroads into the secrets of the long evolutionary path which has led us to our present psycho-social-biological being, with all of our racial and cultural diversities.

The science of the last century or more has seemed a promising course of endeavor. Through it, we have gained some confidence in our ability to nurture human growth and to treat effectively some deviations in the normal course of development. It has become possible for us to define important directions for programs and policies. Yet, few could remain complacent in the face of so many unresolved questions. Many human problems remain at the mercy of future researchers.

Dr. Seymour Lustman addressed himself to this problem in a paper prepared for the Commission. We are presenting it, almost in its entirety, because we feel it represents a significant contribution to the field of research.

If we consider the limitations of our current substantive research knowledge and power, it is abundantly clear that we will have to endure a considerable gap between what we would like and what is possible, and, more than that, we must preserve the soil and plant the trees today which may not flourish for more than a hundred years.

Another way of stating this is the need to consider the area of research from a short and a long range view. More important than that is the inter-relationship between these views and the degree to which they can complement each other and the degree to which they may come into destructive contention. From such an appraisal it may be possible to more clearly approach priorities in terms of recommendations.

A pressing conceptual need is to remain aware of the difference between research and research utilization. It seems necessary to continually restate the difference between basic research, which is process oriented and directed toward new knowledge—and research utilization, or technological development, which is practical, task or product oriented. Under the humanist pressure of the needs of an applied field such as "Mental Health," it is unfortunately easy to forget that the general direction as well as the speed of all technological developments depends on the appropriate current from basic to applied science.

In a simplified schematic sense, we can conceptualize research utilization as an interaction of four complementary sectors. One is a body of substantive research data usually thought of as basic research; the second is the assessment of need; the third is the development of applicable techniques which includes appropriately rigorous assessment; and the fourth is the development of a delivery system by which they can be made available to society.

Viewed from this perspective, the short range view is under the sway of strong humanistic appeals in which needs are stressed and in which the quality of preventive and rehabilitative efforts are to be equally available for all. Such considerations tend to focus on needs and delivery systems and can be considered as one aspect of the work of the Commission that is long overdue. The difficulty lies in the morass of conflicting basic research and development of scientifically-based preventive and interventive techniques. Considering the substantive basic research available, some decisions will be premature in the sense that decisions will be made before research has been done and will be based on professional consensus. Such planning has a different probability of success than the planning which is based on research. One should also remain mindful that planning based on consensus produced the Edsel!

Perhaps this can be made clearer by a brief reference to the history of polio control. The need was clear, the delivery system available, but the production and trial of a vaccine did not stem from this. It had to await the basic research of Enders and the many basic scientists who made possible tissue culture work. Prior to this, the preventive and rehabilitative work in the area was disorderly, if not chaotic, characterized by claims and counter-claims.

In an oversimplified way, we have available to us two strategies for the planning of research. The first of these is in terms of need, and the second is planning, based upon historical knowledge of the way science proceeds.

Having once stated "the need is great," we have in fact made such global description of the research needs of the area of Mental Health that it becomes extremely difficult to explicate any further direction or plan. One such approach might be the mere statistical conceptualization in which planners would have to pit the number of children diagnosed as autistic or schizophrenic against the number of children diagnosed as brain damaged as against the number of children diagnosed as neurotic as against the number of children diagnosed as culturally deprived, etc. Anything other than a statistical approach essentially presents one with the problem of individual value judgments. Accordingly, some people make judgments about need in terms of their own concept of "sickest." By this, is usually meant, those children least accessible to the known and available techniques of intervention or rehabilitation. There is great doubt if the cost and suffering and the loss to society is any greater in an autistic child than in an extremely bright creative youngster who is so phobia-ridden that he cannot get out of his home or function in society. I cannot favor a statistical approach to research planning because it would preclude the heuristic impact and possible breakthrough from relatively insignificant diseases (in terms of incidence). One such example would be the heuristic impact of research on phenylketonuria in spite of the extreme rarity of this condition. Quite likely, as meaningful a way as any of describing need would be to do it alphabetically, starting with A—adoption and autism, all the way to Z—zoophobia.

It is also essential to note that all research planning in terms of need is predicated on a humanistic egalitarian philosophy of life and an equally strong conviction that money and directed effort can produce scientific results. It is as if our political beliefs, our humanism, and our affluence lead us to believe that we can legislate away the troubles of mankind. Or that we can do this by appropriating large enough sums to appropriately designated research areas.

I think this error stems from a stubborn confusion of basic science with development or technology. While there is admittedly an overlap, it exists primarily in those areas of "ripeness." Technology can be heroically mobilized and directed by legislation; science much less so, if at all.

The second strategy stresses the dynamic relationship between available knowledge and technology. To adequately plan for short-range research gains, one must search the basic research data with a view toward what areas for development have been made "ripe" by work such as tissue culture, rather than listing priorities of needs. Painful though it may be, we must bear in mind that the preventative or therapeutic tools for such a condition or conditions as schizophrenia are not at hand because our researchers have not as yet unlocked the nature of the disease. Were we, by some magic, able to increase the number of mental health workers and facilities by ten or one hundred fold, we would be no closer to an understanding, or a treatment or treatments of schizophrenia. This is not to confuse making available the best that is available even if it is ameliorative—while knowing that the definitive intervention can only come from basic research. However, there is a crucial difference between the two and one shouldn't be confused with the other.

SHORT-RANGE RESEARCH

I would like to suggest that two strategic approaches to short-term research are possible. The first, as indicated above, is that the probabilities of pay-off will be enhanced by programming research in those areas where the state of the field (in a research sense) seems "ripe," rather than in those areas where the need seems greatest. This is based on the historical survey of how research usually blends into development. The success of a crash program such as the bomb or a vaccine is not predicated on the need, but rather on the moment of ripeness, how close to a developmental phase the preceding basic research has come.

The second short-range goal would be assessment research, aimed at a closer understanding of existing programs and as an integral part of new programming.

I do not intend . . . to cover all areas of "ripeness" but would like to give an example of what I have in mind. I think it has been substantially documented that the development of the child depends on the availability of a consistent, nourishing, stable, care-taking person. In the usual family, this is the mother. We have abundant and consistent clinical and developmental empiric evidence of the devastating impact of a lack of mothering from over fifty years of research, particularly in certain kinds of institutions. It is clinically documented that certain variations in early mothering will lead to failure to "thrive," to a host of developmental arrests and deviations. I do think that this area of the impact of mothering on development is ripe for concerted and planned research. I would like to contrast this with a condition such as autism where the research goals will be long-range, since not enough is known of the nature of the disease for short-range planning.

In terms of assessment research, we are currently struggling with the results of decades of following a humanist-activist model rather than a research model. Without appropriate assessment or evaluative research, "demonstration project" planning can lead to a Tower of Babel. One cannot overestimate the complexity of evaluation or assessment research. While this is undoubtedly true of all intervention or preventive programs, I would like to focus on treatment intervention as one example. The methodological complexities have made it extremely difficult to do convincing research in this area, and an obstinate lack of humility has prevented us from viewing the problem in terms of indications and contra-indications for one or another of a host of therapeutic interventions. Instead, we continue to ask simplistic, inappropriate questions such as: "Does psychotherapy work?," or "Does psychoanalysis work?," or "Does Drug A, B, or C work?"

This error can be illuminated by attending to a number of rather chronic deficiencies in the research to date.

The first, and most overwhelming, is the fact that in using students in research it has always been related to training and that almost no systematic research exists in which the variable of experience has been adequately dealt with. This is most glaring in psychotherapeutic research where sensitivity and skill are not only among the most important of a host of variables, but are also a product of the state of training and the amount of experience the therapist has had. Treatment research using residents in training is research in training and not directly relevant to the effectiveness of a treatment method.

Given the complexity of a paradigm which would run Patient A (with hundreds of variables) in Life Situation B (with hundreds of variables) getting Treatment C (with many variables) from Dr. D. (with innumerable variables) at Time and Place X (with its host of variables), one readily sees the methodological problems involved in manageable simplification. It is noteworthy that attempts still go on to reduce such complex interactions to two or three variable models of research.

Since virtually all short-range project research is funded, it seems imperative to introduce such concepts as "appropriate rigor" and "relevance" to the funding concepts used. The very old continuum of neat but irrelevant, dirty but important, prevail. All our clinical research is complex and will continue to suffer unless cognizance is taken of that complexity. The area should be supported financially if it is "appropriately" rigorous and "systematic." Methodological complexity is a lesser error and is certain to be more productive ultimately than irrelevance.

It is abundantly clear that good assessment programs for existing therapeutic modes are imperative and that if they are sophisticatedly conceived, can yield a great deal of information about indications and contra-indications. It is thoughtless to expect psychotherapy as we currently know it to have much impact on infantile autism, but it is inordinately hazardous to assume that it has *no* impact on hysteria or phobia or other neurotic states.

Perhaps an example will clarify the meaning of this. If one looks at the 1960–1967 statistics from the State of Connecticut, we find that new admissions to the State Hospital system have increased 55% since 1955. Re-admissions have increased 253% and now account for more than half of the total admissions. This is reflective of a massive humanistic therapeutic endeavor which takes an empiric, researchable question as its basic postulate; i.e., people are better off out of hospitals than inside of them. While this proposition in itself has never been demonstrated, evaluation has focused on the patient population, and has not been extended to the impact of such serial hospitalization on family, children, and communities. The values of such a therapeutic endeavor are revealed in such statistics and are laudable humanistic efforts, but can hardly lend support to the idea that this is a scientifically-based therapeutic endeavor.

Although many people are aware of the distressing impact on dependent children of such serial home-to-hospital-to-home psychotic environments, the definitive research has not yet been done. At the same time, there is every reason to suspect that this program brings about grievous disturbances in the development of children. If we were to rephrase this mental health problem arbitrarily in terms of foster parent care, I have no doubt that every professional and non-professional involved would disqualify an ambulatory psychotic mother and/or father who is hospitalized two to six times per year, and with varying degrees of drug control when out of the hospital, as a good candidate for being a foster parent. Yet, we are in effect condoning this with biological parents in our current hospital policies. The assessment of such programs must include the impact on children, families, and the community, as well as the status of the patient himself.

LONG-RANGE RESEARCH PLANNING

An historic view of the progress of science reveals the reasonable thought that one requires a very large scientific establishment consisting of many individuals or small groups of individuals working on their own or related projects. From this broad base, the probability is enhanced that a single individual or a small group of individuals with sufficient creative genius will either conceptualize something completely new or re-synthesize a field anew. It is these "breakthroughs" which represent the best of basic science and are paradigmatic for the subsequent technological developments which come in its wake.

Again, it would be reasonably clear to study *where* such science occurs and in *what* atmosphere it occurs. If one does this, one is led to the central if not exclusive position of the University. Every aspect of science either happens within a university or is closely related to the university—certainly in the sense of people trained in the university. If the United States did not have a large and probably the world's finest university system, it would be appropriate to request funds to set up such a system. It was this university complex which made American Science pre-eminent. Federal funding was to enhance it. Since we are speaking of preserving the atmophere of the university and extending it and the kinds of innovative people it attracts as a calculated risk for science, it is worth paying some attention to the university itself.

The basic, or perhaps I should more appropriately say, the ideal, university, consists of a community of free and independent scholars, each engaged in the acquisition and transmission of knowledge. The great vitality of the American University system has come from its heterogeneity in the sense that it consists of a large number of very different kinds of institutions, each with its own specific charge. This ranges from the extremely practical mission of certain agricultural colleges to the freest kind of scholarly tradition as represented by schools such as Yale, Harvard, and the University of Chicago. That these universities are in a process of great change is self-evident. It is imperative that the appropriate bodies of educators, citizens, and politicians arrive at some basic conception of the primary mission of universities within the United States.

If I may quote Yale President Kingman Brewster, "The survival as well as the quality of civilization depends greatly upon the effectiveness of continuous discovery and learning in our universities. The effectiveness of American universities depends greatly upon free competition for students, faculty, and new ideas among hundreds of ambitious institutions. The effectiveness of this academic competition depends greatly upon the ability of some of the strongest institutions to direct their own destiny, free of political interference, free of dependence upon outside dictate."

I would hold that it is this quality of the self-directed, free academic enterprise—different, diverse, heterogenous, and dedicated to discovery and learning which is crucial to the well being and future of science in the United States. This is certainly true of all fields but particularly of the chaotic state of scientific endeavor in the mental health sciences.

The major part of research relevant to mental health continues to be forthcoming, primarily from medical schools, and secondarily from certain graduate departments in those aspects of the social and biological sciences which are called behavioral sciences. The Medical School has a tradition of its own, which cannot avoid carrying a considerable burden of providing facilities for patient care when this care is an essential part of the experience of medical education and research.

It is quite clear that the modern university can no longer exist without adequate Federal aid for its operations. Since, in recent years, this has become increasingly tied to part of a service demand for the citizenry, one must seriously question the relationship between quantities of service and research. In addition, it would appear that there is some danger of foreclosure in the interests of maximizing equal care—by that I mean foreclosure in direction and area of growth. That is, however, not the only conflict which is potentially harmful for scientific growth. Another is that of the position of the investigator caught between short and long-range goals, particularly as they relate to current funding practices.

FINANCING

There are essentially three sources of research funds and salaries for research people. These are the university facilities themselves, private foundations, and the Federal Government. Of these, the heroically increasing expense involved in operating an appropriate institution and doing research has made it mandatory that Federal aid be perhaps the most crucial aspect.

By current practice, the largest proportion of research is granted to investigators who apply via appropriate study section review for projects. Although such projects are renewable, they tend to average about three years per request and tend to support the salary of the principal investigator and his staff as well as the expenses of conducting the research. This has developed a number of problems.

The first of these is the difficulty of establishing appropriate criteria of scientific merit which can be used with fairness across a tremendous range of studies which have addressed themselves to essentially different phenomenology. In recent years, this has put an unnecessary hardship on those investigators who do clinical research because of the fact that the multivariant phenomena which they approach—if it is to retain its relevance—does not readily lend itself to the somewhat simplistic criteria of scientific rigor which is more appropriate to more sharply circumscribed studies which usually have no or little clinical relevance. As a result of this, we feel that clinical research is in a decline and think that every effort must be made not only to preserve it but to invigorate it and revitalize it.

The second hardship such project research brings about is the fact that principal investigators are forced to circumscribe small, doable projects rather than to concentrate on a career in a programmatic sense. The only exception to this has been the rather successful Career Awards program operated by NIMH.

Another debilitating factor in this model is the uncertainty and instability of the academic or the research setting for the investigator. He must conceive of a project in order to get his salary and the salary of his staff. If he wants to continue, he must prematurely (while the project is in midstream) initiate an additional request for either a supplementary grant, or else conceive of a new project, etc. What this has resulted in is a loss of the time and energy of the principal investigator who functions under the duress and anxiety of this instability. I think it is fair to assume that these represent the best-trained scientific talent available which must now give a great deal of its time to fund-raising and to administration.

To summarize, such short-range or project or product research tends to place investigators under an unnecessary and self-defeating burden of insecurity, necessity to "go where the money is," necessity to delineate small doable project research, all of which tends to vitiate faculty self-determination. This program-ming plus a service orientation will diminish faculty self-determination in terms of the goals set out at the beginning of the last section.

In addition to this, one must consider the fact that since universities can no longer function without Federal aid, they are obliged to go in the direction of where Federal funding dictates. In the current and foreseeable future it will be easier to get service funding than research funding. This will be particularly true of universities which ally themselves with Mental Health Centers or Heart, Stroke, and Cancer Centers. This then, brings about a subtle change in the direction and in the function of the university which tends to produce a homogeneity within the American University system with each medical school being responsible for an appropriately sized catchment area which strains its service responsibilities. Some future historian may chronicle that "before they became Commissioners of Health, Deans of Medical Schools were considered to be Educators, and their institutions were highly esteemed as centers of learning."

I do not for a moment mean that such concerns aren't crucial concerns of citizenry and government; I merely question the priority and the devastating impact of pre-empting the traditional university function for this purpose.

The dangers of such a continued direction are already apparent, particularly in the rather ominous professionalization of the graduate school. The Ph.D. degree, once granted for original contribution to research, is now granted to engineers. If this continues to be the case in all universities, one cannot help but wonder where the future cadre of scientific talent will develop.

The physical sciences already demonstrate the impact of governmental planning and funding. At the same time, they are not as paradigmatic for the general university as are the health sciences—in particular, Medical Schools. The Medical School is prototypical of the emerging University-Federal Govern-ment homogeneity; and Psychiatry is prototypical of that evolving relationship.

What has occurred to university departments of Psychiatry because of Mental Health planning and Mental Health centers, will happen soon to departments of Medicine, and Surgery with the appearance of Heart, Stroke, and Cancer In-stitutes in an identical "pattern." It is abundantly clear that departments of Psychiatry (and soon all Medical Schools) can no longer exist without Federal funding, and the question for me is, "Can they exist *with* Federal funding?" More appropriately, "In what form can they exist?"

Within Psychiatry, as a result of meeting the demands of Federal planning and funding, there has developed a possible leveling—a pedestrian, monotonous, uniformity of departments throughout the country. This is primarily in the service of a larger humanistic movement of helping people and equalizing all care. While much can be said for this, and I am myself sympathetic to it, Science has and will continue to suffer, particularly in terms of the coming generations of scholarly innovators.

If we pre-occupy ourselves with delivery systems, we will continue to lose sight of the more crucial and difficult problem of what is to be delivered. There are some areas, such as polio vaccine and others, where the disparity is not so great and where the priorities may be different. However, these areas are few, and somewhere within the national planning, the first priority must be to innovators.

The Federal Government must address itself to maintaining an optimal climate in which the Einsteins and the Enders can emerge without a loss of developers. By this, I do not intend to demean the contribution of technology; it is more a matter of priorities.

In the past, both aspects have been encouraged within the United States by the great diversity within our educational system. The value to the country of the ferment that comes from such heterogeneity in terms of different kinds of universities can never be under-estimated.

Given the harsh realities of funding practices, the only antidote must be to plan for self-determination on the part of institutions. This has served the country incredibly well in the past, and is the only way to guarantee the ferment so crucial to the educational enterprise.

This does not mean a "parochial elite" but is an antidote to the possibility that each of the Medical Schools, via controlled planning, tends to become a "service station" for the short-range health needs of the country. Some universities must be preserved for the long-range health needs.

What I see as the only hopeful alternative is large block grants to institutions which will permit them the necessary freedom of self-determination in their faculty, teaching, research, and missions.

On a broader level, it is incredible to me that the educational enterprise—which has served the country so well—should have to justify its existence on any other level than the increased benefits to the country of an educated citizenry. The health and welfare of its citizens is a matter of prime priority to government. It would be a tragic and short-range, blind decision to so pre-empt the values of the University.

In summary, the long-range research needs of the country can be approached as one small segment of the larger issue of the function and status of the university in modern life. It calls for a sober reappraisal of the mutual obligations and mutual impact of the university and the "outside world" (government, industry, and the community) upon each other. To date, this is a matter which has concerned educators far more than scientists.

There can be no doubt that the gradual emergence of the university from its classical monastic seclusion has had an enormously beneficial effect on all concerned. One major function of the university must remain that of a reservoir of highly skilled, specialized talent for the practical problems of government, industry, and the community. It is by now obligated to so remain a vital force in civilization.

And yet, one must seriously question the developing concept of the itinerant consultant—which is the lot of many professors of science. I do not know if it is possible to have it both ways—perhaps it is a matter of degree—but it must be possible to function as such a reservoir without completely relinquishing the concept of university as a community of highly individual, independent, free scholars.

If we focus on psychiatry, besieged by service needs, community needs, national mental health, etc., the problem of basic research can seem a luxury rather than a crucial urgency. This is further complicated by the multidisciplinary nature of the enterprise as well as by the multitheoretical characteristics of the field. It can be a bewildering morass which should concern all psychiatrists.

From the viewpoint of the incomplete nature of the research results of *all* theoretical systems, methods, and disciplines, great humility on the part of all thoughtful scientists seems appropriate. Practically, it may call for eclectic departments of psychiatry. This does not mean departments composed of eclectics. At the stage of scientific progress, most scientists would agree that this blunts the probe and blurs the exploration.

I refer rather to an over-all eclecticism arising from a commuity of experts representing their own disciplines with integrity, dedication, and security. In such a department, psychiatry, pediatrics, education, and psychoanalysis can stand, contribute, and grow alongside neurophysiology, biochemistry, neuropharmacology, and the social sciences. In the unconditional freedom of the university tradition, each specialist must be free to immerse himself in the complexities of his own research area.

He must also be free to collaborate—not by assignment but by inner direction. If there is to be fruitful, multidisciplinary collaboration, it would best arise spontaneously from such an intellectual climate rather than from a calculated financial need. It cannot be programmed for it depends too much on the ripeness of the moment, the people, the methods, and the communication.

I do not intend to demean the multidisciplinary studies which have already been done. For one thing, they have forced helpful clarifications and sharpened awareness of similarities and differences. This is no inconsiderable service. To my mind, they raise the consideration that our knowledge is still insufficient to launch many such teams. The progress of science might be best served by pushing individual theory to its limits. I remain convinced that when the time is at hand for basic research collaboration between disciplines, the best of it will come as highly individual, inspired spurts rather than from premeditated calculation. Perhaps the best one can do to enhance the probability is the preservation of the most fertile soil, i.e., the provocative skepticism of university heterogeneity. In such a structure, whether through intrigued interest or irritated awareness, multidisciplinary communication and teaching occur.

Science *and* the university will both lose something very important if the community of free scholars, and the communication so made possible within the university, is altered. The future development of both begs for a tolerant re-evaluation by men of vision (Lustman, 1968).

Some of Dr. Lustman's recommendations can be noted in the principles which follow.

SOME GENERAL GUIDING PRINCIPLES FOR RESEARCH PROGRAMS

1. There is a critical need for stepped-up programs in the research fields related to mental health. *Both basic and applied research are essential.* "Further support of technological development in society without concurrent and extensive expansion of behavioral research may further widen the gap between the well-being of the individual and of the society" (NICHD, 1968).

2. A high priority must be given *to the establishment and preservation of a national research climate which optimizes the productivity and opportunities of individual researchers.* It is assumed that a very broad concept of child development encompasses the basic disciplines of biology, the social sciences, the behavioral sciences, education, and the medical sciences (Lustman, 1968).

3. *Short-range research projects should be planned on the basis of "the ripeness of the moment,"* that is, what aspect of basic research knowledge is close to a developmental phase, rather than some vague concept of "meeting the need" (Lustman, 1968).

4. *Assessment research must be an integral part of existing action programs.* It seems crucial "to redefine demonstration projects as innovative efforts which include evaluation and assessment as a central orientation. To prevent the spawning of a massive proliferation of demonstration projects which present us with the dangers of a Tower of Babel, it is necessary to stress that no demonstration project should be funded without appropriate rigor and relevant assessment techniques" (Lustman, 1968).

Universities might develop special centers for action-related research which employs the skills of investigators whose particular talents and interests lie in evaluation and assessment of action programs. Such centers might be particularly effective in carrying out action experiments with built-in research and in training nonprofessionals and professionals for practitioner and administrative careers in mental health and related fields. A diversity of approaches by different universities would seem to be the appropriate solution to this matter.

Basic knowledge stands to gain from program research when it is wisely planned. Action programs involve social experimentation which provides an opportunity for examining the effects of many factors on social and behavioral problems (Campbell, 1969).

5. *Multidiscipline collaboration* between researchers in both basic and applied fields should receive increased support. Fruitful collaboration would best be achieved if it arose spontaneously from a free, intellectual climate rather than from a calculated financial need. It is imperative that such a climate be maintained to promote frequent interaction between practitioners and the social scientists (*Report of Task Force IV,* 1968). It is also im-

portant that biologists and researchers from social science areas collaborate closely in their investigations of human development and behavior (NICHD, 1968). Furthermore, there needs to be closer cooperation among economists, political scientists, and philosophers working with other social and behavioral scientists in the development of innovative approaches and new concepts, especially in reference to improving the mental health climate of communities (Gioscia *et al.*, 1968).

In view of the multidisciplinary nature of research in this field and with a view toward preserving a national eclecticism, it is necessary to explore such concepts as "appropriate rigor" and "appropriate relevance" of the phenomena being studied (Lustman, 1968).

6. There is a drastic need for *longitudinal studies of human development that cover the entire life-span*. Cross-sectional studies which investigate the behavior and development of human beings at different ages and developmental periods fail to provide the information that we need on such factors as: the origins of disorders in human development, the continuity of such disorders throughout the life-span, the factors that affect these disorders in both positive and negative directions over a period of time, and the timing and sequence of various behaviors. Presently available studies of human development are particularly lacking on children between the ages of one and three years and on adults between the ages of twenty-one and fifty-five.

Longitudinal studies are very difficult and expensive, but they are crucially needed. New techniques are emerging which promise to reduce some of the difficulties associated with longitudinal studies. These involve the inclusion in the study sample of different age cohorts who will be followed through for five years or so. Thus, a study of child development might include several groups of children of varying age spans, such as birth to five years; five to ten; ten to fifteen, and so on.

7. It is strongly recommended that greater support be granted for *multivariate analyses*. We now have statistical techniques which make it possible to systematically hold a number of variables constant while examining the effects of each separately. If we are to gain the requisite understanding of the causes of human dysfunctions, their prevention, and their treatment, we must simultaneously study a number of factors in relation to their interaction, multiple influences, and differential effects on various kinds of individuals and in relationship to the various components of individual development, such as intellectual, social, physical, and emotional. According to a recent summary of related research (NICHD, 1968), a central gap in the knowledge of human behavior relates to the impact of the social, psychological, physical, and economic environment on the human being— a gap which points to the need for multivariate analyses.

8. We need more basic research knowledge regarding the *nature of social structures and their impact on people*. More experimental studies are

needed which involve planned changes in these structures and an assessment of the impact of these changes. If we do not change many aspects of the social environment, "mental health treatment and prevention programs focused on individuals and small groups will accomplish little" (Gioscia *et al.*, 1968).

9. *Experimental research and development centers employing a multidisciplinary team to study the development of children and families are strongly recommended.* Such centers should undertake carefully planned intervention approaches with provision for replication of these studies. Such centers should be jointly planned by personnel from universities, action programs, and federal and state governments. These centers need to be coordinated with other somewhat similar operations which are already in progress, such as the Regional Educational Laboratories under the sponsorship of the Office of Education (Title IV, Elementary and Secondary Education Act, 1965).

10. It is further recommended that *ways be explored to further coordinate the federal research activities related to children and families.* These are currently being diversely planned and sponsored in a number of federal agencies, such as the Office of Education, the Social and Rehabilitation Service (including the Children's Bureau), NIMH, NICHD, the Departments of Labor and Agriculture, and OEO. The present arrangement leads to numerous difficulties. For example, researchers are forced to "shop around" for support for their studies with little, if any, direction as to where they might find such support. While there is much to recommend in the present diversity of programs, careful thought should be given to better overall coordination of these activities and the development of a central information resource about these programs.

The development and funding of experimental research and development centers, the overall coordination of federal research programs related to child and family development and mental health, and provision for the coordinated review and dissemination of relevant research findings logically might be tied to the advocacy system recommended in this report.

11. *We recommend that the NIMH sponsor, in connection with its clearinghouse activities, studies which would develop techniques for evaluating material which should be quickly retrieved and more rapidly disseminated to the relevant professional practitioners.*

A similar project was designed independently to review recent literature. This task was to be accomplished by an interdisciplinary team, seeking "dimensions" and "innovations." It ran head-on into what has been called the information explosion. We do not think that a policy of occasional, *ad hoc* position papers written by a small group of experts who selectively review the published literature is a particularly good way to keep abreast of dimensions and innovations (*Report of Task Force IV*, 1968).

12. Further efforts are needed to increase and upgrade the *training of research manpower*. Such manpower is a valuable and scarce national resource and requires national support (see Chapter XII).

13. *Epidemiological studies of populations in need of various kinds of services are essential.* If we are to plan appropriately for services, we must know much more about the nature, prevalence, and interaction of problems related to poor physical and mental health. Such studies should be combined with surveys of the availability, nature, and quality of relevant public and private services. These investigations should also include analyses of social and economic conditions affecting the population studies.

At present, service data are available for separate programs, but the information does not disclose what we need to know about people and varying community conditions. These data are variously gathered by many different governmental and voluntary organizations and relate to the specific missions of specific agencies. Thus, it is next to impossible to obtain a comprehensive picture of the needs of all the people and the degree to which programs are meeting these needs.

Through epidemiological studies we would have much clearer information regarding the etiological factors in human malfunctioning; the interaction of these factors; the existence of high-risk populations and the conditions associated with these high risks; and the availability and efficacy of services (*Report of Task Force V*, 1968).

14. Far more work should be done in relation to the *development of better definitions, research methods, and instruments for research in the mental health field*. At present, there is lack of clarity and agreement regarding the definitions of mental illness, emotional disorders, and mental health in general and how these apply to various stages of human development.

Much of the research in the mental health field has been seriously lacking in scientific rigor. This is related to the relative newness of the field and the exceptional research difficulties that are encountered.

Further efforts should be directed toward the development of objective methods of assessing human behavior and functioning. It is important that this assessment be carried out simultaneously in a number of behavioral settings in which the individual operates, such as within the family, the school, and the neighborhood. At present, there is a tendency to study a child's behavior in only one of these settings, such as in a laboratory or treatment situation.

In all studies, the two sexes should be considered independently of each other. Generally speaking, such pervasive psychological differences have been found to exist between the sexes that research findings are confounded unless males and females are considered as separate groups.

15. *Cross-cultural studies* are greatly needed. The perspectives that can be gained from the natural laboratory provided by extreme cultural differ-

ences have not been adequately exploited. Cross-cultural studies provide wider ranges of variation in normative practice than can be found in any single society. They provide a crucial test for distinguishing what is programmed in genetic human nature and what is culturally induced.*

SOCIAL AND PSYCHOLOGICAL ASPECTS
OF CHILD AND ADOLESCENT BEHAVIOR AND DEVELOPMENT

Multivariate Research Directed Toward Multiple Criteria

Challenging as it may be, there is a great need for multivariate research directed toward the multiple criteria of the mentally healthy child or adolescent. Efforts must be directed toward discovering the clustering of factors associated with the various but interrelated aspects of an individual's mental health status.

Most of our research regarding social and psychological aspects of child and adolescent development and behavior has been highly specialized. In general, it has been addressed to single factors and has considered only a limited number of variables. Valuable as this research may be, it tells us very little about how children grow and develop—or fail to grow and develop—in physically and/or mentally healthy ways. This research has led to a situation similar to that fostered by current mental health and related community programs addressed to the needs of children and youth. Earlier in this report we stressed the difficulties arising from the present poor coordination and the proliferation of highly specialized services, as well as the large gaps in needed services. If we are to provide the coordinated, effective, full programs for children and youth which the Commission recommended, it is important that we have a coordinated body of related knowledge on which to base our efforts and assess their effectiveness.

In short, we must enlarge the scope of many of our studies. As Adelson (1969) remarks, "The field of personality these days is marked by abundance, diffuseness, and diversity." He goes on to comment that research in personality may be described as a "disconcerting sprawl." "What we have is a loose collation of topics—an achievement literature, an anxiety literature, and so on—each of which more or less goes its own way. . . . For better or worse, the movement of the field is centrifugal—that is, toward the detailed exploration of empirical domains. The impulse for synthesis, for finding unities, has for the moment been set aside."

In addition to being limited to specific areas of concern, most studies have considered the influence of only one set of variables associated with the attitudes or behavior under investigation. Research also has been

* Written communication to the Commission by M. Brewster Smith, April 9, 1969.

limited by the tendency to select specific age and population groups, primarily because certain groups are readily available for study.

Ideally, multivariate, multiple-criterion studies should be based on carefully selected samples of young people who vary in age and ethnic and social class membership. Research should be undertaken in a wide range of settings. Studies should be designed along the following lines:

1. What relationships exist between age-appropriate competence in mastery of verbal and motor skills, adequate impulse control, capacity for reality perception and appropriate behavior, satisfactory and satisfying social relationships?

2. What association is there between levels of mental health as rated and tested on the above criteria and such factors as the following: physical health, family composition and functioning, socioeconomic status of family, school and neighborhood situation, sex, and ethnicity?

Admittedly, this is a complicated form of research, one which presents a large number of problems such as the difficulties of measurement and ratings, the need for multiple observation in various settings, and possible errors of rating and judgment which make it difficult to arrive at satisfactory operational definitions.

Some research has already been carried out which furnishes guidelines for studying the whole child in his multifaceted environment, such as the studies of Barker and Wright (1959), Escalona et al. (1953), and Yarrow (1968). Greater support is needed for studies of these types.

Some of these multivariate studies might be launched in association with ongoing programs, such as those in preschools or in the experimental research and development centers which were recommended previously (see point 10 above). Such settings may provide ready access to information on children and their families which flows naturally from the operation of the programs and offers the advantage of access to naturalistic settings. There is growing recognition that experimental laboratory studies have a number of drawbacks, including their artificiality and the ethical questions involved in the planned manipulation of human beings. There is also an economic advantage, since it is extremely expensive to set up action programs for the purposes of research only. Moreover, researchers are not generally prepared by training and experience to plan and administer action programs and might function more effectively in programs which are already in progress.

Researchers working within the setting of ongoing programs could provide valuable information by assessing program effectiveness. However, multivariate, naturalistic research should not be limited to program assessment because the multiple restraints frequently placed on assessment research may inhibit the design and operations of multivariate studies. (See also section on program research and evaluation, p. 458.)

Since the basic concept of multivariate, multiple-criterion research applies equally well to any age group, it can be incorporated in a cross-sectional study. This would provide a counter to the present tendency to study only one specific form of behavior among a certain age group.

Specific Fields of Investigation

It is impracticable, and probably undesirable, to undertake only such global studies as those just described. More specific fields of investigation related to the social and psychological aspects of child and youth development and behavior might well be focused on such problem areas as the following:

1. It is important that we identify and gain a deeper understanding of the *many factors that are potentially responsible for damage to the unborn child* (see sections on biological research and program research).

2. We greatly need *more studies on the infant and very young child*, especially children between the ages of one and three. "Perhaps in no other area is there such a pressing need for both basic and applied research, drawing for its direction on the many disciplines involved in the comprehensive care of infants and children" (*Report of Task Force I*, 1968). Particular attention should be paid to parent-infant interaction and to the influence which behavioral models set by the parents have on the child's development.

It is also important that there be more studies of the "toddler" (the child between the ages of one and three years), since this is probably a crucial period in psychological development, when life trajectories are set and perhaps irreversible trends are established. Normal developmental processes during this period—cognitive, social, physical, and emotional—need to be studied in detail. Moreover, short-term longitudinal studies are badly needed to link the phases of infancy, toddlerhood, early childhood, and the school age. In the absence of such studies, we are still not in a position to judge the effects of deprivation or enrichment or of particular patterns of relationship at particular stages.*

3. Advances in the *study of linguistics and early language* should make possible, in the near future, major gains in our understanding of verbal learning in children. Developmental psycholinguistics has advanced enough to develop methods which will further our understanding of the actual strategies and tactics that children use in verbal learning and memory. Gains in this area could be of great use to educators in remedial programs and would add to our general understanding of children, since their use of language is so closely related to their emerging psychological status.

4. Intensive and productive *studies of self-attitudes* are beginning to

* Written communication to the Commission by M. Brewster Smith, April 9, 1969.

emerge and should receive further support. It seems clear that attitudes toward the self bear a direct relationship to constructive or unconstructive behavior, such as whether the person feels that he is a victim of fate or can take an effective role in making the most of his life. We need not only to understand the importance of these attitudes but also how we might change unhealthy self-attitudes.

5. Studies aimed at learning more about the *processes of child development* have important theoretical and practical implications. At present, there are two major schools of thought in this field, with one school taking its lead from Piaget, who sees development as a series of progressive stages through which a child moves, and those who see development as a process by which the child is molded by the demands and rewards which he experiences in his social environment. Both views need further exploration.

6. *Creativity and the capacity to use one's imagination* is an important inner resource for planning, defense against anxiety, and impulse control. Findings from research to date indicate that creativity in children is associated with parental warmth, rich verbal interaction in the home, parental acceptance of a child's interests in fantasy, opportunities for privacy, and parental support of the child's education. It appears that disadvantaged children have less opportunity than other children to fully develop their imaginations. Fundamental research is yet to be done in this area (NICHD, 1968).

7. Research is critically needed on the *"failure to thrive syndrome."* It is recommended that the many factors associated with this syndrome, such as child abuse, physical deficits, and child-rearing behaviors, be taken into consideration and that apparently normal, healthy children be compared to those with the disability under investigation.

8. More research is needed on *individual behavior tendencies which seem apparent at birth* so that we may clarify the origin and the *impact of these tendencies and their modifiability.*

9. We also need to know more about the *effects of discrimination and labeling* on a child's development and behavior. Such studies should include the effects of ethnic and social class discrimination as well as the effects of being labeled a delinquent, a slow learner, emotionally disturbed, mentally ill, and the like.

10. In the field of *adolescent psychology* we need to know more about such factors as the *development of work orientation, the transition from school to work, the development of adult roles and identities, the impact of increasing demands for higher education, the impact of war and the draft, the effects of drug use, the processes of addiction to drugs, and the conditions associated with student protest and riots in junior highs, high schools, and colleges.* Some studies have been centered on the characteristics of those who protest. We also need studies of the "protest" characteristics of

different schools and of the responses of the school, the community, and the mass media to these protests. Under what conditions do these protests occur, under what conditions do they escalate, under what conditions are they resolved?

We also need to know: *Is adolescent rebellion inevitable and necessary in our society?* What are the characteristics of those families in which parent-child relationships continue to be positive and relatively serene during adolescence and those in which there are communication failures and conflicts? Does a relatively "calm" adolescence entail a loss of true individuality and richness of personality?

In addition, we need information on the *factors associated with the tendency to marry early. What factors are associated with "successful" and "unsuccessful" early marriages?*

11. Systematic knowledge is needed on *adult behavior and development*, including the adaptation of adults to their marital and parental roles at different points in the family life cycle. This neglected area of research is clearly significant and intimately associated with the mental health and general well-being of children and youth (Chilman, 1968).

MENTAL ILLNESS AND EMOTIONAL DISORDERS

The Commission strongly urges that research efforts be increased on the study of mental illness and emotional disorders, particularly on the areas discussed below and on the assessment of treatment methods which will be presented in a later section (see "Program Research").

Research Methodologies

There is a critical need for improvement in research methodologies related to clinical issues. At the present time, there is a vast confusion and lack of agreement about diagnostic criteria and classfication systems. (See also Chapter VI.) Assessment of the effects of various forms of therapy has been markedly lacking in appropriate scientific rigor, as will be discussed later in this chapter. According to Meyer Sonis of the University of Pittsburgh School of Medicine:

Unless the clinician and clinical facilities are willing to evolve methods for testing out the effectiveness of various modalities of treatment utilized, the "newer" models of treatment based on current theories will be utilized as the "panacea" for all problems in children. New models of approach, without an equal opportunity for evaluation of programs offered, may produce, at some later time, an even greater number of chronically disturbed children as a result of temporary measures.[*]

[*] Written communication to the Commission from Dr. Meyer Sonis, April 16, 1969.

Better Coordination of Studies

As in other fields, there has been a tendency for clinical investigators to focus on only one variable at a time. According to Haddad (1964):

. . . investigators must avoid concentrating solely on single variables—whether it is urine, blood, mother, or community. Instead of chopping the patient into bits in order to study the variables in isolation, the trend is now toward the study of the many variables involved—physiological, psychological, and social—in their interaction.

Presently, studies on psychiatric issues related to children tend to be conducted by researchers of different theoretical orientations. There is little communication between researchers in these different programs. Further problems are created by the lack of common criteria and agreement on methods of study. Ways must be found to increase "appropriate rigor" in clinical research (*Report of Task Force IV*, 1968).

Psychoses: Autism and Schizophrenia

Very little is known about the causes and treatment of schizophrenia and autism despite several years of intensive research. "There are no assurances on the basis of current research that the schizophrenic illnesses which have challenged the best scientific minds for 2,000 years will be solved within the next year or two. There are, however, a gratifying number of new and interesting observations of considerable potential significance which demand further exploration" (NIMH, 1964).

Workers in the field of schizophrenia and in the areas of the major psychoses have been struggling with a number of basic issues, including the diversity and variability of these disorders and their possible relation to brain damage. Research on schizophrenia today encompasses many sciences—including medical, biological, psychological, and social. Studies range from the most molecular of the biological sciences to the broadest of the behavioral sciences.

It cannot be too often emphasized that significant contributions to an understanding of a clinical disorder such as schizophrenia will in the last analysis depend upon a vast armamentarium of basic information about the workings of the nervous system and of behavior.

The schizophrenia process can hardly be understood, nor can the schizophrenic patient be adequately treated, without recourse to such factors as childhood experiences, patterns of family interaction, and culturally determined attitudes and values. It is these kinds of psychological and social variables that produce the specific, learned behaviors seen among schizophrenics and that mediate the quality, quantity, and contents of the symptoms suffered. In the opinion of some, these factors actually trigger the occurrence of overt, frankly schizophrenic behavior, given the presence of genetically determined neurological and biochemical abnormalities (NIMH, 1964).

Obviously, support is needed for a complex of studies, if we are to understand the causes of schizophrenia and devise effective ways of treating this disorder.

Commenting on research needed in reference to the mentally ill child, Sonis* makes the following points:

a) As yet, no conclusive scientific knowledge exists as to the specific etiology of this disorder or disorders.

b) This disorder has brought with it extensive clinical experience and a body of knowledge about the disorder, the children, the diagnostic issues, the treatment possibilities, but also a myriad set of explanations, theories, diagnostic categories, and inconclusive follow-up studies.

c) This disorder in children has also brought clinical child psychiatry, clinical child psychology, and other professions into close approximation, but not agreement to the issues of: nature-nature, brain-behavior; the significance of neonatal and infant development; the importance of the past versus the present; symptom relief versus cure; defining the role and responsibility of the professional, nonprofessional, and technical staff needed, and the lack of clarity in the profession of child care.

d) The limited clinical facilities available, the myriad approaches, the inconclusive knowledge, the heat of the proponents of one theory over another as opposed to the light shed, the extensive clinical experience gained, the limited manpower: as measured against the estimated number of children with this disorder *pose a serious crisis requiring a national concerted effort.*

Learning Disorders

There is a great need for increased support of learning disorders. At present, there is a widespread lack of agreement over the origins, causes, and treatment of this disorder or group of disorders (Lustman, 1968), and not enough is known about their organic, emotional, and experiential components. It is crucial that these disorders be identified at an early stage in order to prevent or minimize later learning problems that the child is likely to have in school. It is also important that there be more experimental remedial programs and that these be designed to include built-in evaluation. It is also recommended that research in this field include comparisons of children who have learning disorders with children who apparently do not.

In commenting on learning disorders in childhood, Sonis† writes:

* Written communication to the Commission from Dr. Meyer Sonis, April 16, 1969.
† Ibid.

The disorder in childhood subsumed under the rubric of minimal brain damage, learning disorders, perceptual motor dysfunction, and children whose collective repertoire of symptoms has brought clinical child psychiatry, clinical child psychology, pediatrics, pediatric neurology, speech pathology, and educators into close approximation to each other, has also brought with it similar issues as exist for the child diagnosed as mentally ill. The estimated number of children with learning disorders, with even more potentially uncounted, in light of the myriad issues which exist also poses a *serious crisis*.

Other Clinical Research Issues

Among the clinical issues that require further study are the following:

1. The effects of earlier sex maturity on the mental health of children and youth, especially in the case of early-maturing youngsters whose physical maturity is often far ahead of psychological growth. How may such young people be helped to handle this disparity?

2. It has been observed that males are more psychologically and physically vulnerable than females during the early years of development but that females have higher rates of psychoneurosis in adolescence. This suggests that our cultural expectations and general treatment of females may have an adverse effect on them which manifests itself as they reach adolescence. To what extent is this true, and if so, what are the associated factors?

3. Tolerance for anxiety is of central importance in the healthy development of the child. What factors are associated with different levels of anxiety tolerance, especially in the very early years of life?

4. Critical periods in development need to be defined and studied more precisely. As discussed in Chapter VI, there appear to be stages in human growth and development during which specific new learnings most readily occur. If these learnings do not occur at these times there may be lasting damage to the child. To what extent is this formulation true? What are the specific learnings involved? What is the nature of the damage? What are its causes?

5. Are there individual differences among infants and children regarding their capacity to withstand the effects of emotional deprivation, such as inadequate maternal care? To what extent are infants and young children able to recover from such deprivation? Are there individual differences in this regard? What time limit is there during which an infant or very young child can suffer such deprivation and recover from its effects?

6. Are there critical periods in which behavioral patterns of violence and aggression are established with the result that such patterns cannot be altered? What are the origins of these patterns? With what factors are they associated?

7. Psychoanalysis has long been a rich source of hypotheses for the understanding of human behavior. Psychoanalysts and others should test these hypotheses experimentally to produce facts and understandings as well as contributions to theory.

8. Further research is needed on *mental retardation*. We need a greater understanding of those environmental conditions which produce retardation in children who show no organic damage. Studies should be centered on both the preventive and remedial aspects of this disorder (see also section on biological research).

DISADVANTAGED CHILDREN AND YOUTH

There is ample information to indicate that poverty and discrimination adversely affect the physical, intellectual, emotional, and social development of children and youth. However, more detailed research is needed along the following lines:

1. We need more information regarding the impact which life styles of various disadvantaged minority groups and poverty have on physical growth and development, language development and learning skills, emotional and social development, achievement and work attitudes, moral development and values, and attitudes toward the disadvantaged individual's own subgroup and the larger society.

2. More knowledge is needed concerning the life styles and the impact of poverty and discrimination on various subgroups, including individuals and families in small cities, villages, and rural areas in different regions of the country (since most data, to date, is on the urban disadvantaged in the Northeast and Middle West).

3. More information is needed regarding the differential impact of poverty and discrimination on males and females.

4. Studies on the disadvantaged should focus on the strengths of these groups as well as their particular problems.

5. It is important that we gain a deeper understanding of the processes and effects of the adoption of a bicultural pattern, including the adoption of English as a second language. At present, it is not known whether education would be more effective if Standard English were presented as a second language, although this is the feeling proposed and adopted by some educators. Nor is it known what impact this approach would have on the child's value system, sense of identity, and capacity to smoothly integrate within himself these various approaches to living.

6. It is clear that some persons who suffer from poverty and discrimination "make it" in terms of educational and vocational achievement. What factors are associated with these kinds of achievements? What is the

effect of "upward mobility" on the physical and mental health of those who achieve in these ways, in spite of the multiple handicaps of their environment?

7. As we noted earlier, some life styles of the "subcultures of poverty" tend to interact with other factors of the poverty situation to adversely affect the individual's chances for an escape from poverty. In addition, cultural attitudes of the more advantaged operate to prevent the poor from successfully participating in the larger society. We need to know the extent to which the cultural patterns of these various groups change and under what circumstances they change. What effects do cultural change have on the mental health and social and family relationships of those who change? Only by a proper understanding of such problems can we promote effective social change.

8. We need a deeper understanding of the family patterns of disadvantaged groups, including the various patterns of parent-child interaction and the effects of this interaction on the child's cognitive, emotional, and social development.

What are the factors associated with well-organized, stable family life in disadvantaged groups compared to those families which are disorganized? We also need to know the impact of other "socializing agents," such as older children and adults in the neighborhood, the school, the church or temple, and youth-serving organizations.

BIOLOGICAL RESEARCH RELATED TO MENTAL HEALTH

Genetics

The way is open for a new set of advances in the genetics of human behavior, including the important interactions between genetic and environmental inputs. In recent years, the heredity-versus-environment controversies of a generation ago have been productively reformulated. Substantial gains have been made in the understanding of genetic mechanisms and of the important effects of very early experience. But there has not yet been the needed concentration of effort on possible genetic involvements in psychological development. Of particular interest and importance are genetic constitutional differences between children that affect their adaptation both to particular environments and to preventive and remedial programs.

Although there is growing evidence that biological factors play a role in the causation and development of schizophrenia, there are conflicting theories as to whether these factors are related to genetic components. There is considerable evidence that this may be so but that genetic factors interact with a variety of life experiences in very complex ways. It is important that studies on this issue consider various subcategories of schizophrenia and employ genetic criteria along with studies of individuals' biochemistry and life experiences.

Question is being raised as to whether or not there are genetic differences between the races. Most available studies have not been controlled well enough for the impact of socioeconomic factors, discrimination, and the like on the various ethnic groups (NICHD, 1968). Such studies should focus on the implications which any possible ethnic differences might have for planning more effective educational, vocational, and related programs.

The work on genetics is fast becoming a crucial horizon for our research money and energy (*Report of the Committee on Clinical Issues*, 1969):

This should by all means be fostered but along with it a tremendous effort needs to be made to study the implications of these emerging data. For example, let us consider the recent issues around the XYY chromosome aberration, the "super male" so-called: many men institutionalized for violent behavior have been found to carry this particular abnormality. It would seem important to study their off-spring—is this transmitted? Or to study large populations of babies and if some are found to show such a chromosomal pattern to observe their development. Do they develop as other babies do or are they different in some ways? If we can identify children with XYY constitution, how do they study in school? What is their psychological and neurological profile like? If subjected to child analysis, what are the findings? This one discovery opens the universe of basic research studies with enormous implications for mental health.

Other Biological Studies

Much more research is needed on the functioning and development of the brain, both before and after birth. We particularly need more information on normal and aberrant functions, on the neurochemistry of the brain, and on the effects of enriched or deprived prenatal and postnatal environments on brain growth (NICHD, 1968).

Further study is needed on the interaction of the individual and his environment. We need to know more about the impact of the environment and acquired human behaviors on the individual's physiological functioning, including the functions of the nervous system and the endocrinological functions. For example, studies show that physiological functioning can be conditioned to react in certain patterns as a result of behavior patterns that have been established by the individual (NICHD, 1968).

Further study is required on the biological aspects of mental retardation. We also need studies on the effects of stimulation and sensory deprivation on the development and functioning of the nervous system, including its neurochemical aspects. There are clues that maternal deprivation constitutes physical and sensory deprivation and that such behavior difficulties as hyperexcitability, increased violence and aggression, apathy, and some autistic forms of behavior are associated with this deprivation and with neurological deficits in the central nervous system and the brain.

The effects of maternal malnutrition both before conception and during pregnancy require further study, along with careful consideration of possible genetic factors that also may be involved in the outcomes of pregnancy and the condition of the newborn child. We also need more evidence on the effects of poor nutrition on the infant and young child. It is important that multidisciplinary field research be directed toward studies of different human populations to determine the circumstances and manner in which malnutrition influences intellectual and physical development. This must be research that distinguishes differences between temporary effects of acute hunger and the long-term consequences of chronic malnutrition. Studies of the preschool child must also distinguish between the temporary effects of an acute disease process on test performance and behavior and the long-term consequences of chronic malnutrition (Scrimshaw, 1967).

Other important areas of biological research involve the assessment of the effects of the neuro-psycho-pharmacological drugs on the developing nervous system. It is strongly recommended that biologists, social and behavioral scientists, and clinicians work closely together in research activities, so that knowledge from these various fields can be pooled and tested in laboratory and action settings.

PROGRAM RESEARCH AND EVALUATION

The need for evaluation is clear. Time, talent, and other resources can no longer be wasted on ill-planned, non-theoretically based, non-evaluated intervention programs when it seems more crucial than ever that we begin to move in appropriate directions with a minimum of waste motion. . . . It is essential that the success or lack of success of a program be known in order to provide a bench mark for future program policy decision. Part of the skills of both the social scientist and practitioner must be devoted to research and evaluation in field settings. . . . (NICHD, 1968).

The evaluation of programs is highly complex, and we can present only a few highlights here.

Clinical Issues

Psychotherapy: evaluation of its effectiveness. There is a pressing demand for far more extensive and systematic research in the field of psychotherapy. We have already noted that the majority of our youngsters in need of skilled help are not getting it owing to severe shortage of treatment personnel and treatment facilities. However, even if these service deficiencies were overcome, there is an apparent lack of success in the treatment of many mental and emotional disorders, especially those related to infant autism. Research-based evidence is critically needed to determine the most effective way of treating and caring for these children and young people with their different kinds and degrees of emotional and mental disorders.

Question is being raised as to the effectiveness and/or the relevance of many of the current psychotherapeutic approaches. Research aimed at a rigorous assessment of the effects and impact of various forms of psychotherapy is strongly recommended by many experts in the mental health field. This area of research presents many problems. For instance, there is lack of agreement as to what therapy is and what criteria should be used to measure its effects. In addition, there are many factors which cannot be controlled or readily measured that may affect the outcomes of therapy. These include the many influences that impinge on the child's life in his family, school, and neighborhood.

Research in psychotherapy has been difficult, discouraging, and until recently, generally nonrewarding (Gioscia *et al.,* 1968). Most of the studies in this field have been carried out with college students or adults, partly because children are less readily accessible for study and because of the confounding factors of different stages in child development.

There are few studies of the results of psychotherapy with children. It is estimated (Phillips, 1960) that between 80 and 90 percent of published reports on child therapy concern interesting cases and syndromes. Available evaluations usually consist of tabulations of improvement rates at some interval following termination of treatment at a given child guidance center. The more sophisticated analyses of method or outcome have usually been based on adult samples.

Review of assessment studies. In general, evaluative research on the effects of various forms of therapy has been weak, regardless of the age group studied. A review of the literature on the evaluation of psychotherapy with children (Levitt, 1963) shows ratings of "improved" were noted for two-thirds of these children at termination of treatment and for three-fourths at follow-up. The same ratios of reported improvements seemed to apply regardless of therapeutic method, duration, or other factors. Psychoanalytic centers have abandoned this type of evaluation. However, child guidance clinics continue to conduct and publish studies of this nature, although in fewer numbers recently. They appear undeterred by critics, such as Levitt, who have reported that the overall rate of improvement for children who have completed treatment is no different from that noted for control groups who were accepted for but did not receive treatment at the same clinic.

Ratings of improvement published by separate treatment centers are subject to criticism on several grounds. The characteristics of the patient and of the therapist are seldom defined, so it is unclear how far one can generalize from such findings. The identity of the raters is also undetermined, as is the extent of their objectivity in rating. Moreover, the basis of ratings is not stated in most cases (Gioscia *et al.*, 1968). In general, reporting about change rates based on designs of this sort is of questionable validity and provides limited data regarding the effects of psychotherapy.

In the decade following World War II a number of studies were carried out to test patients, usually adults, before and after psychotherapy. Extensive use was made of projective tests, such as the Rorschach. Such studies were generally nonproductive. In more recent years there has been an increasing recognition of the need for a multiple approach to the complex therapeutic process and outcome. There are growing indications that the characteristics of the patient and of the therapist and the nature of their interaction are of critical importance. For example, social class has been found to be an important factor in determining the availability, quality, and outcome of psychotherapy.

There is also emerging evidence that therapists differ in their personal characteristics and in the kinds of skills and capacities which they bring to therapy. Thus, the characteristics of the therapist as well as those of the patient and his total situation must be taken into account when assessing whether or not therapy is effective.

In general, future outcome studies will have to address themselves to the interaction of the patient, therapist, treatment variables, and the appropriate selection of each. It becomes necessary to ask what treatment, by whom, is most effective for this individual with his specific problem. While no single study can answer this question, separate aspects can be dealt with and knowledge accumulated across separate but comparable studies (Gioscia *et al.*, 1968).

In addition, it is important to consider the total life situation of the person who is in treatment, his situation at the beginning and termination of treatment, and his development and functioning at later points in time. It has been noted frequently that therapy often does not have immediate and observable results but may, at a much later point, reveal its long-term effects in more distinct and observable outcomes.

We must determine the effects of various kinds of psychotherapy generally available at clinics on such groups as slow learners among school children, children brought to court for delinquent behavior, drug addicts, and so forth. In a sense, the mental health field has over-extended itself in the public mind and consequently is often assigned tasks which it may be unable to handle. Thus, courts, schools, welfare departments, and recreational programs often seek psychotherapeutic services when, in fact, psychotherapy has not been demonstrably effective for the population groups involved. Indeed, it is becoming apparent that the population groups most in need of large-scale assistance in adapting their behavior to cope with prevailing social expectations are the groups who profit least from psychotherapy as traditionally conducted. There are, however, exceptions to this generalization and these areas need intensive study (Gioscia *et al.,* 1968).

It is also important to determine the effects of psychotherapy on *all* members of the family, not simply on the family member who is in treatment. Although most psychotherapists realize the psychological changes in one member of the family may affect other members in various ways, assessment of these factors is frequently overlooked in the evaluation of therapy outcomes.

Experimental approaches combined with carefully designed assessment research are drastically needed in therapeutic endeavors with low-income individuals or groups. Since studies show that disadvantaged people are less likely to receive psychiatric services, to accept referral to them, and to stay in therapy after they have been accepted for treatment, it is apparent that new strategies are needed which take account of the cultural patterns, the life situations, and the expectancies of such patients.

Other Issues in Program Research

Treatment programs for mental and emotional disorders. The Commission has made several recommendations urging the establishment or expansion of a variety of treatment facilities (see Chapter I, Section II-A).

Our recommendations were based on the best currently available knowledge and clinical judgment. We realize, however, that these various types of treatment facilities have not been rigorously tested for their effectiveness. We urge that such assessments be made and that studies be based on the principles outlined in the beginning of this chapter.

Assessment of Child Development Councils. The leading recommendation of the Commission calls for the establishment of Child Development Councils at the neighborhood level and for other advocate structures at the local governmental, state, and national levels. This recommendation has also been based on the best available judgment and knowledge of experts in the field. It is not known how effectively such councils will actually work. However, the situation is far too grave to delay the establishment of these councils until pilot projects have been developed and thoroughly tested. In order to meet immediate needs and yet not overlook the necessity for assessment, we recommend the establishment of Evaluation Centers. We hope that large-scale evaluation and program research will be considered a "must." We believe that different models of these councils should be tried in various communities. One focus of research, then, should be on the relative effectiveness of these different models.

The assessment of the effectiveness of these councils will be extremely complex. They should be carried out at predetermined points in time, such as *before* the council is established and every year thereafter. They should include the following research operations:

1. A careful description of the program components, including the council's location, the nature of its staff, its sources and amount of financing, the nature of its board, the structure of its facilities, and its program content and goals.

2. A naturalistic history of the founding and operation of the council.

3. The kind of community in which the council is located and the characteristics of the population that it is designed to serve.

4. The number of people reached and their characteristics, together with a systematic comparison of those who are not reached.

5. The effectiveness of the services rendered or the services to which individuals and families are referred. These services should be assessed in relation to such factors in the target population as the following: physical health of children and parents; changes in rates of identified psychoses and other serious disorders, emotional and learning disorders, and behavior problems, as identified and reported by the schools, arrests and commitments for juvenile delinquency, and the like; changes in levels of educational achievement; changes in the effectiveness of child welfare services, such as identification and evidence of treatment of battered and/or neglected children, numbers, auspices, and characteristics of adoption and foster home placements, the use of homemakers, day-care centers, group homes, family counseling services, and the like; changes in employment, wage rates, and training and education programs, especially for youth and for disadvantaged groups; improvements in family income, public assistance levels and policies, and availability and use of other economic assistance programs such as surplus foods and Medicaid; and changes in development, coordination, and use of needed community services. Assessment should also be made of the degree and nature of involvement in the council's operations of different community groups including religious, business, industrial, labor, government, and young people and parents from disadvantaged neighborhoods. The nature of community attitudes and information regarding the council's program and goals should be tested from time to time through the use of opinion-polling techniques directed toward a representative sample of the community's population.

We recognize that this type of program research is extremely complicated and would require a large-scale effort. There are many inherent difficulties, including the fact that some or all of the rates of the kind discussed above might increase rather than decrease in apparent association with the council's program. Yet, such an increase might well occur simply because the problems which had hitherto been unknown and untreated might be discovered through the development of the council and its services. There are, in fact, many variables at work in a community. As any researcher knows, these can readily create an increase in the incidence of mental health and related problems in spite of the establishment of better coordinating and service programs. It is important to design a careful study which involves a thorough analysis of the population characteristics of the community plus a running history of the program and of the community itself.

It is recommended that program assessment not be limited to the overall impact on the total population that the council is attempting to serve. It is also important to look at subgroups within the population. For example, a day-care program might well have positive effects on some children, negative effects on others, and no measurable effects on yet another group. By simply taking the average of assessment scores and ratings, one would miss the evidence that such a program might well be extremely helpful to some children although not helpful to all children.

It is further recommended that a number of communities be studied in similar fashion, including communities with *no* Child Development Councils as well as a variety of communities that employ different Council models. Such comparisons would greatly facilitate the determination of the relative effectiveness of a variety of approaches.

Evaluation of Specific Service Programs

1. Particular attention should be paid to further careful study of *infant and early childhood enrichment programs*. We need to experiment with various models of these programs and to test their relative effectiveness so they will truly benefit our young. It is hoped that programs for infants can be continued, at least through the age of eight. If so, it is crucial that we assess their impact over time.

These studies should take into account the physical, emotional, social, and intellectual development of the child. Murphy (1969) urges that a broader and more imaginative approach be taken to the assessment of the child's intellectual development. She points out that a child needs such traits as curiosity and drive to explore; capacity for organization, planning, and creativity; and resourcefulness. All of these qualities are at the root of intellectual activity and development.

The learning aspects of social experiences also should be studied. As Murphy notes: "Such processes as learning to take turns, to work together on joint tasks, to explain feelings of anger instead of beating up or biting the offender, to plan a joint block-building project, all involve cognitive efforts of varying degrees of complexity of understanding, verbal skill, sequential ideation, organization of objects and people, and useful fantasy."

Murphy further points out that we need to consider the individual physiological, social, and emotional context of both negative and positive changes in cognitive development. Thus, we cannot ignore the careful study of individual children. Simply assessing a program in terms of obtained averaged measures for groups of children is not sufficient.

In the assessment of program effectiveness, it is important to take into account the demographic and related characteristics of the children and parents involved in the program, the training and personal characteristics of staff members, the ecology of the preschool center (for example, arrangement of play yards, room for small groups, and the like), the basic approaches used by the staff (for instance, democratic or authoritarian styles of administration), program components, kinds of materials and curricula used, and so on.

2. It is important that we experiment with *new approaches to the care of infants and children* who cannot get the kind of care they need in their own families. There is mounting evidence that foster care frequently is not effective and that not enough high-quality foster homes can be found. It is time that we experiment with high-quality care of infants and children in small groups with a large enough staff to ensure that the needs of these children are met. In such projects, it is imperative that carefully designed studies be carried out to assess the impact of such care on all aspects of the child's development over a long period of time. It would be highly desirable to compare the results of such care with those obtained for children in other kinds of settings.

3. *Parent education* is recommended with increasing frequency as a way of improving the home environment of children, especially disadvantaged children. However, as we noted in Chapter VII, a recent overview of parent education projects shows that they have many shortcomings. The findings suggest, among other things, that measurement of changes in parents be approached through such strategies as depth interviews and planned observation of parent-child interaction at various points in time rather than through the use of such instruments as information and attitude surveys and questionnaires.

4. It is important that the *effects of day care* be tested in relation to different kinds of children, all aspects of the child's development, and in various kinds of day-care settings and programs. It is also important to assess what effects these programs have on the child's parents, especially on his mother.

5. We also need research to determine the *effect of work training and employment* on low-income mothers and their families, especially as these concern one-parent families, individuals in different kinds of family situations, child-care arrangements, and training and employment settings.

6. Research is needed to determine which *family planning program models* are most effective in reaching people in need of family planning services. A number of questions remain unsettled. For example, how

effective is family planning counseling and/or education in reference to both males and females at various age levels? What effect does the ready availability of contraceptives have on the behavior, values, and attitudes of young people, both male and female? What are the psychological effects of contraceptive use and limitation of family size? What effect does family planning have on the marriage relationship? What impact does smaller family size have on the self-concept and role behavior of low-income men and women whose family values have largely been directed toward their parental functions?

We have recommended that family planning services include *services in genetic counseling and counseling regarding fertility problems.* To what extent are those services available? How might these services be carried out with sensitive regard to mental health as well as physical health issues? What is the effect of mental health counseling in this area?

The Commission recognizes that there are many other research issues related to family planning. We have been concerned with only those that are most closely related to social and psychological issues.

7. There are many research questions regarding *the selection, placement, education, training, and supervision of nonprofessional aides in the human services field.* Although we have strongly recommended that such aides be trained and employed, there is only scanty research-based evidence to support this recommendation. It is important to evaluate the effectiveness of these aides, the impact which training and employment have on them and on the programs in which they work, their opportunities for career development, and the use that they make of these opportunities.

8. We have recommended that *parents, children, and young people be much more actively involved in programs* that affect them, such as those in the school and in many parts of the larger community. We have also recommended that older children and parents work as employees or volunteers in a number of programs, including those designed for younger children. We have little, if any, research-based evidence as to how well such programs work. These projects, as well as programs that involve people at the neighborhood level in policy-making and program planning, should be assessed.

9. Other service programs which have been recommended but which still demand further research assessment include the following: family and personal counseling including premarital and divorce counseling; consumer education and counseling, including nutritional education and counseling; sex education and counseling; various approaches to income maintenance and public assistance; and vocational education, counseling, and employment of disadvantaged youth.

10. *Changes in the social and economic structures of the community* have also been recommended by the Commission. It has been remarked

that services to individuals and families are likely to be of little avail as long as serious problems persist in the environment, such as segregation, poor housing, inadequate transportation, lack of full employment opportunities, inadequate community services and facilities, and the like. Further experiments are called for in the development and assessment of improved community programs, such as the Model Cities Program and New Towns, which are being developed in various parts of the country.

11. *Educational research.* The Commission recommends that a National Institute for Research in Education be established. This institute would have responsibility for planning and developing a research program which would include such provisions as: basic research in learning in the educational setting; research in the area of the teacher-pupil relationship; and the development, assessment, and comparative evaluation of alternative educational strategies, particularly for those children who are high educational and mental health risks (see Chapter I, Section IV-F).

SUMMARY

We urgently need to establish and preserve a national research climate which optimizes the productivity and opportunities of individual researchers. Both basic and applied research are needed in the social, behavioral, and biological sciences if we are to effectively promote the healthy development of children and adolescents, prevent problems of emotional and mental dysfunction, and adequately treat those who are suffering from related disorders.

There must be a constant interweaving between action programs and research so that observations and clues from the action field can be referred to research fields for theory-building and testing, and so that findings from the research can be fed back into action and training programs.

In these research programs we need a multidisciplinary team approach directed toward specific problems. It is also recommended that multivariate research be developed and addressed to the multiple criteria of positive mental health; that longitudinal research projects be undertaken with sufficiently large samples to permit adequate study of children from various kinds of backgrounds; and that applied research programs be designed to study the effectiveness, impact, and possible side effects of various forms of program strategies.

Among the various areas that particularly require further study are the following:

1. The prevalence in the population of moderate to severe emotional and mental disorders and the factors within the individual and the community which are associated with varying levels of behavioral dysfunction.

2. The origins and development of schizophrenia (including autism), learning disorders, and failure to thrive.

3. The development of various levels of behavioral functioning over a period of time. In these studies, particular emphasis might well be given to the neglected age periods of one to three years and ages twenty-one through fifty-five.

4. Basic research in such fields as genetics, neurophysiology, neuro-psychology, processes of child development, and similarities and differences between cultural groups is essential if applied research is to flourish. Program research should include many more carefully designed studies, especially on the relative impact and effect of various forms of therapeutic endeavors on the individual and his family, and on the various approaches to most of the services and programs recommended in this report. Such research should include long-term evaluation components and should encourage a number of planned experimental projects accompanied by sophisticated evaluation components.

5. The results of research findings should be analyzed and made available for the development of policies and legislation as well as for the improvement of programs and training.

6. Research manpower in these fields is extremely scarce, and we need a far larger investment in manpower training for research and for the support of researchers in basic and applied fields related to mental health.

7. Large-scale research and development centers are needed to test out a variety of approaches to the prevention and treatment of behavioral dysfunctions and emotional and mental disorders in children and youth. These centers should be linked to one another so that experimental approaches can be tested and replicated in different parts of the country under a variety of conditions with a variety of staff personnel and treatment populations. Such an approach is essential so that we can arrive at more generalized knowledge in these important fields.

Human Resources for Human Services

1. INTRODUCTION: THE MANPOWER SHORTAGE

Whatever their fields, their premises, and their data sources, for the past ten years or so most experts in the mental health manpower field have come to the same conclusion: We do not have enough properly trained professional personnel to meet the mental health needs of our nation—and probably never will unless we as a nation take some rather drastic steps to change the situation (Albee, 1959). This expert unanimity does not, unfortunately, encompass agreement as to the extent of the shortage, the chances of overcoming it, and the means of reversing the trend, since there are innumerable definitions of mental health and illness, and varied conceptions of what health care means and ought to mean, and what human skills and numbers it demands.

For the moment, if we accept the fact that the shortage exists, then clearly, attempts to upgrade our current and future mental health care for children are in jeopardy. If we haven't enough mental health personnel to staff existing facilities, how will we ever provide the manpower to meet new demands? And how can we fulfill the recommendation of the Commission that we establish numerous Child Development Councils throughout the country?

The traditional answer to the shortage is to train more professionals. But the traditional answer, with its inherent limitations, is by no means possible to implement. After more than ten years of trying to catch up through private and public support of expansion and improvement of traditional training of physicians, nurses, social workers, and psychologists, we have significantly increased our supply of these core professionals, but the increase is by no means sufficient to meet rising demands for their services. Given the voluntary nature of participation in professional training (and strong competition from other professional fields), the limited ability of existing educational facilities to expand continually yet maintain high standards and quality, the time and expense of establishing new training facilities, and the inherent resistance of the professions themselves to intervention and change, simply trying to train more professionals is not the answer. These training efforts must be continued and expanded, but they cannot be the sole focus of attack.

And herein lies a paradox which may contain our greatest cause for hope. Precisely *because* the traditional answer to our manpower problems has not worked well enough, we must now look more systematically and creatively at what we have and what we need. And precisely *because* it is impossible to have the numbers of professionals we need, we must look to make better use of those we do and will have, and must find other ways of providing for the mental health needs of our nation, particularly our children. And precisely *because* we must open ourselves up to new ways of thinking and acting, we stand to gain, in the long run, a far better system of mental health care than the patchwork quilt that has been our traditional pattern.

2. AN ASSESSMENT OF OUR HUMAN RESOURCES: PRESENT AND FUTURE

The Commission has issued an audacious call for mental health of our nation's children. It calls not for merely the absence of mental disease (which is an almost overwhelming task in itself), but for the mental well-being of all children—mental health in its most positive and life-enriching sense:

The Joint Commission strongly urges better treatment for the mentally ill, the handicapped, the retarded, the delinquent, and the emotionally disturbed. We join forces with those who propose a broader but more meaningful concept of mental health, one which is based on the developmental view with prevention and optimum mental health as the major goal. We contend that the mentally healthy life is one in which self-direction and satisfying interdependent relationships prevail, one in which there is meaning, purpose, and opportunity. We believe that lives which are uprooted, thwarted, and denied the growth of their inherent capacities are mentally unhealthy, as are those determined by rigidity, conformity, deprivation, impulsivity, and hostility. Unfulfilled lives cost us twice —once in the loss of human resources, in the apathetic, unhappy, frustrated and violent souls in our midst, and again in the loss of productivity to our society, and the economic costs of dependency. We believe that, if we are to optimize

the mental health of our young and if we are to develop our human resources, every infant must be granted:
— the right to be wanted . . .
— the right to be born healthy . . .
— the right to live in a healthy environment . . .
— the right to satisfaction of basic needs . . .
— the right to continuous loving care . . .
— the right to acquire the intellectual and emotional skills necessary to achieve individual aspirations and to cope effectively in our society. . . .
    For those who need remedial services, we must ensure:
— the right to receive care and treatment through facilities which are appropriate to their needs and which keep them as closely as possible within their normal social setting. . . .

To assure fulfillment of these basic rights, the Commission has recommended the creation of a network of comprehensive services, programs, and policies which will guarantee to every American child, from conception through age twenty-four, the opportunity to develop to his maximum potential.

In conjunction with this recommendation, the Commission advocates the establishment of Child Development Councils in almost every neighborhood throughout the country, so that needed mental health services, both preventive and therapeutic, can be coordinated and delivered effectively at the local level.

The feasibility of providing such services, and their ultimate quality if provided, will obviously depend upon the availability of manpower for the child mental health care system. There will have to be enough people in the right places with the right skills if the Commission's goals are to be even approached, let alone achieved. Yet what is meant by "enough people," or "the right places," or "the right skills"? And how can this be determined? And once these basic questions have been considered, how can we move from the system we presently have to one that more properly suits our present and future needs?

It is the task of this chapter to explore some of these manpower considerations, and to suggest a conceptual framework within which they may be approached constructively, efficiently, and realistically.

A. A Rational Approach to Manpower Planning

In the book *Manpower for Mental Health,* Arnhoff, Rubenstein, and Speisman (1969) have suggested that manpower planning first requires thoughtful assessment of needs and manpower provision, stressing specification of the functions to be performed. Further, study must be given to the total social system within which mental illness arises and manpower is developed and deployed for the delivery of mental health services:

While in no way demeaning the importance of past and continuing efforts directed towards manpower production, the time is propitious for a proper perspective on the locus of manpower problems in the total scheme of things. As has been stated before . . . manpower concerns are the last, not the first steps in the mental health conceptual chain: rational planning, assessment, and future directions only follow from prior specification of goals and resources. The current and continuing American social welfare revolution makes it mandatory that this be done.

Thus, while manpower continues to occupy a critical role in all health planning, it can only be meaningfully addressed and maximally utilized when the goals are specified for target populations.

A similar point has been raised by the Commission's *Report of Task Force IV* (1968) on Research, Manpower, Rehabilitation and Treatment, and Prevention. In their consideration of the manpower planning, they chose as their major theme the rational utilization of manpower:

If a major focus is upon how manpower is to be used, in what settings, and for which populations, then one can examine the available manpower pools, and assess the likelihood of obtaining candidates for those jobs which need to be performed and, equally important, the possibilities of training resources (and) expanding and/or revising their present operations in order to equip new manpower pools with required knowledge and skills.

As suggested by these and other observers and participants in the process of manpower planning for mental health, the first essential step is to specify the general goals for which the manpower is needed. In addition, subgoals must be identified with sufficient clarity and specificity to permit manpower tasks to be determined.

If, as the Commission has recommended, every child is to be provided with "the opportunity to develop to his maximum potential," then manpower planning to meet this goal must consider the mental health requirements of the total child population of mentally ill children.

B. The Target Population

There are currently more than 93,000,000 young people in this country under age twenty-four, a figure which has doubled since 1957 (U.S. Bureau of the Census, 1969). In a country in which the median age is just under twenty-eight, almost half of our nation's population of nearly 200,000,000 is the concern of the Commission. Thus, when we talk about mental health manpower for children and youth we are really asking how we can provide for the needs of the psychologically most dependent and vulnerable half of our population.

In considering the special needs of this population, we must recognize that while we may talk about children en masse, we must provide a multifaceted type of mental health care program that can meet the special needs of children at every stage of development. And we must also understand the socioeconomic, cultural, and geographic factors that determine the expectations of various communities and their demands for and acceptance of mental health care for their children.

When we study the differential risks of mental illness among members of the total child population, three large groups can be singled out: the "overt mentally ill," the "mental health problem population," and the "normal population." These groups require three different types of mental health programs, and may require different types of personnel as well.

The first two groups have been identified by von Mering and Carpenter (1967), who have also analyzed their special needs for health care, personnel, and settings. They state: "It is neither possible *nor* feasible to plan and implement manpower development programs without gearing them to researchable or known variations in the 'target' populations and differentials in available and potential local resources."

1. *The overt mentally ill.* The first group identified by von Mering and Carpenter consists of the seriously disturbed and identified mentally ill or impaired child. Such children, according to most estimates, represent a relatively small proportion of the entire child population—probably between 1 and 3 percent—yet they total between 1,000,000 and 3,000,000 persons. And their problems, "treatable in the framework of existing and modifiable patterns of institutionalized care given in the community," are, according to these investigators, of such intensity or severity "as to require intensive or episodic professional care over prolonged periods, whether this be at home or in institutions."

The following statistics from the National Institute of Mental Health (1965a; 1968) suggest the current prevalence of overt mental illness among children, as well as likely future trends. It is estimated that up to 500,000 children in the United States have psychoses and borderline psychotic conditions, and about 1,000,000 have personality and character disorders. About 1,000,000 children are presently institutionalized (*Report of Task Force IV, 1968*).

According to NIMH, there are about 78,000 child residents in institutions for the mentally retarded; about 13,000 are admitted yearly for the first time. These figures have been gradually increasing over the last decade. Retarded children as well as those suffering from acute and chronic brain syndromes make up almost 30 percent of the approximately 30,000 public mental hospital resident patients under twenty-four. Of the remainder, 43 percent are diagnosed as psychotic, and about 27 percent as having personality disorders.

A particularly distressing trend has been noted over the past few decades and is expected to continue. While the child population is expanding at a rapid rate (about 3 percent a year), the rate at which seriously disturbed children are admitted to mental hospitals is far greater, as we have indicated previously. For example, while between 1950 and 1965 the number of boys between ten and fourteen almost doubled, there was an almost sixfold increase in their numbers in mental hospitals. And this was occurring at a time when the residential patient rates in American mental hospitals as a whole were declining. Between 1965 and 1975 the population of children under eighteen is expected to increase by 10 percent, but their number in mental hospitals for the same period is expected to triple. Further, during the same period, while the proportion of ten- to fourteen-year-olds in the population is expected to increase by 15 percent, their proportion in the mental hospital population is expected to increase by 116 percent. Similarly, while the proportion of children fifteen to twenty-four is expected to increase by 36 percent in the general population, it is expected to undergo a 70 percent rise within the mental hospital patient population. These figures should, however, be considered in the light of improved detection and diagnosis of mental illness; greater hospital turnover, permitting greater volume of patients admitted; and the reduced stigma of hospitalization. All of these factors contribute to greater demand for services without necessarily implying increased disease incidence.

In discussing the health care personnel needed for this target population, von Mering and Carpenter (1967) propose that:

. . . manpower planning for the 3% may largely consist of reducing the present acute shortage of professional health personnel . . . [by increasing] the percentage of M.D.'s, R.N.'s, Ph.D.'s M.S.W.'s, M.A.'s and L.P.N.'s . . . [but merely] increasing the absolute number of professional personnel will not solve the problem. Not only must the professional be trained to work with new categories of workers, but their own talents must be put to the most efficient use.

(For further discussion of the supply of professionals and their efficient use, see Sections II-C and III-B.) Von Mering and Carpenter state that we can meet the manpower needs for this population: "Only by restricting professional efforts to specific tasks and specific age-graded socio-economic, ethnicity related populations will we better be able to meet the needs of the 3% 'overtly ill'."

2. *The mental health problem population.* The second target population identified by von Mering and Carpenter consists of "as many as 24 percent of people at any given time in the community" who "may be troubled and hampered by mental health distresses of a transitional or recurrent 'crisis' nature . . . and may receive attention and support in various formal and informal ways."

Included among this quarter of the child population are those whose problems range from "persistant learning and behavior problems, who are at the bottom of the normal group," through "children [who] have recurrent and fixed problems," to those with "severe problems, such as borderline psychosis."

The percentage of school-age children showing "at least mild sub-clinical problems" for which professional care is not needed is probably as high as 20 percent, according to the literature study by Glidewell and Swallow (1968). "Interpersonal distress and tension (subclinical)," found in 5 percent to 23 percent of children, "was more prevalent in boys, and showed no social class difference." "Interpersonal ineptitude," found in 10 percent to 30 percent of the children studied, was more prevalent in boys, manifested by "inappropriate aggression," and less prevalent in girls, manifested by "inappropriate withdrawals." In addition, as noted earlier, approximately 10 percent of the elementary school population, at any given time, have problems sufficiently severe to require professional help.

Glidewell and Swallow also found that:

The age differences in the prevalence of maladjustment are not great. There is some increase in anti-social behavior as adolescence is approached, and some decrease in developmental problems. The rates for boys are about three times as high as those for girls. Social class differences are difficult to isolate, but the lower class shows somewhat higher rates.

Even those sources, such as NIMH (1968), which suggest smaller estimates than those of the von Mering or Glidewell studies, have proposed that between 10 and 12 percent of the 50,000,000 school-age children, or more than 500,000 children, are emotionally disturbed and in need of psychiatric guidance, and that an additional 250,000 have less severe disorders which nonetheless require services at mental health centers.

Although the relationship between juvenile delinquency and mental illness is not without psychiatric and legal controversy, such antisocial behavior is usually considered to be either indicative of or related to underlying emotional problems. Almost 700,000 children are brought before the juvenile courts yearly for antisocial acts, and the numbers are increasing at a disturbing rate. Between 1960 and 1967, although the population between the ages of eleven and seventeen increased by only 22 percent, the number of juvenile delinquency court cases increased by about 58 percent. According to the FBI, during the same period police arrests of juveniles increased 69 percent, and in 1967 alone the number of juvenile court cases increased by 9 percent over previous years (*Federal Programs Assisting Children and Youth,* 1968).

When one considers the spectrum of problems encompassed within the term "mental health problem population," it is obvious that different services and personnel are needed to meet their varied needs. Thus, as several Commission task force members have suggested, drawing examples from the school-age population, while a normal child can benefit from the total school curriculum, a child at the bottom of the normal group, with persistent learning and behavior problems, could use parent-group counseling as well as school screening programs. A child with recurrent and fixed problems might need remedial programs and systematic mental health consultation while remaining in the normal school environment, while one with a severe problem, such as borderline psychosis, might benefit from special day school. As for the personnel required to provide care for this population, von Mering and Carpenter (1967) suggest that:

> Except for providing the necessary teaching cadre, and supervisory corps, it is wholly unreasonable to speak of the relevance of the mental health professional manpower pool to a problem of such magnitude. If we expect to make a measurable impact in this area, it is reasonable to consider manpower development only in certain alternative support *and* cumulative care senses. . . . Thus, for example, it may be possible by appropriate means to draw more teachers to work with children in a "mental health way"; more clergymen to work with the entire family, and especially young married couples; more nursery and kindergarten teachers to work with troubled as well as "normal" children, etc.

Before proceeding to the next target group, let us consider what services we presently provide to meet the overt needs of the two basic populations which together make up almost 30 percent of our child population. According to NIMH (1968): "It is estimated that approximately 5 percent of the children in the United States who need psychiatric help are getting it; and of those who are treated, less than one-half receive help that is of the kind, quality, and duration needed."

NIMH has noted that of the approximately 300,000 children seen in outpatient psychiatric clinics each year, only one in three receives more than a diagnosis. And the clinics themselves are in short supply. Of the nation's approximately 1,800 mental health clinics, somewhat less than one-fourth are child guidance clinics. Two-thirds of all the clinics do not have a single full-time psychiatrist on their staff, and a few have no psychiatrist at all. In addition, a large proportion of all counties in the United States are without mental health clinics altogether and have no other alternative agencies. In the school setting, according to von Mering and Carpenter (1967), although approximately 10 to 12 percent of the school-age population need some form of special education, "only about 13 percent of the estimated number of seriously maladjusted children receive special education."

In summary, we are not, at present, meeting the mental health needs of the one-quarter to one-third of the child population that obviously requires intervention, whether by mental health professionals or by others with mental health training.

3. *The potentially vulnerable: the "normal" population.* As indicated by

the previous estimates of von Mering and Carpenter, better than two-thirds of our nation's children are presumably "normal," that is, able to function reasonably well at home, in school, and in the community at large despite the inevitable crises of growing up (particularly those at sensitive life stages such as early infancy and adolescence). At least they do not appear to be abnormal. Yet how many of these children will become adults whose lives are ones in which "self-direction and satisfying interdependent relationships prevail," and in which there is "meaning, purpose, and opportunity"? How many lower-class children hardy enough to remain emotionally intact through childhoods of poverty, deprivation, and often racism will find their techniques of adjustment appropriate to a larger society demanding trust, affability, and openness? And how many middle-class and upper-class children, protected from physical stress and want, shielded from the sights of death and deprivation, and isolated from the problems of their hungry peers can cope with the realities of adulthood and the responsibility and resiliency it demands?

By setting as its goal the establishment of positive mental health in the child population, the Commission has a dual interest in the "normal" population. First, since one major concern is to prevent mental illness from occurring, the normal population must be given the conditions which will support and maintain its capacity to cope with crisis and disruption. From the point of view of manpower needs, there must be individuals available in the society competent to identify potential trouble, because of a child's emotional fragility, a developmental stage of particular sensitivity, or an especially disruptive external event. Either the same person or other persons must be able to counsel those in the child's immediate environment, such as parents and teachers, to help them help the child. Similarly, such persons are needed as resources for parents, particularly those who seek practical guidance in child-rearing, whether during periods of crisis or everyday development. So long as these persons are linked to child mental health professionals through teaching and referral networks, they need not be such professionals themselves. If mental health training is provided throughout the community for parents, teachers, community leaders, and all those who come in contact with children or are sought to advise on their behavior, then, as G. T. Barrett-Lenard has called them, a series of "helping relationships" for children can be established in which "one person facilitates the personal development or growth of another, where he helps the other to become more mature, adaptive, integrated, and open to his own experience" (in von Mering and Carpenter, 1967). Conceived of in this way, steps toward the prevention of mental illness may also be steps toward the creation of positive mental health.

A second concern of the Commission is the creation of a societal milieu in which mental illness is minimized and positive mental health is possible. Although this is primarily a societal task, the society requires the help of mental health experts and the impetus of those concerned about mental health if it is to initiate the kinds of changes needed.

C. *The Available Personnel: The Basic Pool*

The most time-consuming and demanding mental health care for children is required for those whose problems are so severe that neither parents nor school personnel can cope with them—that is, the severely disturbed 2 to 3 percent of the population. Whether on an inpatient, outpatient, or residential basis, however, such care usually consists largely of diagnosis, with only cursory psychotherapy. Four professions have provided the core of personnel for this effort: medicine (particularly psychiatry), nursing, social work, and clinical psychology. Within each, areas of subspecialization have developed, devoted specifically to the mental health care of children and their families. Thus, we now have child psychiatrists, child clinical psychologists, child psychiatric nurses, and psychiatric social workers specializing in therapeutic work with children. The supply of these child specialists is very limited, however. Thus, most children who receive mental health care do so from practitioners who were probably either not specifically trained to deal with children or, in the case of other personnel such as pediatricians, not specifically trained to deal with mental health problems.

Within recent years, basic training in all of these professions increasingly has included exposure to the basic principles of community mental health and child psychiatry, thus better preparing trainees for their future role in the mental health care of children. But regardless of their training, these professionals may have little time to provide children with the type of mental health care they require, and even less time to proceed through the long years of training required for specialization in the care of children. If one examines the picture for all health professions and related occupations from various sources, despite estimated increases in all health manpower of more than 1,000,000 between 1965 and 1975, the demand will continue to outstrip the supply and thereby will seriously impair the delivery of all health services. The general shortage will be especially severe among researchers and teachers.

Taking an example from the medical manpower pool, a recent estimate of physician shortages and needs by Fein (1967) suggests that between 1965 and 1975 there will be a 19 percent growth in numbers of physicians (from 305,000 to 362,000, assuming continued foreign-born immigration as well). While this increase will exceed population growth by about 6 percent, income growth will continue to result in health care demands exceeding the supply. As the National Goals Project of the National Planning Association has estimated, about 402,000 physicians will be needed in 1975. We will probably fall short of this figure by about 40,000 physicians.

1. *Psychiatrists.* As in most professional hierarchies, the longest-trained and highest paid members of the "core" mental health professions—psychiatrists—are also the fewest in number. There are currently about 23,000 psychiatrists in the United States. About 17,000 are specifically trained in psychiatry, and about 6,000 are physicians who limit their practice to psychiatry (American Psychiatric Association, 1969). The ratio of psychiatrists to the population has risen steadily over the 20 years from 1946 to 1966, from 2.8 per 100,000 to 10.0 per 100,000 (Arnhoff, Rubenstein, and Speisman, 1969). But despite this increase, according to most assessments of current demands for their services, psychiatrists are in acutely short supply. In 1967 it was estimated that between 10,000 and 15,000 additional psychiatrists were needed.

The rising demand for psychiatric services arises primarily from improved detection of mental health problems, more efficient systems of referral, and a reduced social stigma attached to seeking psychiatric help. Also, as new roles for psychiatrists are being developed in industry, government, education, and other fields, additional demands are created for their services. The development of new community mental health services and of expanded academic and clinical training facilities in psychiatry has also raised manpower demands for psychiatrists.

The supply of psychiatrists is directly dependent upon the supply of medical students from which they are drawn. By all calculations, the future production of physicians cannot possibly rise to meet the total shortage in the field. For example, according to Van Matre (1967), "to reach the 402,000 physicians estimated as required by 1975, U.S. medical and osteopathic schools would have to graduate 153,000 physicians in the 10 years 1966–1975. This would be 15,300 per year, or almost double the 7,890 graduated in 1965." Thus, the basic medical manpower pool for psychiatry will be severely taxed by other medical specialties as well. At present, about 10 percent of medical school graduates go into the field of psychiatry. Assuming that this figure is unlikely to rise—due to recruitment competition within medicine—the chances of significantly increasing the population of psychiatrists in the near future are extremely small; the chances of catching up with ever-increasing demands for their services are practically nil.

Of the approximately 23,000 psychiatrists, it is estimated that about 1,500 are child psychiatrists. The numbers of psychiatrists in this sub-specialty and in adolescent psychiatry have remained relatively stable in recent years, although those primarily in mental retardation work have declined slightly (Whiting, 1968). It has been estimated that possibly half of the child psychiatrists treat emotionally disturbed children. The rest are in administration, teaching, research, or consultation as a primary activity.

The increasing scarcity of psychiatrists, coupled with the many demands for their services in roles other than direct patient care, makes it imperative that their time and energy be used effectively and that they perform only those functions that require their special training and skills (see Section III-B).

2. *Psychologists.* The American Psychological Association (APA) reports a 1969 membership of about 28,800 psychologists. While clinical counseling and school psychology are the subspecialties most usually associated with mental health, 61 percent of all psychologists surveyed by the National Science Foundation report their work and activities to be related to the field of mental health. Since 1950, APA membership has more than tripled, and the psychologists in mental health work have increased more than fivefold (Arnhoff, Rubenstein, and Speisman, 1969).

Clinical psychologists are most commonly thought of as mental health care personnel within their profession, but their roles usually include teaching and research activities as well as diagnosis and treatment. According to a 1966 survey by the American Association of Psychiatric Clinics for Children (AAPCC) (1968), the absolute numbers, the percentage, and the total hours available of clinical psychologists in clinics serving children (particularly in child psychiatric guidance clinics) have remained quite stable between 1955 and 1966. Since this stability occurs despite the continually increasing production of PhD psychologists generally (currently about 1,300 a year) (Arnhoff, Rubenstein, and Speisman, 1969), it suggests that many of the clinically trained psychologists return to academic settings, while the new entrants into clinical settings barely make up for the attrition.

According to an NIMH survey conducted in 1966 (Arnhoff and Shriver, 1966) and a 1967 APA study (Brayfield, 1967), more than 90 percent of the "mental health" psychologists work in public or nonprofit settings. Of these, most clinical psychologists work in mental hospitals and psychiatric clinics.

Of all the mental health professions, psychologists continue to be the most active in research. Almost one-quarter of all psychologists regard this as their most important activity, and a 1966 survey of psychologists revealed that 79 percent are involved in research (Arnhoff and Shriver, 1966).

As for the present and future supply of psychologists, Arnhoff, Rubenstein, and Speisman (1969) note that:

The manpower problems of psychology have been drastically exacerbated by ... recent developments within the field itself and by increased societal demand. It has recently been estimated that the entire doctoral output of psychology for the next five years could be absorbed into the teaching faculties of colleges and universities alone. . . . Projections and estimates made by the National Institute of Mental Health indicate a need for over 2,000 additional professionally trained psychologists for research and services to staff the Community Mental Health Centers by 1970. Since current and anticipated production of psychologists so obviously cannot meet these demands, the search continues for alternative approaches to a solution, focusing primarily on more efficient utilization of manpower.

3. *Social workers.* In 1965–66, the National Association of Social Workers (NASW) reported a membership of 42,500 social workers, of whom 28,850 were certified (NASW, 1967). If those with no graduate training who nonetheless function in the capacities of graduate social workers are included, there are currently an estimated 125,000 to 150,000 social workers in the United States.

In a 1965 survey, the National Institute of Mental Health (1965b) identified about 7,500 social workers employed in 2,500 mental health institutions. About three-quarters of them had master's degrees, and 13 percent had some graduate training but no advanced degree. More than half of the social workers (4,000) were employed in outpatient clinics, better than a quarter in public and private hospitals, and the remainder in public and private institutions for the mentally retarded.

The growth of the social work profession and the numbers of psychiatric social workers has been considerable. Between 1956 and 1966, NASW membership has nearly doubled—from 22,330 to 42,500 (NASW, 1967). Similarly, the number of psychiatric social workers has more than doubled in the decade between 1950 (2,253) and 1960 (5,171). In a scant four years between 1960 and 1964 the number of psychiatric social workers with graduate training doubled, from 3,717 to 7,359 (U.S. Dept. of Health, Education, and Welfare, 1965).

But, as in the other professions, despite this growth, the demand has far outstripped the supply. Of the approximately 2,800 social workers who graduate each year, about one-fourth, or 700, go into psychiatric social work (U.S. Dept. of Health, Education, and Welfare, 1965). Yet NIMH has estimated that 1,305 psychiatric social workers will have to be trained each year for the next five years to reach minimally its mental health manpower goals.

The Departmental Task Force on Social Work Education and Manpower anticipated that about 100,000 fully trained social workers will be needed by 1970, as well as a "vast increase in the number of social workers with baccalaureate level education and the development of several categories of technical and ancillary personnel" (U.S. Dept. of Health, Education, and Welfare, 1965).

French, in a 1964 study, dealt with some of the problems affecting the field of social work manpower which have equal impact on the other mental health professions. As summarized by Arnhoff, Rubenstein, and Speisman (1969), D. G. French has pointed out that:

. . . the source of demand for social welfare personnel stems from the dislocations resulting from technological advances in our society. . . . In addition, the social welfare institutions are themselves changing, leading to changes in the types and numbers of personnel needed to staff them. Expansion of two-year social work schools will not be sufficient as a solution to shortages, and other solutions will have to be found; such as restricting positions to enable subprofessional personnel to perform defined functions, or revising the method of dealing with the given problem. "The task posed to administrators and educators is one of job analysis and creative experimentation with alternative approaches to meeting welfare needs."

4. *Psychiatric nurses.* In 1962, about 550,000 registered nurses were employed in the United States in all types of employment settings, including psychiatric and mental health settings. An NIMH study in 1963 identified about 18,000 nurses as being employed in mental health establishments such as outpatient psychiatric clinics, hospitals for the mentally ill, and institutions for the mentally retarded (Eldridge, 1964). By 1967 the number of employed registered nurses had risen to 640,000 in the United States (Marshall, 1967). According to a 1966 inventory of registered nurses, conducted by the American Nurses Association, there were about 27,000 nurses who reported their area of practice as mental health or psychiatric nursing, out of a total of 593,694 employed RN's.

Estimates of the number of psychiatric nurses working with children have ranged from 5,000 to 8,000. Specific training in child psychiatric nursing has been offered as a major subject in seven of the forty-four graduate programs in psychiatric nursing in 1967.

Psychiatric nursing differs from the other three core professions in being almost exclusively located in hospital settings and residential treatment institutions. It also differs in having the close support of a related nonprofessional group: psychiatric aides. In 1963, about 96,000 of these personnel in state and county hospitals alone contributed to the psychiatric nursing function. In a study conducted in 1966 by the American Hospital Association and the U.S. Public Health Service, Bureau of Health Manpower, it was estimated that a total of 117,629 aides, orderlies, and attendants were employed in psychiatric hospitals.

Despite the help of aides and the large number of nurses trained each year a severe national nursing shortage nonetheless exists. The problem is particularly acute since many recent trainees marry and leave the field. The Surgeon General's Consultant Group on Nursing (1963) projected that by 1970, 850,000 professional nurses and 350,000 practical nurses would be required to provide services which are safe and therapeutically effective.

In the program Review Report of the Nurse Training Act of 1964, it is estimated that 1,000,000 registered nurses will be needed by 1975. To meet this goal, graduations from basic nursing programs would have to be increased to 81,000. The estimate of need did not include a breakdown by type of employment setting.

D. Other Professionals

Beyond the four core mental health professions, there are many others whose practitioners provide treatment or advice concerning actual or potential mental health problems of children. For example, nonpsychiatric nurses serve an important role in providing child health care and often preventive mental health care in settings within hospitals, schools, clinics, and homes throughout their communities. Within the medical profession, three nonpsychiatric groups are particularly vital members of the mental illness primary prevention team: pediatricians, general practitioners, and obstetricians. It is their care that guides the physical development of children prenatally and postnatally, and often affects their early mental and emotional development as well.

1. *Pediatricians.* The number of pediatricians has generally increased at a rapid rate which compares well with other specialties. For example, between 1931 and 1962, while internists increased from 4,800 to 28,000, and surgeons from 5,000 to 22,000, pediatricians increased from 1,600 to 10,500. Despite this rise at a rate of approximately 2.6 percent per year, the child population has been expanding at an even more accelerated rate of 3.3 percent per year. Thus, although the ratio of pediatricians to the child population under fifteen years of age rose from 7.3 per 100,000 in 1940 to 16.3 by 1961, it fell to 12.2 by 1965 (Knowles, 1968).

Despite the key role of pediatricians in guiding child development physically and psychologically, specific training in psychological growth and development and principles of human behavior is still, however, minimal in the pediatric educational process. This generalization is true for all of medical education.

2. *General practitioners.* The number of general practitioners, whose responsibilities include both the delivery of babies and the treatment of children, is on the decline as physicians generally become increasingly specialized. For example, while in 1950, 64 percent of physicians in private practice were GP's, by 1963 only 39 percent of these physicians were GP's (Van Matre, 1967). The ratio of general practitioners to the population of children under fifteen years of age fell from about 345 per 100,000 in 1940 to 135 per 100,000 in 1961 (Knowles, 1968).

Despite their shrinking numbers, general practitioners continue to play an important role in providing pediatric and obstetrical care, particularly in rural areas where specialists are largely unavailable. About a quarter of their time is devoted to the care of children. A 1967 study in Iowa (Knowles, 1968) showed that almost 64 percent of the deliveries were made by general practitioners, while only about 22 percent were by qualified obstetricians. Undoubtedly, general practitioners also serve as the primary mental health and child-rearing consultants in these same areas, despite minimal preparation for such roles.

3. *Obstetricians.* According to the Council of the Association of Professors of Gynecology and Obstetrics (Knowles, 1968), some 13,000 to 16,000 physicians are listed as limiting themselves to the practice of obstetrics and gynecology, although only about 7,380 are certified obstetricians (Gurin *et al.,* 1960). Their numbers are growing steadily, as in most other medical specialties. For example, the number of obstetricians certified yearly almost doubled between 1962 and 1968, rising from 356 to more than 600. Yet, as in other fields of medicine, the growth is short of the demand. Thus, with more than 2,900 residents in training yearly, residency positions are only 89 percent filled, and 30 percent of the positions are occupied by foreign graduates. To complicate the obstetrician shortage, anesthetists are also in short supply to serve with them during deliveries. The net result of these shortages is that of the 3,500,000 births per year in this country, an estimated 500,000 mothers receive inadequate or no prenatal care, and 200,000 deaths occur yearly in the perinatal period (Knowles, 1968).

4. *Nonmedical professionals.* From the point of view of those seeking help for their children's problems, the core mental health professionals tend to be among the last ones they approach. One study of professional aid sought by people for their personal problems revealed that 42 percent went to their clergyman and 29 percent to their nonpsychiatric physician for help. Most of the remaining 29 percent went to lawyers, teachers, judges, and policemen rather than to psychiatrists, psychologists, or social workers (Gurin *et al.,* 1960). The noncore professionals, particularly those outside of medicine, are an important resource for early detection and treatment of mental illness.

The nation's approximately 2,500,000 schoolteachers are clearly in the front line in the perception of problems and the sensitive management of potentially mentally ill children. Their cooperation with school guidance personnel and psychologists, as well as with special education personnel, is an essential part of the child mental health care network. Programs to improve and expand the mental health role of teachers are discussed in Chapter IX.

When children's emotional problems lead to antisocial behavior, they also bring themselves and their families into contact with a number of personnel in law enforcement and corrections professions such as lawyers, judges, policemen, probation and parole officers, and correctional institutional staff. The sensitivity these persons bring to their roles in dealing with young offenders is crucial to the subsequent emotional and social development of the children.

Recently, the importance of mental health training for all these noncore professionals has gained increasing recognition. While training programs, particularly under NIMH sponsorship, have grown rapidly to provide at least the rudiments of mental health knowledge and skills to students and practitioners in many of these fields, they reach only a fragment of this population.

3. OLD AND NEW ROLES

A. *Some Weaknesses of Our Present Child Mental Health Care System*

To summarize key problems of the child mental health care network as it now exists, we presently have a system that is largely oriented toward providing diagnosis and treatment for the severely disturbed 3 percent and crisis care for the less severely disturbed 24 percent of the child population. Preventive measures are few and far between, and mechanisms for early detection of problems and needs are almost nonexistent. Parents rear their children largely with the help and advice of their families and neighbors, with some aid from busy, overtaxed physicians (generally untrained in mental health), augmented by the mass-media advisers who write paperback books, newspaper columns, and articles in women's magazines. When a child has behavior problems within the family, physicians and clergymen are first sought; referral to psychiatric clinics and specialists is generally used only for major crises. Other types of child problems such as learning and behavior difficulties in school or antisocial behavior are often first detected through the school and legal systems; referral to mental health specialists means that even for the extremely troubled child, in many areas needed services are entirely unavailable or waiting lists are painfully long, with the lag between diagnosis and treatment often forever.

According to Whiting (1968), the provision of effective child mental health service "consists of the creation of a confluence of four vital streams":

1. Research   to clarify the requirements for community service.
2. Education   to develop both appropriate competencies among those who provide the service and appropriate utilization of services by families.
3. Administration to synthesize the logistical elements of men, money, and materials so that services are delivered at the right time and place in optimal quality and quantity.
4. Service   the actual satisfaction of community requirements at the point of contact with the child and his family.

Currently, while individuals often function in all four roles, there is insufficient systematic coordination among the "streams" themselves, and inadequate preparation for such diversified functions.

The training of most core mental health personnel consists largely of conventional academic professional education for traditional health care roles, with little specific preparation for teaching, research, or administration. Teachers in these professions are usually drawn from the ranks of practitioners, thus depleting the supply of those available to provide care. Efforts at on-the-job training of subprofessionals have educated new groups of health-care workers but have drawn largely upon the same scant supply of professionals for the design and administration of such programs. Similarly, expanded mental health training for students and practitioners in mental health-related occupations has fortified their ability to deal with emotional and behavioral problems in the community but has drawn heavily upon the pool of core mental health personnel to do so.

The burden of administering mental health care also rests upon professionals who were trained as practitioners. Although there is a tendency to train high-level administrative personnel specifically for work in the health field, the changeover is slow. As mental health services are now organized and administered, they are often inefficient, hard-pressed for coordination among the multiple service organizations and personnel working with the same populations, fraught with professional and geographic jurisdictional problems, and severely hampered by lack of adequate data on the characteristics of present and future demands and services and the impact of past and current programs. Present deployment of financial and human resources is largely unplanned, and rational planning for future change is difficult, if not impossible.

Research in the mental health care field, except for basic scientific studies, is mainly a part-time activity of the same mental health professionals who function in rehabilitative, teaching, and administrative roles. Studies are prompted largely by crises, sampling procedures are inadequate, and the data base in the field is remarkably full of inconsistencies and conflicts. The efforts of the professional, governmental, and voluntary organizations conducting much of the research are usually uncoordinated and meet frequently with little public cooperation, due to public ignorance of the benefits that might ultimately result from such studies. In addition, the practitioners themselves often prefer to preserve the status quo rather than risk the changes such studies might provoke.

In the next section, the report of one such study provides a close-up view of some manpower utilization problems within one core profession—psychiatry—and clarifies the kinds of questions that must be asked throughout the mental health care system if adequate care is to be given in both the present and the future.

B. *Manpower Utilization*

In a working paper for the Commission's Task Force IV, Whiting, Carper, and Feldman (1967) noted:

To safeguard the profession, some professionals, at least so the present practice is, take on the necessary bureaucratic political and administrative tasks. Every hour spent in these activities is an hour taken away from direct service. As suggested by [a study by] the American Psychiatric Association (APA), the time spent by professionals in activities other than direct service is sizable. Perhaps a first step for those concerned with manpower problems in the field of mental health for children is to promote studies of the actual utilization of current manpower. Such studies could suggest some rearrangements of bureaucratic arrangements, possibly some agreements between warring professions, and perhaps some more efficient models for delivery of services. Even if these studies only indicated how the professional was misusing his time, they would be a worthwhile input for overall planning for the future.

The Whiting (1968) study to which the authors referred, based on a 1965 national survey sample of 88 percent of all psychiatrists, revealed that psychiatrists devote about 67 percent of their energy to direct patient care and about 22 percent to "keeping the system of psychiatric services intact and viable" through a combination of administration and consultation, as the authors reported in another paper (Whiting *et al.,* 1967), which notes that "a real question can be raised concerning the efficiency of an operation which requires approximately one quarter of its available energy to keep it going" and continues:

. . . perhaps implying an even more telling criticism of the present mechanism of psychiatric services is the 2–1 ratio between the amount of energy devoted to the combination of administration-consultation (22% of total available energy) and the [amount of energy devoted to the] teaching and research combination (11% of total available energy). Might it not be that if this relationship was reversed that a quantum leap in both quantity and quality of work performed (and available energy) for delivery of mental health services would be achieved?

Whiting reports that 58 percent of all available psychiatric service hours in 1965 were performed within an institutional setting rather than private practice. The setting, he has noted, has a striking effect on the proportion of time psychiatrists spend providing direct patient care or performing administrative-consultative duties:

At one end of the scale, we have private practice where 15.3 hours of direct service to patients is delivered by psychiatrists for every hour spent in administration or consultation. By contrast, even in the best institutional settings (mental hospitals, clinics, and general hospitals) psychiatrists deliver only 2 hours of direct service to patients for every hour spent in administration and/or consultation. Thus, the cost of institutionalization is indeed a heavy one in terms of service rendered to patients to say nothing of the deterioration of morale in psychiatric practitioners engendered by this essential "deprofessionalization" process.

Compared to the information available for the other core health professionals, the APA study is a model of rational self-assessment. Yet far more study is needed. For example, an increasing number of psychiatrists recognize that even if they were to spend more time conducting therapy, the usual one-to-one relationship, the 50-minute hour, and the usual duration of therapy severely limit their capacity to provide treatment on the massive scale required. The search is under way for new forms of brief therapy, both individual and group, that can supplement the traditional psychotherapeutic approach, but it is just a beginning.

A related cluster of vital questions concerns the relevance of psychiatric education for actual practice, and the effectiveness of current treatment methods in reducing at least the presenting symptoms of mental illness for which therapy is sought. This area is fraught with problems of both definition and dogma, but these questions must at least be confronted if we are to make the best use of a highly valued and very scarce resource.

When we think of the limited availability of our current mental health manpower, and consider the differing demands of the three general populations of children identified earlier, a further question arises. Are patients now being seen in any priority based upon their degree of severity of illness and need? Arnhoff has suggested that according to current evidence, this is not the case. A relatively specific group of upper-middle-class patients receives a disproportionate amount of treatment—disproportionate to both their overall need and their numbers when compared with other segments of society.

The strong middle-class orientation of present mental health services has meant also that those services provided increasingly for lower-class populations have often been based on inappropriate assumptions. As Whiting, Carper, and Feldman (1967) have noted:

The first assumption that mental illness is related to poor adjustment to the environment and can be corrected by treatment does not apply when dealing with the poor. The environments in which they live make "normal" adjustment impossible. A second assumption that with treatment an individual can leave an impossible environment or take part in changing it cannot apply. The poor need a variety of services before they can move into the mainstream of society.

Arnhoff, Jenkins, and Speisman (1969) have made a similar point:

A further factor of increasing influence in pressing for alternate methods of solution has been growing acceptance of the various studies and writings regarding the limited effectiveness of traditional approaches to treatment and

their applicability, even if they were universally available to all population segments. . . .

Certainly it has not been demonstrated that all forms of disturbed behavior
and mental illness are best treated by, nor do they respond best, to traditional
methods of psychotherapy, most commonly illustrated by the one-to-one
verbal approach, which usually is quite costly of time. The effectiveness of
these methods for the total range of people and social classes is also in question,
since it has been shown that many patients actually reject such a treatment
approach. Members of the lower socioeconomic groups in particular often demand direction and medication and will leave treatment if these are not forthcoming. . . . As to the large number of borderline mentally ill, that is, those
who return to the community after hospitalization and may well require future
hospitalization, they most often profit from vocational and social rehabilitation
rather than traditional psychotherapy . . . Findings such as these, coupled with
an obvious and increasing inability of the traditional professional groups to deal
with the magnitude of the tasks presented by society, have led to increased
consideration and effort to seek new, different, and less costly types of personnel who can be drawn from a different segment of the total potential labor
pool than is usual for mental health occupations.

C. New Types of Personnel

It is abundantly clear by now that new and alternative systems and new
types of personnel are needed for the provision of mental health care for
children in our country. We simply do not have and will not have enough
professionals to meet our needs. If we intend, as the Commission recommends, to broaden and strengthen our mental health coverage by providing
comprehensive services and Child Development Councils which will ensure
needed services to the child through outreach efforts to families and
collaborative links with agencies, we will urgently have to develop new
types of paraprofessionals and nonprofessionals with which to staff both
the councils and the service institutions.

1. *The potential pool.* If new types of child mental health manpower are
to be developed, what populations are and will be available for such training? A study of national population trends reveals that because of the World
War II baby boom, our country will have an accelerating rate of growth in
its labor force, which will, however, level off in the 1970's (U.S. Bureau of
the Census, 1969). Between 1965 and 1970, it will have grown by 7,500,-
000, which is 50 percent greater than the increase that occurred between
1960 and 1965. Moreover, of the 7,500,000 increase, youth and Negroes
will constitute the largest share. Youths between eighteen and twenty-four
will increase by more than 3,000,000, and nonwhites of all ages will
increase by more than 1,500,000. If current trends continue, both groups
are likely to contribute significantly to the nation's future unemployment
problems. Older adolescents and young adults presently have the highest

unemployment rate of any age group, and nonwhite workers of all ages are more than twice as likely to be unemployed as white workers. For both social and economic reasons, unemployed members of both populations, and particularly individuals belonging to both groups, deserve primary consideration in future planning for new training programs. These training candidates are often hard to employ and require careful preparation, but they also have unique contributions to make. Young adults, being relatively close in age to the young population, are potentially more understanding of youth crises (particularly of adolescence) than older workers. Similarly, the experience of many Negroes in coping with their own problems of poverty may make them sympathetic and adept in dealing with the problems of others, particularly the nonwhites and the poor.

Between 1965 and 1980, the population of those over sixty-five will increase by 27 percent, a growth rate higher than that for either those under fifteen years of age (21 percent) or those between fifteen and sixty-four (26 percent). Thus, large numbers of retired persons will be potentially available for mental health work. With improved health among the elderly, those who are retired are often ready for second careers, or at least able and willing to take on part-time paid or voluntary work with children.

A third group of potential mental health workers consists of married women and widows. Both groups are natural choices for work with children, although many probably would prefer to work on a part-time basis. With proper planning and provision of day-care facilities for young children, many mothers, including those with college backgrounds or with partial or full training in the core mental health professions, could be recruited or returned to the manpower pool.

A fourth group from which new trainees might be drawn consists of individuals who themselves have undergone rehabilitation. Persons who have received treatment and have recovered might be particularly motivated to contribute to the recovery of others.

Every member of the community has a stake in the mental health of children, and potentially, all members could contribute to child mental health either through full- or part-time work in a mental health-related occupation or through their roles as parents, neighbors, volunteers, or citizens.

2. *Potential roles.* The Commission has suggested a spectrum of personnel who might participate in service programs for children, either directly or in contracted service arrangements. These personnel range from full-fledged professionals of both old and new types to part-time community volunteers and even ex-mental patients:

> People from existing professional groups, and especially from the newer technician levels being developed, such as those in pediatrics, psychology, etc.

A new professional group trained in child development. These should be trained at a number of levels (BA, MA, PhD, EdD, etc.) for varying degrees and types of responsibility in the center programs. These professional child workers would include:

educationally oriented child-care specialists to supervise day care and preschool facilities;

child-parent counselors to visit homes, to demonstrate new strategies for child care in homes, and to train and supervise subprofessional workers in home visiting.

A new subprofessional group of child-care workers, aides, "upbringers," etc., approximately at the level of the high school graduate, who might make a life career of work with children or who might with further education move into the professional roles. A large corps of these workers is needed to serve as caretakers in various institutions and service facilities, to serve as "teachers," "teacher's aides," and home visitors.

Adolescents, in large numbers, for both service and training, to work with children in various types of programs and to perform other services in the community.

Volunteers, paid and otherwise, who are employed as full-time or part-time people. These might be drawn from a number of different groups: parents; "foster grandparents"; college men and women (presumably students); hobbyists; "indigenous workers"; Junior League; church groups; former alcoholics, mental patients, delinquents, and criminals purposefully seeking a centering point for their lives; retired teachers; etc.

With an eye toward the development of full-time paraprofessional workers in the field of child mental health, the Committee on Clinical Issues of the Commission has listed some relevant paraprofessional roles, all of which are already under development. These include:

Psychiatric technician: Young people, mostly high school graduates, may be given six months of training in a state hospital in preparation for work with disturbed youth under careful supervision.

Case aide in social work: Following a two- to four-month training period, this high school graduate helps the social worker, but does not usually provide therapy.

Foster grandmother: This older female works in home settings where the mother is ill and provides supportive nontherapeutic care to children in hospital wards. Some initial training and ongoing supervision are required.

Semiprofessional foster parent: This role requires training for work with children in individual and group foster-care settings. The foster parent, while having no psychotherapeutic role, is trained to be a sophisticated parent with some understanding of child behavior, and can also work with mental health professionals.

Child health associate: For this role, a college graduate would require two years of further training providing him with knowledge of mental illness prevention; he could then work in the office of a pediatrician or in an institutional setting.

Child-care worker: While this high school graduate has no formal therapeutic role, he may use the life-space interview approach under intensive supervision, after a few months of on-the-job training.

Nurse practitioner: This paraprofessional role requires training in preparation for conducting physical examinations, providing some anticipatory guidance and counseling for parents, and performing some developmental screening, both physical and psychological.

Homemaker: The woman in this role provides support in the home when the mother is sick or the family is broken or unable to function effectively (*Report of the Committee on Clinical Issues,* 1969).

Although the effort has been unsystematic, the development of new paraprofessional and semiprofessional roles has already begun. Throughout the country, colleges, community colleges, mental hospitals, and mental health clinics are undertaking new, often experimental, programs aimed at training special populations to perform needed services. The following examples, taken mainly from those cited by Arnhoff, Jenkins, and Speisman (1969) in *Manpower for Mental Health,* provide a sampling of training programs for general mental health personnel as well as for specialists in the care of children.

Through the Hospital Staff Development Program sponsored by the NIMH, a massive effort is being made to recruit and provide in-service training for hospital aides and attendants in mental institutions. These nursing staff members, who have extensive patient contact, are given a graded sequence of courses designed to increase their sensitivity and competence in providing patient care and to establish a career ladder which encourages individual growth while upgrading the aide and attendant roles.

At the Philadelphia State Hospital, training for the higher-level role of "social interaction therapist" is being provided for college graduates. They are given courses in personality therapy, psychopathology and treatment, group dynamics, social institutions, activity skills, and social interaction therapy in preparation for working with chronic schizophrenics to modify their behavior toward more socially acceptable responses. These therapists may work in day-care programs, halfway houses, sheltered workshops, and community clinics as well as in mental institutions.

A similar year-long master's degree program at the Rockford Zone Center in Illinois trains "mental health reentry expediters," who work with a team helping ex-patients with a high hospitalization risk adjust to their community.

Another program providing a new group of rehabilitation workers is conducted at Albert Einstein College of Medicine of Yeshiva University. Mature housewives are given nine months of part-time training as "mental health rehabilitation counselors." Their duties are to provide support to discharged mental patients by helping them with their housing, social life, work, and daily living problems.

Many of the new roles under development are specifically related to the care of children. For example, at the Devereux Foundation, a Pennsylvania institution for disturbed and retarded children, a multidisciplinary program provides training in child care for prospective house parents and certification upon their completion of the year-long course. Training personnel also study the predictive criteria for success as a house parent.

At the Western Psychiatric Institute, two levels of personnel are prepared to work with retarded or disturbed children. High school graduates may earn a certificate in child care after two years of training, including a one-year internship. An interdisciplinary master's degree program in child development is offered to college graduates with appropriate backgrounds in behavioral science, social work, education, nursing, or child care.

The Wurzweiller School of Social Work of Yeshiva University in New York, in cooperation with eleven social service agencies, is conducting a program to educate foster parents in child development and psychology. The program is directed toward helping such parents understand the reactions of their foster children—both to them and to the children's natural parents.

To fill the large gap between the unskilled aides and the highly trained professionals working with child inpatients and outpatients, Knox College, in Illinois, offers an undergraduate program in human development stressing training in both psychology and education. The "child care specialists" thus trained can provide therapeutic services understandingly, with a minimum of supervision.

Two allied programs have been conducted at the National Institute of Mental Health for "mature" college-educated women to prepare them for semiprofessional counseling roles. One well-known program by Margaret Rioch and Charmian Elkes prepared housewives to serve in outpatient clinics as "mental health counselors," while a related program prepared similar women to be "child development counselors" in such child-care settings as well-baby clinics and nursery schools.

A notable recent trend in the development of paraprofessional personnel has been the effort to fill needed roles with the needy—that is, to train the poor to serve as "indigenous nonprofessionals" in the mental health field. Pearl and Riessman, in *New Careers for the Poor* (1965), estimated that at least 1,000,000 of the poor should be employed in these roles.

Such persons, it was suggested, could bridge the communications gap between the poor client and the professional. For example, men could serve as role models in the schools, where they could work directly with children suffering "surface disorders." Both men and women could serve in child-oriented social agencies, as helpers in day care centers, sympathetic interviewers, companions, neighborhood developers, aides in juvenile courts, and in scores of other capacities related to child and family mental health.

In one program for the poor, a nine-month project was conducted in Baltimore to train 30 poor persons as psychiatric aides. Most of the program's $70,000 cost was funded by the New Careers program administered by the U.S. Department of Labor. Those who completed the training were to be placed in state mental institutions in positions paying from $4,451 to $5,386.

A joint project of the Albert Einstein College of Medicine of Yeshiva University and the Lincoln Hospital of New York is training deprived, unemployed, or low-income community residents to become "community mental health aides." After training in various social agencies, aides are placed in the hospital's Neighborhood Service Centers (NSC)—storefront satellites which Riessman has described as "neighborhood-based mental health clinics." At each NSC, staffed by six trainees and one mental health professional, the aides provide services for their fellow poor ranging from the primary preventive activities of giving practical advice in social and job skills and conducting youth programs to the more therapeutic activities in which they "intervene in critical situations, engage comparatively pathological people in meaningful relationships, stimulate them to take action on their own behalf, mobilize community resources, and serve as a bridge between the client in need and the professional service."

Members of another needy population—adolescent, high school dropouts—have been trained to serve as "human service aides"; as such, they may staff child-care centers, neighborhood recreation centers, and social research projects, and may serve as peer-group leaders.

Although most of the programs described here provide training on a full-time basis for paraprofessional personnel who will serve in full-time paid positions, many others are designed to prepare volunteers for part-time service, particularly in the child-care area. Such volunteers are used in pediatric wards, in preschool and school situations, and in work with disturbed children. Some adolescent and college student volunteers have been employed successfully to work supportively with children.

D. *Problems and Prospects in the Use of Paraprofessionals*

The programs that have been discussed, and many others like them, are exciting harbingers of future growth in the field of child mental health care. They point the way toward new development of available manpower and suggest that our limited production of professional personnel may not thoroughly hinder future efforts to provide improved preventive and rehabilitative services for children.

To date, most of these programs are essentially in their pilot phases; enthusiasm runs high, and experience is limited. Yet some problems are already apparent. As noted by Arnhoff, Jenkins, and Speisman (1969):

> [Elkes and] Rioch's Mental Health Counselors, although they are all working, had some problem of acceptance by their agencies and the paths to promotion and salary increases are far from clear. A "Mental Health Re-Entry Expediter" may look very much like a social worker, but he has no strong organization to back him in his struggle for advancement. The problem of rewriting job classifications and finding suitable employment for these types is a large one, and if the rewards are not commensurate with their training and abilities, they will leave the field—often to enter graduate school in a more recognized specialty. In short, this new type is dangerous if he competes with the professional, and disillusioned and dissatisfied if he doesn't. As yet, his expectations may be quite unclear, and as a result many of these training programs have vacancies.

The authors have also noted a basic problem in the development of new manpower:

> In our zeal to provide services for those who need help, a rather unsystematic proliferation of manpower approaches has suddenly emerged, but certainly not enough attention has been paid to the people we are training. If they are taught irrelevant or obsolescent skills, what is their future employment picture? Where can they see themselves ten years after training?
>
> Questioning the new trends and roles is not necessarily an argument for maintenance of the status quo and current professional prerequisites. There is a most definite need for a reevaluation of the present professional roles and functions. There is certainly the possibility to consider, however, that if the new careers are not properly designed, if they are not really careers, service may not improve and employment may be a temporary thing. . . .

Members of the Commission's Task Force IV have made several suggestions for consideration in the design of new training programs for paraprofessionals. The first responsibility, of course, is to specify those tasks for which new mental health specialists are needed and to devise appropriate types of training. Pollak (1968) has observed:

> Obviously, a specific set of information and skills is required for persons whom we essentially use for relationship therapy, who are intended to give empathic presence to patients and clients in crises, whom we ask to furnish the continuity of relationship for prolonged periods of time, i.e., object constancy that will assist children in weathering developmental crises. For persons who are supposed to use confrontation or interpretation in interaction with the child, for persons who use play therapy, for persons who work with autistic children, other skills and other types of information will be required.

As a corollary to this suggestion, Pollak notes that:

> The task of all division of labor in complex organizations is fractionalization and coordination. Training programs will have to be developed not only for personnel from the new manpower resources who will be asked to do these fractional jobs, but also for the members of the established professions who will be called upon to coordinate and supervise these fractional activities. In other words, we will also need new training programs for consultants and supervisors.

A second consideration must be a careful matching of the tasks to be performed with the capabilities of those available to perform them. Arnhoff, Rubenstein, and Speisman (1969) have observed: "Often there seems little choice of who is to be trained, particularly, in as low-paid an area as mental health service has traditionally been." Efforts to use the abilities of the underprivileged, the elderly, the unskilled, and the dropout must recognize both their strengths and their weaknesses. Thus, for example, the authors note that the sensitivity and compassion of many of these individuals are particularly appropriate to working in "custodial institutions, often with children and usually with the retarded," but working with such patients as disturbed adults may demand more sophisticated technical and intellectual skills.

A third suggestion is that within each type of subprofessional training, clearly visible career ladders must be made available so that the more highly motivated may reach out toward broader horizons and greater economic and psychic rewards, and those who are lacking in education and initial motivation may find a starting rung. As Pollak (1968) observes: "Ours is a dynamic society which takes change and improvement as a sign of health. Terminal positions have all the implications of professional failures." Another source has proposed that the career ladder should stop short of full professional status but should permit entry into professional areas by appropriate training, if desired. Standards will have to be developed for both training and role performance to assure quality control in the development of these new occupations. The cooperation of professional groups will be necessary, although possibly difficult to obtain, for establishment and sponsorship of licensing, certification, and other formal types of credentials. As the new roles become more recognized, state certification should also be sought.

An additional consideration has been suggested for the design of paraprofessional development training programs: namely, that the training time required be relatively short—from three months to a year, ideally. Longer programs represent little economy, since trainees could become professionals in the same amount of time. Von Mering and Carpenter (1967) have reported on Riessman's three-phase design for rapid on-the-job training of a large number of nonprofessionals:

First, a pre-service period of four weeks enables the trainees to learn two or three selected tasks useful to the agency where they will be placed. Phase two is a transition where the trainee will work half a day and discuss on-the-job experiences the remaining time. It is also proposed that the trainee get special training for one fifth of the week in addition to receiving daily supervision on the job. The rationale behind this type of training is: "The notion is *jobs first, training built in;* that is, the job becomes the motivator for further development on the part of the non-professional."

A final recommendation has been made by several observers of the mental health manpower problem that, given the changing patterns of present and future health care in our country, particularly the growing orientation toward comprehensive health-care service, both professional and nonprofessional training will have to provide mental health workers with flexible skills and a readiness to accept continuing education or retraining as a natural part of their career growth.

The child mental health professionals have an awesome responsibility for the structuring of new care occupations, particularly at the paraprofessional level. They must clarify the tasks that belong in the paraprofessional domain; help to determine the educational · and personality requirements for such jobs; and assume responsibility for training and creative employment.

Paraprofessional manpower, volunteer or paid, must not be wasted through overlap, lack of provisions for advancement, inadequate training, or preparation for irrelevant occupations or already obsolescent skills. Unless these elements are structured into emerging manpower development, trained workers will walk in and out of child mental health occupations through doors that swing in both directions.

⊂ NEEDED: A COMMITMENT TO THE FUTURE

The preceding discussion has been focused on the mental health needs of three major groups within the child population and on the manpower available to fulfill these needs. It has started with the assumption that there is and will be a shortage of professional manpower and has examined how we might better use what manpower we have, and might augment our supply with new types of personnel, particularly those who might carry on the work of the new Child Development Councils throughout the country, either as staff or as service workers through council contracts.

This is a pragmatic approach. If implemented, it might even improve the mental health care given to children—particularly if greater thought is given to the analysis of tasks to be done, the optimal matching of personnel and tasks, and the coordination of training, administration, research, and the delivery of services.

This pragmatic approach, however, is by no means a solution to the basic difficulties confronting the child mental health care system. It would be narrow and shortsighted to assume that the problem of providing manpower to serve mental health needs can be isolated meaningfully from the larger social context within which the problems occur. Nor can mental illness itself be understood or treated significantly without understanding the social pressures and conflicts that appear to contribute to its etiology. The problems of preventing and treating mental illness and of developing and deploying appropriate and sufficient manpower to carry out the tasks needed cannot be met realistically so long as we assume that all we need is more people, more money, and more centers. We may well need all of these, but even more essential is a rational assessment of our needs and a systematic means of assuring that those measures that are in our best national interest receive top national priorities.

There can be little doubt that the mental health of children, our greatest national resource, is vital to our country's future. Yet we do not act as if this were the case. In the name of children we are willing to raise some money, establish some commissions, train some new personnel, but we are uncomfortable when conflicts arise between their best interests and vested interests, between the familiarity of tradition and the need for innovation, between our belief in free enterprise and our recognition that federal funds, and often federal coordination, can spell the difference between good intentions and actual social change.

We have recognized that the training of manpower for mental health is a problem of sufficient magnitude to warrant extensive public concern and financial commitment, both federal and local. For example, in 1967, $95,-600,000 was appropriated for training activities by the National Institute of Mental Health—about 36 percent of the NIMH budget (Arnhoff, Rubenstein, and Speisman, 1969). This figure for training funds represents an increase of more than 769 percent beyond 1948 appropriations, and a twenty-year growth which is more than double that of all mental health appropriations. Yet despite these funds, mental health manpower training has been largely inadequate to meet national needs.

Many potential professional trainees have been put off by the long training required for professional qualification, and by the financial sacrifices required of them to undergo graduate training—particularly in fields such as medicine. Often, they have been drawn into competing manpower pools such as the armed services or voluntary service activities such as the Peace Corps or Vista or have entered other more lucrative or glamorous professions or non-mental health areas of the health professions.

The pool of manpower for mental health will continue to be insufficient as long as the national development of manpower remains a largely irrational process determined by the tug and pull of innumerable parties and uncoordinated factions. As the National Manpower Policy Task Force (1969) noted recently:

> As the scope of manpower policy is broad, so the policy-makers are many and diverse—including employers, unions, school boards, local, state and federal agencies, colleges and voluntary organizations. As a result, no single, consistent, or cohesive strategy has emerged—or perhaps can emerge—for developing and utilizing human resources in the United States. Manpower policy comes in pieces, and pieces do not fit easily into a neat pattern.

If we accept the fact that, as Lester has stated in *Manpower Planning in a Free Society* (1966), ". . . long range and more comprehensive economic planning by the central government . . . raises fears of centralization, bureaucratic domination and industrial regimentation . . ." and if we thus fail to confront the more basic issues underlying any manpower planning, then a moderate improvement in the status quo is the best we can expect from the Commission's recommendations. We owe our children more.

SUMMARY

For a decade or more, experts in the mental health manpower field have recognized that, under the traditional system, we have not, do not, and probably never will have enough properly trained professional personnel to meet the mental health needs of our nation. The traditional answer has been to train more professionals; and while we have increased our supply of the core professionals—physicians, nurses, social workers, and psychologists—in the past few years, the increases have not been sufficient to meet rising demands for services. The problem is further compounded by the uneven geographic distribution of highly trained personnel, which leaves many communities with few, if any, services.

Limitations inherent in our traditional answer to manpower problems make it imperative that we look more systematically and creatively at the existing situation and the accompanying problems. We do need to train more professionals; however, we also need to develop means for making better use of our highly trained personnel. It is equally important that we develop new supporting manpower roles to provide for the mental health needs of our children, such as the training and employment of paraprofessionals as well as specialists trained at the BA and MA levels. We will need to continually expand existing educational and training facilities in ways that will maintain high standards and quality, and we will have to face the inherent resistance of the professions themselves to intervention and change. But change itself can be creative; and it is possible that, in the long run, we may develop a much better system of services. Certainly the needs of our children cannot be met under the existing mental health care network.

APPENDIX

I

LEGISLATION

PUBLIC LAW 89–97

89th Congress, H. R. 6675
July 30, 1965

Social Security Amendments of 1965

Health Study of Resources Relating to Children's Emotional Illness

Sec. 231. (a) The Secretary of Health, Education, and *Program grants*
Welfare is authorized, upon the recommendation of the
National Advisory Mental Health Council and after securing the advice of experts in pediatrics and child welfare,
to make grants for carrying out a program of research into
and study of our resources, methods, and practices for diagnosing or preventing emotional illness in children and of
treating, caring for, and rehabilitating children with emotional illnesses.

(b) Such grants may be made to one or more organizations, but only on condition that the organization will
undertake and conduct, or if more than one organization is
to receive such grants, only on condition that such organizations have agreed among themselves to undertake and conduct, a coordinated program of research into and study of
all aspects of the resources, methods, and practices referred
to in subsection (a).

(c) As used in subsection (b), the term "organization" means a nongovernmental agency, organization, or commission, composed of representatives of leading national medical, welfare, educational, and other professional associations, organizations, or agencies active in the field of mental health of children.

(d) There are authorized to be appropriated for the fiscal year ending June 30, 1966, the sum of $500,000 to be used for a grant or grants to help initiate the research and study provided for in this section; and the sum of $500,000 for the succeeding fiscal year for the making of such grants as may be needed to carry the research and study to completion. The terms of any such grant shall provide that the research and study shall be completed not later than two years from the date it is inaugurated; that the grantee shall file annual reports with the Congress, the Secretary, and the Governors of the several States, among others that the grantee may select; and that the final report shall be similarly filed.

APPENDIX
II

THE JOINT COMMISSION ON MENTAL
HEALTH OF CHILDREN, INC.

OFFICERS

REGINALD S. LOURIE, M.D.
    President and Chairman
    Director, Department of Psychiatry
    Children's Hospital—Hillcrest Children's Center, Washington, D.C.

JULIUS B. RICHMOND, M.D.
    First Vice-President
    Dean, The Medical Faculty
    State University of New York, Syracuse, New York

NICHOLAS HOBBS, Ph.D.
    Second Vice-President
    Director, John F. Kennedy Center for Research on Education and Human
    Development
    Peabody College, Nashville, Tennessee

HARRIET MANDELBAUM
    Third Vice-President
    Council on Childhood Mental Illness, National Association for Mental Health
    Brooklyn, New York

CHARLES SCHLAIFER, F.A.P.A. (Hon.)
    Secretary Treasurer, New York, New York

WALTER E. BARTON, M.D.
    Assistant Secretary
    Medical Director, American Psychiatric Association
    Washington, D.C.

BOARD OF DIRECTORS

ROBERT A. ALDRICH, M.D.
Professor of Pediatrics and Head, Division of Human Ecology
School of Medicine
University of Washington, Seattle, Washington

JOSEPH P. ANDERSON, M.S.W.
Executive Director, National Association of Social Workers
New York, New York

WILLIAM S. ANDERSON, M.D., F.A.A.P.
Clinical Professor of Pediatrics
School of Medicine, George Washington University
Washington, D.C.

HOWARD V. BAIR, M.D.
Superintendent and Medical Director
Parsons State Hospital and Training Center, Parsons, Kansas

WALTER E. BARTON, M.D.
Medical Director
American Psychiatric Association, Washington, D.C.

DAVID L. BAZELON
Chief Judge, U.S. Court of Appeals
U.S. Court House, Washington, D.C.

IRVING N. BERLIN, M.D.
Professor of Psychiatry and Pediatrics and Head, Division of Psychiatry
School of Medicine, University of Washington
Seattle, Washington

VIOLA W. BERNARD, M.D.
Clinical Professor of Psychiatry and Director, Division of Community Psychiatry
Columbia University, New York, New York

ELIZABETH M. BOGGS, Ph.D.
State College, Pennsylvania

THOMAS BRADLEY
Councilman, Tenth District
City Council, City Hall, Los Angeles, California

ORVILLE G. BRIM, Ph.D.
President, Russell Sage Foundation, New York, New York

E. H. CHRISTOPHERSON, M.D.
Clinical Professor of Pediatrics, School of Medicine
University of California, San Diego, California

HENRY V. COBB, Ph.D.
Dean, College of Arts and Sciences
University of South Dakota, Vermillion, South Dakota

ROBERT I. DAUGHERTY, M.D.
Committee on Mental Health
American Academy of General Practice, Lebanon, Oregon

ADA E. DEER, M.S.W.
Social Work Consultant
Minneapolis School System, Minneapolis, Minnesota

LEON EISENBERG, M.D.
Professor of Psychiatry
Massachusetts General Hospital, Boston, Massachusetts

DANA L. FARNSWORTH, M.D.
Director, Harvard University Health Services
Cambridge, Massachusetts

LORENE FISCHER, M.A.
Director, Graduate Programs in Adult and Child Psychiatric Mental Health
Nursing, College of Nursing, Wayne State University, Detroit, Michigan

V. REV. MSGR. ROBERT E. GALLAGHER
Administrative Director, Catholic Charities Counseling Service
Archdiocese of New York, New York, New York
(Deceased October 6, 1968)

GEORGE E. GARDNER, M.D., Ph.D.
Director, Judge Baker Guidance Center, Boston, Massachusetts

MIKE GORMAN
Executive Director, National Committee Against Mental Illness
Washington, D.C.

JAMES L. GROBE, M.D.
Chairman, Commission on Mental Health
American Academy of General Practice, Phoenix, Arizona

NICHOLAS HOBBS, Ph.D.
Director, John F. Kennedy Center for Research on Education and Human De-
velopment
Peabody College, Nashville, Tennessee

PHILIP A. HOLLAND
Former Director of Campus Environmental Studies
U.S. National Student Association, Arvada, Colorado

RABBI I. FRED HOLLANDER
Associate Director, The New York Board of Rabbis, Inc.
New York, New York

EDWIN S. KESSLER, M.D.
Clinical Associate Professor and Director, Children's Psychiatric Services
Georgetown University Medical Center, Washington, D.C.

REV. LEO N. KISROW
Editor, Children's Publications, Board of Publication
The United Methodist Church, Nashville, Tennessee

HYMAN S. LIPPMAN, M.D.
 Consultant Child Psychiatrist, Department of Child Psychiatry
 St. Paul-Ramsey Hospital, St. Paul, Minnesota

NORMAN V. LOURIE, A.C.S.W.
 Executive Deputy Secretary, Pennsylvania Department of Public Welfare
 Harrisburg, Pennsylvania

REGINALD S. LOURIE, M.D.
 Director, Department of Psychiatry
 Children's Hospital—Hillcrest Children's Center, Washington, D.C.

JOSEPH P. MALDONADO, A.C.S.W.
 Deputy Director, Regional Office of Economic Opportunity
 San Francisco, California

HARRIET MANDELBAUM
 Council on Childhood Mental Illness
 National Association for Mental Health, Brooklyn, New York

JOHN L. MILLER, Ph.D.
 Superintendent of Schools
 Great Neck Public Schools, Great Neck, New York

MILDRED MITCHELL-BATEMAN, M.D.
 Director, West Virginia Department of Mental Health
 Charleston, West Virginia

WILLIAM C. MORSE, Ph.D.
 Professor of Education and Psychology
 University of Michigan, Ann Arbor, Michigan

JAMES M. NABRIT, JR., J.D., LL.D.
 President, Howard University
 Washington, D.C.

JOHN J. NOONE, JR., E.D.
 Executive Director, American Association on Mental Deficiency
 Washington, D.C.

JOSEPH D. NOSHPITZ, M.D.
 Washington, D.C.

K. PATRICK OKURA
 Administrative Director, Division of Preventive and Social Psychiatry
 Nebraska Psychiatric Institute, Omaha, Nebraska

ARNOLD PICKER
 Chairman, Executive Committee
 United Artists Pictures Corporation, New York, New York

DANE G. PRUGH, M.D.
 Professor of Psychiatry and Pediatrics
 Chief, Child Psychiatry Division
 University of Colorado Medical Center
 Denver, Colorado

Kurt Reichert, Ph.D.
Director, Division on Standards and Accreditation
Council on Social Work Education, New York, New York

Joseph H. Reid, A.C.S.W.
Executive Director, Child Welfare League of America, Inc.
New York, New York

Eveoleen N. Rexford, M.D.
Professor and Director of Child Psychiatry
Boston University School of Medicine, Boston, Massachusetts

Julius B. Richmond, M.D.
Dean, The Medical Faculty
State University of New York; Upstate Medical Center
Syracuse, New York

Mrs. Winthrop Rockefeller
Morrilton, Arkansas

Alan O. Ross, Ph.D.
Professor of Psychology and Director, Child Development Unit
State University of New York at Stony Brook, Stony Brook, New York

Charles Schlaifer, F.A.P.A. (Hon.)
New York, New York

Meyer Sonis, M.D.
Executive Director, Pittsburgh Child Guidance Center
Pittsburgh, Pennsylvania

Percy H. Steele Jr., A.C.S.W.
Executive Director, Bay Area Urban League, Inc., San Francisco, California

Robert Lee Stubblefield, M.D.
Professor and Chairman, Department of Psychiatry
Southwestern Medical School, University of Texas, Dallas, Texas

George Tarjan, M.D.
Professor of Psychiatry, Program Director, Mental Retardation
Neuropsychiatric Institute, University of California
Los Angeles, California

Mary Alice White, Ph.D.
Professor of Psychology and Education
Teachers College, Columbia University
New York, New York

Leonard Woodcock
Vice President, International Union, UAW
Detroit, Michigan

BOARD OF DIRECTORS' LIAISON REPRESENTATIVES

FROM FEDERAL AGENCIES*

ARTHUR LESSER, M.D.
KATHERINE B. OETTINGER, M.S.W.
P. FREDERICK DELLIQUADRI, M.D.
Children's Bureau
DHEW, Washington, D.C.

ROBERT E. DREW
Division of Indian Health
USPHS, Silver Springs, Maryland

ELDON L. EAGLES, M.D.
National Institute of Neurological
Diseases and Stroke
NIH, USPHS, Bethesda, Maryland

ALBERT C. FREMONT, M.D., M.P.H.
Division of Mental Retardation
Rehabilitation Services Administration
Arlington, Virginia

WILLIAM E. JOHNSTON, Ed.D.
Office of Disadvantaged and Handicapped
Office of Education, DHEW, Washington, D.C.

WAYNE A. KIMMEL
Office of Assistant for Planning and
Evaluation
Office of Secretary, DHEW, Washing-
ton, D.C.

ELI M. BOWER, Ed.D.
E. JAMES LIEBERMAN, M.D.
Center for Studies of Mental Health of
Children and Youth
NIMH, Chevy Chase, Maryland

KATHLEEN E. LLOYD, M.D.
Social and Rehabilitation Service
Rehabilitation Services Administration
DHEW, Washington, D.C.

JOSEPH M. BOBBITT, Ph.D.
DONALD HARTING, M.D.
DWAIN N. WALCHER, M.D.
FRANK T. FALKNER, M.D.
National Institute of Child Health and
Human Development
NIH, USPHS, Bethesda, Maryland

JAMES OSBERG, M.D.
Community Research and Services
Division
NIMH, Bethesda, Maryland

MARY WEAVER
Office of the Secretary of the Department of Health, Education, and Welfare
Washington, D.C.

* In most cases listings show successive liaison designations.

MEMBER ORGANIZATIONS AND THEIR DESIGNATED REPRESENTATIVES TO THE JCMHC

American Academy of Child Psychiatry
Robert C. Prall, M.D., Secretary, Merion Station, Pennsylvania
Sidney Berman, M.D., Pres.-Elect, Washington, D.C.

American Academy of General Practice
Mac F. Cahal, M.D., Executive Director, Kansas City, Missouri
James Grobe, M.D.*

* Member, Board of Directors, JCMHC.

American Academy of Pediatrics
Robert G. Frazier, M.D., Executive Director, Evanston, Illinois

American Association for Children's Residential Centers
Samuel P. Berman, M.D., President, New York City
Joseph Noshpitz, M.D.*

American Association of Psychiatric Clinics for Children
Jacqueline L. Friend, M.S.W., Executive Director, New York City

American Association on Mental Deficiency
John J. Noone, M.D., Executive Director, Washington, D.C.

American College Health Association
James W. Dilley, Executive Secretary, Evanston, Illinois
Dana Farnsworth, M.D.*

American Humane Association
Vincent De Francis, Denver, Colorado
Wilson D. McKerrow

American Legion
Fred T. Kuszmaul, Assistant Director, National Child Welfare Division
Indianapolis, Indiana

American Medical Association
F. J. C. Blasingame, M.D., Executive Vice President, Chicago, Illinois

American Nurses Association
Judith Whitaker, Executive Director, New York City
Julia C. Thompson

American Occupational Therapy Association
Frances Helmig, Executive Director, New York City
R. L. Tillman

American Orthopsychiatric Association
Marion F. Langer, Ph.D., Executive Secretary, New York City
Benjamin Pasamanick, M.D.

American Parents Committee
Barbara D. McGarry, Executive Director, Washington, D.C.

American Personnel and Guidance Association
Willis E. Dugan, Executive Director, Washington, D.C.

American Psychiatric Association
Walter E. Barton, M.D., Medical Director, Washington, D.C.*

American Psychoanalytic Association
Helen Fischer, Executive Secretary, New York City
Seymour Lustman, M.D., Ph.D.

American Psychological Association
Arthur H. Brayfield, Ph.D., Executive Officer, Washington, D.C.
Kenneth Goodall, Ph.D.

* Member, Board of Directors, JCMHC.

American Public Health Association
  Berwyn F. Mattison, M.D., Executive Director, New York City

American Public Welfare Association
  Guy R. Justis, Director, Chicago, Illinois
  Harold Hagen

American Social Health Association
  Earle Lippincott, Executive Director, New York City

American Sociological Association
  Edmund H. Volkart, Ph.D., Executive Officer, Washington, D.C.

American Speech and Hearing Association
  William E. Castle, Ph.D., Associate Secretary, Washington, D.C.

Association for Childhood Education International
  Alberta Meyer, Executive Secretary, Washington, D.C.
  Sylvia Sunderlin

Child Study Association of America
  A. D. Buchmueller, Executive Director, New York City

Council for Exceptional Children
  William C. Geer, Executive Secretary, Washington, D.C.

Council of Jewish Federation & Welfare Funds, Inc.
  Maurice Bernstein, Director Community Planning, New York City
  Elsie Seff

Council of State Governments
  Brevard Crihfield, Executive Director, Lexington, Kentucky

Day Care and Child Development Council of America, Inc.
  Mrs. Richard M. Lansburgh, President, Washington, D.C.

Family Service Association of America
  Clark Blackburn, Executive Director, New York City

Interprofessional Research Commission on Pupil Personnel Services
  Gordon P. Liddle, Ph.D., Executive Director, Silver Spring, Maryland

National Association for Mental Health
  Brian O'Connell, Executive Director, New York City
  D. Douglas Waterstreet

National Association for Retarded Children
  Luther Stringham, Executive Director, New York City

National Association of Social Workers
  Joseph Anderson, Executive Director, New York City*

National Association of State Mental Health Program Directors
  Harry Schnibbe, Executive Director, Washington, D.C.

National Conference of Catholic Charities
  Msgr. Lawrence J. Corcoran, Secretary, Washington, D.C.
  Sr. Maria Mercedes

  * Member, Board of Directors, JCMHC.

National Committee for Children and Youth
   Isabella J. Jones, Executive Director, Washington, D.C.

National Congress of Parents and Teachers
   Irwin E. Hendryson, President, Chicago, Illinois
   William Baisinger

National Council on Crime and Delinquency
   Milton G. Rector, Director, New York City
   Robert E. Trimble

National Education Association
   William G. Carr, Executive Secretary, Washington, D.C.
   Edward Mileff

National League for Nursing
   Inez Haynes, General Director, New York City
   Lucy L. Knox

National Rehabilitation Association
   E. B. Whitten, Executive Director, Washington, D.C.

National Society for Autistic Children
   Ruth Sullivan, President, Albany, New York
   Mooza V. P. Grant, Past President

The Orton Society, Inc.
   Roger E. Saunders, President, Ruxton, Maryland
   Margaret B. Rawson, Past President

Planned Parenthood/World Population
   Dorothy Millstone, Associate Director, New York City

United States National Student Association
   Edward Schwartz, Past President, Washington, D.C.
   Carol Milano

COMMITTEES OF THE BOARD
OF DIRECTORS

Executive Committee

REGINALD S. LOURIE, M.D., Chairman
JOSEPH P. ANDERSON, M.S.W.
WALTER E. BARTON, M.D.
E. H. CHRISTOPHERSON, M.D.
NICHOLAS HOBBS, PH.D.
NORMAN V. LOURIE, A.C.S.W.

HARRIET MANDELBAUM
JOHN L. MILLER, PH.D.
JULIUS B. RICHMOND, M.D.
CHARLES SCHLAIFER, F.A.P.A. (Hon.)
MARY ALICE WHITE, PH.D.

Liaison representative from the Committee on Children of Minority Groups:
Mr. Alex Mercure

Committee on Nominations

JOSEPH P. ANDERSON, M.S.W., Chairman
HOWARD V. BAIR, M.D.
E. H. CHRISTOPHERSON, M.D.
LEON EISENBERG, M.D.
HYMAN S. LIPPMAN, M.D.

NORMAN V. LOURIE, A.C.S.W.
HARRIET MANDLEBAUM
JOHN L. MILLER, PH.D.
MARY ALICE WHITE, PH.D.

Committee on By-Laws and Procedures

GEORGE TARJAN, M.D., Chairman
JOSEPH P. ANDERSON, M.S.W.
WILLIAM S. ANDERSON, M.D., F.A.A.P.
HENRY V. COBB, PH.D.
DANA FARNSWORTH, M.D.

HARRIET MANDELBAUM
WILLIAM C. MORSE, PH.D.
ALAN O. ROSS, PH.D.
ROBERT L. STUBBLEFIELD, M.D.

Committee on Finance

CHARLES SCHAIFER, F.A.P.A. (HON.)
  Chairman
VIOLA W. BERNARD, M.D.

DANE G. PRUGH, M.D.
MRS. WINTHROP ROCKEFELLER
ALLAN O. ROSS, PH.D.

Committee on Studies

NORMAN V. LOURIE, A.C.S.W., Chairman
JUDGE DAVID L. BAZELON
VIOLA W. BERNARD, M.D.
ELIZABETH N. BOGGS, PH.D.
GEORGE E. GARDNER, M.D., PH.D.
JAMES L. GROBE, M.D.

NICHOLAS HOBBS, PH.D.
MILDRED MITCHELL-BATEMEN, M.D.
JOHN J. NOONE, JR., ED.D.
EVEOLEEN N. REXFORD, M.D.
JULIUS B. RICHMOND, M.D.
MEYER SONIS, M.D.

Editorial Committee

IRVING N. BERLIN, M.D., Chairman
  Board of Directors

NORMAN V. LOURIE, A.C.S.W.
  Board of Directors

WILLIAM C. MORSE, PH.D., Co-chairman
  Board of Directors

EVEOLEEN N. REXFORD, M.D.
  Board of Directors
  * Until March 1, 1969.

*MICHAEL AMRINE
  Washington, D.C.

*LEONARD S. COTTRELL, PH.D.
  Chapel Hill, North Carolina

*OSCAR JAGER
  Washington, D.C.

*GREER WILLIAMS
  Hingham, Massachusetts

Special Consultants to the Editorial Committee

MIKE GORMAN
  Board of Directors

ALBERT J. SOLNIT, M.D.
  Task Force V

TASK FORCE COORDINATING COMMITTEE

WILLIAM C. MORSE, PH.D., Chairman
Board of Directors

NORMAN V. LOURIE, A.C.S.W.
Board of Directors

EVEOLEEN N. REXFORD, M.D.
Board of Directors

PETER B. NEUBAUER, M.D.
Task Force I, Chairman

MARY ENGEL, PH.D.
Task Force II, Chairman

EDWARD J. SHOBEN, PH.D.
Task Force III, Chairman

SEYMOUR L. LUSTMAN, M.D., PH.D.
Task Force IV, Chairman

HAROLD M. VISOTSKY, M.D.
Task Force V, Chairman

ROBERT H. FELIX, M.D.
Task Force VI, Chairman

ROBERT H. ALWAY, M.D.
Task Force VI, Co-chairman

TASK FORCES OF COMMISSION

Task Force I: Studies of Infancy Through Age Five

PETER B. NEUBAUER, M.D., Chairman
Director, Child Development Center
New York, New York

RUTH ABBOTT, R.N.
Visiting Nurses Assoc. of Hartford
Hartford, Connecticut

MILLIE ALMY, PH.D.
Professor of Psychology and Education
Teachers College, Columbia University
New York, New York

HERBERT G. BIRCH, M.D., PH.D.
Research Professor
Albert Einstein College of Medicine
Yeshiva University, Bronx, New York

PARK S. GERALD, M.D.
Associate Professor of Pediatrics
Harvard Medical School
Chief, Clinical Genetics Division
Children's Hospital Medical Center
Boston, Massachusetts

LOUIS M. HELLMAN, M.D.
Chairman, Department of Obstetrics
and Gynecology
State University of New York
Downstate Medical Center
Brooklyn, New York

HYLAN LEWIS, PH.D.
Fellow
Metropolitan Applied Research
Center, Inc.
New York, New York

*RICHMOND S. PAINE, M.D.
Professor of Pediatric Neurology
George Washington University
School of Medicine
Washington, D.C.

NORMAN A. POLANSKY, PH.D.
Professor of Sociology and
Social Work
Child Research Field Station
Asheville, North Carolina

SALLY PROVENCE, M.D.
Professor of Pediatrics
Yale Child Study Center
New Haven, Connecticut

HALBERT B. ROBINSON, PH.D.
Department of Psychology
University of Washington
Seattle, Washington

NIMH Liaison Representatives: †

LOUIS WIENKOWSKI, PH.D.

ROBERT REICHLER, PH.D.

* Deceased.
†Represents successive liaison designations.

*Task Force II: Studies of Children from Kindergarten
Age Through Eighth Grade*

MARY ENGEL, PH.D., Chairman
Associate Professor
Department of Psychology
City College of New York
New York, New York

HERMAN S. BELMONT, M.D.
Professor and Head
Child Psychiatry Section
Hahnemann Medical College
Philadelphia, Pennsylvania

BARBARA BIBER, PH.D.
Distinguished Research Scholar
Bank Street College of Education
New York, New York

GEORGE B. BRAIN, PH.D.
Dean, College of Education
Washington State University
Pullman, Washington

ROBERT E. COOKE, M.D.
Given Foundation Professor of
Pediatrics
The Johns Hopkins University School
of Medicine
Baltimore, Maryland

CLAIRE M. FAGIN, PH.D.
Director of the Graduate Programs in
Psychiatric Mental Health Nursing
New York University
New York, New York

RICHARD L. FOSTER, PH.D.
District Superintendent of San Ramon
Valley Unified School District
Danville, California

LAWRENCE KOHLBERG, PH.D.
Professor of Education
School of Education
Harvard University
Cambridge, Massachusetts

SALVADOR MINUCHIN, M.D.
Professor of Child Psychiatry
University of Pennsylvania
Director, Philadelphia Guidance Clinic
Philadelphia, Pennsylvania

SAMUEL M. WISHIK, M.D.
Director, Division of Program
Development and Evaluation
International Institute for Study of
Human Reproduction
Columbia University
New York, New York

MARTIN WOLINS, D.S.W.
Professor of Social Welfare
University of California
Berkeley, California

NIMH Liaison Representatives*

ELI M. BOWER, ED.D.
NED GAYLIN, PH.D.

* Represents successive liaison designations.

Consultants to Task Force II

Conference on Special Education July 10–11, 1967

WESLEY BECKER, PH.D.
Bureau of Educational Research
University of Illinois
Urbana, Illinois

LLOYD M. DUNN, PH.D.
Peabody College
Nashville, Tennessee

WILLIAM GEER
Executive Director
Council for Exceptional Children
Washington, D.C.

LESTER MANN, PH.D.
Superintendent of Schools
Montgomery County, Pennsylvania

MICHAEL MARGE, PH.D.
Bureau for the Handicapped
U.S. Office of Education

TONY MILAZZO, PH.D.
University of Michigan
Ann Arbor, Michigan

WILLIAM MORSE, PH.D.
Board of Directors

JAMES MOSS, PH.D.
Bureau of the Handicapped
U.S. Office of Education

WILLIAM C. RHODES, PH.D.
Professor of Psychology
University of Michigan
Ann Arbor, Michigan

DAVID SHAPIRO, PH.D.
Childrens Village School
Dobbs Ferry, New York

JAMES TOMPKINS
Bureau of the Handicapped
U.S. Office of Education

Consultants in Clinical Child Psychology

RAYMOND J. BALESTER, PH.D.
National Institute of Mental Health
Chevy Chase, Maryland

C. ALAN BONEAU, PH.D.
American Psychological Association
Washington, D.C.

STUART E. GOLANN, PH.D.
American Psychological Association
Washington, D.C.

MRS. JANE HILDRETH
American Psychological Association
Washington, D.C.

LOVICK C. MILLER, PH.D.
Professor of Clinical Psychology
Department of Psychiatry
University of Louisville, School of
   Medicine
Louisville, Kentucky

DAVID RIGLER, PH.D.
National Institute of Mental Health
Chevy Chase, Maryland

SEBASTIAN SANTOSTEFANO, PH.D.
Department of Psychiatry
Boston University
Boston, Massachusetts

STANLEY SCHNEIDER, PH.D.
National Institute of Mental Health
Chevy Chase, Maryland

JEROME L. SINGER, PH.D.
Professor of Psychology
Director of Clinical Psychology
   Training Program
City College
City University of New York
New York, New York

JOSEPH SPEISMAN, PH.D.
National Institute of Mental Health
Chevy Chase, Maryland

ZANWIL SPERBER, PH.D.
Chief Psychologist
Department of Child Psychiatry
Cedars-Sinai Medical Center
Los Angeles, California

MARY ALICE WHITE, PH.D.
Professor of Psychology and
Education
Teachers College
Columbia University
New York, New York

ROBERT WIRT, PH.D.
Professor of Psychology
Department of Psychology
University of Minnesota
Minneapolis, Minn.

Special Meeting on Foster Care/JCMHC
October, 1967, New Orleans, Louisiana

DAVID FANSHEL, PH.D.
School of Social Work, Columbia
University
New York, New York

MORRIS A. HARMON
State Department of Child Welfare
Frankfort, Kentucky

REV. PHILIP JARMACK
National Conference of Catholic
Charities
Washington, D.C.

IRVING KAUFMAN, M.D.
Newtonville, Massachusetts

H. B. M. MURPHY, PH.D.
McGill University
Montreal, Canada

LLOYD RICHARDSON
Children's Aid Society of Toronto
Ontario, Canada

SISTER SERENA, A.C.S.W.
Gonzaga Home
Philadelphia, Pennsylvania

FLORENCE SILVERBLATT, M.S.W.
Philadelphia Department of Public
Welfare
Philadelphia, Pennsylvania

MARVIN B. SUSSMAN, PH.D.
Case Western Reserve University
Cleveland, Ohio

Task Force III: Studies of Adolescents and Youth

EDWARD JOSEPH SHOBEN, JR., PH.D., Chairman
Council on Higher Education Studies
State University of New York
Buffalo, New York

JUNE CHARRY, PH.D.
School Psychologist
Hartsdale Public Schools
Hartsdale, New York

JAMES P. DIXON, PH.D.
President
Antioch College
Yellow Springs, Ohio

W. EUGENE GROVES
Past President
U.S. National Student Association
Baltimore, Maryland

FELIX P. HEALD, M.D.
Professor of Pediatrics
George Washington University
Chief, Adolescent Medicine
Children's Hospital
Washington, D.C.

KENNETH KENISTON, PH.D.
Associate Professor
Department of Psychiatry
Yale University School of Medicine
New Haven, Connecticut

WILLIAM C. KVARACEUS, PH.D.
Professor of Education and Sociology
Chairman of the Education
Department
Clark University
Worcester, Massachusetts

JOE P. MALDONADO, A.C.S.W.
Deputy Director
Regional Office of Economic
Opportunity
San Francisco, California

MORRIS F. MAYER, PH.D.
Executive Director
Bellefaire Treatment Center
Cleveland, Ohio

BERNICE MILBURN MOORE, PH.D.
Hogg Foundation for Mental Health
University of Texas
Austin, Texas

NORMAN E. ZINBERG, M.D.
Assistant Clinical Professor of
Psychiatry
Faculty of Medicine
Harvard University
Cambridge, Massachusetts

NIMH Liaison Representative:

E. JAMES LIEBERMAN, M.D.

Consultants to Task Force III

LEON D. BRAMSON, PH.D.
Swarthmore College
Swarthmore, Pennsylvania

DONALD J. EBERLY, M.D.
National Service Secretariat
Washington, D.C.

PHILIP A. HOLLAND
U.S. National Student Association
Fairbanks, Alaska

*Task Force IV: Programs of Prevention
and Rehabilitation, Research and
Its Uses, and Manpower*

SEYMOUR L. LUSTMAN, M.D., PH.D., Chairman
Professor of Psychiatry
Yale University Child Study Center
New Haven, Connecticut

ALFRED BUCHMUELLER, M.S.W.
Past Executive Director
Child Study Association of America
New York, New York

G. FRANKLIN EDWARDS, PH.D.
Professor of Sociology
Howard University
Washington, D.C.

RAYMOND FELDMAN, M.D.
Director, Mental Health Programs
Western Interstate Commission for
Higher Education
Boulder, Colorado

CARL FENICHEL, ED.D.
Director
League School for Seriously Disturbed
Children
Brooklyn, New York

MORRIS GREEN, M.D.
Professor of Pediatrics
Indiana University School of Medicine
Indianapolis, Indiana

DALE B. HARRIS, PH.D.
Professor and Head
Department of Psychology
Pennsylvania State University
University Park, Pennsylvania

JEWELDEAN JONES, M.S.W.
Associate Director for Health and
Welfare
National Urban League
New York, New York

DOROTHY H. MILLER, D.S.W.
Social Research Laboratory
State of California
Department of Mental Hygiene
San Francisco, California

OTTO POLLACK, PH.D.
Professor of Sociology
Wharton School
University of Pennsylvania
Philadelphia, Pennsylvania

OTTO VON MERING, PH.D.
Professor of Anthropology
University of Pittsburgh School of
Medicine
Western Psychiatric Institute and
Clinic
Pittsburgh, Pennsylvania

NIMH Liaison Representatives*
RAYMOND BALESTER, PH.D.
HARVEY TASCHMAN, PH.D.
MICHAEL FISHMAN, M.D.

Consultants to Task Force IV

JAMES W. CARPER, M.D.
Washington, D.C.

B. OTIS COBB, M.D.
Institute for Research in Childhood
Health and Education
Walnut Creek, California

JAMES P. COMER, M.D.
Child Study Center
Yale University
New Haven, Connecticut

MARIO FANTINI
Division of Education
Ford Foundation
New York, New York

DOUGLAS FERGUSON
Program Officer
Ford Foundation
New York, New York

JOSEPH P. FITZPATRICK, S.J., PH.D.
Institute for Social Research
Fordham University
Bronx, New York

VICTOR GIOSCIA, PH.D.
Jewish Family Service of New York
New York, New York

CHLOETHIEL W. SMITH
Washington, D.C.

JOSEPH F. WHITING, PH.D.
Director, Division of Manpower
Research
American Psychiatric Association
Washington, D.C.

* Represents successive liaison designations.

*Task Force V: Organization, Administration, and Financing of
Services for Emotionally Disturbed Children*

HAROLD M. VISOTSKY, M.D., Chairman
Past Director
Illinois Department of Mental Health
Chicago, Illinois

MORTIMER BROWN, PH.D.
Assistant to the Director
Department of Mental Health
Springfield, Illinois

HOWARD ROME, M.D.
Professor of Psychiatry
Mayo Clinic
Rochester, Minnesota

HYMAN M. FORSTENZER
Second Deputy Commissioner
New York State Department of
Mental Hygiene
Albany, New York

VERA D. RUBIN, PH.D.
Director
Research Institute for the Study
of Man
New York, New York

WILLIAM P. HURDER, M.D.
Institute for Research on
Exceptional Children
University of Illinois
Urbana, Illinois

ALBERT J. SOLNIT, M.D.
Professor of Pediatrics and Psychiatry
Director, Child Study Center
Yale University
New Haven, Connecticut

ALFRED J. KAHN, PH.D.
Professor of Social Work
Columbia University
School of Social Work
New York, New York

HOMER CLARK WADSWORTH
President
Kansas City Association of Trusts
and Foundations
Kansas City, Missouri

FRANK T. RAFFERTY, M.D.
Professor of Psychiatry
Director, Division of Child Psychiatry
University of Maryland School
of Medicine
Baltimore, Maryland

NIMH Liaison Representative:

MORTON KRAMER, PH.D.

Consultants to Task Force V

WILLIAM M. BOLMAN, M.D.
Department of Psychiatry
University of Wisconsin Medical
Center
Madison, Wisconsin

JAY G. HIRSCH, M.D.
Chief, Division of Preventive
Psychiatry
Institute for Juvenile Research
Chicago, Illinois

JAMES J. GALLAGHER, PH.D.
Associate Commissioner
Bureau of Education for the
Handicapped
Washington, D.C.

HARRY C. SCHNIBBE
Executive Director
National Association of State Mental
Health Program Directors
Washington, D.C.

DONALD A. SCHON, PH.D.
  Organization for Social and
    Technical Innovation
  Cambridge, Massachusetts

ALVIN SCHORR, M.S.W.
  Deputy Assistant Secretary for
    Individual and Family Services
  Department of Health, Education,
    and Welfare
  Washington, D.C.

BEN B. SELIGMAN, PH.D.
  Institute of Labor Relations Research
  University of Massachusetts
  Amherst, Massachusetts

JACK C. WESTMAN, M.D.
  Director, Child Psychiatry Division
  University of Wisconsin Medical
    Center
  Madison, Wisconsin

Task Force VI: Innovation and Social Progress in Relation to Mental Health of Children

ROBERT H. FELIX, M.D., Chairman
Dean, School of Medicine
Saint Louis University
St. Louis, Missouri

ROBERT H. ALWAY, M.D., Co-chairman
Professor of Pediatrics, School of Medicine
Stanford University
Palo Alto, California

CONRAD M. ARENSBERG, PH.D.
  Professor of Anthropology
  Columbia University
  New York, New York

JOSEPH J. DOWNING, M.D.
  Past Program Chief, Mental Health
    Services Division, Department of
    Public Health and Welfare
  San Mateo, California

MRS. FRED R. HARRIS
  President, Oklahomans for Indian
    Opportunity
  Washington, D.C.

MATTHEW HUXLEY, M.S.
  Director, Division of Educational
    Development
  Smithsonian Institution
  Washington, D.C.

ROBERT L. LEON, M.D.
  Professor and Chairman, Department
    of Psychiatry
  University of Texas Medical School
  San Antonio, Texas

RONALD LIPPITT, PH.D.
  Program Director, Center for Re-
    search on the Utilization of Scien-
    tific Knowledge
  University of Michigan
  Institute for Social Research
  Ann Arbor, Michigan

JOHN H. NIEMEYER
  President, Bank Street College of
    Education
  New York, New York

JUSTINE WISE POLIER
  Judge, Family Court of the State of
    New York
  New York, New York

M. BREWSTER SMITH, PH.D.
  Professor and Chairman, Department
    of Psychology
  University of Chicago
  Chicago, Illinois

NIMH Liaison Representatives*

MATTHEW HUXLEY, M.S.
PETER BREGGIN, M.D.
LOUIS WIENCKOWSKI, PH.D.

Consultants to Task Force VI

MICHAEL AMRINE
Washington, D.C.

SAM RABINOVITZ
Michigan State Youth Commission
Ann Arbor, Michigan

JULES SUGARMAN
Associate Director,† Project Head
Start
Washington, D.C.

STEPHEN C. SUTHERLAND
Program Director for Higher
Education
NTL Institute for Applied
Behavioral Science
Washington, D.C.

OTHER COMMITTEES OF THE COMMISSION

Committee on Clinical Issues‡

JOSEPH D. NOSHPITZ, M.D., Chairman
HYMAN S. LIPPMAN, M.D.
DANE G. PRUGH, M.D.
EVEOLEEN N. REXFORD, M.D.

MEYER SONIS, M.D.
ROBERT L. STUBBLEFIELD, M.D.
REGINALD S. LOURIE, M.D., ex officio

Consultants to the Committee

RENA SHULMAN, M.S.W.
Assistant Director
Jewish Board of Guardians
New York, New York

MILTON F. SHORE, PH.D.
Mental Health Study Center
Adelphi, Maryland

JEROME SILVERMAN, M.D.
New York, New York

ZANWIL SPERBER, PH.D.
Chief Psychologist
Department of Child Psychiatry
Cedars-Sinai Medical Center
Los Angeles, California

Committee on Education

JOSEPH M. BOBBITT, PH.D., Chairman

MARTIN DEUTSCH, PH.D.
Department of Education
New York University
New York, New York

JAMES J. GALLAGHER, PH.D.
Associate Commissioner
Bureau of Education for the
Handicapped
U.S. Office of Education
Washington, D.C.

* Represents successive liaison designations.
† Mr. Sugarman is now Acting Chief of the Children's Bureau and Acting Director of the Office of Child Development.
‡ All members of the Board of Directors of the Commission.

NORRIS G. HARING, PH.D.
 College of Education
 University of Washington
 Seattle, Washington

*COMMISSIONER HAROLD HOWE
 U.S. Office of Education
 Washington, D.C.

PHILIP W. JACKSON, PH.D.
 School of Education
 University of Chicago
 Chicago, Illinois

JAMES JARRETT, PH.D.
 Associate Dean, School of Education
 University of California
 Berkeley, California

MORTIMER KREUTER, PH.D.
 Assistant Director for Special
 Educational Practices
 Center for Urban Education
 New York, New York

NADINE LAMBERT, PH.D.
 Division of Educational Psychology
 Department of Education
 University of California
 Berkeley, California

MELVIN ROMAN, PH.D.
 Lincoln Hospital
 Mental Health Services
 Bronx, New York

THOMAS A. SHELLHAMMER
 California State Department of
 Education
 Sacramento, California

ABRAHAM J. TANNENBAUM, PH.D.
 Teachers College
 Columbia University
 New York, New York

FRED WILHELMS, PH.D.
 National Association of Secondary
 School Principals
 National Education Association
 Washington, D.C.

* During his tenure as Commissioner.

Liaison Consultants

IRVING N. BERLIN, M.D.
 Board of Directors

MILLIE ALMY, PH.D.
 Task Force I

BARBARA BIBER, PH.D.
 Task Force II

MARY ENGEL, PH.D.
 Task Force II

WILLIAM C. KVARACEUS, PH.D.
 Task Force III

JOHN H. NIEMEYER
 Task Force VI

NIMH Liaison Representative:

ELI M. BOWER, ED.D.

Committee on Children of Minority Groups

JOE P. MALDONADO, A.C.S.W., Chairman
Board of Directors

INEZ CASIANO
 Social Science Adviser to the
 Secretary of Labor
 Office of Policy Planning and
 Research
 U.S. Department of Labor
 Washington, D.C.

PRICE M. COBBS, M.D.
 San Francisco, California

ADA DEER, M.S.W.
 Board of Directors

MRS. FRED R. HARRIS
 President
 Oklahomans for Indian Opportunity
 Washington, D.C.

PATRICIA LEO
Special Assistant for Intergroup Relations
American Public Health Association, Inc.
New York, New York

RUTH McKAY, PH.D.
Hillcrest Children's Center
Washington, D.C.

ALEX MERCURE
Home Education Livelihood Program
Albuquerque, New Mexico

DANIEL O'CONNELL, M.D.
Executive Secretary
National Committee on Indian Health
Association on American Indian Affairs
New York, New York

K. PATRICK OKURA
Board of Directors

CHESTER PIERCE, M.D.
Professor of Education and Psychiatry
Harvard University
Cambridge, Massachusetts

FREDERIC SOLOMON, M.D.
Assistant Professor of Psychiatry
Howard University
Washington, D.C.

PERCY H. STEELE, JR., A.C.S.W.
Board of Directors

WILLIAM WATERMAN
Director, Offenders Division
United Planning Organization
Washington, D.C.

NIMH Liaison Representatives*

JAMES P. COMER, M.D.
ALVIN GOINS, PH.D.

ROBERT DREW
Division of Indian Health
USPHS Liaison Representative

* Represents successive liaison designations.

Consultants to Committee on Children Minority Groups

IRVING JACOBY
Mental Health Film Board
New York, New York

ALBERTA JACOBY, M.P.H.
Mental Health Film Board
New York, New York

RUFUS MAYFIELD
Washington, D.C.

LEROY WASHINGTON
Washington, D.C.

Committee on Religion

V. REV. MSGR. ROBERT E. GALLAGHER*
Co-chairman, Board of Directors

RABBI I. FRED HOLLANDER
Co-chairman, Board of Directors

REVEREND LEO N. KISROW
Co-chairman, Board of Directors

BEVERLY BIRNS, M.D.
Department of Psychiatry
Albert Einstein College of Medicine
Bronx, New York
* Deceased.

LaDONNA BOGARDUS
Methodist Church Office
Nashville, Tennessee

HARVEY J. TOMPKINS, M.D.
  Chairman
  New York City Mental Health Board
  New York, New York

ISRAEL ZWERLING, M.D.
  Medical Director
  Bronx State Hospital
  Bronx, New York

Committee on Curriculum Development for Early Child Care

FRANC BALZER
  Office of Economic Opportunity
  Washington, D.C.

T. BERRY BRAZELTON, M.D.
  Department of Cognitive Studies
  Harvard University
  Cambridge, Massachusetts

CATHERINE CHILMAN, PHD.
  Social Rehabilitation Services
  Department of Health, Education, and
    Welfare
  Washington, D.C.

IRA GORDON, PH.D.
  College of Education
  University of Florida

DOROTHY HUNTINGTON, PH.D.,
  Committee Chairman
  Children's Hospital
  Washington, D.C.

IRVING LAZAR, PH.D.
  Kirschner Associates, Inc.
  Los Angeles, California

FRANK RAFFERTY, M.D.
  University of Maryland
  School of Medicine
  Baltimore, Maryland

SAM SILVERSTEIN, PH.D.
  Experimental Training Branch
  National Institute of Mental Health
  Chevy Chase, Maryland

JOSEPH STONE, PH.D.
  Department of Psychology
  Vassar College
  Poughkeepsie, New York

DAVID WEIKART, PH.D.
  Ypsilanti Public School
  Ypsilanti, Michigan

DAVID WICKENS, PH.D.
  Peabody College
  Nashville, Tennessee

ELAINE WICKENS
  Bank Street College
  New York, New York

YOUTH PANEL OF THE JOINT COMMISSION ON MENTAL HEALTH OF CHILDREN

Adult Advisers

LACY C. STREETER
  Project Adviser
  Community Action Training School of
    Compeers, Inc.
  Washington, D.C.

WILLIAM WATERMAN
  United Planning Organization
  Washington, D.C.

Panelists

LAWRENCE BRADFORD
Washington, D.C.

MARSHALL BROWN
Washington, D.C.

EDDIE W. GILREATH
Washington, D.C.

BARBARA E. McCOY
Washington, D.C.

MARIE E. POTTER
Washington, D.C.

RUZAILIA RAY
Brooklyn, New York

KENNETH RICHARDSON
Washington, D.C.

CLARENCE SIMON
Washington, D.C.

RONALD SINCLAIR
Washington, D.C.

VINCENT L. SMITH
Washington, D.C.

CARVIN SOLOMON
Washington, D.C.

GEORGE SPRIGGS
Washington, D.C.

DAVID WELLINGTON
Washington, D.C.

JULIUS WHELLER
Washington, D.C.

CLARENCE S. WILLIAMS
Washington, D.C.

STAFF OF THE COMMISSION

Executive and Technical Staff

JOSEPH M. BOBBITT, PH.D.
Executive Director

DOMINIC J. DERISO
Administrative Officer

CATHERINE S. CHILMAN, PH.D.
Senior Writer

ELIZABETH BOGAN, Executive Secretary
LORENA K. JONES, Secretary

BEATRICE H. GUSTAFSON, M.A.
Senior Research Associate

RITA A. PENNINGTON, M.A.
Research Associate

BARBARA SOWDER, M.A.
Research Associate

ELEANOR M. JORDAN, Bookkeeper
SHEILA M. KELLEHER, Receptionist
EVELYN J. WOODS, Secretary

Former Staff

EDWARD D. GREENWOOD, M.D.
Deputy Director

SIDNEY L. WERKMAN, M.D.
Deputy Director

ISRAEL GERVER
Senior Research Coordinator

RUTH M. BARTFELD, B.A.
Research Associate

CATHLEEN M. BLASKO

PAMALA M. BLOCHER

ROSLYN J. COHEN

ANNIE S. COPLAN, M.A.
Research Associate

STANLEY S. GOLDMAN, M.A.*
Research Associate

* Deceased.

FLORENCE S. JACOBSON, B.S.
  Research Associate

PEGGY LAMPL
  Information Officer

ANNETTE G. MOSHMAN, M.S.
  Librarian

FRANCES H. BUCHANAN

BERNICE S. GORDON

MARIA P. PEYSER

KAREN G. RICKER

JOHN SMITH

JAMES BETHEA

EUGENE D. DUGGER

ANN KELLEY

SHEP W. REIDINGER

RODNEY A. ROLLO

JOAN V. TODD

SPECIAL CONSULTANTS TO THE STAFF, JCMHC

JAMES G. KELLY, PH.D. (Program
  Consultant)
  Associate Professor
  Department of Psychology
  University of Michigan
  Ann Arbor, Michigan

WILLIAM RHODES, PH.D. (Program Con-
  sultant)
  Professor of Psychology
  University of Michigan
  Ann Arbor, Michigan

HERBERT H. FOCKLER, M.A., M.S.L.S.
  (Consultant for Library Services)
  National Library of Medicine
  Bethesda, Maryland

SAMUEL GREENHOUSE, PH.D. (Perinatal
  Studies)
  National Institute Child Health and
  Human Development
  National Institutes of Health
  Public Health Service
  Bethesda, Maryland

SOURCES OF FINANCIAL SUPPORT

Major Support from the National Institute of Mental Health
in the Form of a Research Grant

OTHER CONTRIBUTORS

Organizations:

    American Academy of Child Psychiatry
    American Academy of Pediatrics
    American Association for Children's Residential Centers
    American Association of Psychiatric Clinics for Children
    American Child Guidance Foundation
    American Medical Association
    American Nurses Association
    American Orthopsychiatric Association
    American Psychiatric Association
    The Grant Foundation, Inc.
    Milwaukee County Mental Health Association
    National Association for Mental Health
        (Maurice Falk Medical Fund)
    National Association for Retarded Children
    National Association of Social Workers
    National Foundation for Child Mental Welfare, Inc.
    Pittsburgh Child Guidance Center
    Rockefeller Brothers Fund
    Smith, Kline & French Laboratories

Individuals:

Dr. Viola Bernard
Dr. Joseph Bobbitt
Dr. Reginald Lourie
Charles Schlaifer, Esq.
Dr. Meyer Sonis
Mr. and Mrs. David J. Winton

APPENDIX

IV

CONTRACTORS OF THE JOINT COMMISSION ON MENTAL HEALTH OF CHILDREN AND AREAS OF PARTICIPATION

CONTRACTOR	PROJECT
RICHARD J. CLENDENEN National Council of State Committees for Children and Youth Minneapolis, Minnesota	Youth Participation Review
HENRY P. DAVID, PH.D. American Institute for Research Washington, D.C.	International Perspectives in Child Mental Health
JOSEPH P. FITZPATRICK, S.J. Institute for Social Research Fordham University New York City	Mental Health Needs of Spanish-Speaking Children
DONALD S. GAIR, M.D. DEXTER M. BULLARD, M.D. Massachusetts Mental Health Research Corporation Boston, Massachusetts	Psychiatric Problems in the First Five Years of Life: Review of the Literature
VICTOR GIOSCIA, PH.D. Jewish Family Service of New York New York, New York	Dimensions and Innovations in the Therapy of Children
JOHN C. GLIDEWELL, PH.D. MRS. CAROLYN S. SWALLOW University of Chicago Chicago, Illinois	Prevalence of Maladjustment in Elementary Schools

527

STEPHEN GOODMAN
CHARLES HALPERN
  Attorneys-at-Law
  Washington, D.C.

Judicial Review of the Treatment of
Juveniles

ZONA HOSTETLER
  Attorney-at-Law
  Washington, D.C.

Summary of State and Federal Legislation Affecting Mental Health of
Children

IRENE JOSSELYN, M.D.
  Phoenix, Arizona

Adolescence

SAMUEL Z. KLAUSNER, PH.D.
  University of Pennsylvania
  Philadelphia, Pennsylvania

Two Centuries of Child-Rearing
Manuals

JUDGE MARY CONWAY KOHLER, Director
  National Commission on Resources
    for Youth, Inc.
  New York, New York

Selected Youth Participation
Projects

IRVING LAZAR, PH.D.
  Kirschner Associates, Inc.
  Los Angeles, California

To Work With Infants. A Manual for
Trainers

DOROTHY H. MILLER, D.S.W.
  Social Psychiatry Research Associates
  San Francisco, California

An Overview of Mental Health Problems
of American Indian Children

JOSEPH D. NOSHPITZ, M.D.
  American Association of Children's
    Residential Centers
  Washington, D.C.

Residential Treatment Study

NORMAN POLANSKY, PH.D.
NANCY POLANSKY, R.N.
  University of Georgia
  Child Research Field Station
  Asheville, North Carolina

Status of Child Abuse and Child Neglect
in the U.S.

BERT N. REIN
  Attorney-at-Law
  Washington, D.C.

The Confidentiality of Children's Mental Health Records

HARRY SCHNIBBE
  National Association of State Mental
    Health Program Directors
  Washington, D.C.

Survey of State Services for Emotionally
Disturbed Children

DONALD A. SCHON, PH.D.
  Organization for Social and Technical
    Innovation
  Cambridge, Massachusetts

Organization of Children's Services
(Report of Task Force V)

RICHARD A. SEIDEN, PH.D.
  University of California
  Berkeley, California

Youthful Suicide

HARRY SILVERSTEIN
  New School for Social Research
  New York City

Some Themes Expressive of Alienated Youth

WILLIAM SOSKIN, PH.D.
  University of California
  Berkeley, California

Hippie: Bastard Son of the Beat Generation

VICTOR WEINGARTEN
  Victor Weingarten Company, Inc.
  New York, New York

Preparation of Chart Book and Popularized Version of Final Report

JOSEPH F. WHITING, PH.D.
  Division of Manpower Research and
    Development
  American Psychiatric Association
  Washington, D.C.

Community Functioning, Manpower Utilization and Impact Evaluation: Foundation Stones for the Delivery of Effective Child Mental Health Services

CHARLES WINICK, PH.D.
  City College of New York
  New York City

Impact of Mass Media upon Mental Health of Young People

APPENDIX

V

PAPERS PREPARED BY BOARD, TASK
FORCE, AND COMMITTEE MEMBERS, STAFF
SPECIAL CONSULTANTS TO STAFF, JOINT
CONFERENCES AND WORKSHOPS

RUTH D. ABBOTT, R.N.
Task Force I

Public Health Nurse Functions in Child Development Centers

Review of Research re Child and Maternal Health with Implications for Nursing

MILLIE ALMY, PH.D.
Task Force I

Priorities for the Three-to-Six-Year-Old

HERMAN S. BELMONT, M.D.
Task Force II

Common Denominators (of Mental Health Pertinent to Ages Five to Twelve)

Introductory Material Concerning the Area of Psychopathological Disorders in Childhood from Ages Five to Twelve

The Psychotherapies of the School-Age Child

BARBARA BIBER, PH.D.
Task Force II

Steps Essential for Implementing an Expanded Concept of the School's Responsibility for the Education of the Elementary School Child

Education and Mental Health in the Elementary School—Précis for Final Report

Developmental Characteristics in the Middle Years of Childhood

530

Recommendations for the Functioning of the Elementary School in the Interests of Positive Development During the Middle Years of Childhood

The School's Responsibility for the Mental Health of Children Ego Strength and Individuality

WILLIAM BOLMAN, M.D.
JACK WESTMAN, M.D.
Consultants, Task Force V

Planning Services for Mental Health of Children

JUNE CHARRY, PH.D.
Task Force III

Adolescence, Education, and Preventive Mental Health

What Do We Want from Education?

MARY ENGEL, PH.D.
Task Force II

Boys and Teachers—A Discussion of Certain Kind of Imbalance in Public Education

Ideologies and Financial Support in Clinical Child Psychology

CLAIRE M. FAGIN, PH.D.
Task Force II

Providing for Mental Health in Health Services for Children in the Six-to-Twelve Age Group

Outline of Developmental Tasks of the School-Age Child

The Nurse and the School-Age Child

RAYMOND FELDMAN, M.D.
Task Force IV

Present Status of the Clinical Field (Care and Treatment of Children)

CARL FENICHEL, ED.D.
Task Force IV

Rehabilitation of the Seriously Disturbed Child

JAMES J. GALLAGHER, PH.D.
Committee on Education

Mental Health Objectives for the School

PARK S. GERALD, M.D.
Task Force I

Preliminary Report on the Status of Genetics in Understanding Behavioral Problems

W. EUGENE GROVES
Task Force III

Testimony in Favor of the Eighteen-Year-Old Vote

NORRIS G. HARING, PH.D.
Committee on Education

Mental Health Objectives for Teacher Preparation

JEWELDEAN JONES, M.S.W.
Task Force IV

Presentation on Income Maintenance

Welfare Institutions and Their Role in Prevention

ALFRED J. KAHN, PH.D.
  Task Force V

Introduction to the Presentation Organization of Services

KENNETH KENISTON, PH.D.
  Task Force III

The Tasks of Adolescence

Dissent and Deviance in American College Students

LAWRENCE KOHLBERG, PH.D.
JEAN LACROSSE, PH.D.
  Task Force II

Predictability of Adult Mental Health from Childhood Behavior

WILLIAM C. KVARACEUS, PH.D.
  Task Force III

The Adolescent in School

The Disadvantaged Learner: Some Implications for Teachers and Teaching

Guiding the Adolescent in School

SEYMOUR L. LUSTMAN, PH.D., M.D.
  Task Force IV

Research: Issues in Basic and Applied Fields

JOE P. MALDONADO, A.C.S.W.
  Committee on Children of Minority Groups
  Task Force III

The Mental Health of Disadvantaged Adolescents and Young Adults

MORRIS F. MAYER, PH.D.
  Task Force III

The Adolescent in Placement

OTTO VON MERING, PH.D.
  Task Force IV

Needed: Mental Health Manpower Development and Training Patterns

Outline for JCMHC-WPIC Reports

Toward an Understanding of Manpower Pools, Their Training and Development in Relation to Populations with Different Mental Health Risks

Feedback on Joint Commission Priorities

Considerations Regarding Manpower Study (Memos 1, 2, 3)

Focal Concerns of Task Force IV

DOROTHY MILLER, D.S.W.
  Task Force IV

Rehabilitation of Mentally Ill Children: A Position Paper

American Indian Children: To Be or Not to Be

SALVADOR MINUCHIN, M.D.
  Task Force II

Treatment and Services for the Disturbed Child

<table>
<tr><td></td><td>The Slum Family and the Slum School Broadening the Unit of Intervention— The Delivery of Services According to an Ecological Model</td></tr>
<tr><td>DANIEL J. O'CONNELL, M.D.
Committee on Children of Minority Groups</td><td>Assimilation: A Threat to the American Indian</td></tr>
<tr><td>RICHMOND S. PAINE, M.D.
Task Force I</td><td>Organic Factors Affecting the Mental Health of Children</td></tr>
<tr><td>RITA PENNINGTON, M.A.
(JCMHC Staff)
Paper prepared for Task Force III</td><td>Mental Health Services as Related to the Lower-class Adolescent</td></tr>
<tr><td>NORMAN POLANSKY, PH.D.
Task Force I</td><td>The Apathy-Futility Syndrome in Child Neglect</td></tr>
<tr><td></td><td>Changing Concepts of Social Work Treatment of the Multi-Problem Client</td></tr>
<tr><td>OTTO POLLAK, PH.D.
Task Force IV</td><td>Mental Health Goals in Child Rearing and Child Care</td></tr>
<tr><td></td><td>Suggestions for Alleviating Manpower Shortages in the Child Mental Health Services</td></tr>
<tr><td></td><td>Position Paper on Elements of Mental Health in a Corporate Society</td></tr>
<tr><td>SALLY PROVENCE, M.D.
Task Force I</td><td>The First Three Years</td></tr>
<tr><td>DANE G. PRUGH, M.D.
Committee on Clinical Issues</td><td>Psychosocial Disorders in Childhood and Adolescence: Theoretical Considerations and an Attempt at Classification</td></tr>
<tr><td>FRANK T. RAFFERTY, M.D.
Task Force V</td><td>Preface Statements for Report of Task Force V</td></tr>
<tr><td></td><td>Systems Model for the Child-Care Industry</td></tr>
<tr><td>HALBERT B. ROBINSON, PH.D.
Task Force I</td><td>Need for More Comprehensive Programs for Children</td></tr>
<tr><td>HOWARD P. ROME, M.D.
Task Force V</td><td>The Problem of Nomenclature</td></tr>
<tr><td>VERA RUBIN, PH.D.
Task Force V</td><td>Family and Society—Implications for Social Action</td></tr>
<tr><td>LEON J. SAUL, M.D.
WILLIAM LUBOW, M.D.
Prepared for Task Force I</td><td>A Bibliography of 3500 Abstracted References to Recent Literature, Organized Around All Aspects of Childhood Emotional Relationships</td></tr>
</table>

MILTON F. SHORE, PH.D.
Committee on Clinical Issues

Statement on Racism

RENA S. SHULMAN, M.S.W.
Committee on Clinical Issues

Utilization of Paraprofessionals in Clinical Settings

FREDERIC SOLOMON, M.D.
Committee on Children of Minority Groups

On the Disabling Effects of Poverty upon Child Development

MEYER SONIS, M.D.
Committee on Clinical Issues

A Clinician's Overview

BARBARA J. SOWDER, M.A. (JCMHC Staff)
Paper prepared for Task Force III

The Question of Effective Treatment of Adolescents

BARBARA J. SOWDER, M.A. (JCMHC Staff)
Paper prepared for the Committee on Children of Minority Groups

The American Indians: Acculturation or Assimilation?

ABRAHAM J. TANNENBAUM, PH.D.
Committee on Education

Educational Innovation for Mental Health: Some Notes

JOSEPH F. WHITING, PH.D.
JAMES W. CARPER, PH.D.
RAYMOND FELDMAN, M.D.
(Consultants, Task Force IV)

Mental Health Services for the Community: Process, Requirements and Solutions

Needed: A Scientific Base for Manpower Utilization in Mental Health Services

MARTIN WOLINS, D.S.W.
MARY JANE OWEN
Task Force II

Foster Care Assumptions, Evidence and Alternatives: An Exploratory Analysis

NORMAN ZINBERG, M.D.
KENNETH KENISTON, PH.D.
Task Force III

Mental Health Services in American Colleges

NORMAN ZINBERG, M. D.
Task Force III

The Mirage of Mental Health

ALFRED D. BUCHMUELLER
Task Force IV

Preventive Services for Children

SEYMOUR L. LUSTMAN, PH.D.
Task Force IV

Mental Health Research and the University (A Position Paper to the Joint Commission on Mental Health of Children)

JOINT CONFERENCES AND WORKSHOPS

AMERICAN ACADEMY OF CHILD PSYCHIATRY— JCMHC, ANN ARBOR, MICHIGAN, OCTOBER, 1967

Workshop 1: *Infancy Through Age Five Years*
CALVIN F. SETTLAGE, M.D., Chairman
PETER B. NEUBAUER, M.D., Task Force I

Workshop 2: *School-Age Children*
MAURICE R. FRIEND, M.D., Chairman
HERMAN S. BELMONT, M.D., Task Force II

Workshop 3: *Adolescents and Youth*
EVEOLEEN N. REXFORD, M.D., Chairman
VIRGINIA CLOWER, M.D., Co-Chairman
NORMAN ZINBERG, M.D., Task Force III

Workshop 4: *Prevention, Rehabilitation, Manpower and Research*
PIERRE JOHANNET, M.D., Chairman
SEYMOUR L. LUSTMAN, M.D., PH.D, Task Force IV

Workshop 5: *Organization, Administration and Planning of Services*
OTHILDA KRUG, M.D., Chairman
ALBERT SOLNIT, M.D., Task Force V

Workshop 6: *Innovative Approaches to Social Progress*
GASTON BLOM, M.D., Chairman
ROBERT LEON, M.D., Task Force VI

JOINT CONFERENCE ON CHILDHOOD MENTAL ILLNESS, THE NATIONAL ASSOCIATION FOR MENTAL HEALTH, INC., AND THE JOINT COMMISSION ON MENTAL HEALTH OF CHILDREN, INC.

Work Group I—Education and Rehabilitation

CARL FENICHEL, ED.D., Chairman
Director, League School for Seriously
Disturbed Children
Brooklyn, New York

WILLIAM WATTENBERG, PH.D.,
Co-chairman
Assistant Superintendent
Detroit Public Schools
Detroit, Michigan

BERTRAM BLACK, Co-chairman
Altro Health and Rehabilitative
Services, Inc.
New York, New York

MRS. CELIA BENNEY, Co-chairman
Altro Health and Rehabilitative
Services, Inc.
New York, New York

STONEWALL B. STICKNEY, M.D., Recorder
  Director, Division of Mental Health
    Services
  Pittsburgh Public Schools
  Pittsburgh, Pennsylvania

THOMAS-ROBERT AMES
  Young Adult Institute
  New York, New York

ELI BOWER, ED.D.
  National Institute for Mental Health
  Chevy Chase, Maryland

HELMAR MYKLEBUST, PH.D.
  Northwestern University
  Evanston, Illinois

JAMES TOMPKINS
  Bureau of Education for the
    Handicapped
  Department of Health, Education, and
    Welfare
  Office of Education
  Washington, D.C.

ARNOLD VETSTEIN
  League School of Boston for Seriously
    Disturbed Children
  Newton Centre, Massachusetts

Work Group II—Residential and Institutional Centers

RALPH RABINOVITCH, M.D., Chairman
  Hawthorn Center
  Northville, Michigan

BARBARA FISH, M.D., Recorder
  Psychiatrist-in-Charge
  Children's and Adolescent Services
  Bellevue Hospital
  New York, New York

HERBERT BIRCH, M.D., PH.D.
  Research Professor
  Albert Einstein College of Medicine
  Yeshiva University
  Bronx, New York

MARIAN DEMYER, M.D.
  Larue D. Carter Memorial Hospital
  Indianapolis, Indiana

DAVID M. ENGELHARDT, M.D.
  Downstate Medical Center
  Brooklyn, New York

CHARLES FERSTER, PH.D.
  Professor of Psychology
  Department of Psychology
  Georgetown University
  Washington, D.C.

MAURICE W. LAUFER, M.D.
  Director
  Emma Pendleton Bradley Hospital
  Riverside, Rhode Island

CARLO PIETZNER
  Camphill Village U.S.A., Inc.
  Copake, New York

JAMES Q. SIMMONS 3RD, M.D.
  Chief, Children's Inpatient Services
  Neuropsychiatric Institute, UCLA
  Los Angeles, California

Work Group III—Comprehensive Community Planning and Implementing

HAROLD M. VISOTSKY, M.D.
  Chairman, Department of Psychiatry
  Northwestern University
  Chicago, Illinois

MICHAEL FREELUND, Recorder
  National Association for Mental
    Health
  New York, New York

HARVEY J. TOMPKINS, M.D.
  Reiss Mental Health Pavilion
  St. Vincent's Hospital
  New York, New York

MILDRED MITCHELL-BATEMAN, M.D.
  Director, West Virginia Department
    of Mental Health
  Charleston, West Virginia

WILLIAM BEACH, JR., M.D.
Department of Mental Hygiene
Sacramento, California

MRS. ROBERT M. BLUM
New York, New York

MORTON KRAMER, PH.D.
Office of Biometry
National Institute of Mental Health
Chevy Chase, Maryland

MRS. WINTHROP ROCKEFELLER
Little Rock, Arkansas

MARK TARAIL, M.D.
Administrator
Maimonides Mental Health Center
Brooklyn, New York

Work Group IV—Community-Based Partial Hospitalization and Transitional Services

JAMES F. KIPFER, Chairman
Michigan Society for Mental Health,
Inc.
Detroit, Michigan

EDWARD D. GREENWOOD, M.D.,
Recorder
The Menninger Clinic
Topeka, Kansas

ALANSON HINMAN, M.D.
Department of Pediatrics
Bowman Gray School of Medicine
Winston-Salem, North Carolina

NORMAN LOURIE, A.C.S.W.
Executive Deputy Secretary
Pennsylvania Department of Public
Welfare
Harrisburg, Pennsylvania

DANE G. PRUGH, M.D.
Chief, Child Psychiatry Division
University of Colorado Mental Center
Denver, Colorado

ELI RUBIN, PH.D.
Lafayette Clinic
Detroit, Michigan

MRS. RUTH CHRIST SULLIVAN
President, Capital District Chapter
National Society for Autistic Children
Voorheesville, New York

Work Group V—Manpower and Training

WILLIAM C. MORSE, PH.D., Chairman
The University of Michigan
School of Education
Ann Arbor, Michigan

MRS. DAVID PARK, Recorder
Williamstown, Massachusetts

EVERETT BUSBY
Bedford-Stuyvesant Youth in Action
Corp.
Brooklyn, New York

MIKE GORMAN
Executive Director
National Committee Against Mental
Illness
Washington, D.C.

REGINALD S. LOURIE, M.D.
Director, Department of Psychiatry
Children's Hospital
Hillcrest Children's Center
Washington, D.C.

SUMNER ROSEN, PH.D.
New Careers Development Center
New York University
New York, New York

ROBERT L. STUBBLEFIELD, M.D.
Chairman, Department of Psychiatry
University of Texas
Southwestern Medical School
Dallas, Texas

LAWRENCE TAFT, M.D.
  Chief, Pediatric Neurology
  Albert Einstein College of Medicine
  Yeshiva University
  Bronx, New York

JOSEPH F. WHITING, PH.D.
  American Psychiatric Association
  Washington, D.C.

At-Large Group

GEORGE TARJAN, M.D., Conference
  Chairman
  Program Director, Mental Retardation
  The Neuropsychiatric Institute
  Los Angeles, California

NICHOLAS HOBBS, PH.D., Conference
  Co-chairman
  Director, John F. Kennedy Center for
  Research on Education and Human
  Development
  Peabody College, Nashville, Tennessee

HENRY WORK, M.D., Special Consultant
  Department of Psychiatry
  UCLA School of Medicine
  Neuropsychiatric Institute
  Los Angeles, California

JOSEPH M. BOBBITT, PH.D.
  Executive Director
  Joint Commission on Mental Health
  of Children
  Chevy Chase, Maryland

MRS. JAMES FINN
  Staff Member, National Association
  for Mental Health
  New York, New York

MRS. JOSEPH MANDELBAUM
  Chairman, Advisory Council on
  Childhood Mental Illness
  National Association for Mental
  Health
  New York, New York

SIDNEY L. WERKMAN, M.D.
  Deputy Director
  Joint Commission on Mental Health
  of Children
  Chevy Chase, Maryland

CHILDREN IN THE 1970'S—NEW APPROACHES TO THEIR MENTAL HEALTH AMERICAN MEDICAL ASSOCIATION, COUNCIL ON MENTAL HEALTH

MARCH 14–15, 1969, CHICAGO, ILLINOIS *

Workshop Chairmen, Residents, Resource Persons

I. *New Knowledge of Child Development: Basis for Mental Health*
  PETER B. NEUBAUER, M.D. (Chairman)
    Director
    Child Development Center
    New York

* At these sessions, a preliminary report of the findings and the recommendations of the Commission was presented. Planning of the conference was done in consultation with the officers and staff of the Commission.

BERTRAND CRAMER, M.D. (Resident)
Child Development Center
New York

JULIUS B. RICHMOND, M.D. (Resource)

II. *Action Necessary to Insure Optimal Development*
IRVING N. BERLIN, M.D. (Chairman)
Professor of Psychiatry and Pediatrics
University of Washington
Seattle

MURIEL KING, M.D. (Resident)
Division of Child Psychiatry
University of Washington
Seattle

JOHN L. OTTO, M.D. (Resource)

III. *Diagnosis and Treatment: Clinical Issues*
MEYER SONIS, M.D. (Chairman)
Chief, Child Psychiatry
Department of Psychiatry
University of Pittsburgh
Western Psychiatric Institute and Clinic

GEORGE ZITNER, M.D. (Resident)
Western Psychiatric Institute and Clinic
Pittsburgh

JOHN DONNELLY, M.D. (Resource)

IV. *Community Services in Treatment*
GEORGE TARJAN, M.D. (Chairman)
Professor of Psychiatry
UCLA Center for the Health Sciences
The Neuropsychiatric Institute

GLORIA POWELL, M.D. (Resident)
The Neuropsychiatric Institute
Los Angeles

V. *Manpower: Nature and Training*
HAROLD VISOTSKY, M.D.
Chairman, Department of Psychiatry
Northwestern University
Chicago, Illinois

FRANK BOWERS, M.D. (Resident)
Mayo Clinic
Rochester

HOWARD P. ROME, M.D. (Resource)

VI. *Evaluative Research*
SEYMOUR L. LUSTMAN, M.D. (Chairman)
Professor of Psychiatry
Yale University Child Study Center

JOSEPH JANKOWSKI, M.D. (Resident)
Yale University Child Study Center
New Haven

WALTER E. BARTON, M.D. (Resource)

VII. *The Effects of Racism*
CHESTER M. PIERCE, M.D. (Chairman)
Professor of Psychiatry
University of Oklahoma
Oklahoma City

HELENA E. WEBB, B.A. (Resident)
Graduate Student in Education
Harvard Graduate School of Education
Cambridge

HERBERT C. MODLIN, M.D. (Resource)

VIII. *The Effects of a Changing Society*
DANA L. FARNSWORTH, M.D. (Chairman)
Director, University Health Services
Harvard University
Cambridge

ROBERT SHARPLEY, M.D. (Resident)
Assistant Psychiatrist to University Health Services and Teaching Fellow
Harvard University
Cambridge

H. THOMAS MCGUIRE, M.D. (Resource)

Conference Panel Members

LLOYD C. ELAM, M.D.
(Panel Moderator)
President
Meharry Medical College
Nashville, Tennessee

IRVING N. BERLIN, M.D.
Professor of Psychiatry and Pediatrics
University of Washington School of
Medicine
Seattle, Washington

JOSEPH M. BOBBITT, PH.D.
Executive Director
Joint Commission on Mental Health
of Children
Chevy Chase, Maryland

DANA L. FARNSWORTH, M.D.
Director
University Health Services
Harvard University
Cambridge, Massachusetts

REGINALD S. LOURIE, M.D.
Director
Department of Psychiatry
Children's Hospital
Washington, D.C.

DANE G. PRUGH, M.D.
Professor of Psychiatry and Pediatrics
University of Colorado Medical Center
Denver, Colorado

JULIUS B. RICHMOND, M.D.
Dean, Upstate Medical Center
State University of New York
Syracuse, New York

APPENDIX
VI

REFERENCES

I. INTRODUCTION AND RECOMMENDATIONS

AMERICAN COLLEGE OF NURSE MIDWIFERY, 1968.

CHAMBER OF COMMERCE OF THE UNITED STATES, Task Force on Economic Growth and Opportunity. "The Disadvantaged Poor: Education and Employment." Third Report, 1966.

GENERAL REPORT OF THE ADVISORY COUNCIL ON VOCATIONAL EDUCATION. "The Bridge Between Man and His Work," (Publication 1.) Department of Health, Education, and Welfare, Office of Education, 1968.

GIOSCIA, V., RABKIN, R., SPECK, R., et al. Dimensions and Innovations in the Therapy of Children. (A report of the Research Department of Jewish Family Service of New York to Task Force IV of the Joint Commission on Mental Health of Children, Inc.) 1968. (Mimeo.)

Hunger, U.S.A. (A Report by the Citizens' Board of Inquiry into Hunger and Malnutrition in the United States.) Washington, D.C.: New Community Press, 1968.

HUNT, J. McV. A Bill of Rights for Children. (Draft paper prepared for the Group on Early Child Development, 1960 White House Conference on Children and Youth.) 1966. (Mimeo.)

"A Look at Problems in Prenatal Service Programs." Currents in Public Health 5, 1–4 (May, 1966).

MAYER, M., AND GOLDSMITH, J. "The Child Care Worker in Residential Treatment," in A Residential Treatment Study. (Report by the American Association of Children's Residential Centers for the Joint Commission on Mental Health of Children, Inc.) 1968. (Mimeo.)

NATIONAL ASSOCIATION FOR MENTAL HEALTH. "A Comprehensive Program for the Severely Mentally Ill Child and His Family." (10 Columbus Circle, New York, N.Y. 10019) 1968.

NATIONAL LEAGUE FOR NURSING. "Masters Education, 1967." New York: National League for Nursing, 1967.

————. "Some Statistics on Baccalaureate and Higher Degree Programs in Nursing, 1966." New York: National League for Nursing, 1966.

PRESIDENT'S COMMISSION ON LAW ENFORCEMENT AND ADMINISTRATION OF JUSTICE. Task Force Report: Juvenile Delinquency and Youth Crime. Washington, D.C.: Government Printing Office, 1967.

U.S. Department of Health, Education, and Welfare. *Program Analysis: Maternal and Child Care Programs.* October, 1966.
————. Welfare Administration, Children's Bureau. "Adoptions in 1965. Child Welfare Statistics—1965." (*Children's Bureau Statistical Series* No. 84.) Washington, D.C., 1966b.
U.S. House of Representatives, Subcommittee on the War on Poverty Program. Hearings held in Washington, D.C., April 12, 13, 14, 15, and 30, 1965.
U.S. Senate, Subcommittee on Education of the Committee on Labor and Public Welfare. *Notes and Working Papers Concerning the Administration of Programs Authorized Under Title VI of Public Law 89-10, Elementary and Secondary Education Act, as Amended—Education of Handicapped Children.* (90th Congress, 2d Sess., May, 1968.) Washington, D.C.: Government Printing Office, 1968, pp. 2–3.
————. Subcommittee on Employment, Manpower, and Poverty of the Committee on Labor and Public Welfare. *Hunger and Malnutrition in America.* (90th Congress, 1st Sess. on Hunger and Malnutrition in America, July 11 and 12, 1967.) Washington, D.C.: Government Printing Office, 1967.

OTHER SOURCES

Many of the Commission's recommendations were taken from the reports of its various task forces and committees which are listed in Appendix II.

II. CONTEMPORARY AMERICAN SOCIETY: ITS IMPACT ON THE MENTAL HEALTH OF CHILDREN AND YOUTH

Campbell, A. "Population Dynamics and Family Planning," *Journal of Marriage and the Family,* 30 (May, 1968), 202–6.
Cavan, R. "Subcultural Variations and Mobility," in *Handbook of Marriage and the Family,* H. Christensen (ed.). Chicago: Rand McNally, 1964, pp. 535–58.
Chilman, C. *Growing Up Poor.* U.S. Department of Health, Education, and Welfare. Washington, D.C.: Government Printing Office, 1966.
Freedman, R., and Combs, L. "Childspacing and Family Economic Position." Ann Arbor: University of Michigan, Populations Studies Center, 1967. (Mimeo.)
Gans, H. *The Urban Villagers.* New York: The Free Press of Glencoe, 1962, Chap. 11.
Glick, P. "Demographic Analysis of Family Data," in *Handbook of Marriage and the Family,* H. Christensen (ed.). Chicago: Rand McNally, 1964, pp. 300–34.
Glidewell, J., and Swallow, C. *The Prevalence of Maladjustment in Elementary Schools.* (A report prepared for the Joint Commission on Mental Health of Children, Inc.) Chicago: University of Chicago, July 26, 1968.
Herzog, E. "Some Assumptions About the Poor," *Social Service Review,* XXXVII, 4 (December, 1963).
Hollingshead, A., and Redlich, F., *Social Class and Mental Illness: A Community Study.* New York: Wiley & Son, 1958.

KOHN, M. "Social Class and the Exercise of Parental Authority," *American Social Review,* XXIV (1959), 352–66.

KOMAROVSKY, M. *Blue Collar Marriage.* New York: Random House, 1964.

LEWIS, O. *Children of Sanchez.* New York: Random House, 1961.

MILLER, S. M., AND REIN, M. "Poverty and Social Change," *American Child,* National Committee on Employment of Youth (March, 1964).

MILLER, S. M., AND RIESSMAN, F. "The Working Class Subculture: A New View," *Social Problems,* No. 9 (Summer, 1961), 86–97.

MINUCHIN, S., *et al. Families of the Slums.* N.Y.: Basic Books, Inc., 1967.

PAVENSTEDT, E. "A Comparison of the Child-Rearing Environment of Upper-Lower and Very Low Lower-Class Families," *American Journal of Orthopsychiatry,* 35 (January, 1965), 89–98.

RAINWATER, L., AND WEINSTEIN, K. *And the Poor Get Children.* Chicago: Quadrangle Books, 1960.

Report of Task Force I. Joint Commission on Mental Health of Children, Inc. 1968. (Mimeo.)

Report of Task Force III. "The World of Adolescence and Youth." Joint Commission on Mental Health of Children, Inc. 1968. (Mimeo.)

Report of Task Force V. Joint Commission on Mental Health of Children, Inc. 1968. (Mimeo.)

Report of Task Force VI. Joint Commission on Mental Health of Children, Inc. 1968. (Mimeo.)

RIESSMAN, F. *The Culturally Deprived Child.* New York: Harper and Bros., 1962.

RODMAN, H. "The Lower-Class Value Stretch," in *Poverty in America—A Book of Readings.* L. Ferman, J. Kornbluh, and A. Haber (eds.). Ann Arbor: University of Michigan Press, 1965, pp. 270–85.

SEWELL, W., AND HALLER, A. "Social Status and the Personality Adjustment of the Child," *American Social Review,* XXIV (1959), 511–20.

U.S. DEPARTMENT OF AGRICULTURE. *Age of Transition: Rural Youth in Changing Society.* Economic Research Service. (Handbook 347). Washington, D.C.: Government Printing Office, 1967.

U.S. BUREAU OF THE CENSUS. Personal communication. July, 1967.

U.S. DEPARTMENT OF HEALTH, EDUCATION, AND WELFARE. "V.D. Fact Sheet." 1967.

———, Public Health Service, National Center for Health Statistics. *Vital Statistics of the United States.* (Ser. 21, No. 15.) February, 1968.

III. CONTEMPORARY AMERICAN SOCIETY: ITS IMPACT ON FAMILY LIFE

CLAUSEN, J. "Family Structure, Socialization and Personality," in *Review of Child Development Research,* II, H. M. Hoffman and L. Hoffman (eds.). New York: Russell Sage Foundation, 1966.

DOUVAN, E., AND ADELSON, J. *The Adolescent Experience.* New York: John Wiley and Sons, 1966.

DUNCAN, O., AND BLAU, P. *The American Occupational Structure.* New York: John Wiley and Sons, 1967.

FELDMAN, H. *Development of the Husband-Wife Relationship.* Ithaca, N.Y.: Cornell University Press, 1965.

HERZOG, E. *Children of Working Mothers.* Washington, D.C.: Government Printing Office, 1960.

HERZOG, E., AND SUDIA, C. "Fatherless Homes: A Review of Research," *Children,* XV, 5 (September–October, 1968).

HILL, R., AND RODGERS, R. "The Developmental Approach," in *Handbook of Marriage and the Family,* H. Christensen (ed.). Chicago: Rand McNally, 1964.

HOFFMAN, L. "Effects of Maternal Employment and the Child," *Child Development,* 32 (1961), 187–97.

MOORE, B., AND HOLTZMAN, W. *Tomorrow's Children.* Austin: University of Texas, 1965.

Report of Task Force I. Joint Commission on Mental Health of Children, Inc. 1968. (Mimeo.)

Report of Task Force II. "The Mental Health of the School-Age Child." Joint Commission on Mental Health of Children, Inc., 1969. (Mimeo.)

Report of Task Force V. Joint Commission on Mental Health of Children, Inc. 1968. (Mimeo.)

Report of Task Force VI. Joint Commission on Mental Health of Children, Inc. 1968. (Mimeo.)

STOLZ, L. *Influences on Parent Behavior.* Stanford, Calif.: Stanford University Press, 1967.

SUSSMAN, M., AND BURCHINAL, L. "Kin Family Network," *Marriage and Family Living,* No. 24 (1962).

U.S. BUREAU OF THE CENSUS. *Population Characteristics.* (Ser. P-20, No. 170.) "Marital Status and Family Status: March 1967." (February 23, 1968a.)
———. *Population Characteristics.* (Ser. P-20, No. 171.) "Mobility of the Population of the United States: March 1966 to March 1967." (April 30, 1968b.)
———. *Population Estimates.* (Ser. P-25, No. 398.) "Estimates of the Population of the United States and Components of Change: 1940–1968." (July 31, 1968c.)

VINCENT, C. "Mental Health and the Family," *Journal of Marriage and the Family,* XXXIX (1967), 18–39.

WHELPTON, P., CAMPBELL, A., AND PATTERSON, J. *Fertility and Family Planning in the United States.* Princeton, N.J.: Princeton University Press, 1966.

WOMEN'S BUREAU, U.S. DEPARTMENT OF LABOR. "Background Facts on Women Workers in the United States." May, 1967.
———. "Who Are the Working Mothers?" (Leaflet 37.) 1968.

IV. POVERTY AND MENTAL HEALTH

ASSOCIATION ON AMERICAN INDIAN AFFAIRS. Circular. 1968.

BEISER, M. "Poverty, Social Disintegration and Personality," *Journal of Social Issues,* 21, 1 (January 1965), 56–78.

BLAU, P., AND DUNCAN, D. *The American Occupational Structure.* New York: John Wiley & Sons, Inc., 1967.

BRONFENBRENNER, U. "Damping the Unemployability Explosions," *Saturday Review* (January 4, 1969), pp. 108–10.

CAMPBELL, A. "The Role of Family Planning in the Reduction of Poverty," *Journal of Marriage and the Family,* 30, 2 (May, 1968), 236–45.

CARTER, G. "Employment Potential of AFDC Mothers," *Welfare in Review* (July–August, 1968), pp. 1–11.

CHILMAN, C. *Growing Up Poor.* U.S. Department of Health, Education, and Welfare. Washington, D.C.: Government Printing Office, 1966.

DEUTSCH, M. "The Disadvantaged Child and the Learning Process," in *Education in Depressed Areas,* A. Passow (ed.). New York: Bureau of Publications, Teachers College, Columbia University, 1963, pp. 163–79.

FITZPATRICK, J., *et al. Mental Health Needs of Spanish-Speaking Children in the New York City Area.* (A report prepared for Task Force IV, the Joint Commission on Mental Health of Children, Inc.) 1968. (Mimeo.)

GIL, D. "Mother's Wages: One Way to Attack Poverty," *Social Issues Outlook,* 4, 4 (April, 1969).

GLICK, P. "Demographic Analysis of Family Data," in *Handbook of Marriage and the Family,* H. Christensen (ed.). Chicago: Rand McNally, 1964.

GLIDEWELL, J., AND SWALLOW, C. *The Prevalence of Maladjustment in Elementary Schools.* (A report prepared for the Joint Commission on Mental Health of Children, Inc.) Chicago: University of Chicago, July 26, 1968.

GOLENPAUL, D. (ed). *Information Please Almanac Atlas and Yearbook, 1967.* 21st ed. New York: Simon and Schuster, 1966, p. 597.

HARRINGTON, M. "The Technological Revolution: Human and Social Ecology." (Paper presented to the opening general session of the 23rd National Conference on Higher Education, sponsored by the American Association for Higher Education, Chicago, March 3, 1968.) (Mimeo.)

Health Care and the Negro Population. National Urban League, Inc., 1965.

HERZOG, E., AND SUDIA, C. "Fatherless Homes: A Review of Research," *Children,* XV, 5 (September–October, 1968), pp. 178–82.

HOLLINGSHEAD, A., AND REDLICH, F. *Social Class and Mental Illness: A Community Study.* New York: Wiley, 1958.

IRELAN, L. (ed.) *Low Income Life Styles.* U.S. Department of Health, Education, and Welfare. Washington, D.C.: Government Printing Office, 1966.

JAFFE, F., AND POLGAR, S. "Family Planning and Public Policy," *Journal of Marriage and the Family,* 30, 2 (May, 1968), 228–35.

KELLAM, S., AND SCHIFF, S. "Adaptation and Mental Illness in the First-Grade Classrooms of an Urban Community," *Psychiatric Research Report 21,* American Psychiatric Association (April, 1967), pp. 79–91.

KOMAROVSKY, M. *Blue Collar Marriage.* New York: Random House, 1964.

LANGNER, T., *et al.* "A Survey of Psychiatric Impairment in Urban Children." Unpublished manuscript. 1967.

LEIGHTON, A. Prepared statement of Alexander H. Leighton, M.D., Head, Department of Behavioral Sciences, Harvard School of Public Health. *Human Resources Development.* Hearings before the Subcommittee on Government Research of the Committee on Government Operations, United States Senate (90th Congress, 2nd Sess.). Deprivation and Personality—A New Challenge to Human Resources Development. Part 2. April 23–24, 1968. Washington, D.C.: Government Printing Office, 1968.

MALONE, C. "Safety First: Comments on the Influence of External Danger in the Lives of Disorganized Families," *American Journal of Orthopsychiatry,* 36, 1 (1966), 3–12.

———. "Some Observations on Children of Disorganized Families and Problems of Acting Out," *Journal of Child Psychiatry,* 2 (1963), 22–49.

MARRIS, P., AND REIN, M. *Dilemmas of Social Reform.* New York: Atherton Press, 1967.

MINUCHIN, S., MONTALVO, B., GUERNEY, B., *et al. Families of the Slums: An Exploration of Their Structure and Treatment.* New York: Basic Books, 1967.

NATIONAL COMMITTEE AGAINST MENTAL ILLNESS, INC. *What Are the Facts About Mental Illness in the United States?* Washington, D.C.: Government Printing Office, 1966.

O'DONNELL, E., AND CHILMAN, C. "Participation of the Poor on Public Welfare Boards." *Welfare in Review* (July–August, 1969).

PAVENSTEDT, E. "A Comparison of the Child-Rearing Environment of Upper-Lower and Very Low Lower-Class Families." *American Journal of Orthopsychiatry,* 35 (January, 1965), 89–98.

PCMR Message. "The Retarded Victims of Deprivation. (An address by Whitney M. Young, Jr., Executive Director, National Urban League, to the 18th Annual Convention of the National Association for Retarded Children, Portland, Oregon, October 19, 1967.) Washington, D.C.: The President's Committee on Mental Retardation, January, 1968.

RAINWATER, L. "Crucible of Identity and the Negro Lower Class Family," in *The Negro American,* T. Parsons and K. Clark (eds.). Boston: Beacon Press, 1967.

Report of the National Advisory Committee on Civil Disorders. New York: Bantam Books, 1968.

U.S. BUREAU OF THE CENSUS. *Current Population Reports,* "Income in 1966 of Families and Persons in the United States." (Ser. P-60, No. 53.) Washington, D.C.: Government Printing Office, 1967, p. 28.

———. *Current Population Reports, Population Characteristics,* "School Enrollments, October, 1964." (Ser. P-20, No. 148.) Washington, D.C.: Government Printing Office, February 8, 1966a.

———. *Vital and Health Statistics,* "Characteristics of Patients of Selected Types of Medical Specialists and Practitioners. United States, July 1963–June 1964." National Center for Health Statistics. (Ser. 10, No. 28.) May, 1966b.

U.S. DEPARTMENT OF AGRICULTURE. *Age of Transition: Rural Youth in Changing Society.* Economic Research Service. (Handbook 347.) Washington, D.C.: Government Printing Office, 1967.

———. *Family Economics Review,* 1968.

U.S. DEPARTMENT OF LABOR. *News,* "City Worker's Family Budget for a Moderate Living Standard." (USDL-8478.) Washington, D.C.: Bureau of Labor Statistics, October 25, 1968.

U.S. HOUSE OF REPRESENTATIVES. Subcommittee on the War on Poverty Program. Hearings held in Washington, D.C., April 12, 13, 14, 15, and 30, 1965.

The Welfare and Child Health Provisions of the Social Security Amendments of 1967 (PL 90–248), "Legislative History and Summary," *Welfare in Review* (May–June, 1968). (Reprints available from Division of Intramural Research, Social and Rehabilitative Service, U.S. Department of Health, Education, and Welfare, Washington, D.C.)

WHELPTON, P., CAMPBELL, A., AND PATTERSON, J. *Fertility and Family Planning in the United States.* Princeton, N.J.: Princeton University Press, 1966.

V. CHILDREN OF MINORITY GROUPS: A SPECIAL MENTAL
HEALTH RISK

ABLON, J., ROSENTHAL, A., AND MILLER, D. "An Overview of the Mental Health Problems of Indian Children." (Prepared for Joint Commission on Mental Health of Children, Inc.) 1967. (Mimeo., 88 pp.)

BAGDIKIAN, B. "It Has Come to This." *The Saturday Evening Post* (August 10, 1968). Pp. 20–22; 80–83.

BAHN, A. "Methodological Study of Population of Out-Patient Psychiatric Clinics, Maryland, 1958–59." (*Public Health Monograph,* No. 65, Public Health Service Publication, No. 821.) Washington, D.C.: Government Printing Office, 1961.

BENNETT, F. "The Condition of Farm Workers and Small Farmers in 1967." (Report to the Board of Directors of the National Sharecroppers Fund.) (Mimeo.)

CHILMAN, C. *Growing Up Poor.* U.S. Department of Health, Education, and Welfare. Washington, D.C.: Government Printing Office, 1966.

CLARK, K. *Dark Ghetto: Dilemmas of Social Power.* New York: Harper & Row, 1965.

COLES, R. "Psychiatrists and the Poor," in *Poverty in the Affluent Society,* H. Meissner (ed.). New York: Harper & Row, 1966, pp. 181–90.

CONGER, J., AND MILLER, W. *Personality, Social Class, and Delinquency.* New York: John Wiley & Sons, 1966.

DAVID, M., *et al. Educational Achievement: Its Causes and Effects.* Ann Arbor: University of Michigan, Survey Research Center, 1961, p. 2.

ELLISON, R. "The Crisis of Optimism," in *The City in Crisis,* Ellison, Young, and Gans (eds.), with an Introduction by B. Rustin. New York: A. Philip Randolph Educational Fund, 1966, pp. 6–26.

FARB, P. "The American Indian—A Portrait in Limbo," *Saturday Review* (October 12, 1968), pp. 26–29.

FITZPATRICK, J., GOULD, R., FERNANDEZ, M., POLKA, J., *et al. Mental Health Needs of Spanish-Speaking Children in the New York City Area.* (A report prepared for Task Force IV, Joint Commission on Mental Health of Children, April 26, 1968.) (Mimeo., 158 pp.)

GARDNER, E., MILES, H., AND BAHN, A. "A Cumulative Survey of Psychiatric Experience in a Community: Report of the First Year's Experience," *Archives of General Psychiatry,* 9, 4 (1963), 369–78.

GROOTENBOER, E. "The Relation of Housing to Behavior Disorder," *American Journal of Psychiatry,* No. 119 (November, 1962), 469–72.

HEBER, R. "Research on Personality Disorders and Characteristics of the Mentally Retarded." *Mental Retardation Abstracts,* I. U.S. Department of Health, Education, and Welfare, 1964, pp. 304–25.

KENNEDY, W., *et al.* "A Normative Sample of Intelligence and Achievement of Negro Elementary School Children in the Southeastern United States," *Monographs of the Society for Research in Child Development,* 28, 6 (Ser. No. 90.), 1963.

LANGNER, T., *et al.* "A Survey of Psychiatric Impairment in Urban Children." Unpublished manuscript. 1967.

MCDERMOTT, J., *et al.* "Social Class and Mental Illness in Children: Observations of Blue Collar Families," *American Journal of Orthopsychiatry,* No. 35 (1965), 500–8.

MENTAL HEALTH DEVELOPMENT COMMISSION. "Mental Health Services for the Disadvantaged." Los Angeles: Welfare Planning Council, Los Angeles Region, 1967. (A position paper of the Committee on Mental Health Services for the Disadvantaged.)

MILLER, S. "The American Lower Class: A Typological Approach," *Social Research,* No. 31 (1964), 1–22.

MILLER, S. M., REIN, M., ROBY, P., AND GROSS, B. M. "Poverty, Inequality, and Conflict." *Social Goals and Indicators for American Society,* Vol. II, The Annals of the American Academy of Political and Social Science, Vol. 373, September, 1967. Pp. 16–52.

MOYNIHAN, D. *The Negro Family (The Case for National Action).* Washington, D.C.: Department of Labor, Office of Policy Planning and Research, 1965.

ORSHANSKY, M. "Who's Who Among the Poor: A Demographic View of Poverty." Washington, D.C.: Department of Health, Education, and Welfare, Social Security Administration, 1965.

PETERSON, J. "The Comparative Abilities of White and Negro Children," *Comparative Psychology Monographs.* No. 5 (1923), 1–141.

Report of the Committee on Minority Group Children. Joint Commission on Mental Health of Children, Inc., 1968. (Mimeo.)

Report of the National Advisory Commission on Civil Disorders. New York: Bantam Books, 1968.

ROSEN, B., BAHN, A., AND KRAMER, M. "Demographic and Diagnostic Characteristics of Psychiatric Clinic Outpatients in the U.S.A., 1961," *American Journal of Orthopsychiatry,* No. 34 (1964), 455–68.

ROSEN, B., KRAMER, M., REDICK, R., AND WILLNER, S. *Utilization of Psychiatric Facilities by Children: Current Status, Trends, Implications.* (Report prepared for Joint Commission on Mental Health of Children, Inc., 1968.) National Institute of Mental Health, Mental Health Statistics. (Ser. B, No. 1.) 1968.

SCHUEY, A. *The Testing of Negro Intelligence.* Lynchburg, Virginia: Bell, 1958.

SEXTON, P. *Spanish Harlem: Anatomy of Poverty.* New York: Harper & Row, 1965.

SIEGEL, E. "Migrant Families: Health Problems of Children," *Clinical Pediatrics,* No. 5 (1966), 635–40.

SOLOMON, FREDERIC. "On the Disabling Effects of Poverty upon Child Development." (Paper prepared for the Committee on Children of Minority Groups, The Joint Commission on Mental Health of Children, Inc.) 1968.

U.S. BUREAU OF THE CENSUS. *Current Population Reports.* (Ser. P-60, No. 53.) "Income in 1966 of Families and Persons in the United States." Washington, D.C.: Government Printing Office, 1967, p. 28.

———. *Current Population Reports, Population Characteristics.* (Ser. P-20, No. 148.) "School Enrollments, October, 1964." Washington, D.C.: Government Printing Office, February 8, 1966.

U.S. DEPARTMENT OF HEALTH, EDUCATION, AND WELFARE. "America's Children and Youth in Institutions: 1950–1960–1964." (Children's Bureau Publication, No. 435.) 1965.

U.S. SENATE, Subcommittee on Employment, Manpower, and Poverty of the Committee on Labor and Public Welfare. *Hunger and Malnutrition in America.* (90th Congress, 1st Sess. on Hunger and Malnutrition in America, July 11 and 12, 1967.) Washington, D.C.: Government Printing Office, 1967.

WERKMAN, S., SHIFMAN, L., AND SKELLY, T. "Psychosocial Correlates of Iron Deficiency Anemia in Early Childhood," *Psychosomatic Medicine*, No. 26 (1964), 125–34.

YAMAMOTO, J., QUINTON, C., BLOOMBAUM, M., AND HATTEM, J. "Racial Factors in Patient Selection," *American Journal of Psychiatry*, 124, 5 (1967), 84–90.

VI. EMOTIONALLY DISTURBED AND MENTALLY ILL CHILDREN AND YOUTH

ACKERMAN, N. *Treating the Troubled Family*. New York: Basic Books, 1966.

AMERICAN ASSOCIATION OF PSYCHIATRIC CLINICS FOR CHILDREN. *Children and Clinics*. (Survey conducted for the Joint Commission on Mental Health of Children, Inc., 1966.) American Association of Psychiatric Clinics for Children, June, 1968.

AMERICAN PSYCHIATRIC ASSOCIATION. *Planning Psychiatric Services for Children in the Community Mental Health Program*. Washington, D.C., American Psychiatric Association, 1964.

ANTONOSKY, H. "A Contribution to Research in the Area of the Mother-Child Relationship," *Child Development*, No. 30 (1959), 37–51.

ASHBY, W. *An Introduction to Cybernetics*. New York: Wiley & Sons, 1956.

BALDWIN, A. "Socialization and the Parent-Child Relationship," *Child Development*, No. 19 (1948), 127–36.

BALDWIN, A., KALHORN, J., AND BREESE, F. "Patterns of Parent Behavior," *Psychological Monographs*, No. 48 (1945), p. 3.

BATESON, G. "A Note on the Double-Bind," *Family Process*, 2, 154 (1962).

BAUM, O., et al. "Psychotherapy Dropouts and Lower Socioeconomic Patients," *American Journal of Orthopsychiatry*, 36, 629 (1966).

BLOCK, J., PATTERSON, V., BLOCK, J., AND JACKSON, D. "A Study of the Parents of Neurotic and Schizophrenic Children," *Psychiatry*, No. 21 (1958), 387–97.

BRONFENBRENNER, U. "Toward a Theoretical Analysis of Parent-Child Relationships in a Social Context," in *Parental Attitudes and Child Behavior*, J. Glidewell (ed.). Springfield, Illinois: Charles C. Thomas, Inc., 1961.

CALDWELL, B. "The Effects of Infant Care," in *Review of Child Development Research*, I, M. Hoffman and L. Hoffman (eds). New York: Russell Sage Foundation, 1964.

CHILMAN, C. *Growing Up Poor*. U.S. Department of Health, Education, and Welfare. Washington, D.C.: Government Printing Office, 1966.

CLAUSEN, J., AND WILLIAMS, J. "Sociological Correlates of Child Behavior," *Child Psychology*, H. Stevenson, J. Kagan, and C. Spiker (eds). Chicago: University of Chicago Press, 1963, pp. 26–107.

CLEMENTS, S. "Minimal Brain Dysfunction in Children." (*NINDB Monograph*, No. 3.) U.S. Department of Health, Education, and Welfare, Public Health Service Publication No. 1415, 1966.

COLE, V., BRANCH, C., AND ELLISON, R. "Some Relationships between Social Class and the Practice of Dynamic Psychotherapy," *American Journal of Psychiatry*, 18, 10004 (1962).

COLEMAN, M., NELSON, B., AND SHERMAN, M. *Role and Paradigm in Psychotherapy*. New York: Grune & Stratton, 1969.

DAVID, H. "Relevance of Programs for Emotionally Disturbed Youth in Other Lands." (Paper presented at the 1969 Annual Meeting of the American

Orthopsychiatric Association and based on a report prepared under contract with the Joint Commission on Mental Health of Children.) 1969.

DAVIS, A., AND HAVIGHURST, R. "Social Class and Color Differences in Child-Rearing," *American Sociological Review,* No. 11 (1946), 698–710.

DUNHAM, H. "Social Class and Schizophrenia," *American Journal of Orthopsychiatry,* 34, (1964) 634–42.

ERIKSON, K. *The Wayward Puritans.* New York: Wiley & Sons, 1966.

EYSENCK, H., AND RACHMAN, S. *The Causes and Cures of Neurosis.* San Diego, Calif.: Knapp, 1965.

GIOSCIA, V., RABKIN, R., SPECK, R., *et al. Dimensions and Innovations in the Therapy of Children,* p. 43. (A report of the Research Department of Jewish Family Service of New York to Task Force IV of the Joint Commission on Mental Health of Children, 1968.) (Mimeo.)

GLIDEWELL, J., *et al. Parent Attitudes and Child Behavior.* Springfield, Ill.: Charles C. Thomas, Inc., 1961.

GORDON, S. "Are We Seeing the Right Patients?" *American Journal of Orthopsychiatry,* 35, 99 (1965).

GROUP FOR THE ADVANCEMENT OF PSYCHIATRY. *Psychopathological Disorders in Childhood: Theoretical Considerations and a Proposed Classification,* VI, 62. New York: Group for the Advancement of Psychiatry, April, 1967.

HANDEL, G., AND RAINWATER, L. "Working-Class People and Family Planning," *Social Work,* No. 6 (April, 1961), p. 2.

HERZOG, E. "Some Assumptions About the Poor," *Social Service Review,* XXXVII, 4 (December, 1963).

HOBBS, N. "Helping Disturbed Children, Psychological and Ecological Strategies," *American Psychologist,* No. 21 (1966), 1105–15.

HOLLINGSHEAD, A., AND REDLICH, F. *Social Class and Mental Illness.* New York: Wiley & Sons, 1958.

KIRCHOFF, A. "A Theory of Hysterical Contagion." (Paper read before the American Sociological Association.) 1967.

KOHLBERG, L. *The Modifiability of Mental Health in the School Years.* (Paper prepared for Task Force II, Joint Commission on Mental Health of Children, Inc., 1968.) (Mimeo.)

KOMAROVSKY, M. *Blue Collar Marriage.* New York: Random House, 1964.

LAING, K., AND LAING, G. *Collective Dynamics.* New York: Crowell, 1961.

LAING, R., AND ESTERSON, A. *Sanity, Madness, and the Family,* Vol. I of *Families of Schizophrenics.* New York: Basic Books, 1965.

LAW, S. "The Mother of the Happy Child," *Smith College Studies in Social Work,* No. 25 (1954), 1–27.

LEWIS, H. "Child-Rearing Practices Among Low Income Families in the District of Columbia." Washington, D.C.: Health and Welfare Council of the National Capitol Area, 1961. (Paper presented at the National Conference on Social Welfare in Minneapolis, Minnesota, May 16, 1961.)

LEWIS, O. *Children of Sanchez.* New York: Random House, 1961.

LORENZ, K. *On Aggression.* New York: Harcourt, 1966.

LOURIE, R. "Personality Development and the Genesis of Neurosis," *Clinical Proceedings,* 23, 6 (1967), 167–82. (Reprinted with permission from *Psychoneuroses and Schizophrenia,* G. Usdin [ed.], New York: Lippincott, 1966.)

MCDERMOTT, J., HARRISON, S., SCHRAGER, J., AND WILSON, P. "Social Class and Mental Illness in Children," *American Journal of Orthopsychiatry,* 35, 500 (1965).

McKINLEY, D. *Social Class and Family Life.* London: The Free Press of Glencoe, Collier-Macmillan, Ltd., 1964.

MILLER, S. M., AND RIESSMAN, F. "The Working Class Subculture: A New View," *Social Problems,* No. 9 (Summer, 1961), 86–97.

MINUCHIN, S., AND MONTALVO, B. "Techniques for Working with Disorganized Low Socioeconomic Families," *American Journal of Orthopsychiatry,* 37, 5 (1967).

MYERS, J., AND ROBERTS, B. *Family and Class Dynamics in Mental Illness.* New York: Wiley and Sons, Inc., 1959.

NATIONAL ASSOCIATION FOR MENTAL HEALTH. "A Comprehensive Program for the Severely Mentally Ill Child and His Family." (10 Columbus Circle, New York, New York 10019.) 1968.

NATIONAL INSTITUTE OF MENTAL HEALTH. *Mental Health Services for Children, Focus: Community Mental Health Center.* (Public Health Service Publication 1844.) U.S. Department of Health, Education, and Welfare. Washington, D.C.: Government Printing Office, October, 1968.

NEUBAUER, P. "Therapeutic Programs." (Paper presented to the Joint Commission on Mental Health of Children.) 1967. (Mimeo.)

PAPENFORT, D., DINWOODIE, A., AND KILPATRICK, D. "Population of Children's Residential Institutions in the United States." Center for Urban Studies, University of Chicago, 1968.

PAVENSTEDT, E. "A Comparison of the Child-Rearing Environment of Upper-Lower and Very Low Lower-Class Families," *American Journal of Orthopsychiatry,* 35 (January, 1965), 89–98.

PETERSON, D., BECKER, W., HELLMER, L., SHOEMAKER, D., AND QUAY, H. "Parental Attitudes and Child Adjustment," *Child Development,* No. 30 (1959), 119–30.

PORTER, B. "The Relationship Between Marital Adjustment and Parental Acceptance of Children," *Journal of Home Economics,* No. 57 (1955), 176–82.

RADKE, M. "The Relation of Parental Authority to Children's Behavior and Attitudes." University of Minnesota Child Welfare Monographs, No. 22 (1946).

RAINWATER, L., AND YANCEY, W. *The Moynihan Report and the Politics of Controversy.* Cambridge: Massachusetts Institute of Technology Press, 1967.

Report of the Committee on Clinical Issues. Joint Commission on Mental Health of Children, Inc., 1969. (Mimeo.)

Report of Task Force I. Joint Commission on Mental Health of Children, Inc., 1968. (Mimeo.)

Report of Task Force II. Joint Commission on Mental Health of Children, Inc., 1969. (Mimeo.)

Report of Task Force V. Joint Commission on Mental Health of Children, Inc., 1968. (Mimeo.)

REUSCH, J. *Therapeutic Communication.* New York: Norton, 1961.

REXFORD, E. "Children, Child Psychiatry, and Our Brave New World," *Archives of General Psychiatry,* 20 (January, 1969), 25–37.

RIESSMAN, F., COHEN, J., AND PEARL, A. *Mental Health of the Poor: New Treatment Approaches for Low-Income People.* New York: Free Press, 1964.

RODMAN, H. "On Understanding Lower Class Behavior," *Social and Economic Studies,* No. VIII (December, 1959), 441–50.

ROFF, M. "A Factorial Study of the Fels Parent Behavior Scales," *Child Development,* No. 20 (1949), 29–45.

ROSEN, B., KRAMER, M., REDICK, R., AND WILLNER, S. *Utilization of Psychiatric Facilities by Children: Current Status, Trends, Implications.* (Report prepared for Joint Commission on Mental Health of Children, Inc., 1968.) National Institute of Mental Health, Mental Health Statistics. (Ser. B, No. 1.) 1968.

ROSENTHAL, D., AND FRANK, J. "The Fate of Psychiatric Clinic Out-Patients Assigned to Psychotherapy," *Journal of Nervous and Mental Diseases,* 127, 4 (1958), 330–43.

RUDOLPH, C., AND CUMMING, J. "Where Are Additional Psychiatric Services Most Needed?" *Social Work,* 7, 15 (1962).

SCHNEIDERMAN, L. "Social Class, Diagnosis, and Treatment," *American Journal of Orthopsychiatry,* 35, 99 (1965).

SEWELL, W., AND HALLER, A. "Social Status and the Personality of the Child," *Sociometry,* No. XIX (June, 1956), 114–25.

SILVERSTEIN, H. *The Social Control of Mental Illness.* New York: Crowell, 1969.

SKINNER, B. *Science and Human Behavior.* New York: Macmillan, 1953.

SMELSER, N. *Theory of Collective Behavior.* New York: Free Press, 1962.

SPECK, R. "Psychotherapy of the Social Network of a Schizophrenic Family," *Family Process,* 6, 208 (1967).

TARJAN, G. "Community Services and Treatment: Introductory Comments." (Paper given at the 15th Annual Conference of State Mental Health Representatives, American Medical Association, Council on Mental Health.) 1969.

THOMPSON, G. *Child Psychology.* 2nd ed. Boston: Houghton-Mifflin Co., 1962, pp. 621–60.

WATSON, G. "Some Personality Differences in Children Related to Strict or Permissive Discipline," *Journal of Psychology,* No. 44 (1957), 227–49.

WEINBERG, S. (ed.). *The Sociology of Mental Disorders.* Chicago: Aldine, 1967.

WOLPE, J. *Psychotherapy by Reciprocal Inhibition.* Stanford: Stanford University Press, 1958.

WORTIS, H., *et al.* "Child-rearing Practices in a Low Socioeconomic Group," *Pediatrics,* No. 32 (1963), 298–307.

VII. SOCIAL-PSYCHOLOGICAL ASPECTS OF NORMAL GROWTH AND DEVELOPMENT: INFANTS AND CHILDREN

BAYLEY, N. "Mental Growth in Young Children," *Yearbook of the National Society for the Study of Education,* 39, 2 (1940), 11–47.

BERNSTEIN, B. "Social Class and Linguistic Development, A Theory of Social Learning," *Education, Economy, and Society,* A. Halsey, J. Flod, and C. Anderson (ed.). New York: Free Press of Glencoe, 1961.

BIBER, B. Memorandum to Task Force II, Joint Commission on Mental Health of Children, Inc., 1968. (Mimeo.)

BLOOM, B. *Stability and Change in Human Characteristics.* New York: John Wiley and Sons, 1964.

BRODERICK, C. "Sex Interests of the School Age Child," in *The Individual, Sex, and Society.* C. Broderick and J. Bernard (eds.). Baltimore: Johns Hopkins Press, 1969.

CALDWELL, B., AND RICHMOND, J. "Programmed Day Care for the Very Young Child: A Preliminary Report," *Journal of Marriage and the Family,* XXVI, 4 (November, 1964), 481–88.

CHILMAN, C. "Recent Trends in Parent Education and Parent Participation," in *Review of Child Development Research,* III, B. Caldwell and H. Riciutti (eds.). Chicago: University of Chicago Press (in press).

Dairy Council Digest, "Malnutrition in Early Life and Subsequent Mental Performance," 39, 3 (May–June, 1968).

DE FRIES, Z., JENKINS, S., AND WILLIAMS, E. "Foster Family Care for Disturbed Children—A Nonsentimental View," *Child Welfare,* 44, 2 (February, 1965).

ERIKSON, E. "Identity and the Life Cycle," *Psychological Issues,* I, (1959), 1–171.

ESCALONA, S. *The Roots of Individuality.* Chicago: Aldine, 1968.

GIL, D. "Developing Routine Follow-Up Procedures for Child Welfare Services," *Child Welfare,* 43, 5 (May, 1964).

HEBB, D. "Drives and the CNS," *Psychological Review,* LXII (1955), 253–54.

HESS, R., AND SHIPMAN, V. "Early Experiences and Socialization of Cognitive Modes of Children," *Child Development,* 36 (1965), 869–86.

HOFFMAN, L. "Early Processes in Moral Development." New York Social Science Research Council, Conference on Character Development, 1963.

HONZIK, M., MACFARLANE, J., AND ALLEN, L. "The Stability and Mental Performance Between Two and Eighteen Years," *Journal of Experimental Education,* No. 17 (1948), 309–24.

Hunger, U.S.A. (A report by the Citizens' Board of Inquiry into Hunger and Malnutrition in the United States.) Washington, D.C.: New Community Press, 1968.

HUNT, J. McV. *A Bill of Rights for Children.* (Draft paper prepared for the Group on Early Child Development, 1960 White House Conference on Children and Youth.) 1966. (Mimeo.)

INKELES, A. "The Individual and the Community," in *Socialization and Society,* J. Clausen (ed.). Boston: Little, Brown & Co., 1968.

JENKINS, S., AND SAUBER, J. *Paths to Child Placement.* New York: New York City Department of Welfare and the Community Council of Greater New York, 1966.

JETER, H. *Children, Problems and Services in Child Welfare Programs.* Washington, D.C.: Department of Health, Education, and Welfare, 1963.

JOHN, V., AND GOLDSTEIN, L. "The Social Context of Language Acquisition," *Merrill Palmer Quarterly,* X, 3:265–75 (July, 1964).

KAGAN, J., AND MOSS, H. *Birth to Maturity.* New York: John Wiley and Sons, Inc., 1962.

KOHLBERG, L. "Development of Moral Character and Moral Ideology," in *Review of Child Development Research,* I, M. Hoffman and L. Hoffman (eds.). New York: Russell Sage Foundation, 1964.

MAAS, H., AND ENGLER, JR., R. *Children in Need of Parents.* New York: Columbia University Press, 1959.

MACCOBY, E. "Moral Values and Behavior in Childhood," in *Socialization and Society,* J. Clausen (ed.). Boston: Little, Brown Co., 1968.

MURPHY, L. *The Widening World of Childhood.* New York: Basic Books, 1964.

PIAGET, J. *The Origins of Intelligence in Children.* New York: International University Press, 1952.

PRUGH, D. "Psychosocial Disorders in Childhood and Adolescence: Theoretical Considerations and an Attempt at Classification," Joint Commission on Mental Health of Children, Inc., 1968. (Mimeo.)

Report of Task Force I. Joint Commission on Mental Health of Children, Inc., July, 1968. (Mimeo.)

Report of Task Force II. "The Mental Health of the School-Age Child." Joint Commission on Mental Health of Children, Inc., 1969. (Mimeo.)

RICHMOND, J., AND LIPTON, E. "Some Aspects of the New Physiology of the Newborn," *Dynamic Psychology in Childhood,* L. Jessner and E. Pavenstedt (eds.). New York: Grune and Stratton, 1959.

SMITH, M. "Competence and Socialization," in *Socialization and Society,* J. Clausen (ed.). Boston: Little, Brown and Co., 1968.

STINE, O., SARATSIOTIS, J., AND FURNO, O. "Appraising the Health of Culturally Deprived Children," *American Journal of Chemical Nutrition,* 20, 1084–95 (1967).

THOMAS, A., *et al. Behavior and Individuality in Early Childhood.* New York: New York University Press, 1963.

U.S. DEPARTMENT OF HEALTH, EDUCATION, AND WELFARE. "Parents as Partners." Office of the Secretary, U.S. Department of Health, Education, and Welfare, 1968.

WHITE, R. "Motivation Reconsidered: The Concept of Competence," *Psychological Review,* No. 66 (1959), 297–333.

WOODRUFF, C. *Journal of the American Medical Association,* 196, 214 (1966).

VIII. SOCIAL-PSYCHOLOGICAL ASPECTS OF NORMAL GROWTH AND DEVELOPMENT: ADOLESCENTS AND YOUTH

ALSKNE, H., LIEBERMAN, L., AND BRILL, L. "A Conceptual Model of the Life Cycle of Addiction," *The International Journal of the Addictions,* 2 (Fall, 1967), 221–39.

CHEIN, I., GERARD, D., AND LEE, R. *The Road to H.* New York: Basic Books, Inc., 1964.

CLENDENEN, R., VOTAW, R., MCBRIDE, P., AND CASSIDY, R. *The Youth Participation Review,* a cooperative inquiry of the Joint Commission on Mental Health of Children and the National Council of State Committees on Children and Youth. (Paper prepared by the National Council on State Committees on Children and Youth for the Joint Commission on Mental Health of Children, Inc.) May 1, 1968. (Mimeo.)

"Correction in the United States," a survey for the President's Commission on Law Enforcement and Administration of Justice by the National Council on Crime and Delinquency, in *Crime and Delinquency,* 13, 1 (1967), pp. 64–65, 77, 82–86, 131, 252–53.

DOUVAN, E., AND ADELSON, J. *The Adolescent Experience.* New York: John Wiley and Sons, Inc., 1966, p. 351.

ERIKSON, E. "Identity and the Life Cycle," *Psychological Issues,* I (1959), pp. 1–171.

FLACKS, R. "The Liberated Generation: An Exploration of the Roots of Student Protest," *The Journal of Social Issues* (July, 1967), pp. 52–75.

JOSSELYN, I. *Adolescence.* Joint Commission on Mental Health of Children, Inc., 1968.

KENISTON, K. "Heads and Seekers: Student Drug Users." (Paper presented at the Divisional Meeting of the American Psychiatric Association, New York City.) 1967.

KIFNER, J. "The Drug Scene: Marijuana, for Many Students, Has Become a Part of Growing Up," *New York Times* (January 11, 1968).

KIRKENDAL, L., AND LIBBY, R. "Sex and Interpersonal Relationships," in *The Individual, Sex, and Society*. C. Broderick and J. Bernard (eds.), Baltimore: Johns Hopkins Press, 1969.

KRAMER, R. "The State of the Boy, 1969," *New York Times Magazine* (March 30, 1969), pp. 97–110.

NATIONAL SERVICE SECRETARIAT. *Directory of Service Organizations*, 1968. (1629 K St., N.W., Washington, D.C.)

OFFER, D., *The Psychological World of the Teenager*, New York: Basic Books, 1969.

PENNINGTON, R. *Young Suicide*. Unpublished Master's thesis, George Washington University, June, 1968.

POLIER, J. *The Rule of Law and the Role of Psychiatry*. Baltimore: Johns Hopkins University Press, 1968.

REISS, I. "Premarital Sex Standards," *The Individual, Sex, and Society*, C. Broderick and J. Bernard (eds.). Baltimore: Johns Hopkins Press, 1969.

Report of the National Advisory Commission on Civil Disorders. New York: Bantam Books, March, 1968.

Report of Task Force III. Joint Commission on Mental Health of Children, Inc., 1968. (Mimeo.)

Report of Task Force V. Joint Commission on Mental Health of Children, Inc., 1968. (Mimeo.)

Report of Task Force VI. Joint Commission on Mental Health of Children, Inc., 1968. (Mimeo.)

RODMAN, H., AND GRAMS, P. "Juvenile Delinquency and the Family: A Review and Discussion," in Task Force Report: Juvenile Delinquency and Youth Crime. Washington, D.C.: Government Printing Office, 1967, pp. 188–221.

ROSEN, B., KRAMER, M., REDICK, R., AND WILLNER, S. *Utilization of Psychiatric Facilities by Children: Current Status, Trends, Implications*. (Report prepared for Joint Commission on Mental Health of Children, Inc., 1968.) National Institute of Mental Health, Mental Health Statistics. (Ser. B, No. 1.) 1968.

SHORT, J. "Juvenile Delinquency: The Socio-Cultural Context," in *Review of Child Development Research*, II, L. Hoffman and M. Hoffman (eds.). New York: Russell Sage Foundation, 1966. Pp. 423–68.

SILVERSTEIN, H., ROSENBERG, B., AND WEINGARTEN, K. "Some Themes Expressive of Alienated Youth." (Report to Joint Commission on Mental Health of Children, Inc.) November, 1967.

SMITH, M. "Morality and Student Protest." PSI CHI Newsletter (Winter, 1969).

SMITH, KLINE AND FRENCH LABORATORIES, in cooperation with the American Association for Health, Physical Education, and Recreation, a department of the National Education Association. *Drug Abuse: Escape to Nowhere*. NEA, Washington, D.C., 1967.

STUDENT COMMITTEE ON MENTAL HEALTH OF PRINCETON UNIVERSITY. "Psychedelics and the College Student." Princeton N.J., Princeton University Press, 1967.

U.S. DEPARTMENT OF HEALTH, EDUCATION, AND WELFARE. *America's Children and Youth in Institutions: 1950–1960–1964.* (Children's Bureau Publication No. 435–1965.) Washington, D.C., 1965.

——, Public Health Service, National Center for Health Statistics. *Vital Statistics of the United States,* II, Part A. Table 1–8. 1966.

U.S. SENATE, Subcommittee on Employment, Manpower, and Poverty of the Committee on Labor and Public Welfare in the United States. *Juvenile Delinquency Prevention and Control Act.* (90th Congress, September 21, 26, 28, October 19, 20, 25, and 26, 1967.) Washington, D.C.: Government Printing Office, 1967.

IX. EDUCATION AND THE MENTAL HEALTH OF CHILDREN AND YOUTH

BOWER, E. *Early Identification of Emotionally Handicapped Children in School.* Springfield, Ill.: Charles C. Thomas, 1960.

Report of Task Force II. Joint Commission on Mental Health of Children, Inc., 1969. (Mimeo.)

OTHER SOURCES

AMERICAN EDUCATIONAL RESEARCH ASSOCIATION. "Education of Exceptional Children," *Review of Educational Research,* XXXVIX, 1 (February, 1969).

——. "Mental and Physical Health," *Review of Education Research,* XXXVIX, 5 (December, 1968).

BOWER, E., AND HOLLISTER, W. *Behavioral Science Frontiers in Education.* New York: John Wiley and Sons, Inc., 1967.

BRODERICK, C., AND BERNARD, J. *The Individual, Sex, and Society.* Baltimore: Johns Hopkins Press, 1969.

CAPLAN, G. (ed.). *Prevention of Mental Disorders in Children.* New York: Basic Books, 1961.

COWEN, E., GARDNER, E., AND ZAX, M. *Emergent Approaches to Mental Health Problems.* New York: Appleton-Century-Crofts, 1967.

HELLMUTH, J. (ed.). *Educational Therapy.* B. Straub and J. Hellmuth, Co-Publishers. (c) 1965 Special Child Publications of the Seattle Seguin School Inc., Seattle, Washington, 1966.

LAMBERT, N. (ed.). *The Protection and Promotion of Mental Health in Schools.* (U.S. Public Health Service Publication No. 1226.) Washington, D.C.: Government Printing Office, 1964.

Mental Health and Teacher Education. Forty-Sixth Yearbook of the Association for Student Teaching. 1967.

Mental Health in the Schools. Prepared jointly by the Association of State and Territorial Health Officers, the Association of State and Territorial Mental Health Authorities, and the Council of Chief State School Officers. Washington, D.C.: Council of Chief State School Officers, 1966.

MINUCHIN, P. BIBER, B., SHAPIRO, E., AND ZIMILES, H. *The Psychological Impact of the School Experience.* New York: Basic Books, Inc., 1969.

NEWMAN, R. *Psychological Consultation in the Schools.* New York: Basic Books, Inc., 1967.

OJEMANN, R. (ed.). *The School and the Community Treatment Facility in Preventive Psychiatry.* Iowa City: University of Iowa, 1965.

X. EMPLOYMENT: PROBLEMS AND ISSUES RELATED TO THE
MENTAL HEALTH OF CHILDREN AND YOUTH

ABLON, J., ROSENTHAL, A., AND MILLER, D. "An Overview of the Mental Health Problems of Indian Children." (Prepared for Joint Commission on Mental Health of Children, Inc.) 1967. (Mimeo., 88 pp.)

BEALE, C., HUDSON, J., AND BANKS, V. "Characteristics of the U.S. Population by Farm and Non-Farm Origin," *Agricultural Economic Report,* No. 66 (December, 1964).

BERNERT, E. *America's Children.* New York: John Wiley & Sons, Inc., 1958.

BURCHINAL, L., HALLER, A., AND TAVES, M. *Career Choices of Rural Youth in a Changing Society.* (North Central Region Research Bulletin, No. 412.) St. Paul: University of Minnesota, November, 1962.

COLEMAN, J., *et al.* "Equality of Educational Opportunities." Washington, D.C.: U.S. Office of Education, 1966.

ENGEL, M., MARSDEN, G., AND WOODAMAN, S. "Children Who Work and a Concept of Work Style." *Psychiatry,* 30, 4 (November, 1967), 392–404.

———. "Orientation to Work in Children," *American Journal of Orthopsychiatry,* 38, 1 (1968), 137–43.

Federal Programs Assisting Children and Youth. Department of Health, Education, and Welfare, Social and Rehabilitation Service, Children's Bureau, Interdepartmental Committee on Children and Youth. Washington, D.C.: Government Printing Office, rev. 1968.

FOGEL, W. *Mexican-American Study Project.* Advance Report I. Los Angeles: University of California, November, 1965.

FOLGER, J., AND NAM, C. "Trends in Education in Relation to the Occupational Structure," *Sociology of Education,* 38, 1 (Fall, 1964), 19–33.

Fortune (January, 1969), p. 70. This survey was done by the Fortune-Yankelovich combination.

General Report of the Advisory Council on Vocational Education. "The Bridge Between Man and His Work." (Publication 1.) Department of Health, Education, and Welfare, Office of Education, 1968, p. 61.

HALLER, A. "Occupational Choices of Rural Youth," *Journal of Cooperative Extension,* IV, 2 (Summer, 1966), 93–102.

Handbook of Labor Statistics 1968. Department of Labor, Bureau of Labor Statistics. Washington, D.C.: Government Printing Office, 1968, pp. 97–99.

HAVIGHURST, R., AND NEUGARTEN, B. *Society and Education.* Boston: Allyn and Bacon, Inc., 2nd ed., 1962.

HOLLAND, J. "Major Programs of Research on Vocational Behavior," in *Man in a World at Work,* H. Borow (ed.). Boston: Houghton Mifflin, 1964, Chap. 12.

JOINT COMMISSION ON CORRECTIONAL MANPOWER AND TRAINING. "Differences That Make the Difference," R. McNickle (ed.). (Paper presented at a seminar on the implications of cultural differences for corrections in Washington, D.C., August, 1967.)

KLEINBERGER, P. *The Daily Iowan* (April 5, 1968). (Reprinted with permission in a flyer, "Vocations for Social Change," Canyon, California.)

Manpower Report of the President. Department of Labor. Washington, D.C.: Government Printing Office, April, 1967.

———. April, 1968.

———. January, 1969.

NEA RESEARCH DIVISION. "School Dropouts." *Research Summary*, 1967–S–1, p.
5. (Originally appeared in Daniel Schreiber [ed.], "Guidance and the
School Dropout," NEA School Dropouts Project and American Personnel
and Guidance Association joint publishers, 1964, p. 3.)

OFFICE OF EDUCATION. "The Educational Problem of the Mexican-American."
Department of Health, Education, and Welfare, Office of Programs for
the Disadvantaged, 1968.

THE PRESIDENT'S COUNCIL ON YOUTH OPPORTUNITY. "Summer 1968." (A
Summary Report.) n.d.

RAINWATER, L. "Work and Identity in the Lower Class," in *Planning for a
Nation of Cities,* S. Warner (ed.). Cambridge, Mass.: MIT Press, 1966,
pp. 105–23.

Report of Task Force VI. Joint Commission on Mental Health of Children, Inc.,
1968. (Mimeo.)

ROSENTHAL, N., AND HEDGES, J. "Matching Sheepskins with Jobs." *Monthly
Labor Review* (November, 1968), pp. 9–15.

RUKEYSER, W. "How Youth Is Reforming the Business World," *Fortune*
(January, 1969), p. 141.

RUSALEM, H., COHEN, M., AND RUSALEM, R. "Depersonalization Stops Here!"
Social and Rehabilitation Service, Final Report of Project RD–1589–P,
October 1, 1964–September 30, 1967. Federation of the Handicapped,
New York, New York.

SCHREIBER, D. "The Dropout and the Delinquent," *Thi Delta Kappan,* 44, 5
(February, 1963), 215–21.

———. "School Dropouts—A Symposium," *National Education Association
Journal,* 51 (1962), 50.

SHEPPARD, H. *The Nature of the Job Problem and the Role of New Public
Service Employment.* Kalamazoo: The Upjohn Institute, 1969.

SIMON, W. "Working Class Youth: Alienation Without Image." (Paper presented at the American Orthopsychiatric Annual Meeting, March 30–
April 2, 1969, New York City.)

SPARER, E. "Employability and the Juvenile 'Arrest' Record." (Training Series,
Center for the Study of Unemployed Youth.) New York University
Graduate School of Social Work, 1966.

Statistics on Manpower. Department of Labor. Washington, D.C.: Government
Printing Office, March, 1969.

THUROW, L. "The Occupational Distribution of the Returns to Education and
Experience for Whites and Negroes," in *Federal Programs for the
Development of Human Resources,* submitted to the Subcommittee on
Economic Progress of the Joint Economic Committee. Vol. 1. Washing-
ton, D.C.: Government Printing Office, 1968.

U.S. BUREAU OF CENSUS. *Current Population Reports.* (Ser. P-20, 1960–1968.)
(1967–68 unpublished figures.)

XI. RESEARCH

ADELSON, J. "Personality." *Annual Review of Psychology,* 20. Palo Alto, Calif.:
Annual Reviews, Inc., 1969.

BARKER, R., AND WRIGHT, H. *One Boy's Day.* Harper & Row, 1959.

CAMPBELL, D. "Reforms as Experiments," *American Psychologist,* 24, 4
(April, 1969), 409–29.

CHILMAN, C. "Families and Development at Mid-Stage of the Family Life Cycle," *The Family Coordinator* 17, 4 (October, 1968) 297–312.

————. "Recent Trends in Parent Education and Parent Participation," in *Review of Child Development Research*, III, B. Caldwell and H. Riciutti (eds.). Chicago: University of Chicago Press, 1969.

ESCALONA, S., LEITCH, M., *et al. Earliest Phases of Personality Development.* (Child Research Monograph, 17.) 1953.

GIOSCIA, V., *et al. Dimensions and Innovations in the Therapy of Children.* (A report prepared by the Research Department of Jewish Family Service of New York for Task Force IV, Joint Commission on Mental Health of Children, 1968.) (Mimeo.)

HADDAD, R. K., quoted in *Research in Schizophrenia.* (NIMH, Mental Health Monograph, 4.) U.S. Department of Health, Education, and Welfare, 1964.

LEVITT, E. "Psychotherapy with Children: A Further Evaluation," *Behavior Research Therapy*, 1, 45 (1963).

LUSTMAN, S. "Mental Health Research and the University." (Paper prepared for Task Force IV, Joint Commission on Mental Health of Children.) 1968.

MURPHY, L. "Programs for Disadvantaged Pre-School Children," *Children* (March–April, 1969).

NICHD. *Perspectives on Human Deprivation: Biological, Psychological, and Sociological.* U.S. Department of Health, Education, and Welfare. Washington, D.C.: Government Printing Office, 1968.

NIMH. Research in schizophrenia. Public Health Service, 1964.

PHILLIPS, E. "Parent Child Psychotherapy: A Follow-up Study Comparing Two Techniques," *Journal of Psychology*, 49, 195 (1960).

Report of the Committee on Clinical Issues. Joint Commission on Mental Health of Children, Inc., 1969. (Mimeo.)

Report of Task Force I. Joint Commission on Mental Health of Children, Inc., 1968. (Mimeo.)

Report of Task Force IV. Joint Commission on Mental Health of Children, Inc., 1968. (Mimeo.)

Report of Task Force V. Joint Commission on Mental Health of Children, Inc., 1968. (Mimeo.)

Report of Task Force VI. Joint Commission on Mental Health of Children, Inc., 1968. (Mimeo.)

SCRIMSHAW, G. "Malnutrition, Learning, and Behavior," *American Journal of Clinical Nutrition*, 20, 5 (1967), 493–502.

YARROW, L. "Conceptualizing the Early Environment," in *Early Child Care*, L. Dittman (ed.). New York: Atherton Press, 1968.

XII. HUMAN RESOURCES FOR HUMAN SERVICES

ALBEE, G. *Mental Health Manpower Trends.* New York: Basic Books, 1959.

AMERICAN ASSOCIATION OF PSYCHIATRIC CLINICS FOR CHILDREN. *Children and Clinics: A Summary of Findings, Conclusions, and Recommendations.* (A survey conducted for the Joint Commission on Mental Health of Children, Inc.) American Association of Psychiatric Clinics for Children, 1968.

AMERICAN PSYCHIATRIC ASSOCIATION. 1969 membership figures. (Mimeo.)

AMERICAN PSYCHOLOGICAL ASSOCIATION. 1969 membership figures. (Mimeo.)

ARNHOFF, F., AND SHRIVER, B. *A Study of the Current Status of Mental Health Personnel Supported under National Institute of Mental Health Training Grants.* (Public Health Service Publication No. 1541.) Washington, D.C.: Government Printing Office, 1966.

ARNHOFF, F., JENKINS, J., AND SPEISMAN, J. "The New Mental Health Workers," in *Manpower for Mental Health,* F. Arnhoff, E. Rubenstein, and J. Speisman (eds.). Chicago: Aldine, 1969.

ARNHOFF, F., RUBENSTEIN, E., AND SPEISMAN, J. (eds.). *Manpower for Mental Health.* Chicago: Aldine, 1969.

BRAYFIELD, A. *Psychology-Manpower Fact Sheet.* Washington, D.C.: American Psychological Association, 1967.

CARPER, J., WHITING, J., AND FELDMAN, R. *Mental Health Services for the Community: Process, Requirements, and Solutions.* (Paper prepared for the Joint Commission on Mental Health of Children, Inc., 1967.) (Mimeo.)

ELDRIDGE, M. *Selected Characteristics of Nurses Employed in Mental Health Establishments, 1963. Mental Health Manpower Current Statistics and Activities Report No. 7.* Chevy Chase, Md.: National Institute of Mental Health, 1964.

Federal Programs Assisting Children and Youth. Interdepartmental Committee on Children and Youth. Washington, D.C.: Department of Health, Education, and Welfare, Social and Rehabilitation Service, Children's Bureau, 1968.

FEIN, R. *The Doctor Shortage: An Economic Diagnosis.* Washington, D.C.: Brookings Institution, 1967.

GLIDEWELL, J., AND SWALLOW, C. *The Prevalence of Maladjustment in Elementary Schools.* (A report prepared for the Joint Commission on Mental Health of Children, Inc.) Chicago: University of Chicago, July 26, 1968.

GURIN, G., VEROFF, J., AND FELD, S. *Americans View Their Mental Health.* New York: Basic Books, 1960.

KNOWLES, J. *Medical Manpower: Quantity Versus Quality.* (Report to the Association of American Medical Colleges, 1968.) (Mimeo.)

LESTER, R. *Manpower Planning in a Free Society.* Princeton, N.J.: Princeton University Press, 1966.

MARSHALL, E. *Facts About Nursing: A Statistical Summary.* New York: American Nurses Association, 1967.

NATIONAL ASSOCIATION OF SOCIAL WORKERS. Membership Statistics. January 1967. (Mimeo.)

NATIONAL INSTITUTE OF MENTAL HEALTH, Division of Manpower and Training Programs. *Selected Characteristics of Social Workers. Mental Health Manpower Current Statistics and Activities Report No. 6.* Chevy Chase, Md.: National Institute of Mental Health, 1965b.

———, Office of Program Analysis. *Mental Health of Children: The Child Program of the National Institute of Mental Health.* Washington, D.C.: Department of Health, Education, and Welfare. (Public Health Service Publication No. 1396.) 1965a.

———, Public Information Branch, and Center for Studies of Child and Family Mental Health. *Mental Health Services for Children.* (Public Health Service Publication No. 1844.) 1968.

NATIONAL MANPOWER POLICY TASK FORCE. *The Nation's Manpower Programs.* Washington, D.C.: National Manpower Policy Task Force, 1969.

PEARL, A., AND RIESSMAN, F. (eds.). *New Careers for the Poor: The Non-professional in Human Service.* New York: The Free Press, 1965.

POLLAK, O. *Suggestions for Alleviating Manpower Shortages in the Child Mental Health Services.* (Paper prepared for the Joint Commission on Mental Health of Children, Inc., 1968.) (Mimeo.)

Report of the Committee on Clinical Issues. Joint Commission on Mental Health of Children, Inc., 1969. (Mimeo.)

Report of Task Force IV. The Joint Commission on Mental Health of Children, Inc., 1968. (Mimeo.)

SURGEON GENERAL'S CONSULTANT GROUP ON NURSING. *Toward Quality in Nursing Needs and Goals.* U.S. Public Health Service. Washington, D.C.: Government Printing Office, 1963.

U.S. BUREAU OF THE CENSUS. *Current Population Reports: Population Estimates.* (Ser. P-25, No. 416.) Washington, D.C.: Government Printing Office, 1969.

U.S. DEPARTMENT OF HEALTH, EDUCATION, AND WELFARE. *Closing the Gap in Social Work Manpower.* Report of the Departmental Task Force on Social Work Education and Manpower. Washington, D.C.: Government Printing Office, 1965.

VAN MATRE, R. *Statement at Conference on Psychiatry and Medical Education Social Climate Task Force,* 1967. (Mimeo.)

VON MERING, O., AND CARPENTER, G. *Needed: Mental Health Manpower Development and Training Patterns.* (Paper prepared for the Joint Commission on Mental Health of Children, Inc., 1967.) (Mimeo.)

WHITING, J. *Community Functioning, Manpower Utilization, and Impact Evaluation. Foundation-Stones for the Delivery of Effective Child Mental Health.* (Paper prepared for the Joint Commission on Mental Health of Children, Inc., 1968.) (Mimeo.)

WHITING, J., CARPER, J., AND FELDMAN, R. *Needed: A Scientific Basis for Manpower Utilization in Mental Health Services.* (Paper prepared for the Joint Commission on Mental Health of Children, Inc., 1967.) (Mimeo.)

APPENDIX

VII

FORTHCOMING VOLUMES FROM THE JOINT COMMISSION ON MENTAL HEALTH OF CHILDREN

MENTAL HEALTH: *From Infancy Through Adolescence.* A volume combining Task Forces I, II, and III and the Committees on Education and Religion.

THE MENTAL HEALTH OF CHILDREN: *Services, Research, and Manpower.* A volume combining Task Forces IV, V, and the Committee on Clinical Issues.

SOCIAL CHANGE AND THE MENTAL HEALTH OF CHILDREN. A volume combining Task Force VI and the Committee on Children of Minority Groups.

THE MENTAL HEALTH OF CHILDREN: *A Reader.* Selected Papers of the Joint Commission on Mental Health of Children.

ADOLESCENCE, by Irene M. Josselyn, M.D.

CHILD MENTAL HEALTH IN INTERNATIONAL PERSPECTIVE, edited by Henry P. David.

Index

DATE DUE